MCQs in Cardiology
for DM Entrance Examination

MCQs in Cardiology
for DM Entrance Examination

Second Edition

Vinod Sharma
MD DM (Cardiology) FRCP (London) FACC MBA (Healthcare Admn)

Vice-CEO and Head
Cardiology Services
National Heart Institute
East of Kailash, New Delhi, India

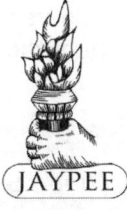

JAYPEE BROTHERS MEDICAL PUBLISHERS
The Health Sciences Publisher
New Delhi | London

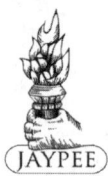 **Jaypee Brothers Medical Publishers (P) Ltd**

Headquarters
EMCA House
23/23-B, Ansari Road, Daryaganj
New Delhi 110 002, India
Landline: +91-11-23272143, +91-11-23272703
+91-11-23282021, +91-11-23245672
E-mail: jaypee@jaypeebrothers.com

Corporate Office
Jaypee Brothers Medical Publishers (P) Ltd.
4838/24, Ansari Road, Daryaganj
New Delhi 110 002, India
Phone: +91-11-43574357
Fax: +91-11-43574314
E-mail: jaypee@jaypeebrothers.com

Overseas Office
JP Medical Ltd.
83, Victoria Street, London
SW1H 0HW (UK)
Phone: +44-20 3170 8910
Fax: +44(0)20 3008 6180
E-mail: info@jpmedpub.com

Website: www.jaypeebrothers.com
Website: www.jaypeedigital.com

© 2023, Jaypee Brothers Medical Publishers

The views and opinions expressed in this book are solely those of the original contributor(s)/author(s) and do not necessarily represent those of editor(s) or publisher of the book.

All rights reserved by the author. No part of this publication may be reproduced, stored or transmitted in any form or by any means, electronic, mechanical, photocopying, recording or otherwise, without the prior permission in writing of the publishers.

All brand names and product names used in this book are trade names, service marks, trademarks or registered trademarks of their respective owners. The publisher is not associated with any product or vendor mentioned in this book.

Medical knowledge and practice change constantly. This book is designed to provide accurate, authoritative information about the subject matter in question. However, readers are advised to check the most current information available on procedures included and check information from the manufacturer of each product to be administered, to verify the recommended dose, formula, method and duration of administration, adverse effects and contraindications. It is the responsibility of the practitioner to take all appropriate safety precautions. Neither the publisher nor the author(s)/editor(s) assume any liability for any injury and/or damage to persons or property arising from or related to use of material in this book.

This book is sold on the understanding that the publisher is not engaged in providing professional medical services. If such advice or services are required, the services of a competent medical professional should be sought.

Every effort has been made where necessary to contact holders of copyright to obtain permission to reproduce copyright material. If any have been inadvertently overlooked, the publisher will be pleased to make the necessary arrangements at the first opportunity.

Inquiries for bulk sales may be solicited at: jaypee@jaypeebrothers.com

MCQs in Cardiology for DM Entrance Examination / Vinod Sharma

First Edition: 2013

Second Edition: **2023**

ISBN: 978-93-5696-115-9

Printed at: Sterling Graphics Pvt. Ltd.

Dedicated to

My Parents
Shri CP Dubey
and
Late Mrs Manoramma Dubey

Late Dr (Prof) S Padmavati
Founder President and Director of All India Heart Foundation and
National Heart Institute
New Delhi, India

Professor M Khalilullah
Former Director, Maulana Azad Medical College and
Associated GB Pant Hospitals and
Chairman, Heart Centre
New Delhi, India

Privileged Support and Special Thanks

My wife Dr Anamika Sharma, a charming gardener who make our soul blossom. She deserves special credit for tolerating my preoccupation happily during the preparation of this book.

My daughter Dr Ruchi Sharma, whose infectious smile brings enthusiasm and affectionate criticism infuses wisdom in me. She deserves special credit for proofreading of entire manuscript.

Preface to the Second Edition

The field of medicine, especially cardiology, is rapidly changing. Newer developments in pathobiology, molecular basis of various cardiovascular diseases, and introduction of percutaneous techniques for the treatment of atherosclerotic coronary artery disease, congenital cardiac defects, and rheumatic valvular lesions have focused the subject of cardiology on mass attention. More and more young postgraduates in medicine are now aspiring for postdoctoral training (DM) in cardiology. Various medical schools in India including All India Institute of Medical Sciences and Maulana Azad Medical College, New Delhi, conduct entrance test for DM Cardiology every year. In spite of availability of several textbooks of cardiology written by eminent authors, there is paucity of a concise multiple choice question-and-answer book. This book is an attempt to overcome this deficiency.

The MCQs in Cardiology with Explanation provides a concise and thorough screening of all the chapters of cardiology in a readily accessible outline format. It is based mainly on "Textbook of Cardiovascular Medicine," edited by Eugene Braunwald, and "The Heart," edited by J Willis Hurst. To be more comprehensive, questions and answers from the "Textbook of the Clinical Recognition of Congenital Heart Disease," by J Perloff, and "Cardiac Catheterization and Angiography," by William Grossman, are also included. To facilitate the readings from the reference books, each answer is studded with reference of the resources.

The book is well suited for postgraduate fellows who are preparing for postdoctoral training in cardiology. I hope this book will prove to be both informative and easy-to-use.

Vinod Sharma

Preface to the First Edition

The field of medicine especially cardiology is rapidly changing. Newer developments in pathobiology, molecular basis of various cardiovascular diseases and introduction of percutaneous techniques for treatment of atherosclerotic coronary artery disease, congenital cardiac defects and rheumatic valvular lesions have focused the subject of cardiology into mass attention. More and more young postgraduates in medicine are now aspiring for postdoctoral training (DM) in cardiology. Various medical schools in India including All India Institute of Medical Sciences and Maulana Azad Medical College, New Delhi, are conducting entrance test for DM Cardiology every year. In spite of availability of several textbooks of cardiology written by eminent authors, there is paucity of concise multiple choice question-and-answer book. This book is an attempt to overcome this deficiency.

The *MCQs in Cardiology with Explanation* provides a concise and thorough screening of all the chapters of cardiology in readily accessible outline format. It is based mainly on *'Textbook of Cardiovascular Medicine'* edited by Eugene Braunwald, and *'The Heart'* edited by J Willis Hurst. To be more comprehensive, questions and answers from the *'Textbook of the Clinical Recognition of Congenital Heart Disease'*, by J Perloff and *'Cardiac Catheterization and Angiography'* by William Grossman are also included.

The book is well suited for postgraduate fellows who are preparing for postdoctoral training in cardiology. I hope this book will prove to be both informative and easy-to-use.

Vinod Sharma

Acknowledgments

Special Thanks to

Dr OP Yadava, CEO, National Heart Institute. A truly **WISE** man, full of **W**isdom, **I**ntellect, **S**acrifice, and **E**mpathy, for his suggestions and constructive criticism in a systematic presentation of this book.

My special gratitude for their *generous cup of suggestions, reflections, and a handful of memories together*:

- Prof (Dr) Shridhar Dwivedi
- Brig (Dr) YK Arora
- Dr Lokesh Chandra Gupta
- Dr Arvind Singh
- Dr Sukriti
- Dr Uday Singh Yadav
- Dr Samina Asfaq
- Dr Vikas Ahlawat
- Dr Amita Yadav
- Dr Arvind Prakash
- Dr Suruchi Ladha
- Dr Vandana Bhardwaj

I would like to specially thank M/s Jaypee Brothers Medical Publishers Pvt Ltd, New Delhi, India, who have granted permission to reproduce various chapters from the first edition of this book.

Last but not least, Mr Sankaranarayanan, my administrative assistant, deserves special mention and sincere thanks. He was responsible for the arduous day-to-day preparation of manuscript. His sense of responsibility and selfless devotion to task cannot be exaggerated.

Vinod Sharma

Contents

Chapter 1: Cardiac Anatomy and Embryology 1
Chapter 2: Cardiac Physiology 10
Chapter 3: Clinical Cardiology 22
Chapter 4: EKG and Stress Test 32
Chapter 5: Cardiac Radiology 50
Chapter 6: Echocardiography and Doppler 62
Chapter 7: Ambulatory Blood Pressure Monitoring 67
Chapter 8: Cardiac Catheterization and Angiography 68
Chapter 9: Hypertension 78
Chapter 10: Hyperlipidemia 92
Chapter 11: Congestive Heart Failure 99
Chapter 12: Sleep Disorder Breathing and Cardiovascular Disease 121
Chapter 13: Atherosclerosis and Coronary Artery Disease 125
Chapter 14: Acute Rheumatic Fever and Infective Endocarditis 159
Chapter 15: Valvular Heart Disease and Prosthetic Heart Valves 175
Chapter 16: Congenital Heart Disease 196
Chapter 17: Acquired Disease of Infants and Childhood 247
Chapter 18: Cardiomyopathies 252
Chapter 19: Cor Pulmonale and Pulmonary Embolism 274
Chapter 20: Cardiac Arrhythmia, Pacing and Electrophysiology 294
Chapter 21: Pulmonary Hypertension 337
Chapter 22: Cardiovascular Changes with Aging 341
Chapter 23: Athlete Heart 342

Chapter 24:	Pericardial Disease	345
Chapter 25:	Cardiac Tumor	358
Chapter 26:	Cardiac Trauma	364
Chapter 27:	Aortic Disease	366
Chapter 28:	Collagen Diseases and Heart	375
Chapter 29:	Cardiovascular Related Disorders	381
Chapter 30:	Preventive Cardiology	393

Index 401

CHAPTER 1

Cardiac Anatomy and Embryology

ANATOMY

1. Which of the following is *not* an intra-pericardial structure?
   a. Ascending aorta
   b. Main pulmonary artery
   c. Pulmonary veins
   d. Ductal artery (ductus arteriosus)

2. Which of the following structure is intra-pericardial?
   a. Right pulmonary artery
   b. Left pulmonary artery
   c. Ductal artery (ductus arteriosus)
   d. Confluence of pulmonary veins in patients with total anomalous pulmonary venous connection

3. Following open heart surgery, the isolated left atrial tamponade is seen due to accumulation of blood within:
   a. Transverse sinus
   b. Oblique sinus
   c. Posterior pericardial space
   d. Anterior pericardial space

4. The oblique sinus is:
   a. A tunnel like passage way behind the great arteries
   b. A posterior midline cul-de-sac along the pulmonary veins and vena cava
   c. Space behind coronary sinus
   d. Space between great arteries and veins

5. "True" statement regarding false tendons in LV cavity is all *except*:
   a. They connect two walls of LV
   b. They can connect two papillary muscles
   c. They are not attached to mitral leaflets
   d. All are true

6. The majority of clinically significant ventricular septal defects involves the:
   a. Inlet ventricular septum
   b. Trabecular septum
   c. Membranous septum
   d. Infundibular septum

7. Atrioventricular portion of atrial septum is clinically important because of:
   a. It is the potential site for left-ventricular to right atrial shunts
   b. It corresponds to the triangle of Koch's
   c. It contains AV node
   d. All of the above

8. Which is *not* a correct match?
   a. Nodule of Arantius—Lambl excrescence
   b. Crista supraventricularis—Muscular ridge separating tricuspid and pulmonary valve
   c. Crista terminalis—Muscle ridge separating right atrium into smooth posterior region and muscular anterior region
   d. Pulmonary veins—Thebesian valves

9. All the following are correct match *except*:
   a. Persistent left superior vena cava—Coronary sinus
   b. Moderator band—Right ventricle
   c. Descending thoracic aorta—Post left atrial wall
   d. Crista terminalis—Left atrium

10. The common site of origin of posterior descending artery is:
    a. Distal right coronary artery
    b. Proximal left anterior descending artery
    c. Distal left anterior descending artery
    d. Distal left circumflex artery

11. The His bundle and proximal left bundle branch receives blood supply through:
    a. Left main coronary artery
    b. Septal branch of right coronary artery
    c. Obtuse marginal branch of left circumflex artery
    d. First septal perforator branch of left anterior descending artery

12. *Incorrect* statement regarding myocardial bridging is:
    a. Its prevalence is 0.5 to 1.6% in the general population
    b. It is reported to be 28% in children and 30–50% in adults with hypertrophic cardiomyopathy
    c. It is associated with poor prognosis in general
    d. It is associated with poor prognosis in patients with hypertrophic cardiomyopathy only

CHAPTER 1 | Cardiac Anatomy and Embryology

13. Large number of patients with which congenital heart disease has left dominant coronary system:
  a. ASD
  b. PDA
  c. VSD
  d. Bicuspid aortic valve

14. The common dominant coronary artery in human heart is:
  a. Right coronary artery
  b. Left coronary artery
  c. Shared dominance
  d. None of them

15. The ostium of coronary sinus is guarded by:
  a. Thebesian valve
  b. Eustachian valve
  c. Semilunar valve
  d. No valve

16. During cardiac operations, cardioplegic solutions are administered into:
  a. Left main coronary artery
  b. Superior and inferior vena cava
  c. Coronary sinus
  d. Great cardiac veins

17. Identify an *incorrect* combination:
  a. Veins of Marshall—Connection between persistent left superior vena cava (LSVC) and coronary sinus
  b. Chiari-net—Fenestrated Eustachian or Thebesian valve
  c. Double chambered right—Large Thebesian valve atrium
  d. Supravalvular aortic stenosis – sinotubular junction

18. Rupture of posterior aortic sinus of Valsalva leads to communication with:
  a. RVOT or right atrium
  b. Left ventricle
  c. Left atrium
  d. Pericardial cavity

19. The ligamentum arteriosum represents vestigial remnant of:
  a. Ductus venosus
  b. Fetal ductal artery
  c. Vein of Marshall
  d. None of them

20. Which of the following statement is *correct*?
  a. The left bundle can be disrupted following surgical myomectomy
  b. The right bundle can be damaged during percutaneous alcohol septal ablation
  c. Following right ventriculotomy for reconstruction of RVOT, the EKG shows RBBB pattern even though the right bundle is not disrupted.
  d. Left bundle is a cord like structure

ANSWERS WITH EXPLANATIONS

1. Ans. d. Ductal artery (ductus arteriosus)

Hurst's 14th Ed; Page 71 & 73

The fibrous (parietal) pericardium is a resilient sack that envelope the heart and attaches onto the great vessel. Almost the entire ascending aorta and main pulmonary artery and portion of both vena cavae and all four pulmonary veins are intrapericardial. In patients with total anomalous pulmonary venous connection, the confluence of pulmonary veins is intrapericardial. In contrast the right and left pulmonary arteries and ductal artery (ductus arteriosus) are extrapericardial structures.

2. Ans. d. Confluence of pulmonary veins in patients with total anomalous pulmonary venous connection

Hurst's 14th Ed; Page 71 & 73

Refer to explanation for Q. No 1.

3. Ans. b. Oblique sinus

Hurst's 14th Ed, Page 73

The serous pericardium forms the delicate inner lining of the fibrous pericardium as well as the outer lining of heart and great vessel (visceral pericardium). Over the heart it is referred as a epicardium. The junction between the visceral and parietal pericardium lie along the great vessel and form the pericardial reflection. The reflection along the pulmonary veins and vena cavae are continuous and form a posterior mid line cul-de-sac known as oblique sinus. Behind the great arteries the transverse sinus forms a tunnel like passage way. After the open heart surgery localized accumulation of blood within the oblique sinus can produce isolated left atrial tamponade. Similarly, a hematoma adjacent to low pressure right atrium can cause isolated right atrial tamponade.

4. Ans. b. A posterior midline cul-de-sac along the pulmonary veins and vena cava

Hurst's 14th Ed, Page 73

Refer to explanation for Q. No 3.

5. Ans. d. All are true

Hurst's 14th Ed, Page 84

Left ventricular false tendons, also referred to as pseudotendons are bands or discrete, thin, cordlike fibromuscular structure that connect two walls, the two papillary muscles or a papillary muscle to a wall usually the ventricular septum. However, false tendons are not attached to the mitral leaflet. False tendons are common anatomic variant of the normal left ventricle occurring in the 50% of the heart and may become calcified with the age. They are frequently observed in the man but their incidence does not appear to be age related. It has been suggested that they may be the cause of innocent systolic musical murmur. Although they are readily detectable by echocardiography, they may be misinterpreted by the inexperience sonographer as pathologic structure such as rupture chordate, mural thrombus or vegetation.

6. Ans. a. Inlet ventricular septum

Hurst's 14th Ed; Page 85-86

Ventricular septum is a complex intracardiac partition that can be considered to comprise of four parts, i.e., inlet, trabecular, membranous and infundibular septum. The ventricular septum may also be divided into muscular and membranous portion. The membranous septum lies beneath the right and posterior (noncoronary), aortic cusps and connect the mitral and tricuspid annuli. The majority of clinically significant ventricular septal defect involve the membranous septum.

The atrial septum is composed of interatrial and atrioventricular regions. The interatrial portion is characterized by fossa ovalis, which is the anatomic hallmark of a morphologic right atrium. The atrioventricular portion of the atrial septum is made up of major muscular and minor membranous component and separates the right atrium from the left ventricle. This explains why there is a potential for left ventricular to right atrial shunt. The atrioventricular septum corresponds roughly to the triangle of Koch, an important anatomic surgical landmark because it contains the AV node and proximal portion of AV bundle (His bundle). During tricuspid annuloplasty procedures and patch closure of membranous ventricular septal defect care must be taken to avoid injury to the conduction system. The muscular component of atrioventricular septum is interposed between the membranous septum anteriorly and internal cardiac crux posteriorly.

7. Ans. b. It corresponds to the triangle of Koch's

Hurst's 14th Ed; Page 85-86

Refer to explanation for Q. No 6.

8. Ans. d. Pulmonary veins—Thebesian valves

Hurst's 14th Ed; Page 79, 82-83 & 92

a.
The aortic valve has three half moon shaped (semilunar) cusps which forms pocket like tissue flaps. Just below the free edge of each cusp is a ridge like closing edge. At the centre of each cusp the closing edge meets a free edge and forms a small fibrous mount which is called the Nodule of Arantius. Age related thickening along the nodule of Arantius and closing edges may be associated with the formation of Whisker-like projection called Lambl's excrescences. Lambl's excrescences can be detected by echocardiography and have been associated with cardioembolic stroke.

b.
Crista supraventricularis is a prominent arch shaped muscle ridge which separate the tricuspid and pulmonary valves. It is made up of three components (parietal band, infundibular septum and septal band) that may appear as distinguish structure or may merge together.

c.
Crista terminalis is a prominent internal muscle ridge, which separates the right atrial free wall into a smooth walled posterior region that receives the vena cava and coronary sinus and a muscular anterior region, i.e., lined by parallel pectinate muscle and from which the right atrial appendages emanates. Pectineus is a Latin for "comb" and the pectinate muscle and crista terminals resembles the teeth and backbone of comb respectively.

d.
The thebesian valve is a crescent shaped valvular remnant which guards the ostium of the coronary sinus.

9. Ans. d. Crista terminalis—Left atrium

Hurst's 14th Ed; Page 79, 82-83 & 92

Refer to explanation for Q. No 8.

10. Ans. a. Distal right coronary artery

Hurst's 14th Ed, Page 91

The right coronary artery runs in the right atrioventricular groove and the left circumflex artery runs in the left atrioventricular groove. The artery that crosses the cardiac crux and gives rise to posterior descending branch represents the dominant coronary artery. Dominance is right in 70% of the human heart, left in 10% and shared in 20%. In patients with a congenitally bicuspid aortic valve, the incidence of left dominance is 25-30%. Therefore, it is the distal right coronary artery which give rise to posterior descending artery in 70% of the heart and it is the dominant artery.

11. Ans. d. First septal perforator branch of left anterior descending artery

Hurst's 14th Ed, Page 90

The left anterior descending artery courses within the epicardial fat of the anterior interventricular grooves, wraps around the cardiac apex and travel a variable distance along the inferior interventricular groove towards the cardiac base. It's septal perforating branches supplies the anterior septum and apical septum. The first septal perforator branch supplies the AV (His bundle) and proximal left bundle branch.

12. Ans. d. It is associated with poor prognosis in patients with hypertrophic cardiomyopathy only

Hurst's 14th Ed, Page 90

Myocardial bridge is a condition where a short segment of left anterior descending artery travels within the myocardium (covered by a so called myocardial bridge). The resulting systolic luminal narrowing is probably benign in vast majority of the people. The prevalence of myocardial bridging is only 0.5–1.6% in general population, it is reported to be 28% in children and 30–50% in adults with hypertrophic cardiomyopathy. More importantly myocardial bridging appears to be associated with poor prognosis (higher incidence of myocardial ischemia and sudden death) in patients with hypertrophic cardiomyopathy regardless of age.

13. Ans. d. Bicuspid aortic valve

Hurst's 14th Ed, Page 91

Refer to explanation for Q. No 10.

14. Ans. a. Right coronary artery

Hurst's 14th Ed, Page 91

Refer to explanation for Q. No 10.

15. Ans. a. Thebesian valve

Hurst's 14th Ed, Page 91–92

The coronary venous circulation is comprised of coronary sinus, cardiac veins, and thebesian venous systems. The great cardiac vein and other cardiac veins such as the left posterior and middle cardiac veins, drain into the coronary sinus, which courses along the posteroinferior aspect of the left atrioventricular groove and empties into the right atrium. The ostium of coronary sinus is guarded by a crescent-shaped valvular remnant, the thebesian valve. Rarely, the coronary sinus drains directly into the left atrium.

16. Ans. c. Coronary sinus

Hurst's 14th Ed, Page 92

During cardiac operation, cardioplegic solution is administered retrogradely into the coronary sinus.

17. Ans. c. Double chambered right—Large Thebesian valve atrium

Hurst's 14th Ed, Page 95–96

The superior vena cava lies anterior to the right pulmonary artery and receives the azygos vein posteriorly before draining into the superior aspect of the right atrium, just posterior to the atrial appendage. The vein of Marshall forms the terminal connection between a persistent left superior vena cava and the coronary sinus. Its vestigial remnant in normal adults is the ligament of Marshall. Both vein and ligament are a potential source of arrhythmias. The ostium of the inferior vena cava is guarded by a crescent-shaped, often fenestrated flap of tissue, the eustachian valve, which is readily seen by echocardiography. Although generally small, the eustachian valve may become so large that it can produce a double-chambered right atrium. Also when either the eustachian or thebesian valve is large and fenestrated, it is referred to as a Chiari net. By echocardiography, a Chiari net may be misinterpreted as a mass. The thoracic aorta arises at the level of the aortic valve and is divided into the three segments: (i) ascending aorta, (ii) aortic arch, and (iii) descending thoracic aorta. The ascending aorta consists of sinus and tubular portions, which are demarcated by the sinotubular junction. This is the site at which supravalvular aortic stenosis is often most severe.

18. Ans. a. RVOT or right atrium

Hurst's 14th Ed, Page 96

Behind the aortic valve cusps are three out pouching or sinuses (of Valsalva). The right aortic sinus abuts against the ventricular septum and right ventricular parietal band and is covered in part by the right atrial appendage. In contrast, the left aortic sinus rest against the anterior left ventricular free wall and a portion of anterior mitral leaflets abuts the left atrial free wall and is covered in part by pulmonary trunk and left atrial appendage. The posterior (noncoronary) aortic sinus overlies the ventricular septum and a part of anterior mitral leaflet, abuts the atrial septum and indents both atrial free walls. Rupture of the right and posterior aortic sinuses of Valsalva may result in a communication with the right ventricular outflow tract or right atrium, whereas rupture of left aortic sinus of Valsalva leads to a communication with left atrium or left ventricular outflow tract.

19. Ans. b. Fetal ductal artery

Hurst's 14th Ed, Page 96

The ligamentum arteriosum (ductal artery ligament) represents the vestigial remnant of the fetal ductal artery which when patent connects the proximal left pulmonary artery to the under surface of aortic arch.

20. Ans. d. Left bundle is a cord like structure

Hurst's 14th Ed, Page 98

The right bundle branch emanates from the distal portion of AV bundle and forms a cordlike structure that travels along the septal and moderator bend towards the anterior tricuspid papillary muscles. In contrast, the left bundle branch represents a broad fenestrated sheet of subendocardial conduction fibre that is spread along the septal surface of the left ventricle. The right and left bundle branch receives dual blood supply from septal perforators of left anterior descending coronary artery and posterior descending coronary arteries. Following right ventriculotomy for reconstruction of right ventricular outflow tract, the electrocardiogram shows a pattern of right bundle branch block even though the right bundle is not disrupted.

CARDIAC ANATOMY

1. **A distensible fibroadipose annulus is unique to:**
   a. Mitral valve
   b. Tricuspid valve
   c. Pulmonary valve
   d. Aortic valve

2. **Left ventricular false Tendon's may attach all *except*:**
   a. Two papillary muscles
   b. Two walls of LV
   c. Papillary muscle to wall
   d. Papillary muscle to mitral leaflets

3. **A prominent internal muscle ridge "The crista terminalis" is located in:**
   a. Right atrium
   b. Left atrium
   c. Right ventricle
   d. Left ventricle

4. **Crista supraventricularis is located in:**
   a. Right atrium
   b. Left atrium
   c. Right ventricle
   d. Left ventricle

5. **What is the prevalence of myocardial bridging in patients with HOCM?**
   a. 5–10%
   b. 10–15%
   c. 25–30%
   d. 30–50%

6. **What is prevalence of myocardial bridge in normal population?**
   a. 1.5–2%
   b. 5–10%
   c. 10–15%
   d. 20–30%

7. **A congenital bicuspid valve is associated with higher incidence of:**
   a. Single coronary artery
   b. Anomalous origin of LCA
   c. Left coronary dominance
   d. Right coronary dominance

8. **Thebesian valve guards the ostia of:**
   a. SVC
   b. IVC
   c. Great cardiac vein
   d. Coronary sinus

9. **Correctly match the following:**
   A. Sinotubular junction
   B. Ligament of Marshall
   C. Chiari net
   D. Thebesian valve
   E. Eustachian valve
   F. Circle of Vieussens

   A. Coronary sinus
   B. IVC
   C. Supravalvular aortic stenosis
   D. Terminal remnant of Marshall vein
   E. Fenestrated Thebesian or eustachian valve
   F. Conus artery

10. **The sinus node artery arises commonly from:**
    a. Right coronary artery
    b. Left anterior descending artery
    c. Left circumflex artery
    d. Posterior descending artery

ANSWERS WITH EXPLANATIONS

1. Ans. b. Tricuspid valve

Hurst's 14th Ed, Page 74

The tricuspid valve is comprised of 5 components (i.e., annulus, leaflets, commissures, chordae tendineae and papillary muscle). The anterior tricuspid leaflet is the larger and most mobile and forms an intracavitary curtain that partially separates the inflow and outflow tract of right ventricle. The posterior leaflet is usually the smallest. The septal leaflet is the least mobile because of its many direct chordal attachment to the ventricular septum. A distensible fibroadipose annulus is unique to the tricuspid valve. Consequently, dilatation of the right ventricle commonly produces circumferential tricuspid annular dilatation that results in variable degree of tricuspid valve regurgitation.

2. Ans. d. Papillary muscle to mitral leaflets

Hurst's 14th Ed; Page 84

Left ventricular false tendons also referred to as pseudo-tendons or bands are discrete thin cordlike fibromuscular structures that connect to wall, the two papillary muscles or papillary muscles to a wall, usually the ventricular septum. However, false tendons are not attached to the mitral leaflet. Cordal attachment between the mitral leaflet and ventricular septum are abnormal and are usually associated with atrioventricular septal defects. False tendons are common anatomic variant of normal left ventricle occurring in 50% of heart and may become calcified with age. They may be the cause of innocent systolic musical murmur. Although they are readily detectable by echocardiography, they may be misinterpreted by the inexperienced sonographer as pathologic structures such as rupture called mural thrombi or vegetation.

3. Ans. a. Right atrium

Hurst's 14th Ed, Page 87

A prominent internal muscle ridge, the crista terminalis separate the right atrial free wall into a smooth walled posterior region that receives the vena cava and coronary sinus and a muscular anterior region, i.e., lined by parallel pectinate muscles and from which the right atrial appendage emanates.

4. Ans. c. Right ventricle

Hurst's 14th Ed, Page 83

The crista supraventricularis is a prominent arch shaped muscular ridge, which separates the tricuspid and pulmonary valves. It is made up of three components (i.e., parietal band, infundibular septum and septal band) that may appear as distinguish structure or may merge together. The parietal band is free wall structure whereas the adjacent infundibular septum is intracardiac and separates two ventricular outflow tracts beneath the right and left cusp of both semilunar valves.

5. Ans. d. 30-50%

Hurst's 14th Ed, Page 90

The left main coronary artery arises from left aortic sinus and travels for a very short distance along the epicardium between the pulmonary trunk and left atrium and then divides into left anterior descending and circumflex artery. The left anterior descending artery courses within the epicardial fat of the anterior interventricular groove, wraps around the cardiac apex and travel a variable distance along the inferior interventricular groove towards the cardiac base. Although the short segment of left anterior descending artery may travel within the myocardium (covered by a so-called myocardial bridge), the resulting systolic luminal narrowing is probably benign in vast majority of people. Whereas the prevalence of myocardial bridging is only 0.5-1.6% in general population, it is reported to be 28% in children and 30-50% in adults with hypertrophic cardiomyopathy. Myocardial bridging appears to be associated with poor prognosis (higher incidence of myocardial ischemia and sudden death) in patient with hypertrophic cardiomyopathy regardless of age.

6. Ans. a. 1.5-2%

Hurst's 14th Ed, Page 90

Refer to explanation for Q. No 5.

7. Ans. c. Left coronary dominance

Hurst's 14th Ed, Page 91

The artery that crosses the cardiac crux and give rise to the posterior descending branch represents the dominant coronary artery. In 70% of the human heart, it is the right coronary artery which give rise to the posterior descending branch and therefore right dominance is seen in 70% of the cases. While in 10% it is the left circumflex artery which give rise to the posterior descending artery and it is shared by both the arteries in remaining 20%. In patients with a congenitally bicuspid aortic valve, the incidence of left coronary dominance is 25-30%.

8. Ans. d. Coronary sinus

Hurst's 14th Ed, Page 91-92

The coronary venous circulation is comprised of coronary sinus, cardiac veins and the thebesian venous system. The great cardiac veins travel in the anterior interventricular groove besides the left anterior descending artery and in the left atrioventricular groove besides the left circumflex artery. The great cardiac veins and other cardiac veins drain into the coronary sinus which courses along the posteroinferior aspect of left atrioventricular groove and empties into the right atrium. The ostium of the coronary sinus is guarded by a crescent shaped valvular remnant, the thebesian valve.

9. Ans. (A—C, D—A, B—D, E—B, C—E, F—F)

Hurst's 14th Ed, Page 89 & 95-96

The subclavian and internal jugular veins merge bilaterally to form the right and left innominate veins. The left innominate vein is two to three times the length of its right sided counterpart. The left innominate vein joins the shorter right innominate vein and forms superior vena cava, which drains into the superior aspect of right atrium. The vein of Marshall forms the terminal connection between a persistent left superior vena cava and coronary sinus. Its vestigial remnant in normal adult is ligament of Marshall. Both vein and ligament are a potential source of arrhythmias. The ostium of the inferior vena cava is guarded by a crescent shaped often fenestrated flap of tissue, the eustachian valve which is readily seen by echocardiography. Although generally small, the eustachian valve may become so large that it can produce a double chambered right atrium. When either eustachian or thebesian valve (valve of coronary sinus) is large and fenestrated, it is referred to as Chiari net. By echocardiography, a Chiari net may be misinterpreted as a mass. The thoracic aorta which arises at the level of aortic valve is divided into three segments, i.e., ascending aorta, arch of aorta and descending thoracic aorta. The ascending aorta consists of sinus and tubular portion which are demarcated by the sinotubular junction. This is the site at which supravalvular aortic stenosis is often most severe. The right coronary artery arises from right sinus of Valsalva and courses within the right atrioventricular groove. In 50-60% of patient of persons, its first branch is the conus artery which supplies the right ventricular outflow tract and forms an important collateral anastomosis (circle of Vieussens) just below the pulmonary valve with an analogous branch from the left anterior descending artery.

10. Ans. a. Right coronary artery

Hurst's 14th Ed, Page 97

The sinus node artery arises commonly from the right coronary artery.

CHAPTER 1 | Cardiac Anatomy and Embryology

EMBRYOLOGY

1. Embryologically the coronary sinus forms from:
   a. Left horn of sinus venosus
   b. Left umbilical vein
   c. The left vitalline vein
   d. Left common cardinal vein

2. Thebesian vein drain which part of the heart chamber:
   a. Right atria
   b. Right ventricle
   c. Left atria
   d. Left ventricle

3. Which is the most common type of anomalous coronary artery origin?
   a. Ectopic origin of left circumflex artery from right sinus of Valsalva
   b. Origin of right coronary artery from left sinus of Valsalva
   c. Origin of left anterior descending artery from separate ostia in the left sinus of Valsalva
   d. Origin of all the three artery from the right sinus of Valsalva

4. Intramyocardial sinusoids communicating with either or both coronary arteries or end blindly is seen in which of the following congenital heart disease:
   a. Tetralogy of Fallots
   b. Supravalvular aortic stenosis
   c. Pulmonary atresia with intact ventricular septum
   d. Congenital coronary artery ectasia

5. The common coronary artery receiving retrograde flow from ductus arteriosus is seen in which of the following congenital heart disease:
   a. Aortic atresia with intact ventricular septum
   b. Pulmonary atresia with intact ventricular septum
   c. Hypertrophic obstructive cardiomyopathy
   d. Supravalvular aortic stenosis

6. Which of the following congenital heart disease is characterized by ventriculocoronary communication?
   a. Aortic atresia with intact ventricular septum
   b. Tetralogy of Fallots
   c. Bicuspid aortic valve
   d. Coarctation of aorta

7. Which of the following is most malignant form of congenital heart disease?
   a. Pulmonary atresia with VSD
   b. Large VSD with PAH
   c. Aortic atresia
   d. Double outlet right ventricle

8. The persistence of connection of the left bundle branch to ventricular septal musculature with abundant Mahaim fibers is a feature of:
   a. Hypertrophic obstructive cardiomyopathy
   b. Pulmonary atresia with VSD
   c. Aortic atresia
   d. Tetralogy of Fallots

9. The most common location of infective endocarditis in cases with coarctation of aorta is:
   a. Site of coarctation
   b. VSD
   c. Circle of Willis
   d. Bicuspid aortic valve

ANSWERS WITH EXPLANATIONS

1. **Ans. a. Left horn of sinus venosus**

   Hurst's 11th Ed; Page 223

   The coronary circulation conveys blood into three separate intercommunicating systems of veins. The larger system of veins terminates in the coronary sinus that drains venous blood from most of the left ventricle. A second system of relatively large veins is separate from the coronary sinus and drains most of venous blood from the right ventricle. A small thebesian veins drain a variable portion of right ventricular venous blood directly into the cavity of right ventricle and right atrium. The coronary sinus is formed in the embryo from the distal part of the left horn of sinus venosus.

2. **Ans. b. Right ventricle**

   Hurst's 11th Ed; Page 223

   Refer to explanation for Q. No 1.

3. **Ans. a. Ectopic origin of left circumflex artery from right sinus of Valsalva**

   Perloff; 3rd Ed; Page 664

   Congenital anomalies of coronary arteries unassociated with congenital heart disease.
   1. Anomalies of aortic origin:
      a. Eccentric ostium within an aortic sinus.
      b. High ostial origin above a coronary sinus.
      c. Conus artery from right aortic sinus.
      d. Left anterior descending and circumflex arteries from separate ostia in the left aortic sinus (absent left main coronary artery).
      e. Left anterior descending coronary artery from right aortic sinus or from right coronary artery.
      f. Circumflex artery from right aortic sinus, from right coronary artery or absent circumflex.
      g. Left main coronary artery from right or posterior aortic sinus or from right coronary artery.

h. Right coronary artery from left aortic sinus, from posterior aortic sinus or from left coronary artery.
i. Single coronary artery (single ostium) from right or left aortic sinus.
2. Anomalous origin of a coronary artery from an extracardiac systemic artery.

4. Ans. c. Pulmonary atresia with intact ventricular septum

Perloff; 3rd Ed; Page 541-542

In pulmonary atresia with intact ventricular septum the presence of small right ventricle results into the flow of blood from a suprasystemic pressure right ventricle retrogradely through intratrabecular channels therefore establishing ventriculocoronary arterial connection. Myocardial ischemia is an important feature of these abnormal communications. A large unobstructed communication functions as a fistulous steal because aortic root blood flows freely during diastole into the right ventricular cavity.

5. Ans. a. Aortic atresia with intact ventricular septum

Perloff; 3rd Ed; Page 653

Similar to the answer 4
The coronary circulation is a matter of interest in patients with hypoplastic left heart syndrome. The hypoplastic ascending aorta act as a common coronary artery receiving retrograde systolic and diastolic flow from the ductus arteriosus. In pulmonary atresia with intact ventricular septum and hypoplastic right ventricle, coronary artery abnormalities includes ventriculocoronary arterial communications, stenosis or interruption of coronary arteries, absent proximal aortocoronary connection and abnormalities of coronary arterial origin and distribution. Anomalous coronary arterial abnormalities are anticipated in patient with aortic atresia, a hypoplastic left ventricle and a hypoplastic perforate mitral valve. In both hypoplastic right ventricle and hypoplastic left ventricle excessive ventricular systolic pressure act as analogous driving force for ventriculocoronary arterial communication. Direct ventriculocoronary arterial communication differ from myocardial sinusoids that connects a ventricular cavity to subepicardial and epicardial coronary arteries and represent an inherently restrictive vascular network that spare the coronary arteries from the impact of high ventricular systolic pressure. In aortic atresia with hypoplastic but perforate mitral valve, the predominate type of ventriculocoronary arterial communication is sinosidal.

6. Ans. a. Aortic atresia with intact ventricular septum

Perloff; 3rd Ed; Page 653

Refer to explanation for Q. No 5.

7. Ans. c. Aortic atresia

Perloff; 3rd Ed; Page 653

The term 'Hypoplastic left heart syndrome' in its most characteristic form is applied to the hypoplasia of left ventricle together with atresia or stenosis of its inflow and outflow valves. In this condition, there is under development – hypoplasia – of the left atrium, mitral valve, left ventricle and aortic valve. In the most extreme expression of hypoplastic left heart both the mitral and aortic valves are atretic and left ventricle is absent or nearly so. In the less extreme form, a hypoplastic left ventricle receives a patent but hypoplastic mitral valve and give rise to an atretic aortic valve. The hypoplastic left ventricle with aortic atresia and mitral hypoplasia predominately seen in the males. The hypoplastic left heart syndrome accounts for 25% of cardiac death in the first week of life and has been called the most malignant form of congenital heart disease. There is an average life span is 5-14 days. The survival in these patients depends upon three precarious variables, i.e., patency of ductus arteriosus, pulmonary vascular resistance and an adequate interatrial communication. The greatest risk of death is at the time of normal ductal closure. An additional important variable is the performance of the right ventricle, whose functional adequacy may be compromised by ischemia in these patients. Ninety-five percent of the infants with hypoplastic left heart syndrome die within first month of life.

8. Ans. c. Aortic atresia

Perloff; 3rd Ed; Page 656

In hypoplastic left heart syndrome, significant changes are found in the branching portion of the bundle of HIS and in the left bundle branch when there is profound abnormality in the development of left ventricle. There are persistent connection of left bundle branch to ventricular septal musculature with abundant Mahaim fibers. Despite abundant Mahaim fibers, Wolff-Parkinson-White bypass tract are rare and despite abnormalities in the left bundle branch, left axis deviation is uncommon and left bundle branch block is unknown. The QRS usually shows pure right ventricular hypertrophy. The relative infrequency of left ventricular hypertrophy in the electrocardiogram despite a thick wall left ventricle in a case of hypoplastic left heart syndrome is a point of clinical importance and interest. Variation in the end diastolic volume affects the magnitude of QRS forces which are generated at the end diastole. An increase in the end diastolic volume, increases the amplitude of early portion of QRS whereas a decrease has the opposite effect. Consistent with this observation are the greater left ventricular forces that results when aortic atresia is associated with ventricular septal defect and an adequately develop left ventricular chamber in hypoplastic left heart syndrome.

9. Ans. d. Bicuspid aortic valve

Perloff; 3rd Ed; Page 132

Infective endocarditis and endarteritis is a potential serious complication in the natural history of coarctation of aorta. Infection tends to occur between ages 10 years and 40 years. Although this complication is unlikely in infants and young children, it not only has been observed in these age group and but has been responsible for saccular mycotic aneurysm. The most common location of the infection is not at the site of coarctation but on the particularly susceptible bicuspid aortic valve.

CHAPTER 2: Cardiac Physiology

1. **Anrep effect includes all *except*:**
   a. A sudden increase in BP is compensated by an increase force of contraction
   b. There is reflex decrease of peripheral resistance mediated by baroreceptors
   c. It is seen in only experimental preparations
   d. It is seen in both normal humans and experimental preparations

2. **Which of the following parameter is taken as measure of afterload in clinical practice?**
   a. Venous pressure
   b. Arterial blood pressure
   c. Aortic impedance
   d. Product of heart rate and blood pressure

3. **Aortic impedance is derived by:**
   a. It is the aortic pressure divided by the aortic flow
   b. It is the aortic flow divided by aortic pressure
   c. It is the aortic pressure multiplied by aortic flow
   d. None of the above

4. **According to Laplace law:**
   a. Wall stress $= \dfrac{\text{Pressure} \times \text{Radius}}{2 \times \text{Wall thickness}}$
   b. Wall stress $= \dfrac{\text{Pressure} \times \text{Radius}}{\text{Wall thickness}}$
   c. Wall stress $= \dfrac{\text{Radius} \times \text{Wall thickness}}{\frac{1}{2}\,\text{Pressure}}$
   d. Wall stress $= \dfrac{\text{Wall thickness}}{\sqrt{\text{Pressure} \times \text{Radius}}}$

5. **In physiological preparation, an increased heart rate progressively increases the force of ventricular contraction, even in isolated papillary muscle preparation—It is called as:**
   a. Frank–Starling mechanism
   b. Anrep effect
   c. Treppe or Bowditch effect
   d. Laplace effect

6. **Which is *correct* regarding coronary blood flow?**
   a. Resting coronary blood flow is normally between 60–90 mL/min/100 g of myocardium
   b. It can increase four to fivefold during exercise
   c. Coronary artery perfusion pressure is an important determinant of coronary blood flow
   d. All are correct

7. **The increase in heart rate associated with atrial distention is known as:**
   a. Bezold–Jarisch reflex
   b. Bainbridge reflex
   c. Anrep effect
   d. Frank–Starling effect

8. **Ventricular distention producing depressor reflex is called as:**
   a. Bezold–Jarisch reflex
   b. Bainbridge reflex
   c. Anrep effect
   d. Frank–Starling effect

9. **Increasing left ventricular end diastolic volume increases stroke volume in ejecting beats is:**
   a. Frank–Starling effect
   b. Anrep effect
   c. Bowditch effect
   d. Bainbridge reflex

10. **Echocardiographically depressed regional wall motion, the hypocontractile segment that still have a sustain glucose extraction as shown by positron emission tomography (PET) is suggestive of:**
    a. Stunned myocardium
    b. Ischemic preconditioning
    c. Hibernating myocardium
    d. Myocardial embalment

11. **Bernheim effect (when a large left ventricle compresses the right ventricle, the volume on the left side being so great that right side is unable to fill properly) is as a:**
    a. Systolic ventricular interaction
    b. Diastolic ventricular interaction
    c. Systolic ventricular interference
    d. Diastolic ventricular interference

12. **Which statement is *not* correct regarding the relation of tension, pressure and radius?**
    a. Tension is directly related to thickness of wall
    b. Tension is inversely related to thickness of wall
    c. Tension is directly related to pressure
    d. Tension is directly related to radius

13. A nonproductive cough is a patient with heart failure is called as:
 a. Dyspnea
 b. Dyspnea equivalent
 c. Orthopnea equivalent
 d. Trepopnea

14. Orthopnea limited to one lateral decubitus position is named as:
 a. Dyspnea equivalent
 b. Orthopnea equivalent
 c. Trepopnea
 d. Paroxysmal nocturnal dyspnea

15. Which of following is *not* a mechanism for occurrence of paroxysmal nocturnal dyspnea?
 a. Sudden expansion of thoracic blood volume due to resorption of interstitial fluid from the periphery and dependent portion
 b. Sudden elevation of thoracic blood volume and of diaphragm on assuming recumbency
 c. Enhanced adrenergic flow to support LV function during sleep
 d. Normal nocturnal depression of the respiratory center

16. Paroxysmal nocturnal dyspnea reflects the presence of:
 a. Pulmonary venous congestion
 b. Interstitial edema
 c. Alveolar edema
 d. Reduction in vital capacity

17. Trepopnea means:
 a. Breathlessness coming on brisk walking
 b. Breathlessness that develops in the recumbent position and is relieved by elevation of the head with pillows
 c. Breathlessness which develops on climbing stairs
 d. Orthopnea limited to one lateral decubitus position

18. Enzyme neprilysin is responsible for breakdown of:
 a. Natriuretic peptides
 b. Bradykinin
 c. Angiotensin II
 d. All of the above

19. Which statement is *correct* regarding use of Sacubitril/Valsartan combinations?
 a. At least 36 hours washout period should be allowed when switching from an ACEI before starting Sacubitril/Valsartan
 b. Patient must be able to tolerate an ACEI or an ARB prior to being started on Sacubitril/Valsartan
 c. Brain natriuretic peptide (BNP) will be elevated in patients taking this drug
 d. All of the above

20. Which of the following should be utilized in patient on Sacubitril/Valsartan combination to assess heart failure exacerbation?
 a. Brain natriuretic peptide (BNP) level
 b. NT-proBNP
 c. Serum creatinine level
 d. Serum potassium level

21. Which of the following are chief contractile proteins in myocyte?
 a. Actin and myosin
 b. Troponin C
 c. Titin
 d. None of them

22. Which is the functional contractile unit of cardiac muscle?
 a. Cardiac myocyte
 b. Sarcomere
 c. Actin and myosin
 d. Myofibril

23. Which of the following is known to be a stretch sensor, that transmit the signals resulting into the myocyte growth pattern characteristics of volume overload condition?
 a. Titin protein
 b. LIM protein (MLP)
 c. Adenosine gynaculate
 d. ATP

24. Conditions in which contraction of cardiac muscle is strengthen independent of sarcomere length is labelled as:
 a. Frank–Starling effect
 b. Positive Inotropic states
 c. Lusitropy
 d. All

25. Enhanced conduction velocity through the conduction system is called as:
 a. Positive chronotropy
 b. Positive inotropy
 c. Positive lusitropy
 d. Positive dromotropy

26. All the following are the main determinants of ventricular mechanical performance *except*:
 a. Preload and afterload
 b. Contractility
 c. Heart rate
 d. Peripheral resistance

27. The cardiac cycle was assembled and conceived by:
 a. Schmaroth
 b. Braunwald
 c. Forssman
 d. Lewis and Wiggers

28. The phase of LV contraction after mitral valve closure and before aortic opening when the LV volume is fixed is referred as:
 a. Isovolumic contraction
 b. Isovolumic relaxation
 c. Phase of reduced ejection
 d. None of the above

CHAPTER 2 | Cardiac Physiology

29. In cardiac cycle Diastasis occurs during:
   a. End of left ventricular filling phase
   b. In the mid part of left ventricular filling phase
   c. The beginning of left ventricular ejection
   d. At the end of left ventricular ejection

30. Atrial systole or left atrial kick is important for left ventricular filling during:
   a. High heart rate   b. During exercise
   c. In LV hypertrophy   d. All

31. The interval between the first heart sound (M1) to the closure of aortic valve (second heart sound A2) is called as:
   a. Cardiologic systole   b. Physiologic systole
   c. Physiologic diastole   d. Proto diastole

32. Physiologic systole lasts from:
   a. Start of isovolumic contraction to the peak of the ejection phase
   b. The start of isovolumic contraction to the end of ejection phase
   c. Between the first heart sound (M1) and the second heart sound (A2)
   d. None of the above

33. The degree of myocardial stretch or distention before contraction starts is called as:
   a. Inotropic state   b. Preload
   c. Afterload   d. Wall stress

34. The component of Frank–Starling effects are:
   a. Only positive inotropic effect
   b. Only increased lusitropic effect
   c. Both positive inotropic effect and increased lusitropic effect
   d. None of the above

35. The slow force response or adaptation of left ventricular inotropy in response to the elevation of aortic pressure is called as:
   a. Frank–Starling effect   b. Anrep effect
   c. Treppe phenomenon   d. Staircase phenomenon

36. Which state is *correct* regarding cardiac mechanics?
   a. Preload is represented by the LV end diastolic volume (EDV).
   b. Preload and afterload are interlinked
   c. When preload increases the stroke volumes rises conversely when afterload increases stroke volume drops
   d. All of the above

37. According to Laplace's Law left ventricular wall stress is:
   a. Directly proportional to the product of pressure and radius and inversely proportional to the double of wall thickness
   b. It is directly proportional to the double of wall thickness and inversely proportional to the product of pressure and radius.
   c. It is directly proportional to the product of wall thickness and radius and inversely proportional to the double of pressure.
   d. It is directly proportional to the double of wall thickness and inversely proportional to the double of radius.

38. Peak systolic wall stress reflects which components of afterload?
   a. Peripheral resistance
   b. Arterial compliance
   c. Peak intraventricular pressure
   d. All of the above

39. Bowditch staircase phenomenon is:
   a. A larger heart volume increases the initial length of muscle fiber, to increase stroke volume at the cardiac output.
   b. An increased heart rate progressively enhances the force of ventricular muscle contraction.
   c. When the aortic pressure is elevated abruptly it limit ejection and tend to increase end diastolic volume, which acutely increases force and pressure at next beats.
   d. None of the above

40. Which of the following is the best Index of cardiac work or O_2 uptake?
   a. Double product (systolic blood pressure × heart rate)
   b. External work (pressure × volume)
   c. Minute work (SBP × SV × HR)
   d. Pressure volume area

41. The wall stress in right ventricular function is lower due to which of the following factor?
   a. Different chamber geometry of right ventricle.
   b. Lower pressure in the right ventricle and pulmonary circulation
   c. Lower right ventricular wall thickness
   d. All the factors are contributory

42. Which chamber of the heart is called as "blood volume sensor"?
   a. Left ventricle   b. Left atrium
   c. Right ventricle   d. Right atrium

43. Which of the following cellular process plays important role in progressive cardiac dysfunction and LV remodelling in failing myocardium?
   a. Necrosis   b. Apoptosis
   c. Autophagy   d. All of the above

ANSWERS WITH EXPLANATIONS

1. Ans. c. It is seen in only experimental preparations

Braunwald 11th Ed; Page 435-436

Anrep effect: During the systole of cardiac cycle, the left ventricle contract against the afterload (the load after the onset of contraction, against which LV contracts during LV ejection). It was studied in experimental animal that abruptly increasing the blood pressure of the heart lung preparation, the left ventricular performance increases to overcome the greater peripheral resistance. Both systolic and diastolic LV volumes rises indicating that left ventricle did not empty completely. The increased diastolic volume 'x' in a manner similar to an increase preload to prevent the stroke volume from falling as the afterload increased. Such an afterload dependent myocardium is probably the result of experimental condition in which the left ventricle is in a state of incipient failure. In experimental preparations and in normal humans, a sudden increase in the blood pressure is compensated for by an increase force of contraction, i.e., anrep effect and by a reflex decrease in the peripheral vascular resistance mediated by the baroreflexes.

When the aortic pressure is elevated abruptly a positive inotropic effect follows within 1-2 minutes. This is called as Homeometric autoregulation because it is apparently independent of muscle length and by definition it is a true inotropic effect. Stress develop in the ventricle when tension is applied to a cross sectional area and the units are force per unit area. According to Laplace law, wall stress equal to pressure into radius divided by 2 × wall thickness.

This equation emphasizes two points: (1) The bigger the left ventricle and greater its radius, the greater is the wall stress. (2) At any given radius (LV size) the greater the pressure developed by the left ventricle, the greater is the wall stress. An increase in the wall stress achieved by either of these two mechanism (LV size or intraventricular pressure) increases myocardial oxygen uptake. This is because a greater rate of ATP used is required, as the myofibrils develop greater tension.

2. Ans. b. Arterial blood pressure

Braunwald 11th Ed; Page 435-436

Wall stress, preload and afterload: Preload can be defined as the wall stress at the end of diastole and therefore at the maximal resting length of sarcomere. Measurement of wall stress in vivo is difficult because the radius of left ventricle neglects the confounding influence of the complex anatomy of left ventricle. Surrogate measurement of indices of preload include LV diastolic pressure or dimension. The afterload, being the load on the contractile myocardium is also the wall stress during left ventricle ejection. Increased afterload means that an increased intraventricular pressure has to be generated first to open the aortic valve and then during the ejection phase. These increases translate themselves into an increased myocardial wall stress which can be measured either as an average value or at a given phase of systole such as end systole. Systolic wall stress reflects the two major components of the afterload, namely the arterial blood pressure and the arterial compliance. Decreased arterial compliance and increase afterload can be anticipated when there is a aortic dilatation as in severe systemic hypertension or in elderly person. In clinical practice, it is a sufficient approximation to take the arterial blood pressure as a measure of afterload provided there is no significant aortic stenosis or change in arterial compliance.

The aortic impedance also term the arterial input impedance, gives another accurate measure of afterload. The aortic impedance is the aortic pressure divided by the aortic flow at that instance, so that this index of the afterload varies at each stage of contraction cycles. Factors reducing aortic flow such as high arterial blood pressure or aortic stenosis or loss of aortic compliance increases impedance and hence the afterload.

3. Ans. a. It is the aortic pressure divided by the aortic flow

Braunwald 11th Ed; Page 435-436

Refer to explanation for Q. No 1.

4. Ans. a. $$\text{Wall stress} = \frac{\text{Pressure} \times \text{Radius}}{2 \times \text{Wall thickness}}$$

Braunwald 11th Ed; Page 435-436

Refer to explanation for Q. No 1.

5. Ans. c. Treppe or Bowditch effect

Braunwald 11th Ed; Page 437

Treppe or Bowditch effect: An increased heart rate progressively increases the force of ventricular contraction, even in an isolated papillary muscle preparation. This is also called as Treppe phenomenon or positive inotropic effect of activation or force frequency relation. Conversely, a decreased heart rate has a negative staircase effect. When stimulation becomes too rapid force decreases. It is proposed that during rapid stimulation more sodium and calcium ions enter the myocardial cells than can be handled by the sodium pump and the mechanism for calcium exit. Opposing the force frequency effect is the negative contractile influence of the decreased duration of ventricular filling at high heart rate. The longer the filling interval the better ventricular filling and the stronger subsequent contraction. This phenomenon is also seen in patient with mitral stenosis and atrial fibrillation with a variable filling interval.

6. Ans. d. All are correct

Hurst's 14th Ed; Page 120

Resting coronary blood flow is normally between 60 and 90 ml/min/100 gm of myocardium and can rapidly increase four to five folds during exercise or other conditions requiring augmented flow. The coronary flow rate is determined by the coronary artery perfusion pressure and by the resistance to flow exaggerated by forces generated within and outside the coronary vascular bed. The complexity of these forces is highlighted by the unexpected finding that the coronary diastolic pressure at the time of zero flow is greater than coronary sinus pressure. Control of coronary blood flow is metabolic, mechanical, autonomic and endothelial. The exact local feedback control mechanism that match coronary blood flow to myocardial oxygen consumption is still poorly understood.

7. Ans. b. Bainbridge reflex

Hurst's 14th Ed; Page 123

Mechanoreceptors are there in the heart, which possess both vagal and sympathetic efferent. Sensors on the atria and ventricle receive vagal efferent and sensors on pulmonary veins and coronary vessel receives sympathetic efferents. Atrial A and B receptors are located at the venoatrial junctions and have distinct function. Type 'A' receptors react primarily to heart rate but adapt to long-term changes in atrial volume. Type 'B' receptors increase their discharge during atrial distention. C-fibers arise from receptors is scattered throughout through the atria and these discharge with a low frequency and respond with increased discharge to increase in atrial pressure. The A and B receptors are thought to mediate the increase in heart rate associated with atrial distention (as it occurs with intravenous infusion) known as Bainbridge reflex. In contrast, activation of atrial C-fibers produces a vasodepressor effect (bradycardia and peripheral vasodilatation). Ventricular mechanoreceptor efferent discharge decreases periodically with inspiration. Ventricular C-fibers are primarily located in the epicardium and discharge more rapidly in response to increase in both systolic and diastolic blood pressure. Ventricular distention can produce a powerful depressor reflex called Bezold–Jarisch reflex. Vagal efferent of this cardiopulmonary reflex are also activated by chemical stimulation, e.g., cytokines, serotonin and classically veratrum alkaloids.

8. Ans. a. Bezold–Jarisch reflex

Hurst's 14th Ed, Page 123

Refer to explanation for Q. No 7.

9. Ans. a. Frank–Starling effect

Hurst's 14th Ed; Page 113

The influence of preload on measures of ventricular performance defines the LV function curve known as the Frank–Starling curve. Increasing LV end diastolic volume increases stroke volume in ejecting beats an increase peak LV pressure in isovolumic beats. The modulation of ventricular performance by changes in the preload is termed as heterometric regulation, operates on a beat by beat basis and is responsible for matching output of the right and left ventricle as with the changes in posture and breathing. The Frank–Starling curve also represents and important compensatory mechanism that maintains left ventricular stroke volume when left ventricular shortening is impaired, owing either to myocardial contractile dysfunction or due to excessive afterload. The atria also exhibit a Frank–Starling curve that becomes clinically important during exercise and when there is resistance to early diastolic left ventricular filling.

10. Ans. c. Hibernating myocardium

Hurst's 11th Ed; Page 710

The hibernating myocardium like the hibernating animal is temporarily asleep and can wake up to function normally when blood supply is fully restored. It is proposed that the fall of myocardial function to a lower level copes with the reduced myocardial oxygen supply and leads to self-preservation, the so called smart heart. Hibernation is a complex clinical situation without a good animal model. When ischemia in patient is delineated echocardiographically as depressed regional wall motion, the hypocontractile segment that still have a sustained glucose extraction has shown by positron emission tomography (PET), have a high chance of recovery after coronary artery bypass surgery. In contrast those segments with the decreased glucose extraction almost uniformly fail to recover. It has also been proposed that hibernation can occur even when the resting coronary blood flow is normal despite the presence of coronary artery disease. The proposed mechanism is that recurrent episode of ischemia leave behind stunned myocardium so that hibernation is the sum of repetitive and cumulative stunning.

11. Ans. b. Diastolic ventricular interaction

Hurst's 11th Ed; Page 710

The left ventricular function is intimately linked to that of right ventricle; both functionally and anatomically. The cardiac output of left ventricle must equal that of the right ventricle unless there is state of imbalance, as in condition of acute left ventricular failure when blood may accumulate in the lungs to cause pulmonary edema. In general, the right ventricle is working against a low resistance circuit and afterload is not a major problem in physiological condition. What the right ventricle received by means its filling pressure in the venous system, it empties in response to the Starling effect. The amount of pressure work generated by the right ventricle is relatively low and therefore the right ventricle is of thin wall. Anatomically, the two ventricles are interlinked. They share a common septum. That septum constitutes part of the load against which each ventricle must work. In the left ventricular hypertrophy, which includes the septum the right ventricle must work harder and tends to become hypertrophied. This is systolic ventricular interaction. One type of diastolic ventricular interaction is the 'Bernheim effect', whereby a large left ventricle compresses the right ventricle, the volume on the left side being so great that the right side is unable to fill properly. A converse ventricular interaction can occur in severe heart failure, when the dilated right ventricle may impinge on the left. When the right ventricle is unloaded by the venodilator agents (nitroglycerine) it can decrease in size and allow the left ventricular function to improve. When there is a physical impairment of mechanical function on the other as a result of volume overloading with blood the result is diastolic ventricular interference.

12. Ans. a. Tension is directly related to thickness of wall

Braunwald 11th Ed; Page 435–436

Refer to explanation for Q. Nos 1 to 4.

13. Ans. b. Dyspnea equivalent

Braunwald 11th Ed; Page 404–405

In patients with congestive heart failure, cough may be caused by pulmonary congestion, occurs under the same circumstances as dyspnea (i.e., during exertion or recumbency), and is relieved by treatment of heart failure. Thus a nonproductive cough in patients with heart failure is often a dyspnea equivalent, whereas a cough on recumbency may be considered an orthopnea equivalent. Patients with severe chronic obstructive lung disease sometime complain of orthopnea. Trepopnea is a rare form of orthopnea limited to one lateral decubitus position. It has been attributed to distortions of the great vessel in one position but not in the other.

14. Ans. c. Trepopnea

Braunwald 11th Ed; Page 404–405

Refer to explanation for Q. No 13.

15. Ans. c. Enhanced adrenergic flow to support LV function during sleep

Braunwald 11th Ed; Page 404–405

Paroxysmal nocturnal dyspnea: Attacks of paroxysmal dyspnea usually occur at night. The patient awakens, often quite suddenly and with a feeling of severe anxiety and suffocation, sits bolt upright and gasps for breath. Bronchospasm, which may be caused by congestion of the bronchial mucosa and by interstitial pulmonary edema compressing the small bronchi, increases ventilator difficulty and the work of breathing and is a common complicating factor of paroxysmal nocturnal dyspnea. In contrast to orthopnea, which may be relieved immediately by sitting upright at the side of the bed with the legs dependent, attacks of paroxysmal nocturnal dyspnea may require 30 minutes or longer in this position for relief. The reason for the common occurrence of these episodes at night is not clear, but it seems likely that the combination of: (1) The slow resorption of interstitial fluid from the dependent portion of the body and the resultant expansion of thoracic blood volume, (2) Sudden elevation of thoracic blood volume and of the diaphragm which occurs immediately on assuming recumbency (3) Reduced adrenergic support of left ventricular function during sleep, and (4) Normal nocturnal depression of the respiratory center. All the factors play major roles.

The mechanism of dyspnea: Increase awareness of respiration or difficulties in breathing is commonly associated with pulmonary capillary hypertension caused by an elevation of left atrial or left ventricular filling pressure. Patients with left ventricular failure typically exhibit restrictive ventilatory defect, characterized by a reduction of vital capacity as a consequence of replacement of the air in the lung with blood are interstitial fluid or both. Dyspnea during exertion and orthopnea are usually the clinical expression of pulmonary venous or capillary congestion. Paroxysmal nocturnal dyspnea reflect the presence of primarily interstitial edema, whereas pulmonary edema in which there is transudation and expectoration of blood tinged fluid is often a manifestation of alveolar edema.

16. Ans. b. Interstitial edema

Braunwald 11th Ed; Page 404–405

Refer to explanation for Q. No 15.

17. Ans. d. Orthopnea limited to one lateral decubitus position

Braunwald 11th Ed; Page 404–405

Refer to explanation for Q. No 13.

18. Ans. d. All of the above

Hurst's 14th Ed; Page 1709

The drug LCZ696 used in heart failure is composed of the ARB valsartan and the neprilysin inhibitor sacubitril. Valsartan blocks the AT1 receptor. Sacubitril is converted to the active neprilysin inhibitor, which inhibits neprilysin, an enzyme that breaks down atrial natriuretic peptide, BNP, and C-type natriuretic peptide, as well as other vasoactive substances such as bradykinin, angiotensin II, substance P.

CHAPTER 2 | Cardiac Physiology

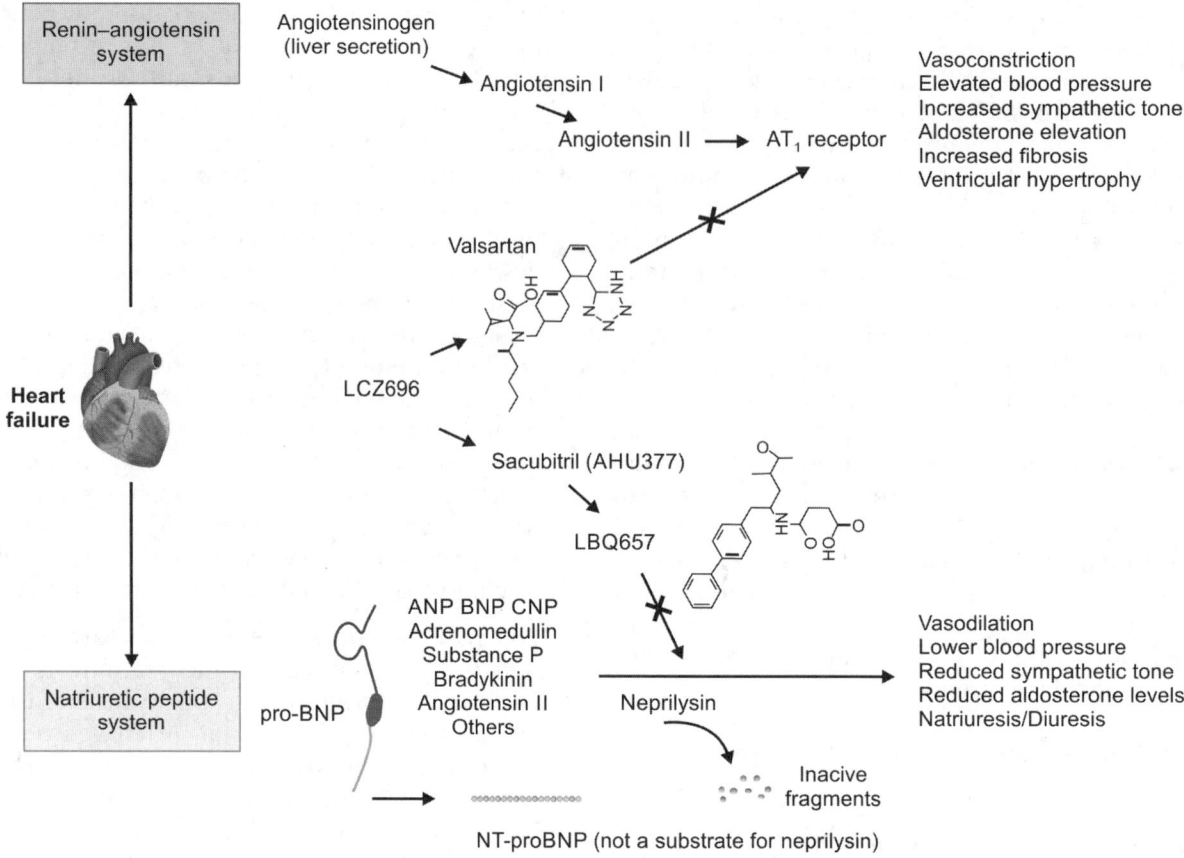

Schematic showing the mechanism of action of LCZ696

---

19. Ans. d. All of the above

ACC/AHA Guidelines for diagnosis and management of Heart Failure 2022

Oral neprilysin inhibitors, used in combination with angiotensin converting enzyme inhibitor, can lead to angioedema, and concomitant use is contraindicated and should be avoided. This adverse effect is thought to occur because ACE inhibitor and neprilysin break down bradykinin, which can directly or indirectly cause angioedema. An ARNI should not be administered within 36 hours of switching from or to an ACEI.

20. Ans. b. NT-proBNP

ACC/AHA Guidelines for diagnosis and management of Heart Failure 2022

B-type natriuretic peptide (BNP), atrial natriuretic peptide (ANP), and C-type natriuretic peptide (CNP) are the three main natriuretic peptides. They share a common structure and ultimately mediate their action by activating cyclic guanosine monophosphate (cGMP). ARNI therapy results in a decrease of N-terminal pro-BNP (NT-proBNP) and increase of BNP levels respectively and therefore, NT-proBNP should be utilized to assess heart failure exacerbation.

21. Ans. a. Actin and myosin

Braunwald, 12th Ed; Page 892–893 & 895

The two chief contractile proteins are the motor protein myosin on the thick filament and the actin on the thin filament. Calcium ions initiates the contraction cycle by binding to the thin filament regulatory protein Troponin-C to relieve the inhibition, otherwise exerted by this Troponin complex. The thin actin filaments are connected to Z-line at the either end of Sarcomere which is the functional contractile unit that is repeated through the filaments.

Titin is a large protein molecule. It is extraordinarily long, elastic, and slender. Titin extends from Z-line into thick filament approaching the M-line and connect the thick filament to Z-line. Titin has two distinct segments an inextensible anchoring segment and an extensible elastic segment that stretches as sarcomere length increases. Titin has multiple functions. First, tethers myosin and thick filaments to the Z-line therefore stabilizing sarcomeric structure. Second, as it stretches and relaxes, its elasticity contributes to the stress-strain relationship of cardiac muscles. Similar to spring, it helps in re-lengthening the sarcomere and aid early diastolic filling. Third, the increased diastolic stretch of the titin as the length of sarcomere in cardiac muscle is increased causes the unfolded part of titin molecules to straighten. This stretched molecular spring limits overstretching of

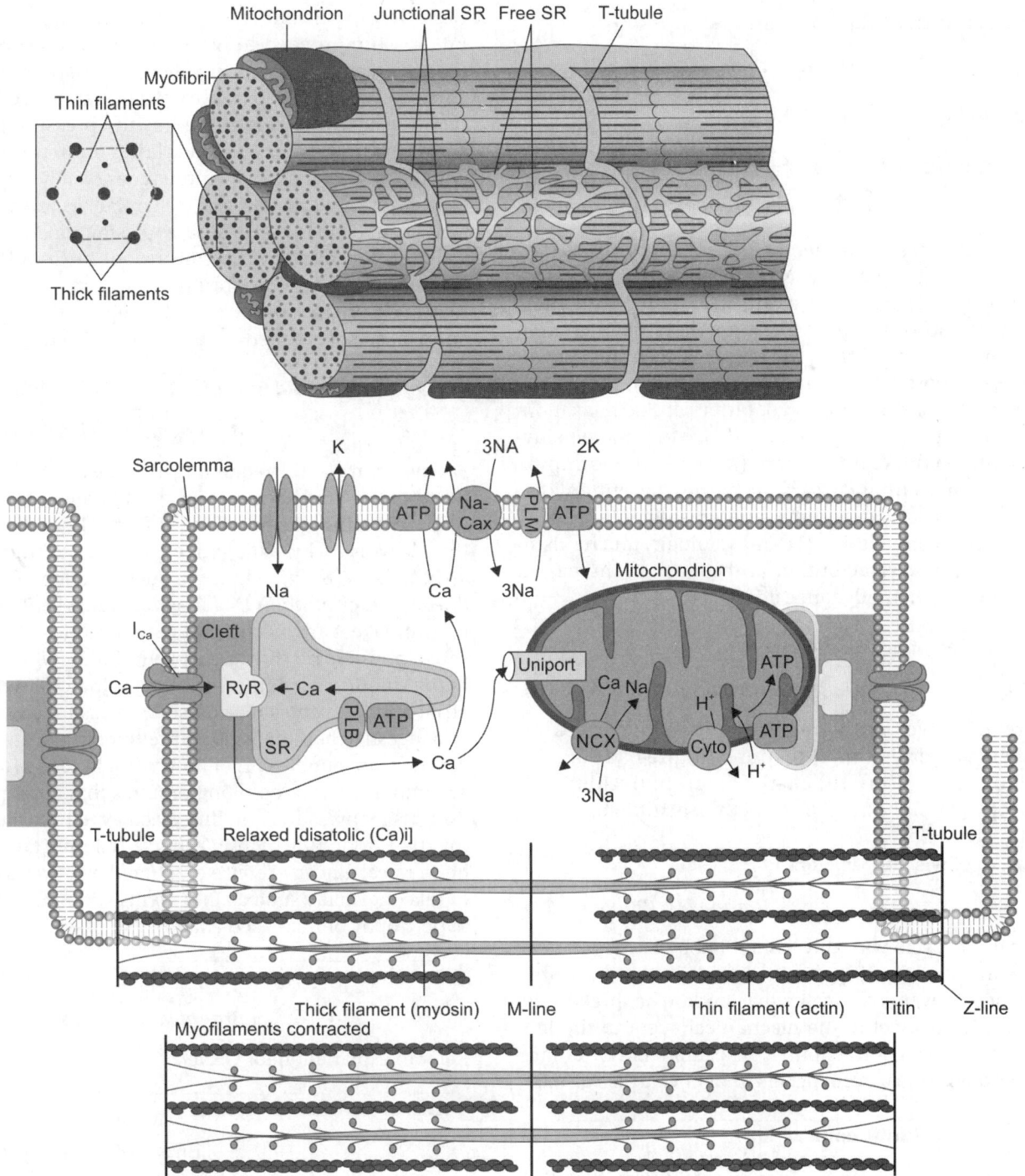

sarcomeres and end-diastolic volume. Fourth, titin may transduce mechanical stretch into the growth signals. Sustained diastolic stretch, as in volume overload condition can cause titin dependents signalling to muscle LIM protein (MLP) attached to the Z-line end of titin. MLP is known to be a stretch sensor that transmits the signal that results in the myocyte growth pattern characteristic of volume overload. This mechanism is defective in a subset of dilated cardiomyopathy patients.

When changes in diastolic length (or preload) are the cause of altered contractile-strength, it is called as Frank–Starling effect. Conditions in which contraction is strengthen independent of sarcomere length (typically by increased Calcium ion transient amplitude) are referred to as positive inotropic states or enhanced contractility.

22. Ans. b. Sarcomere

Braunwald, 12th Ed; Page 892–893 & 895

Refer to explanation for Q. No 23.

23. Ans. b. LIM protein (MLP)

Braunwald, 12th Ed; Page 892–893 & 895

Refer to explanation for Q. No 23.

24. Ans. b. Positive Inotropic states

Braunwald, 12th Ed; Page 892-893 & 895

Refer to explanation for Q. No 23.

25. Ans. d. Positive Dromotropy

Braunwald 12th Ed; Page 899-900

During the classic adrenergic fight or flight response, cardiac myocyte beta-adrenergic receptors are activated which leads to increased cAMP production and PKA activation and consequent phosphorylation and altered function of numerous myocyte targets. This results iin an increased heart rate (positive chronotropy), increased contractility (positive inotropy), faster cardiac relaxation (positive lusitropy) and enhanced conduction velocity through the conduction system (positive dromotropy). These events enhance cardiac output by enhancing the heart rate, stroke volume, and diastolic filling. The adrenergic response is a key physiologic mechanism for increasing cardiac output in response to increased metabolic and hemodynamic demands.

26. Ans. d. Peripheral resistance

Braunwald 12th Ed; Page 904

There are five main determinants of ventricular mechanical performance, they are: (a) preload (Frank-Starling mechanism), (b) afterload; (c) contractility; (d) Lusitropy (Diastolic function) and € the heart rate.

27. Ans. d. Lewis and Wiggers

Braunwald 12th; Page 904

The cardiac cycle was fully assembled by Lewis but was first conceived by Wiggers. It describes the temporal sequence of events during cardiac cycle. The three basic events with respect to the mechanical event in the left ventricle are, LV contraction, LV relaxation and LV filling. Similar mechanical event occurs in right ventricle also.

28. Ans. a. Isovolumic contraction

Braunwald 12th Ed; Page 904

Left ventricular contraction begins with the LV pressure increased as calcium ion arrives at contractile protein after cellular depolarization triggers actin myosin interaction. This occurs soon after the upstroke of ventricular action potential indicated by QRS complex of electrocardiogram. When LV pressure exceeds that in left atrium (normally 8 to 15 mm Hg), the mitral valve closes, causing the mitral components of first heart sound. Right ventricular pressure changes are usually slightly delayed because of the electrical conduction such that tricuspid valve closure (T1) follows M1. The phase of LV contraction after mitral valve closure and before aortic opening when the LV volume is fixed is referred to as Isovolumic Contraction. As more myofibers become activated, LV pressure proceed to increase until it exceeds aortic pressure, causing the aortic valve to open. Opening of the aortic valve is followed by the phase of rapid ejection. The rate of ejection is determined by the pressure gradient across aortic valve, as well as elastic properties of aorta and the arterial tree, which undergoes systolic expansion. LV pressure rises to peak and to start fall. As myocytes Ca^{2+} starts to decline because of sarcoplasmic calcium uptake. Calcium ion dissociates from troponin C and thereby preventing further cross-bridge formation. As this state of relaxation progresses the rate of LV ejection of blood into aorta falls, that is called as "phase of reduced ejection".

29. Ans. b. In the mid part of left ventricular filling phase

Braunwald 12th Ed; Page 433-434

Following mitral valve opening the phase of rapid or early filling occurs and accounts for most of the increase in LV volume during diastole. Under normal circumstances, this is caused by a negative pressure gradient from atrium to LV apex, creating a suction effect, especially during exercise, when LV filling rate must be augmented to increase cardiac output. Such rapid filling may cause physiologic third heart sound (S3), when there is hyperkinetic circulation or a pathologic S3 when left atrial and left ventricular diastolic pressure are elevated in congestive heart failure. As pressure in the atrium and ventricle are equalize, LV filling virtually stops (diastasis, separation). Renewed filling requires that atrial pressure exceeds LV pressure, and this is achieved by atrial systole (or the LA kick), which is especially important at high heart rates, during exercise or when the left ventricle fails to relax normally such as in patients with left ventricular hypertrophy or increased chamber stiffness.

30. Ans. d. All

Braunwald 12th Ed; Page 433-434

Refer to explanation for Q. No 29.

31. Ans. a. Cardiologic systole

Braunwald 12th Ed; Page 905

The start of ventricular systole can be regarded as the beginning of isovolumic contraction, when left ventricular pressure exceeds the atrial pressure so as to bring mitral valve closure. Physiologic systole lasts from the start of isovolumic contraction to the peak of ejection phase. Physiologic diastole commences as calcium ion is taken back into sarcoplasmic reticulum, so that myocyte relaxation dominates over contraction, and as the LV pressure start to fall. Cardiologic systole is longer than physiologic systole and is demarcated by the interval between the first heart sound to the closure of aortic valve (A2). The remainder of the cardiac cycle automatically becomes cardiologic diastole. Proto diastole is the early phase of rapid filling, the time when S3 can be heard.

32. Ans. a. Start of isovolumic contraction to the peak of the ejection phase

Braunwald 12th Ed; Page 905

Refer to explanation for Q. No 33.

33. Ans. b. Preload

Braunwald 12th Ed; Page 906

Contractility or the inotropic state is the inherent capacity of the myocardium to contact independently of changes in preload or afterload. At the molecular level, an increased inotropic state is usually explained by either enhanced calcium ion transients or enhanced myofilament calcium sensitivity and typically means a greater rate of contraction to reach a greater peak force. The preload describes the degree of myocardial stretch or distention before contract has started and is best represented at the chamber level by LV end-diastolic volume (EDV). Because, volume is difficult to measure accurately and precisely in practice, preload is often estimated by LV end-diastolic pressure. Afterload refers to the forces opposing LV ejection. Afterload is usually equal to aortic blood pressure but more accurately described as aortic impedance or elastance, which incorporates steady and oscillatory components of cardiac load. LV afterload can also be expressed by the wall stress that exists during systole.

Wall stress developed when the tension is applied to a cross sectional area and the unit are force per unit area.

34. Ans. c. Both positive inotropic effect and increased lusitropic effect

Braunwald 12th Ed; Page 906

If a larger heart volume increases the initial length of muscle fiber, to increase stroke volume and thus cardiac output, diastolic stretch of left ventricle (and increased sarcomere length) increases the force of contraction. Frank initially reported that the greater the initial LV volume, the more rapid the rate of rise, the greater the peak pressure reached, and the faster rate of relaxation. He described both positive inotropic effect and an increased lusitropic effect. These complimentary findings of Frank and Starling are often combined into Frank–Starling Law. Thus an increase in the strength of contraction can generally be categorized as either a Frank–Starling effect (increased sarcomere length) or an inotropic effect (altered calcium transient or myofilament calcium sensitivity), although both effects can occur simultaneously as during physical exercise.

35. Ans. b. Anrep effect

Braunwald 12th Ed; Page 906

When the aortic pressure is elevated abruptly, it limits ejection and tends to increase end diastolic volume, which acutely increases force and pressure at the next beat by the Frank–Starling effect. However, in a slower adaptation that takes seconds to minutes, the inotropic state of the heart increases (and calcium transients are larger). This slow force response or adaptation is referred to as the Anrep effect.

36. Ans. d. All of the above

Braunwald 12th Ed; Page 906

The preload describes the degree of myocardial stretch or distention before contraction has started and is represented at the chamber level by LV end diastolic volume. Afterload refers to the forces opposing LV ejection. Afterload is more accurately described as aortic impedance or elastance. When preload increases stroke volume rises according to Starling's law, if all other factors are held constant. Conversely, when afterload increases, stroke volume drops. The preload and afterload influence each other. By the Frank–Starling Law, an increased LV volume leads to increase contractile function which in turn will increase systolic aortic pressure and thus the afterload in the subsequent contraction cycle. During LV ejection, sarcomere length progressively declines, decreasing both myofilament calcium and sensitivity and maximal force, which along with progressive calcium decline, reduces the contractile force. Afterload also dynamically changes during ejection and decline as ejection wanes.

37. Ans. a. Directly proportional to the product of pressure and radius and inversely proportional to the double of wall thickness

Braunwald 12th Ed; Page 907

Wall stress develops when the tension is applied to a cross-sectional area, and the units are force per unit area. According to Laplace's law, wall stress = (pressure × radius)/(2 × wall thickness). According to this equation,

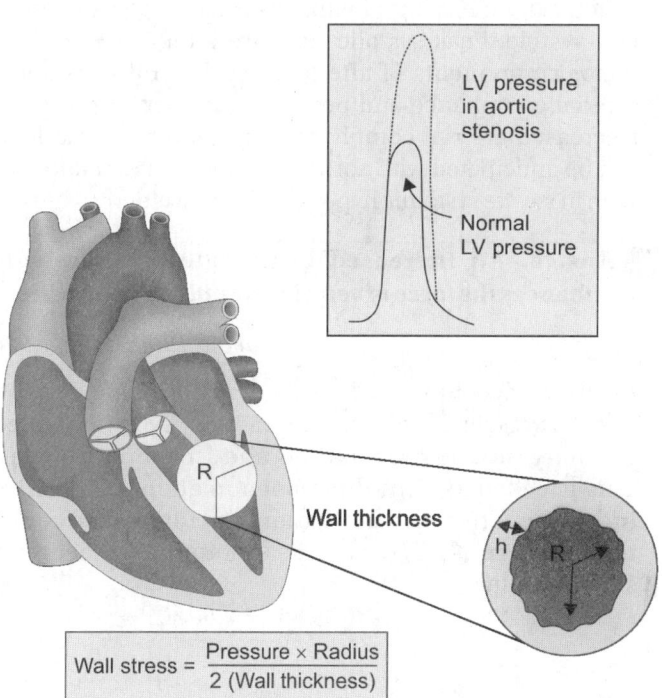

the larger the LV size and radius, the higher is the wall stress. Secondly, at any given radius (LV size), greater the pressure developed by the left ventricle, greater is the wall stress. An increase in wall stress is achieved either by increasing the LV size or increasing intraventricular pressure. Both of this will increase myocardial oxygen uptake because a greater rate of ATP use is required for the myofibrils to develop more tension. In cardiac hypertrophy, Laplace's law explains the effect of changes in wall thickness on wall stress. The increased wall thickness from hypertrophy balances the increased pressure, and wall stress remains unchanged during the phase of compensatory hypertrophy. Similarly, in congestive heart failure, the heart dilates so that increased radius will elevates wall stress. Moreover, in patient with congestive heart failure, the quantum of ejected blood is inadequate, the radius stays too large throughout the contractile cycle, and both end-diastolic and end-systolic wall stress is higher. This decreases LV efficiency, increases myocardial oxygen demand, and augments release of natriuretic peptide levels. The overall reduction in heart size decreases wall stress and improves LV function.

38. Ans. d. All of the above

Braunwald 12th Ed; Page 907

Preload is defined as the wall stretch at the end of diastole and therefore at the maximal resting length of sarcomere. The surrogate marker of preload is LVEDP or dimensions (the dimensions being the major or minor axis of the heart in 2-D Echocardiographic view). Afterload being the load on the contractile myocardium is the wall stress during LV ejection. Increased afterload means that increased intraventricular pressure is to be generated to open the aortic valve and then during the ejection phase. This increase is translate into increased myocardial wall stress, which can be measured either as an average value or at end-systole. Peak systolic wall stress reflects the three major components of afterload, peripheral resistance, arterial compliance and peak intraventricular pressure. Decreased arterial compliance and increased afterload can be anticipated with aortic remodeling and dilation, as seen in severe systemic hypertension or in elderly patients.

39. Ans. b. An increased heart rate progressively enhances the force of ventricular muscle contraction.

Braunwald 12th Ed; Page 908

An increased heart rate progressively enhances the force of ventricular muscle contraction, even in isolated papillary muscle preparations and isolated myocytes. This is called as "Bowditch phenomenon" or positive inotropic effect of activation or force frequency relationship. A decreased heart rate has a negative staircase effect.

40. Ans. c. Minute work (SBP × SV × HR)

Braunwald 12th Ed; Page 909

There are three determinants of myocardial oxygen uptake, they are: Preload, afterload and heart rate. External work (pressure × volume) is done by the heart, with stroke volume (cardiac output) being the volume moved against the arterial blood pressure. Volume work (associated with increased stroke volume) requires less oxygen than pressure work. Minute work can be defined as the product of systolic blood pressure, stroke volume and heart rate (SBP × SV × HR). This pressure work index takes into accounts both the double product (SBP × HR) and HR × SV (cardiac output). The pressure volume areas is another useful index of cardiac work or O_2 uptake but it requires invasive monitoring for accurate measurements.

41. Ans. b. Lower pressure in the right ventricle and pulmonary circulation.

Braunwald 12th Ed; Page 911

Right ventricular myocytes are fundamentally the same as those in left ventricle, with some minor quantitative differences in their ion channel, calcium ion handling, electrophysiology, and myofilament properties. The most important functional differences are in the chamber geometry related to Laplace's law and normal levels of pressure developed. The pressure in the right ventricle and pulmonary circulation is much lower than the left sided circulation. The right ventricle has a larger radius of curvature which would tend to increase wall tension, but it normally develops much lower pressure, which greatly reduces wall tension. Right ventricular wall thickness is also lower such that the normal characteristics of right ventricular shape and size are functionally matched to the different prevailing conditions on right ventricle. Once there is a pathophysiological condition like pulmonary hypertension where the afterload dependent is heightened, the right ventricle being poorly suited to eject against high pressure, it leads to right heart failure.

42. Ans. b. Left atrium.

Braunwald 12th Ed; Page 911

The left atrium has several important functions.
1. The left atrium functions as a blood receiving reservoir chamber;
2. It is a contractile chamber that by presystolic contraction helps to complete left ventricular filling with an atrial kick;
3. The left atrium function as a conduit that empties its contents into the left ventricle down a pressure gradient after the opening of mitral valve;

4. It is called as "blood volume sensor" of the heart and releases atrial natriuretic peptide (ANP) in response to stretch so that ANP induced diuresis can help restore blood volume to normal;
5. Left atrium contains receptors for a afferent arms of various reflexes including mechanoreceptors that increase the sinus discharge rate, thereby contributing to the tachycardia of exercise as venous return increases (Bainbridge reflex).

43. Ans. b. All of the above.

Braunwald 12th Ed; Page 926

In failing myocardium, there are several changes occurs both in volume of cardiac myocytes and also in the volume and composition of the extra cellular matrix. Progressive myocytes loss occurs through process of necrosis, apoptosis or autophagic cell death.

Chapter 3: Clinical Cardiology

1. **Which variety of interrupted aortic arch is associated with subclavian steal syndrome?**
   a. Type A interrupted aortic arch
   b. Type B interrupted aortic arch
   c. Type C interrupted aortic arch
   d. All of the above

2. **The balloon atrial septostomy was first performed by:**
   a. Rashkind
   b. DeBakey
   c. Blalock–Taussig
   d. Kirklin

3. **Which of the following is commonest type of cyanotic congenital heart disease?**
   a. Total anomalous pulmonary venous return
   b. Truncus arteriosus
   c. Pulmonary atresia
   d. Tetralogy of Fallot

4. **Pulsatile exophthalmos (pulsation of eyeballs) are seen in:**
   a. Severe aortic regurgitation
   b. Thyrotoxicosis
   c. Advanced congestive heart failure
   d. Severe tricuspid regurgitation

5. **Beading of the retinal artery may be seen in:**
   a. Infective endocarditis
   b. Left atrial myxoma
   c. Hypercholesterolemia
   d. Malignant Hypertension

6. **Type II hyperlipoproteinemia is characterized by?**
   a. Tuberoeruptive xanthomas
   b. Xanthoma striatum palmare
   c. Xanthoma tendinosum
   d. Eruptive xanthoma

7. **Tuberoeruptive Xanthoma is a feature of:**
   a. Type I hyperlipoproteinemia
   b. Type II hyperlipoproteinemia
   c. Type III hyperlipoproteinemia
   d. Type IV hyperlipoproteinemia

8. **Eruptive xanthoma and xanthoma striatum palmare is a feature of:**
   a. Type I and V hyperlipoproteinemia
   b. Type I and IV hyperlipoproteinemia
   c. Type I and III hyperlipoproteinemia
   d. Type II and V hyperlipoproteinemia

9. **The right internal jugular vein is chosen for analyzing venous pulse because left internal jugular vein:**
   a. Is not in straight line to RA
   b. May be kinked or compressed by mediastinal structures
   c. Have venous valves located at the caudal end
   d. All of the above

10. **A paradoxical rise in the height of Jugular venous pressure during inspiration is most commonly seen in:**
    a. Tricuspid stenosis
    b. Chronic constrictive pericarditis
    c. Congestive heart failure
    d. COPD

11. **The recommended width of cuff for measuring blood pressure in the lower extremities is:**
    a. 5 inch
    b. 8 inch
    c. 7 inch
    d. 9 inch

12. **Regular canon A wave in JVP is suggestive of:**
    a. Ventricular tachycardia
    b. Complete AV block
    c. Sinus tachycardia
    d. Junctional tachycardia

13. **Which is *not* correct regarding pulsus alternans?**
    a. Often there is systolic pressure alteration by more than 20 mm Hg
    b. There is alteration in the intensity of Kortkoff sounds
    c. There is alteration in intensity of heart sound
    d. There is electrical alternans also

14. **Reversed pulsus paradoxus may occur in:**
    a. Aortic regurgitation
    b. Hypovolumic shock
    c. Restrictive cardiomyopathy
    d. Hypertrophic obstructive cardiomyopathy

15. Bisferiens pulse is seen in:
a. Aortic regurgitation
b. Hypertrophic obstructive cardiomyopathy
c. Hyperkinetic circulatory state
d. All of the above

16. The Water-Hammer pulse of aortic regurgitation is characterized by all *except*:
a. Abrupt upstroke followed by rapid collapse later in systole
b. Abrupt upstroke followed by rapid collapse later in diastole
c. Absence of dicrotic notch
d. Increased pulse pressure

17. Pectus excavatum is commonly observed in all *except*:
a. Ankylosing spondylitis
b. Homocystinuria
c. Mitral valve prolapse
d. Ehlers-Danlos syndrome

18. Elevation of JVP due to RVF is differentiated from that of superior vena cava obstruction by which of the following measures?
a. Neck veins pulsation
b. Hepatojugular reflux
c. Both are present
d. Both are absent

19. Which is *true* regarding the hepatojugular reflux?
a. During pressure patient should not hold breath or strain
b. The pressure may be exerted anywhere in the abdomen
c. To be positive, venous pulsation should ascend > 1 cm in neck
d. All are true

20. An approximation of AV conduction is best done with
a. A—C interval
b. A—V interval
c. X—Y interval
d. A—Y interval

21. Which of the following is *true* regarding JVP in tricuspid stenosis?
a. A wave is prominent
b. Y descent is slow
c. Inspiration exaggerates both A and Y waves
d. All are true

22. Prominent 'A' wave is *not* expected in:
a. Corpulmonale
b. Mitral stenosis
c. Pulmonary embolism
d. Fallot's tetralogy

23. Possible underlying cause suggested for absent A wave in Fallot's tetrology is:
a. Occurrence of overriding aorta
b. Occurrence of VSD
c. Pulmonic stenosis is mild
d. RV is compliant

24. A large irregular A wave is produced by which of the following condition?
a. Complete heart block
b. Atrial premature beat/junctional
c. Ventricular premature beat
d. All of the above

25. Pistol shot sound on auscultation over the femoral artery are found in:
a. Aortic regurgitation
b. Tricuspid regurgitation
c. Ebstein's anomaly
d. Right ventricular failure

26. The most characteristic sign in patient's of tricuspid regurgitation with AF is:
a. Large A wave
b. Prominent X descent
c. Large CV wave
d. Prominent Y descent

27. Which of the following is *true* regarding CV waves?
a. It is the only venous pulse seen in cases of tricuspid regurgitation with AF
b. In a febrile patient's it is the only clue to the presence of tricuspid valve endocarditis when murmur of tricuspid regurgitation is inconspicuous
c. With CHF—CV wave occur with minor degree of tricuspid regurgitation
d. All are true

28. Kussmaul's sign is found in:
a. Tricuspid stenosis
b. CHF
c. Constrictive pericarditis
d. All

29. Which of the following murmur reduces in intensity following amyl nitrite inhalation?
a. Systolic murmur of aortic stenosis
b. Murmur of tricuspid regurgitation
c. Mid systolic murmur of TOF
d. Functional systolic murmurs

30. Sudden assumption of lying from standing or sitting position decreases which of the following murmur?
a. Murmur of aortic stenosis.
b. Murmur of pulmonary stenosis
c. Murmur of VSD
d. Murmur of hypertrophic obstructive cardiomyopathy

31. Standing decreases the murmur of all the following conditions *except*:
a. Aortic stenosis
b. Pulmonary stenosis
c. Mitral regurgitation
d. IHSS

32. Murmur of all *except* following is diminished by rapid standing from a lying position:
   a. Murmur of aortic stenosis
   b. Murmur of aortic regurgitation
   c. Functional murmurs
   d. Murmur of mitral valve prolapse

33. All the following murmurs are reduced by amyl nitrite inhalation *except*:
   a. Murmur of aortic regurgitation
   b. Murmur of small VSD
   c. Murmur of mitral regurgitation
   d. Murmur of large VSD with hyperkinetic pulmonary circulation

34. Which of the following maneuver amplifies the murmur of hypertrophic obstructive cardiomyopathy?
   a. Valsalva maneuver
   b. Sudden assumption of lying from standing position
   c. Squatting
   d. Isometric exercise

35. In a known case of VSD if systolic murmur becomes louder with amyl nitrite then it indicates possibility of:
   a. Small VSD with aneurysm of membranous septa
   b. Large VSD with hyperkinetic pulmonary hypertension
   c. Large VSD with severe pulmonary vascular obstructive disease
   d. A + B

36. Paradoxical splitting of second heart sound is found in which of the following condition?
   a. Right bundle branch block
   b. Left ventricular pacemaker
   c. Complete left bundle branch block
   d. None of the above

37. The term Pancake heart is used in reference to:
   a. ASD
   b. Mild pulmonary stenosis
   c. Idiopathic dilatation of the pulmonary artery
   d. Straight back syndrome

38. The common most congenital anomaly associated with coarctation of aorta is:
   a. Bicuspid aortic valve
   b. Ventricular septal defect
   c. Patent ductus arteriosus
   d. Parachute mitral valve

39. Corkscrew tortuosity and Serpentine Pulsations is the characteristic fundoscopic finding in:
   a. Hypertensive retinopathy
   b. Eclampsia of pregnancy
   c. Takayasu's disease
   d. Coarctation of aorta

40. Which of the following is *not* a correct match?
   a. Pistol-shot sound—Corrigan's sign
   b. Basic blanching of the nail bed—Quincke's sign
   c. Systolic pressure in the lower extremity exceeding that of arm by more than 20 mm—Hill's sign
   d. Visible pulsation of the retinal arteriole—Becker's sign

41. Unilateral clubbing of finger is seen in:
   a. Cirrhosis of liver
   b. Pulmonary AV fistula
   c. Coarctation of aorta
   d. Aortic aneurysm

42. W-shaped JVP (jugular venous pressure) is characteristic of:
   a. Restrictive cardiomyopathy
   b. Constrictive pericarditis
   c. Cardiac tamponade
   d. Hypertrophic cardiomyopathy

43. Systolic retraction of the chest, particularly of the ribs in the left axilla is seen in:
   a. Cardiac tamponade
   b. Hypertrophic obstructive cardiomyopathy
   c. Mitral valve prolapse
   d. Constrictive pericarditis

44. Systolic retraction of chest particularly of the ribs in the left axilla is known as:
   a. Muller's sign   b. Broadbent's sign
   c. Traube's sign   d. Levine sign

45. The sound produced by the abrupt seating of a pedunculated mobile atrial myxoma (Tumor plop) is a:
   a. Early systolic sound   b. Early diastolic sound
   c. Mid diastolic sound   d. Late diastolic sound

46. Muller's maneuver augments all *except*:
   a. It exaggerate the inspiratory effort
   b. Widens the split second heart sound
   c. Augments murmur and filling sounds originating in the right side of the heart
   d. Augment the murmur and filling sounds originating in the left side of the heart

CHAPTER 3 | Clinical Cardiology

47. The finding of left bundle branch block pattern in limb leads and right bundle branch block pattern in chest lead is known as:
   a. Nonspecific intraventricular conduction defect
   b. Masquerading bundle branch block
   c. Bilateral bundle branch block
   d. Bundle branch block alternans

48. Ashman phenomenon (Aberrancy due to changes in the preceding cycle length) is seen in:
   a. Atrial fibrillation
   b. Repetitive atrial tachycardia
   c. Atrial tachycardia with Wenckebach type I AV block
   d. All of the above

49. Which of the following cardiac chamber is *not* border forming in frontal projection of a X-ray and cannot be directly viewed?
   a. Right atrium   b. Right ventricle
   c. Left atrium   d. Left ventricle

50. Pericardial calcification are rarely seen in:
   a. Right atrial pericardium   b. Atrioventricular groove
   c. Right ventricular border   d. Left atrium

51. Myocardial calcification is usually localized to:
   a. Left atrium   b. Left ventricle
   c. Right atrium   d. Right ventricle

52. Selective right upper lobe pulmonary edema has been described radiologically in patients with:
   a. Patent ductus arteriosus
   b. AV fistula
   c. Pulmonary embolism
   d. Acute or chronic mitral regurgitation

53. Secundum atrial septal defect maybe incorrectly diagnosed clinically as:
   a. VSD   b. Pulmonary stenosis
   c. Mitral stenosis   d. Tricuspid stenosis

ANSWERS WITH EXPLANATIONS

1. Ans. b. Type B interrupted aortic arch

Perloff 3rd Ed; Page 148

Interruption of aortic arch is a rare malformation characterized by complete anatomic discontinuity or less commonly by an atretic fibrous remnant between the arch or isthmus and the descending aorta. The classification of Celoria and pattern remains in current use. Interruption between the left common carotid and left subclavian arteries (Type B) is slightly commoner than isthmic interruption distal to the left subclavian artery (Type A), whereas the list common site is between the innominate and left carotid arteries (Type C). Congenital subclavian still occurs when both subclavian arteries arise distal to the interruption.

2. Ans. a. Rashkind

Hurst's 14th Ed; Page 1385

The balloon atrial Septostomy was first performed by Rashkind.

3. Ans. d. Tetralogy of Fallot

Hurst's 11th Ed; Page 1821

The tetralogy of Fallot is the most common cyanotic congenital heart disease found in the population. The overall incidence of this anomaly is around 10% of all forms of congenital heart disease.

4. Ans. d. Severe tricuspid regurgitation

Hurst's 11th Ed; Page 249

Exophthalmos and stare occurs in cases with hyperthyroidism which can cause high output cardiac failure but it is also seen in advance congestive heart failure in which there is pulmonary venous hypertension and weight loss. The stare is probably due to lid retraction caused by increased adrenergic tone that accompanies heart failure. Severe tricuspid regurgitation can cause pulsation of eyeballs (Pulsatile exophthalmos) as well as of the ear lobe.

5. Ans. c. Hypercholesterolemia

Hurst's 11th Ed; Page 249

The examination of the fundi allows classification of arteriolar disease in patient with hypertension and may also be helpful in the recognition of arteriosclerosis. Beading of the retinal artery may be present in patient with hypercholesterolemia.

6. Ans. c. Xanthoma tendinosum

Hurst's 11th Ed; Page 237

Several types of xanthomas, i.e., cholesterol filled nodules are found either subcutaneously or over tendons in patients with hyperlipoproteinemia. Premature atherosclerosis frequently develops in these individuals.

Tuberoeruptive xanthomas present subcutaneously or on the extensor surface of extremity or xanthoma striatum palmer which produces yellowish, orange or pink discoloration of the palmer and digital creases occurs most commonly in patients with type III hyperlipoproteinemia. Patient with xanthoma tendinosum, i.e., nodular swelling of the tendons especially of the elbows, extensor surface of the hands and Achilles tendon usually have type II hyperlipoproteinemia. Eruptive xanthomas are tiny yellowish nodules 1-2 mm in diameter on an erythematous base, which may occur anywhere on the body and associated with hyperchylomicronemia and are therefore often found in patient with *Type I and Type V* hyperlipoproteinemia.

7. Ans. c. Type III hyperlipoproteinemia

Hurst's 11th Ed; Page 237

Refer to explanation for Q. No 6.

8. Ans. a. Type I and V hyperlipoproteinemia

Hurst's 11th Ed; Page 237

Refer to explanation for Q. No 6.

9. Ans. d. All of the above

Braunwald 9th Ed; Page 110

Important information regarding the dynamics of the right side of the heart can be obtained by the observation of jugular venous pulse. The internal jugular vein is ordinarily employed in the examination. The venous pulse can usually be analyzed more readily on the right than on the left side of the neck because the right is innominate and jugular veins extends in an almost straight line cephalad to the superior vena cava. Thus favoring transmission of the hemodynamic changes from the right atrium while the left innominate vein is not in a straight line and may be kinked or compressed by a variety of normal structure, by a dilated aorta or by an aneurysm.

10. Ans. b. Chronic constrictive pericarditis

Braunwald 9th Ed; Page 110

Elevation of jugular venous pressure reflects and increases in right atrial pressure and occurs in heart failure, reduce compliance of right ventricle, pericardial disease, hypervolemia, obstruction of tricuspid orifice and obstruction of superior vena cava. During inspiration, the jugular venous pressure normally declines but the amplitude of pulsation increases. Kussmaul's sign is a paradoxical rise in the height of the jugular venous pressure during inspiration which typically occurs in patient with chronic constrictive pericarditis and sometime in congestive heart failure and tricuspid stenosis.

11. Ans. b. 8 inch

Braunwald 9th Ed; Page 972

Sphygmomanometer is used to obtain an indirect measurement of blood pressure. The cuff should fit snugly around arm with its lower edge at least 1 inch above the antecubital space and diaphragm of the stethoscope should be placed close to or under the edge of sphygmomanometer cuff. The width of the cuff selected should be at least 40% of the circumference of the limb to be used. The standard size with a 5 inch white cuff is designed for adults with an arm of average size. When this cuff is applied to a large upper arm or a normal adult thigh, arterial pressure is overestimated leading to spurious hypertension in the obese. When it is applied to a small arm, the pressure is underestimated. The cuff width should be approximately 1½ inches in infants and small children, 3 inches in young children (2-5 years) and 8 inches in the obese individuals.

12. Ans. d. Junctional tachycardia

Braunwald 9th Ed; Page 110

The cannon (amplified) *A* waves are noted in patients with atrioventricular dissociation when the right atrium contracts against a closed tricuspid valve. Irregular cannon wave can be seen in complete AV block and in patient with ventricular tachycardia while regular cannon A wave is seen in junctional tachycardia.

13. Ans. d. There is electrical alternans also

Hurst's 11th Ed; Page 241

Pulses alternans (alternating strong and weak pulses) is a sign of severe depression of myocardial function. Although more readily recognized on sphygmomanometry when the systolic pressure alternates by more than 20 mm Hg. The alternans can be detected by palpation of a peripheral pulse more frequently than by a central pulse. Pulses alternans generally accompanied by alternation in the intensity of Korotkoff's sounds and occasionally by alternation in the intensity of heart sound. Rarely pulses alternans is so marked that the weak beat is not perceived at all. Aortic regurgitation, systemic hypertension and reducing venous return by administration of nitroglycerin or by tilting the patient into the upright position, all exaggerate pulses alternans and helps in its perception. Pulses alternans is not accompanied by electrical alternans.

14. Ans. d. Hypertrophic obstructive cardiomyopathy

Braunwald 9th Ed; Page 113

Pulsus paradoxus is an exaggerated reduction in the strength of arterial pulse during normal inspiration or an exaggerated inspiratory fall in systolic pressure more than 10 mm Hg during quite breathing. When marked, i.e., an inspiratory reduction of pressure greater than 20 mm Hg, the paradoxical pulse can be detected by palpation of brachial arterial pulse. Pulsus paradoxus represent an exaggeration of normal decline in systolic arterial pressure with inspiration. It results from the reduced left ventricular stroke volume and the transmission of negative intrathoracic pressure to the aorta. It is a frequent characteristic finding in patient with cardiac tamponade, occurs less frequently in patients with chronic constrictive pericarditis and is also found patient with emphysema and bronchial asthma, as well as in hypovolemic shock and pulmonary embolism, pregnancy and extreme obesity. Aortic regurgitation tends to prevent the development of pulsus paradoxus despite the presence of cardiac tamponade. Reverse pulsus paradoxus (an inspiratory rise in arterial pressure) may occur in hypertrophic obstructive cardiomyopathy.

15. Ans. a. Aortic regurgitation

Hurst's 11th Ed; Page 244

A bisferiens pulse is characterized by two systolic peaks, the percussion and tidal wave is separated by a distinct mid systolic dip. The peak may be equal or may be larger. This type of pulse is detected most readily by palpation of carotid and less commonly of the brachial artery. It occurs in condition in which a large stroke volume is ejected rapidly from the left ventricle and is observed most commonly in patient with pure aortic regurgitation or with a combination of aortic regurgitation and stenosis. It may disappear as heart failure supervenes. A bisferiens pulse also occurs in patients with hypertrophic obstructive cardiomyopathy and occasionally a bisferiens pulse is observed in hyperkinetic circulatory states and very rarely it occurs in normal individuals.

16. Ans. b. Abrupt upstroke followed by rapid collapse later in diastole

Hurst's 11th Ed; Page 244

The Corrigan's or waterhammer pulse of aortic regurgitation consist of an abrupt increase of stroke, i.e., percussion wave followed by a rapid collapse later in the systole but not dicrotic notch. Water, hammer pulse reflects low resistance in the reservoir into which the left ventricle rapidly discharges an abnormally elevated stroke volume and it can be exaggerated by raising the patient's arm. In acute aortic regurgitation, the left ventricle may not be significantly dilated and premature closure of mitral valve may occur and limit the volume of aortic ejection. Therefore the aortic diastolic pressure may not be very low, the arterial pulse not bounding and pulse pressure not widen despite a serious abnormality of valve function.

17. Ans. a. Ankylosing spondilytis

Hurst's 11th Ed; Page 226

Pectus excavatum, a condition in which the sternum is displaced posteriorly, is commonly observed in Marfan syndrome, homocystinuria, Ehlers-Danlos syndrome, Hunter-Hurler syndrome and a small fraction of patient with mitral valve prolapse. This thoracic deformity rarely compresses the heart or elevates the systemic and pulmonary venous pressure and the signs of heart disease are more often apparent rather than real.

18. Ans. d. Both are absent

Braunwald 5th Ed; Page 19

Refer to answer from the chapter on Congestive Heart Failure Q. No 4.

19. Ans. d. All are true

Braunwald 5th Ed; Page 19

Refer to answer from the chapter on Congestive Heart Failure Q. No 4.

20. Ans. a. A—C interval

Hurst's 11th Ed; Page 247

Abnormal Venous Pulse—Elevated Venous Pressure

The most common cause of an elevated jugular venous pressure is an increased RV pressure such as occurs in patients with PS, PH or RV failure secondary to left-sided heart failure or RV infarction. The venous pressure also is elevated when obstruction to RV inflow occurs, as with tricuspid stenosis (TS) or RA myxoma, or when constrictive pericardial disease impedes RV inflow. It also may result from vena cava obstruction and, at times, an increased blood volume. Patients with obstructive pulmonary disease may have an elevated venous pressure only during expiration.

Kussmaul's sign: Normally, during inspiration, there is an increase in a wave of the JVP but a decrease in the mean JVP as a result of the increased filling of the right-sided chambers associated with the decrease in intrathoracic pressure. Kussmaul's sign denotes an inspiratory increase in the venous pressure, which may occur in patients with severe constrictive pericarditis when the heart is unable to accept the increase in RV volume without a marked increase in the filling pressure. Although Kussmaul's sign was first described in patients with constrictive pericarditis, its most common cause is severe right-sided heart failure, regardless of etiology. The presence of Kussmaul's sign is also useful in the diagnosis of RV infarction.

Abnormalities of the 'A' wave: The 'A' wave in the JVP is absent when there is no effective atrial contraction, such as in atrial fibrillation. In certain other conditions, the 'A' wave may not be apparent. In sinus tachycardia, the 'A' wave may fuse with the preceding 'V' wave, particularly if the PR interval is prolonged. In some patients with sinus tachycardia, the jugular 'A' wave may occur during the 'V' or 'Y' descent and may be small or absent. In the presence of first-degree AV block, a discrete 'A' wave with ascending and descending limbs is often completed prior to the first heart sound, and the 'ac' interval is prolonged. Large 'A' waves are of considerable diagnostic value. When giant 'A' waves are present with each beat, the right atrium is contracting against an increased resistance. This may result from obstruction at the tricuspid valve (TS or atresia, right atrial myxoma) or conditions associated with increased resistance to RV filling. A giant 'A' wave is more likely to occur in patients with PS or PH in whom both the atrial and ventricular septa are intact.

Cannon 'A' waves occur when the right atrium contracts while the tricuspid valve is closed during RV systole. Cannon 'a' waves may occur either regularly or irregularly and are most common in the presence of arrhythmia.

Abnormalities of the 'X' wave: The most important alteration of the normally negative systolic collapse (X wave) of the JVP is its obliteration or even replacement by a positive wave, usually due to TR. Although atrial relaxation may contribute to the normal 'X' descent, the development of atrial fibrillation does not obliterate the 'X' wave except in the presence of TR. Accordingly, the occurrence of a positive wave in the JVP during ventricular systole is strong evidence of TR. Mild TR lessens and shortens the downward 'X' wave as the regurgitation of blood into the right atrium procedures a positive wave that diminishes the usual systolic fill in venous pressure. In some patients with moderate TR, there is a fairly distinct positive wave during ventricular systole between the 'C' and 'V' waves. This abnormal systolic waveform is usually referred to as a 'V' or 'CV' wave, although it has also been referred to as an 'R' (regurgitant) or an 'S' (systolic) wave. In patients with constrictive pericarditis, the x-descent wave during systole is often more prominent than the early diastolic y wave.

Abnormalities of the 'v' wave: The positive, late systolic 'V' wave results from the increasing RV blood volume during ventricular systole when the tricuspid valve normally is closed. With mild TR, the 'V' wave and the obliteration of the 'X' descent result in a single, large positive systolic wave (ventricularization). Normally in the JVP the 'V' wave is lower in amplitude than the 'A' wave. In patients with an ASD, however the 'A' and 'V' waves are often equal in the right atrium and the JVP. In patients with constrictive pericarditis and sinus rhythm, the RA 'A' and 'V' waves also may be equal, but the venous pressure is increased, which is unusual with isolated ASD. In patients with constrictive pericarditis who are in atrial fibrillation, the 'cv' wave is prominent and the y descent rapid.

21. Ans. d. All are true

Hurst's 11th Ed; Page 247

Refer to explanation for Q. No 20.

22. Ans. d. Fallot's tetralogy

Hurst's 11th Ed; Page 247

The jugular pulse is normal or nearly so and there is good reason why this is the case. The normal neonatal right ventricle has the inherent capacity to eject against systemic resistance without extra help from its atrium. In Fallot's tetralogy, resistance to right ventricular discharge remains at but does not exceed the systemic level because the nonrestrictive ventricular septal defect permits free decompression into the aorta. The right ventricle maintains its neonatal capacity to eject at systemic levels without elevating its filling pressure. Accordingly, the right atrium is not required to increase its contractile force, so the jugular venous pulse remains normal in both wave form and height. There are two important variations on this theme. Accessory tricuspid leaflet tissue may partially occlude the ventricular septal defect, so right ventricular systolic pressure exceeds the systemic level. The A wave then become prominent. 'A' more common and therefore more important variation on the theme occurs in adult survivors who develop systemic hypertension. The elevated aortic pressure provokes an equivalent rise in right ventricular systolic pressure. The right ventricle contracts from an increased end diastolic fiber length in response to forceful right atrial systole. The result is an increase in amplitude of the jugular venous 'A' wave.

23. Ans. b. Occurrence of VSD

Hurst's 11th Ed; Page 247

Refer to explanation for Q. No 22.

24. Ans. d. All of the above

Hurst's 11th Ed; Page 247

Refer to explanation for Q. No 20.

25. Ans. a. Aortic regurgitation

Hurst's 11th Ed; Page 2819

Exaggerated or bounding arterial pulses may be observed in patients with an elevated stroke volume, with sympathetic hyperactivity, and in patients with a rigid, sclerotic aorta. In aortic regurgitation, there is a very brisk rate of rise with an increased pulse pressure.

The Corrigan or water hammer pulse of aortic regurgitation consists of an abrupt upstroke (percussion wave) followed by rapid collapse later in systole, but no dicrotic notch.

Signs characteristic of severe chronic aortic regurgitation include "pistol-shot" sounds heard over the femoral artery when the stethoscope is placed on its (Traube's sign); a systolic murmur heard over the femoral artery when the artery is gradually compressed distally (Duroziez's sign) and Quincke's sign (phasic blanching of the nail bed) of these, Duroziez's sign is the most predictive. Bounding arterial pulses are also present in patients with patent ductus arteriosus or large arteriovenous fistulas; in hyperkinetic states such as thyrotoxicosis, pregnancy, fever, and anemia; in severe bradycardia; and in arteries proximal to coarctation of the aorta. In Hill's sign of aortic regurgitation (or any condition leading to an increased stroke volume, or the hyperkinetic circulatory state) the indirectly recorded systolic pressure in the lower extremities exceeds that in the arms by more than 20 mm Hg. Other signs of increase pulse pressure include Becker's sign (visible pulsations of the retinal arterioles) and Mueller's sign (pulsating uvula).

26. **Ans. c. Large CV wave**

Hurst's 11th Ed; Page 247

Refer to explanation for Q. No 20.

27. **Ans. d. All are true**

Hurst's 11th Ed; Page 247

Refer to explanation for Q. No 20.

28. **Ans. d. All of the above**

Hurst's 11th Ed; Page 247

Refer to explanation for Q. No 20.

29. **Ans. c. Mid systolic murmur of TOF**

Hurst's 11th Ed; Page 261-264

Please refer to the answer of Q. No 31.

30. **Ans. d. Murmur of hypertrophic obstructive cardiomyopathy**

Hurst's 11th Ed; Page 261-264

Please refer to the answer of Q. No 31.

31. **Ans. d. IHSS**

Hurst's 11th Ed; Page 261-264

Dynamic Auscultation

Postural changes and exercise: Sudden assumption of the lying from the standing or sitting position or sudden passive elevation of both legs results in an increase in venous return, which augments first right ventricular and, several cardiac cycles later, left ventricular stroke volume. The systolic murmurs of pulmonic valve stenosis and aortic stenosis, the systolic murmurs of mitral and tricuspid regurgitation and ventricular septal defect, and most functional systolic murmurs are augmented. On the other hand, because left ventricular end diastolic volume is increased, the systolic murmur of hypertrophic obstructive cardiomyopathy is diminished and the midsystolic click and late systolic murmur associated with mitral valve prolapses are delayed and sometimes attenuated. Rapid standing or sitting up from a lying position or rapid standing from a squatting posture has the opposite effect. The decrease in venous return reduces stroke volume and innocent pulmonary flow murmurs as well as the murmurs of semilunar valve stenosis and of AV valve regurgitation. The auscultatory changes in hypertrophic cardiomyopathy and mitral valve prolapse are opposite to those on assumption of the lying posture described above.

Pharmacological agent (inhalation of amyl nitrite): The drug produces marked vasodilatation, resulting in the first 30 seconds in a reduction of systemic arterial pressure, and 30 to 60 seconds later in a reflex tachycardia, followed in turn by a reflex increase in cardiac output, velocity of blood flow, and heart rate. The systolic murmurs of aortic valve stenosis, pulmonary stenosis, hypertrophic obstructive cardiomyopathy, tricuspid regurgitation, and functional systolic murmurs are all accentuated.

The reduction of arterial pressure increases the right-to-left shunt and decreases the blood flow from the right ventricle to the pulmonary artery and diminishes the mid systolic murmur in patients with tetralogy of Fallot. The increase in cardiac output augments the diastolic murmurs of mitral and tricuspid stenosis and of pulmonary regurgitation and the systolic murmur of tricuspid regurgitation. However, as a result of the fall in systemic arterial pressure, the systolic murmurs of mitral regurgitation and ventricular septal defect, the diastolic murmurs of aortic regurgitation and the Austin Flint murmur as well as the continuous murmurs of patent ductus arteriosus and of systemic arteriovenous fistula are all diminished. The reduction of cardiac size results in an earlier appearance of the mid systolic click and late systolic murmur of mitral valve prolapse; the intensity of the systolic murmur exhibits a variable response.

32. **Ans. d. Murmur of mitral valve prolapse**

Hurst's 11th Ed; Page 261-264

Please refer to the answer of Q. No 31.

33. **Ans. d. Murmur of large VSD with hyperkinetic pulmonary circulation**

Hurst's 11th Ed; Page 261-264

Response of murmur of VSD to intervention:
a. Small defect with pulmonary hypertension—Fades with amyl nitrite; increases with isometric handgrip or phenylephrine.
b. Large defect with hyperkinetic pulmonary hypertension—Louder with amyl nitrite; fades with phenylephrine.
c. Large defect with severe pulmonary vascular disease—little change with any of above interventions.

34. Ans. a. Valsalva maneuver

Hurst's 11th Ed; Page 261-264

Please refer to the answer of Q. No 31

35. Ans. b. Large VSD with hyperkinetic pulmonary hypertension

Hurst's 11th Ed; Page 261-264

Refer to explanation for Q. No 33.

36. Ans. c. Complete left bundle branch block

Hurst's 11th Ed; Page 261-264

Paradoxical splitting of the second heart found: This term refers to a reversed sequence of semilunar valve closure, the pulmonary component (P2) preceding the aortic component (A2). Common causes of paradoxical splitting are complete left bundle branch block or a right ventricular pacemaker, both of which are associated with initial activation of the right side of the ventricular septum and delayed activation of the left ventricle owing to transseptal (right-to-left) depolarization. When the second heart sound splits paradoxically, its two components separate during exhalation and become single (synchronous) during inspiration.

37. Ans. d. Straight back syndrome

Hurst's 11th Ed; Page 337

The term Pancake heart is used in reference to straight back syndrome where as a result of straightening of the spine heart is compressed anteroposteriorly and produces flattening and enlargement of heart shadow in posteroanterior view of X-ray chest.

38. Ans. a. Bicuspid aortic valve

Perloff; 3rd Ed; Page 127

a. There is a strong association between typical coarctation of aorta and bicuspid aortic valve. Bicuspid valve is the usual cause of aortic stenosis and coarctation. Subaortic obstruction is relatively uncommon and occurs as one component of Shone's complex (supravalvular mitral ring, parachute mitral valve, subaortic stenosis and coarctation of aorta).
b. Shunt lesions often coexist with coarctation of aorta, i.e., patent ductus arteriosus and ventricular septal defect.

39. Ans. d. Coarctation of aorta

Perloff; 3rd Ed; Page 130

There is a low incidence of vascular disease in coarctation of aorta and the frequency of toxemia of pregnancy is lower in women with coarctation than in pregnant women with other forms of hypertension. Eye grounds rarely show hypertensive retinopathy but instead occasionally display 'U' shaped or Corkscrew retinal arteries.

40. Ans. a. Pistol-shot sound—Corrigan's sign

Hurst's 11th Ed; Page 2819

Please refer to answer of Q. No 25.

41. Ans. d. Aortic aneurysm

Perloff; 6th Ed; Page 292

Clubbing of digits is characteristic of general cyanosis (cyanotic congenital heart disease or pulmonary disease with hypoxia). It may also appear within a few weeks of the development of infective endocarditis. These are usually bilateral. Unilateral clubbing of the fingers is rare but can occur when an aortic aneurysm interfere with the arterial supply of one arm.

42. Ans. b. Constrictive pericarditis

Hurst's 11th Ed; Page 247

Refer to explanation for Q. No 20.

43. Ans. d. Constrictive pericarditis

Braunwald 9th Ed; Page 1662-1663

Constrictive pericarditis is characterized by systolic retraction of the chest, particularly of the ribs in the left axilla (Broadbent's sign). This inward movement results from interference with the descent of the base of the heart and the compensatory exaggerated motion of the free wall of the left ventricle during ventricular ejection.

44. Ans. b. Broadbent's sign

Braunwald 9th Ed; Page 1662-1663

Refer to explanation for Q. No 43.

45. Ans. b. Early diastolic sound

Hurst's 11th Ed; Page 2083

Heart sounds are relatively brief, discrete auditory vibrations of varying intensity (loudness), frequency (pitch), and quality (timbre). The first heart sound identifies the onset of ventricular systole, and the second heart sound identifies the onset of diastole. These two auscultatory events establish a framework within which other heart sounds and murmurs can be placed and timed.

An early systolic sound might be an ejection sound (aortic or pulmonary) or an aortic prosthetic sound. Mid and late systolic sounds are typified by the click(s) of mitral valve prolapse but occasionally are 'remnants' of pericardial rubs. Early diastolic sounds are represented by opening snaps (usually mitral), early third heart sounds (constrictive pericarditis, less commonly mitral regurgitation), the opening of a mechanical inflow prosthesis, or the abrupt seating of a pedunculated mobile atrial myxoma ('tumor plop'). Mid diastolic sounds are generally third heart sounds or summation sounds (synchronous occurrence of third and fourth heart sounds). Late diastolic or presystolic sounds are almost always fourth heart sounds, rarely pacemaker sounds.

46. Ans. d. Augment the murmur and filling sounds originating in the left side of the heart

Braunwald 11th Ed; Page 1446

This maneuver is the converse of the Valsalva maneuver but is less frequently employed because it is not as useful. The maneuver is continued for about 10 seconds as the patient forcibly inspires while the nose is held closed and the mouth firmly sealed. The Muller maneuver exaggerates the inspiratory effort, widens the split second sound, and augments murmurs and filling sounds originating in the right side of the heart.

47. Ans. b. Masquerading bundle branch block

J Clin and Diagnostic Research 2016, Sept 10, Vol 9

This form of BBB is rare. It is manifest by RBBB, marked left-axis deviation, and absence of a significant S wave in leads I, aV1, and V6. In essence, it can be described as LBBB in the limb leads and RBBB in the chest leads. In contrast to the ordinary RBBB with left anterior fascicular block, or bifascicular block, the masquerading BBB is usually associated with significant heart disease and a relatively poor long-term prognosis.

48. Ans. d. All of the above

BMJ Case Report 2013, May 24

Ashman phenomenon: The duration of refractory period is a function of the immediate preceding cycle length. The longer the preceding cycle the longer is the refractory period that follows. Consequently with a relatively constant heart rate sudden prolongation of the immediately preceding cycle length may result in aberration. This relationship of aberrancy to changes in the preceding cycle length is known as Ashman phenomenon. It usually exhibit RBBB morphology and may be associated with left anterior or rarely with left posterior division block. This is seen in the presence of irregular supraventricular rhythm such as atrial fibrillation, repetitive atrial tachycardia or atrial tachycardia with Wenckebach's (Type I) AV block.

49. Ans. b. Right ventricle

Hurst's 11th Ed; Page 333

The right border of heart is formed in upper part by superior vena cava and the right atria forms the lower portion of right border in frontal projection. The right ventricle is not bordered forming in the frontal projection and cannot be directly viewed.

50. Ans. d. Left atrium

Hurst's 11th Ed; Page 333

Pericardial calcification occurs most often in association with previous pericarditis are trauma. Pericardial calcification are most abundant along the right atrial and ventricular borders and in the area of atrioventricular groove. The pericardium adjacent to the left ventricle is usually free of calcification probably because of its vigorous pulsations and calcification rarely occurs in the left atrial pericardium because of the absence of pericardium behind the left atrium. On the other hand, myocardial calcification is usually localized to the left ventricle and is rare in the right atrium or ventricle.

51. Ans. b. Left ventricle

Hurst's 11th Ed; Page 333

Please refer to the Answer of Q. No 50.

52. Ans. d. Acute or chronic mitral regurgitation

Hurst's 11th Ed; Page 333

Acute mitral regurgitation may be related to the rupture cardi tendineae, rupture of papillary muscle, ischemic dysfunction are infective endocarditis. While the heart may not be enlarged in acute mitral regurgitation, severe pulmonary edema is frequently present as a result of left sided cardiac failure. Although pulmonary edema secondary to mitral regurgitation is usually symmetrical, selective right upper lobe pulmonary edema has been described in as many as 9% of patients with acute or chronic mitral regurgitation. It is probably due to selective retrograde flow from the mitral valve to the right upper lobe pulmonary veins.

53. Ans. c. Mitral stenosis

Hurst's 11th Ed; Page 333

A secundum atrial septal defect may be incorrectly diagnosed as mitral stenosis because of the similar physical sign. The split second sound may be misinterpreted as the opening snap. The diastolic rumble due to increase flow through a normal tricuspid valve may mimic the murmur of mitral stenosis. The X-ray sign of two NTTs however are quite different and helps in differentiating these two conditions.

CHAPTER 4

EKG and Stress Test

EXERCISE STRESS TESTING

1. All the parameters increases at maximal exercise, *except*:
   a. Oxygen extraction
   b. Peripheral resistance
   c. Mean arterial pressure
   d. Diastolic blood pressure

2. What is the maximal extent of increment in cardiac output during strenuous exercise in the upright position?
   a. 100%
   b. 200%
   c. 400%
   d. 600%

3. A change from supine to upright position causes decrease in all, *except*:
   a. Left ventricular end diastolic volume
   b. Stroke volume
   c. End systolic volume
   d. Cardiac index

4. 1 MEt is equivalent to _____ of VO_2.
   a. 1.5 mL/min/kg
   b. 3.5 mL/min/kg
   c. 2.6 mL/min/kg
   d. 4.5 mL/min/kg

5. What is the prevalence of abnormal exercise electrocardiogram in middle aged asymptomatic men?
   a. 1–2%
   b. 4–6%
   c. 5–12%
   d. 10–15%

6. What is the prevalence of an abnormal exercise ECG in middle aged asymptomatic women?
   a. 4–5%
   b. 5–10%
   c. 10–20%
   d. 20–30%

7. What is the approximate predicted 1 year mortality in a post MI patient who could complete 5–6 MET's of exercise without any abnormal ECG in treadmill test?
   a. 1–2%
   b. 2–4%
   c. <10%
   d. Can't be predicted

8. What is the prevalence of repetitive ventricular premature beats during treadmill stress test in an asymptomatic patient?
   a. 0–1%
   b. 0–5%
   c. 2–10%
   d. 15–20%

9. Which is *not* true regarding ventricular arrhythmia during exercise testing?
   a. Exercise induced ventricular arrhythmia is not a useful diagnostic marker of CAD
   b. Suppression of ventricular arrhythmia during exercise rules out CAD
   c. In a post MI patients exercise induced ventricular arrhythmia predicts increased risk of cardiac events.
   d. Exercise induced ventricular arrhythmias are more frequent in recovery phase of exercise

10. The most important factor to influence the heart rate response to exercise is:
    a. Age
    b. Medication use
    c. Blood volume
    d. Body position

11. *Incorrect* statement about stroke volume is:
    a. The product of stroke volume and heart rate determines the cardiac output
    b. The stroke volume is equal to the difference between end diastolic and end systolic volume
    c. A increase in preload increases stroke volume
    d. A increase in after load increases stroke volume

12. During dynamic exercise, despite a fivefold increase in cardiac output, the mean arterial pressure increases only moderately because of:
    a. Increase in preload
    b. Increase in afterload
    c. Increase in contractility
    d. Decrease in peripheral resistance

13. Which of the following is neural control mechanism responsible for the cardiovascular response to exercise?
    a. Bainbridge reflex
    b. Bezold–Jarisch reflex
    c. Exercise pressor reflex
    d. None of them

14. Which is a *correct* statement regarding autonomic modulation during exercise
  a. During light exercise, the plasma norepinephrine level do not increase significantly
  b. During the first minute of recovery, the plasma norepinephrine concentration remains constant or even increases
  c. A delay in heart rate recovery is a marker of autonomic dysfunction
  d. All are correct

15. Which of the following is an absolute contraindication to stress testing?
  a. Left main coronary stenosis
  b. High-risk unstable angina
  c. Severe arterial hypertension
  d. High degree AV block

16. Which of the following is *not* an absolute contraindication to exercise testing?
  a. High-risk unstable angina
  b. Symptomatic severe aortic stenosis
  c. Left main coronary stenosis
  d. Acute aortic dissection

17. Which is *incorrect* regarding stress testing?
  a. The physical examination including assessment of systolic murmurs should be performed before all stress tests
  b. Pretest standard 12 lead EKG are necessary in both supine and standing positions
  c. Hyperventilation should be avoided before testing
  d. Hyperventilation should be performed to identify false (+) ve response

18. During stress test, a cool down walk is advisable for:
  a. When a patient with an ischemic cardiomyopathy exhibits severe chest pain due to ischemia
  b. When a patient with a history of sudden death or collapse develops frequent premature ventricular contraction
  c. When a patient exhibits ST segment elevation
  d. a + b

19. Which is *incorrect* regarding stress testing by bicycle ergometer versus treadmill method?
  a. The bicycling is an isometric exercise
  b. Most individual perform more work on treadmill than bicycle
  c. The maximal heart rate values are similar in two methods
  d. The maximal oxygen uptake is shown to be up to 25% greater during treadmill exercise

20. Exercise induced ST segment depression loses its diagnostic power in patients with:
  a. LBBB
  b. WPW syndrome
  c. Resting ST depression of >1 mm
  d. All of the above

21. ST segment changes isolated to which of the following is more likely to be false positive:
  a. Anterior precordial leads
  b. Inferior leads
  c. Only lateral leads
  d. Lead I and aVL

22. *Incorrect* statement is:
  a. The lead II is known to have high false positive rate
  b. Exercise induced ST segment depression in inferior lead is a poor maker of CAD
  c. ST segment depression limited to recovery period does not generally represent a false positive response
  d. All are correct

23. In evaluation of result of stress test:
  a. There is increasing sensitivity of the test as more vessels are involved
  b. More false negatives are found in cases with single vessel disease especially if disease vessel was not LAD
  c. There is reciprocal relationship between sensitivity and specificity
  d. a + b + c

24. The primary predictor of prognosis in all categories of cardiac patients is:
  a. Heart rate   b. ST-T changes
  c. BP response   d. Exercise capacity

25. In a post MI patient, which of the following parameter is predictive of adverse cardiac event and poor outcome?
  a. Exercise induced ischemia
  b. Lower exercise capacity
  c. Abnormal SBP response
  d. b + c

26. *Incorrect* statement regarding use of stress test for screening asymptomatic individual is:
  a. False positive tests are common among asymptomatic individuals especially women
  b. Exercise treadmill test should be used for screening only in groups with a higher estimated prevalence of the disease
  c. An add-on imaging modality (Echo or nuclear studies) should be the first choice is evaluating asymptomatic individuals with abnormal exercise test
  d. A positive test result should lead to invasive testing

27. Which of the following can produce heart rate turbulence?
   a. Respiration
   b. Thermoregulation
   c. Premature beats
   d. All

28. Which is *not* true regarding QT interval?
   a. It is longer in men than women
   b. It is affected by catecholamines and autonomic tone
   c. It shows circadian rhythm
   d. This interval is related to heart rate

29. Bazett formula is used for calculation of:
   a. Ventricular gradient
   b. ST-T vector
   c. Corrected QT interval
   d. Heart rate turbulence

30. Which is *true* regarding the reperfusion following acute myocardial infarction:
   a. ST segment resolution is an acceptable surrogate for tissue level reperfusion
   b. Persistent ST segment elevation suggest an occluded infarct related artery
   c. Patent artery with failure of myocardial and microvascular reperfusion leads to persistent ST segment elevation
   d. All are true

31. In pericarditis, ST segment elevation can be seen in all leads, *except*:
   a. Lead II, III, aVF
   b. aVR
   c. aVL
   d. V_5–V_6

32. Which of the following increases the ST segment elevation of early repolarization?
   a. Exercise
   b. Hyperventilation
   c. Isoproterenol
   d. Propranolol

33. Epsilon wave in ECG is found in:
   a. Hypothermia
   b. Hypomagnesemia
   c. Hypokalemia
   d. Arrhythmogenic right ventricular dysplasia

34. Which of the following is an indication of old myocardial infarction with left bundle branch block?
   a. Presence of small q wave in Lead I, V_5 and V_6
   b. Late notching of s wave in lead V_3–V_5
   c. Notching of the upstroke of R wave in lead I, aVL, V_5–V_6
   d. All of the above

35. An ECG pattern similar to that of hypokalemia can be produced by which antiarrhythmic drug:
   a. Quinidine
   b. DL—Sotalol
   c. Both a and b
   d. None of them

36. All are correct regarding ECG changes of hypothermia, *except*:
   a. QT interval is prolonged
   b. Positive Osborn wave is seen in leads facing the left ventricle
   c. Osborn wave is due to delayed depolarization
   d. The size of Osborn wave is directly related to body temperature

37. The term inter heart dissociation is an ECG finding in cases with:
   a. Pacemakers
   b. Bundle branch block
   c. Orthotopic heart transplantation
   d. Heterotropic heart transplantation

ANSWERS WITH EXPLANATIONS

1. Ans. b. Peripheral resistance

Braunwald 9th Ed; Page 168

Anticipation of dynamic exercise result in an acceleration of ventricular rate due to vagal withdrawal, increase in the alveolar ventilation and increase venous return as a result of sympathetic vasoconstriction. In normal subject, the net effect is an increase in resting cardiac output before the start of exercise. The magnitude of hemodynamic response during exercise depends on the severity and amount of muscles involved. In the early phase of exercise, in the upright position cardiac output is increased by an augmentation in stroke volume mediated through the use of the Frank-Starling mechanism and heart rate. The increase in cardiac output in the later phase of exercise is primarily due to an increase in ventricular rate. During maximal exertion, sympathetic discharge is maximal and parasympathetic stimulation is withdrawn resulting in vasoconstriction of most circulatory body system except for that in exercise muscle and in the cerebral and coronary circulation. Venous and arterial nor-epinephrine release from sympathetic nerve ending is increased and epinephrine levels are increase at peak exertion. This enhances ventricular contractility. As exercise progresses, skeletal muscle blood flow is increased, oxygen extraction increases by as much as 3 folds, total peripheral resistance decreases and systolic blood pressure, mean arterial pressure and pulse pressure usually increases. Diastolic blood pressure is unchanged or may increase or decrease by approximately 10 mm Hg. The pulmonary vascular bed can accommodate as much as a 6 folds in cardiac output with only modest increase in pulmonary artery pressure, pulmonary capillary wedge pressure and right atrial pressure. Cardiac output is increased by 4 to 6 folds above basal level during maximal exertion in upright position depending on genetic endowment and level of training. The maximum heart rate and cardiac output are decreased in older individuals related in part to the decreased beta- adrenergic responsivity.

At rest, cardiac output and stroke volume are higher in supine than in upright position with exercise, in normal supine subject, the elevation of cardiac output result almost entirely from increase in heart rate with little augmentation of stroke volume. In the upright position increase in cardiac output in normal subject result from a combination of elevation in stroke volume and heart rate. A change from supine to upright posture causes decrease in venous return, left ventricular end diastolic volume and pressure, stroke volume and cardiac index. End systolic volume and ejection fraction are not significantly changed. A normal individual end systolic volume decreases and ejection fraction increases to a similar extent from rest to exercise in supine and upright position.

2. Ans. d. 600%

Braunwald 9th Ed; Page 168

Refer to explanation for Q. No 1.

3. Ans. c. End systolic volume

Braunwald 9th Ed; Page 168

Refer to explanation for Q. No 1.

4. Ans. b. 3.5 mL/min/kg

Braunwald 9th Ed; Page 168-169

Cardiopulmonary exercise testing involves measurement of respiratory oxygen uptake (VO_2), CO_2 production (VCO_2) and ventilatory parameters during a symptom limited exercise test. The relationship between work output, oxygen consumption, heart rate and cardiac output during exercise is linear. VO_2 max is the product of maximal arterial venous oxygen difference and cardiac output. The term metabolic equivalent (MET) refers to the resting VO_2 for a 70 kg, 40-year-old male and 1 MET is equivalent to 3.5 mL/min/kg of body weight. Work activities can be calculated in multiples of METs. This measurement is useful to determine exercise prescription, assesses disability and standardized the reporting of submaximal and peak exercise workload when different protocol are employed. An exercise workload of 3-5 METs is consistent with activities such as light carpentry, golf and walking at 3-4 miles/hour. Workload of 5-7 METs are consistent with exterior carpentry, tennis playing and light backpacking. Workload in excess of 9 METs are compatible with heavy labor, hand ball, squash and running at 6 miles /hour.

5. Ans. c. 5-12%

Braunwald 9th Ed; Page 180

The prevalence of an abnormal exercise electrocardiogram in middle aged asymptomatic man ranges from 5 to 12%. The risk of developing a cardiac event such as angina, myocardial infarction or death in a man is 9 times greater when the test is abnormal as when it is normal. However, over 5 years of follow-up only one in four such men will suffer a cardiac event and this will most commonly due to the development of angina. The risk is slightly greater when the test is strongly positive. The prevalence of an abnormal exercise ECG in middle aged asymptomatic woman ranges from 20-30%. In general, the prognostic value of an ST segment shift in women is less than in the men.

6. Ans. d. 20-30%

Braunwald 9th Ed; Page 180

Refer to explanation for Q. No 5.

7. Ans. a. 1-2%

Braunwald 9th Ed; Page 182

A low level exercise test (achievement of 5-6 METs or 70-80% of age predicted maximum) is frequently performed before hospital discharge to establish the hemodynamic response and functional capacity for exercise prescription, to identify serious ventricular arrhythmias and to identify patient at increased risk of cardiac event. The ability to complete 5-6 METs of exercise or 70-80% of age predicted maximum in the absence of abnormal ECG or blood pressure abnormality is associated with a one year mortality of 1-2%. Parameters associated with increased risk includes inability to perform the low level predischarge exercise test, poor exercise capacity, inability to increase or decrease in exercise systolic blood pressure and angina or exercise induced ST segment depression at low workload.

8. Ans. b. 0-5%

Braunwald 9th Ed; Page 184

The genesis of cardiac arrhythmias during exercise includes re-entry, delayed after potential and enhance automaticity of ectopic foci. Increased catecholamines during exercise accelerates impulse conduction velocity, shortens the myocardial refractory period, increase the amplitude of delayed after potentials. Other potentiators of cardiac rhythm disturbances include metabolic acidosis and exercise induced myocardial ischemia. Ventricular premature beats occur frequently during exercise testing and increases with age. Repetitive forms occur in 0 to 5% of asymptomatic subjects without suspected cardiac disease and are not associated with an increased risk of cardiac death. Exercise induced ventricular ectopic activity is not a useful diagnostic marker of ischemic heart disease in the absence of ischemic ST segment depression. Suppression of ventricular ectopic activity during exercise is a nonspecific finding and may occur in patient with coronary artery disease as well as in normal subject. The prognostic importance of ventricular arrhythmias in patients with chronic ischemic heart disease after adjustment for baseline, clinical and left ventricular function characteristic is small. Approximately 20% of patients with known heart disease and 50-70% of sudden cardiac death survivors have repetitive ventricular beats induced by exercise. In patient with a recent myocardial infarction the presence of exercise induced repetitive forms of ventricular arrhythmia is associated with an increased risk of subsequent cardiac event. Exercise induced ventricular arrhythmias tend to be more frequent in the recovery phase of exercise because peripheral plasma norepinephrine levels continue to increase for several minutes after cessation of exercise and vagal tone is high in the immediate recovery phase. Beta-adrenergic blocking drugs may suppress exercise induced ventricular arrhythmias.

9. Ans. b. Suppression of ventricular arrhythmia during exercise rules out CAD

Braunwald 9th Ed; Page 184

Refer to explanation for Q. No 8.

10. Ans. a. Age

Hurst's 14th Ed; Page 320

Sympathetic and parasympathetic nervous system influences underlie the cardiovascular system first response to exercise, i.e., increase in the heart rate. Vagal withdrawal is responsible for the initial 10-30 beats per minute changes, whereas the remainder is thought to be largely caused by increased sympathetic outflow. Of the two major components of cardiac output, heart rate and stroke volume, heart rate is responsible for most of the increase in cardiac output during exercise particularly at high level. Heart rate increases linearly with workload and oxygen uptake. The heart rate response to exercise is influenced by several factors including age, type of activity, body position, fitness, presence of heart disease, medication use, blood volume and environment. Of these, the most important factor is age. A significant decline in maximal heart rate occurs with increasing age. This decline appears to be a result of intrinsic cardiac changes rather than neural influences.

11. Ans. d. A increase in after load increases stroke volume

Hurst's 14th Ed; Page 320

The product of stroke volume (the volume of blood ejected per heartbeat) and heart rate determines cardiac output. Stroke volume is equal to the difference between end-diastolic and end-systolic volume, thus a greater diastolic filling (preload) will increase stroke volume. Alternatively factor that increases arterial blood pressure will resist ventricular outflow (afterload) and results in a reduce stroke volume. During exercise, stroke volume increases up to approximately 50-60% of maximal capacity, after which increases in cardiac output are caused by further increase in heart rate.

12. Ans. d. Decrease in peripheral resistance

Hurst's 14th Ed; Page 320

During dynamic exercise, the force resisting ejection in the periphery (total peripheral resistance) is reduced by vasodilatation, owing to the effect of local metabolites on the skeletal muscle vasculature. Thus, despite even a five-fold increase in cardiac output among normal subjects during exercise, the mean arterial pressure increases only moderately.

13. Ans. c. Exercise pressor reflex

Hurst's 8th Ed; Page 424-427

The neural control mechanism responsible for the cardiovascular response to exercise occurs through two processes that initiate and maintain the response: 1. Central command—neural impulses, arising from the central nervous system, recruit motor units, excite medullary and spinal neuronal circuit and caused the cardiovascular changes during exercise, 2. Muscle afferents—muscle contraction stimulate afferent endings within the skeletal muscle which in turn reflexively evoke the cardiovascular changes. This mechanism is called exercise pressor reflex comprising all of the cardiovascular changes reflexively induced from contracting skeletal muscle that cause changes in efferent sympathetic and parasympathetic output to the cardiovascular system, that in turn are responsible for increase in arterial blood pressure, heart rate, myocardial contractility, cardiac output and blood flow distribution.

14. Ans. d. All are correct

Hurst's 8th Ed; Page 424-427

Autonomic physiology during recovery from acute episode of exercise involves reactivation of the parasympathetic system and deactivation of sympathetic activity. The decline in heart rate after cessation of exercise is the variable. A delay in the heart rate recovery has been used as a marker of autonomic dysfunction and/or failure of the cardiovascular system to respond to the normal autonomic response to exercise. During light exercise with work loads of 25-40% of VO_2 max or while heart rate remains within 30 beats/min over baseline, plasma norepinephrine level do not significantly increase, confirming that the sympathetic nervous system is more important with higher level of exercise. Rather than declining plasma norepinephrine concentration during first minute of recovery remains constant or even increase immediately after exercise.

15. **Ans. a. Left main coronary stenosis**

Contraindication to Exercise Testing
Absolute
- Acute myocardial infarction (within 2 d)
- Unstable angina not previously stabilized by medical therapy*
- Uncontrolled cardiac arrhythmias causing symptoms or hemodynamic compromise. Symptomatic severe aortic stenosis
- Uncontrolled symptomatic heart failure
- Acute pulmonary embolism or pulmonary infarction Acute myocarditis or pericarditis
- Acute aortic dissection

*Relative**
- Left main coronary artery stenosis. Moderate stenotic valvular heart disease. Electrolyte abnormalities
- Severe atrial hypertension#. Tachyarrhythmias or bradyarrhythmias
- Hypertrophic cardiomyopathy and other forms of outflow tract obstruction. Mental or physical impairment leading to inability to exercise adequately. High-degree atrioventricular block
- * Appropriate timing of testing depends on level of risk of unstable angina, as defined by the Agency for Health Care Policy and Research Unstable Angina Guidelines
- ** Relative contraindications can be superseded if the benefits of exercise outweigh the risks
- # In the absence of definitive evidence, the committee suggests a systolic blood pressure of >200 mm Hg and/or diastolic blood pressure of >110 mm Hg.

Hurst's 14th Ed; Page 1176

16. **Ans. c. Left main coronary stenosis**

Hurst's 14th Ed; Page 1176

Refer to explanation for Q. No 15.

17. **Ans. d. Hyperventilation should be performed to identify false (+) ve response**

Hurst's 14th Ed; Page 324

Hyperventilation should be avoided before testing. Subject with and without disease can exhibit ST- segment changes with hyperventilation, thus hyperventilation to identify false positive responder is no longer considered useful.

18. **Ans. d. a + b**

Hurst's 11th Ed; Chapter 16, Page 467–479

To ensure the safety of exercise testing in exercise laboratory following dangerous circumstances should be recognized and the operator needs to remain vigilant:
1. When patient exhibit ST segment elevation (without baseline diagnostic Q wave) this can be associated with dangerous arrhythmias and infarction. The incidence is approximately 1 in 1000 clinical tests and usually occurs in leads V2 or aVF rather than V5.
2. When a patient with ischemic cardiomyopathy exhibit severe chest pain because of ischemia (angina pectoris, a cool down walk is advisable).
3. When a patient develops exertional hypotension accompanied by ischemia (angina or ST segment depression) or when it occurs in a patient with history of congestive heart failure, cardiomyopathy or recent myocardial infarction, safety is a serious issue.
4. When a patient with history of sudden death or collapse during exercise develop ventricular premature depolarizations that become frequent, a cool down walk is advisable.

19. **Ans. d. The maximal oxygen uptake is shown to be up to 25% greater during treadmill exercise**

Hurst's 11th Ed; Chapter 16, Page 467–479

Bicycle Ergometer versus Treadmill
The bicycle ergometer usually cost less, takes up less space and makes less noise than a treadmill. Although bicycling is a dynamic exercise, most individual perform more work on a treadmill because a greater muscle mass is involved, and most subjects are more familiar with walking than cycling. In most studies comparing exercise on an upright cycle ergometer versus a treadmill exercise, maximal heart rate values have been demonstrated to be roughly similar, whereas maximal oxygen uptake has been shown to be up to 25% greater during treadmill exercise.

20. **Ans. d. All of the above**

Hurst's 11th Ed; Chapter 16, Page 467–479

ST segment depression is representation of global subendocardial ischemia, with a direction determined largely by the placement of the heart in the chest. ST segment does not localize coronary artery disease. ST segment depression in the inferior lead (II, aVF) is most often caused by atrial repolarization wave. Exercise induced ST segment depression loses its diagnostic power in patient with left bundle branch block, WPW syndrome, electronic pacemakers, intraventricular conduction defects (IVCDs) with inverted T wave and in patient with more than 1 mm of resting ST depression. ST segment changes isolated to the inferior leads are more likely to be false positive responses unless profound (i.e., >1 mm). Precordial lead V_5 alone consistently out performs the inferior leads are a combination of leads V_5 with II, because lead II has been shown to have a high false positive rate. Exercise induced ST segment depression in inferior lead is a poor marker for CAD by itself. In patient without prior myocardial infarction and normal resting electrocardiogram, ST segment depression in lead V_5 along with V_4 and V_6 are reliable marker for coronary artery disease and the monitoring of inferior limb leads adds little diagnostic information but elevation in these inferior leads should not be ignored.

21. Ans. b. Inferior leads

Hurst's 11th Ed; Chapter 16, Page 467–479

Refer to explanation for Q. No 20.

22. Ans. d. All are correct

Hurst's 11th Ed; Chapter 16, Page 467–479

Refer to explanation for Q. No 20.

23. Ans. d. a + b + c

Hurst's 11th Ed; Chapter 16, Page 467–479

It has been found that there is increase in sensitivity of the exercise test as more vessels are involved. The most false negative have been found among patient with single vessel disease, particularly if the diseased vessel was not the left anterior descending artery. Irrespective of the techniques used, there is a reciprocal relationship between the sensitivity and specificity. The more specific a test is (i.e., the more able it is to determine who is disease free) the less sensitive it is and vice versa.

24. Ans. d. Exercise capacity

Hurst's 11th Ed; Chapter 16, Page 467–479

Exercise capacity is the primary predictor of prognosis in all categories of patients. With each decrease in the MET value achieved there is a 10–20% increase in overall mortality.

25. Ans. d. b + c

Hurst's 11th Ed; Chapter 16, Page 467–479

The benefit of performing an exercise test in post MI patients are numerous including it helps in optimizing discharge, it helps in recognizing exercise induced ischemia and dysarrhythmia and also helps in prognostication. Review of the post MI exercise studies have showed that normal systolic blood pressure response or a low exercise capacity during exercise test is consistently associated with a poor outcome and is a more predictive of adverse cardiac event after MI than measures of exercise induced ischemia.

26. Ans. d. A positive test result should lead to invasive testing

Hurst's 11th Ed; Chapter 16, Page 467–479

Screening for asymptomatic coronary artery disease has become a topic of increasing interest because of the remarkable efficacy of the statins in reducing the risk of cardiac events even in asymptomatic individuals. If the exercise treadmill test is to be used for screening, it should be done in the group with the higher estimated prevalence of disease using the Framingham score or another predictive model. In addition, a positive test result should not immediately lead to the invasive testing. In most of circumstances an add on imaging modalities (Echo or nuclear study) should be the first choice in evaluating asymptomatic individuals with an abnormal exercise test. False positive tests are common among asymptomatic adults especially women and can lead to unnecessary diagnostic testing, over treatment and labeling.

27. Ans. d. All

Hurst's 11th Ed; Chapter 16, Page 467–479

In normal individuals, intervals between sinus beats show different degree of variation because of respiration, blood pressure regulation, thermoregulation, action of the renin-angiotensin system, circadian rhythms, premature beats and so on. This is called as heart rate variability or heart rate turbulence.

28. Ans. a. It is longer in men than women

Hurst's 11th Ed; Chapter 16, Page 467–479

QT interval is considered as a surrogate of action potential duration. QT interval is slightly longer in women than in men, is affected by autonomic tone as well as catecholamine and it shows circadian variation. QT interval has a relation with heart rate. A large number of formula have been proposed to establish a rule allowing conversion of a pair of QT and RR duration into a standardized QTc value corresponding to a basal RR interval of one second. Bazett a most commonly used formula in which QTc equal to 'k' $\sqrt{QT/R-R}$ interval (second).

The 'k' value as modified is 0.397 for men and 0.415 for women. Values of 0.46 seconds for men and 0.47 seconds for women apply only when rates are within normal range, because this formula tends to overcorrect at rapid rate and under-correct at slower rate. The mean value ranges from 0.40–0.44 seconds at of 60/min, and 0.31–0.34 seconds at of 100/min.

29. Ans. c. Corrected QT interval

Hurst's 11th Ed; Chapter 16, Page 467-479

Refer to explanation for Q. No 28.

30. Ans. d. All are true

Hurst's 11th Ed; Chapter 16, Page 467-479

The typical electrocardiographic sequential changes in a nonintervened patient is appearance of hyper acute T wave to ST segment elevation to abnormal Q wave to T wave inversion. Commonly two or more of these findings appear together depending on the timing of the first recorded static ECG. Acceleration of these phases is now common with the elective interventional reperfusion. The time course of regression of ST segment elevation is a good predictor of reperfusion. ST segment resolution is an acceptable surrogate for tissue level reperfusion. Persistent ST segment elevation suggest either an occluded infarct related artery or a patent artery with failure of myocardial and microvascular reperfusion.

31. Ans. b. aVR

Hurst's 11th Ed; Chapter 16, Page 467-479

The electrocardiographic changes of acute pericarditis may mimic acute myocardial infarction especially if there is ST segment elevation. In pericarditis ST segment can be elevated in all leads except aVR and rarely in V_1. Symmetric T wave inversion usually develops after the ST segment have return to the baseline. Neither reciprocal ST segment changes nor abnormal Q waves are seen as it is in acute myocardial infarction. In most cases of acute pericarditis, the PR segment is depressed. Average ECG resolution occurs in close to two weeks. Sometimes acute pericarditis can be difficult to differentiate from that of normal variant refer to as early repolarization.

32. Ans. d. Propranolol

Hurst's 11th Ed; Chapter 16, Page 467-479

Early repolarization: In its classical form there is 'J' point elevation (of no >3 mm) with an upwardly concave ST segment. R waves can be tall and at times have a distinct notch and slur on the downs row. ST segment elevation is more frequent in chest lead but can occur in lead I and II. These dynamic ECG changes can be affected by exercise and hyperventilation. Isoproterenol reduces and propranolol increases ST segment elevation.

33. Ans. d. Arrhythmogenic right ventricular dysplasia

Hurst's 11th Ed; Chapter 16, Page 467-479

Very slight ST segment elevation with an incomplete right bundle branch block (RBBB) pattern showing an epsilon wave has been described in arrhythmogenic RV dysplasia.

34. Ans. d. All of the above

Hurst's 11th Ed; Chapter 16, Page 467-479

Diagnosis of old myocardial infarction especially anteroseptal is difficult in presence of complete left bundle branch block. In presence of anteroseptal myocardial infarction, the initial vector point towards the free wall of right ventricle because the right ventricular free wall forces are not neutralized by the normally preponderant septal and/or initial LV free wall forces. Thus a small 'q' wave will be recorded in leads I, V_5 and V_6 (where it is not normally present in complete LBBB). Similar finding can be seen in paced beat when in lead I, the spike is followed by a well-defined 'Q' wave. Late notching of 'S' waves in V_3 through V_5 has been found to have moderate to high specificity and moderate-to-low sensitivity. Notching of upstroke of 'R' wave in lead I, aVL, V_5 and V_6 has a sensitivity of 21% and a specificity of 82% to diagnose anteroseptal myocardial infarction.

35. Ans. c. Both a and b

Hurst's 11th Ed; Chapter 16, Page 467-479

The abnormal and delayed depolarization that occurs in hypokalemia is best expressed as QU interval. As the serum potassium level fall 'U' wave become prominent and with further lowering the ST segment becomes progressively more depressed and there is a gradual blending T wave into what is appear to be a tall 'U' wave. An ECG patterns similar to that of hypokalemia can be produced by some antiarrhythmic drugs, especially Quinidine and experimentally DL—Sotalol.

36. Ans. d. The size of Osborn wave is directly related to body temperature

Hurst's 11th Ed; Chapter 16, Page 467-479

Subnormal temperature of the body has been defined as temperature below 97°F (36°C). The QT interval becomes prolonged. In addition, a deflection called as "Osborn wave" appears in a place set to be located between the end of QRS complex and beginning of ST segment. This deflection has been attributed to the delayed depolarization, to a current of injury or to early repolarization. In leads pacing the left ventricle, the deflection is positive and its size is inversely related to body temperature.

37. Ans. d. Heterotropic heart transplantation

Hurst's 11th Ed; Chapter 16, Page 467-479

In a patient with heterotopic heart transplantation, there is an 'inter heart' dissociation during which the ventricular activity of the recipient heart is totally independent from that of the donor's heart. If there is a ventricular ectopic beat, then there is a difficulty in diagnosis.

ECHOCARDIOGRAPHY AND DOPPLER

1. Which of the following is *incorrect* regarding color flow doppler imaging?
   a. It is a pulse wave Doppler based technique
   b. It is subjected to aliasing
   c. It helps in semiquantitative assessment of blood flow velocity
   d. All are correct

2. Doppler echocardiography measures:
   a. Velocity
   b. Flow
   c. Pressure
   d. All

3. What is the Nyquist limit for pulse wave Doppler?
   a. <1 m/sec
   b. <1.5 m/sec
   c. <2 m/sec
   d. <2.5 m/sec

4. M-mode echocardiography is inaccurate in assessment of which of the following:
   a. Rheumatic mitral stenosis
   b. Mitral valve prolapse
   c. Systolic anterior motion of mitral valve
   d. LV aneurysm

5. What is the average speed of ultrasound through the body tissue?
   a. 1000 m/sec
   b. 1240 m/sec
   c. 1440 m/sec
   d. 1540 m/sec

6. Which of the following value of LV mass index is considered as abnormal?
   a. >65 g/m^2 for women and 100 g/m^2 for men
   b. >75 g/m^2 for women and >100 g/m^2 for men
   c. >95 g/m^2 for women and >115 g/m^2 for men
   d. >110 g/m^2 for women and >125 g/m^2 for men

7. Which of the following is *not* the component for assessment of myocardial performance index or Tei index?
   a. Isovolumic relaxation time
   b. Isovolumic contraction time
   c. Ejection time
   d. Ejection fraction

8. What is the usual wall motion score index (WMSI) in patients with heart failure?
   a. >1.0
   b. >1.2
   c. >1.5
   d. >1.7

9. Which of the following is the gold standard method for assessment of left ventricular diastolic dysfunction?
   a. Mitral inflow pattern and mitral inflow Doppler
   b. Doppler tissue imaging
   c. Pulmonary venous Doppler flow pattern
   d. Invasively obtained pressure volume loop

10. Tricuspid annular plane systolic excursion (TAPSE), a measures of RV contractility is usually measured with:
    a. Two-dimensional imaging
    b. Tissue Doppler imaging
    c. M-mode imaging
    d. Spectral echocardiography

11. What would be estimated right atrial pressure based on inferior vena cava diameter and collapse if the IVC diameter is <2.1 cm and respirophasic collapse is <50%?
    a. 0 to 5 mm
    b. 5 to 10 mm
    c. 10 to 15 mm
    d. >15 mm

12. Which of the following is best imaged with transesophageal echocardiography (TEE)?
    a. Mitral valve and mitral prostheses
    b. Aortic valve and aortic prostheses
    c. Thoracic aorta
    d. Abdominal aorta

13. Presence of which of the following diminishes the sensitivity and specificity of stress echocardiography?
    a. Multi vessel disease
    b. Presence of previous infarcted segment
    c. Left bundle branch block
    d. All of the above

14. Which of the following diagnostic modality is helpful in delineating anatomic and physiological consequences of constrictive pericarditis?
    a. CT
    b. CMR
    c. X-ray chest
    d. Echocardiography

15. On echocardiography, what is the normal increase in the radial distance between the epicardial and endocardial borders during systole?
    a. 10%
    b. 20%
    c. 30%
    d. 50%

16. Which of the following defines scar on echocardiography?
    a. Thinning of walls to <6 mm
    b. Echo brightness
    c. Dyskinesis
    d. All of the above

17. Pseudoaneurysm appear more often in which of the following location of infarct?
    a. Anterior infarct
    b. Lateral infarct
    c. Inferior infarct
    d. Apical infarct

18. Extravasation of intravenous echocardiographic contrast from the LV cavity into pericardial effusion suggest the diagnosis of:
   a. Tamponade
   b. Pseudoaneurysm
   c. Free wall rupture
   d. All

19. A distinctive gel like appearance of pericardial fluid on echocardiography is suggestive of:
   a. Serous pericardial effusion
   b. Hemopericardium
   c. Biopericardium
   d. Constrictive pericarditis

20. Which of the following is the index of left ventricular remodeling?
   a. TAPSE
   b. Ejection fraction
   c. Myocardial performance index or Tei index
   d. Sphericity index

21. Dilated cardiomyopathy caused by which of the following pathological process shows discrete area of hypokinesis or akinesis?
   a. Postpartum
   b. Chemotherapy induced
   c. Toxic metabolic causes
   d. Sarcoidosis

22. Wall motion abnormality depicted on echocardiography that do not follow a coronary distribution and associated thickening secondary to edema points toward the diagnosis of:
   a. Viral myocarditis
   b. Chemotherapy induced cardiomyopathy
   c. Discrete inflammatory process
   d. All of the above

23. Spongy appearance of the inner layer of myocardium is characteristic echocardiographic findings of:
   a. Hypertrophic cardiomyopathy
   b. Restrictive cardiomyopathy
   c. Left ventricular noncompaction
   d. Arrhythmogenic cardiomyopathy

24. The most commonly associated abnormality in arrhythmogenic cardiomyopathy is:
   a. RVOT long axis dimension of more than 30 mm
   b. RV global hypokinesia
   c. Segmental wall motion abnormality
   d. Thinning and aneurysm of RV

25. "Scintillating" echo bright appears of myocardium in association with preserved LVEF is characteristic echocardiographic finding of:
   a. Hypertrophic cardiomyopathy
   b. Arrhythmogenic cardiomyopathy
   c. Cardiac amyloidosis
   d. Viral myocarditis

26. Formation of prominent diffuse thrombi along the endocardium in one or both LV apices is characteristic echocardiographic finding of:
   a. Hemochromatosis
   b. Fabry disease
   c. Endomyocardial fibrosis
   d. Cardiac amyloidosis

27. The specificity of stress echocardiography is higher for:
   a. Single vessel disease
   b. Double vessel disease
   c. Left main disease
   d. Left main and triple vessel coronary artery disease

28. What should be an increase in stroke volume to indicate significant contractile reserve during dobutamine stress echocardiography in patients with low gradient, low output aortic stenosis?
   a. At least 5%
   b. 10%
   c. 15%
   d. 20%

29. Mitral valve area calculation by pressure half time is invalid in which of the following conditions?
   a. Immediate post valvuloplasty setting
   b. In presence of significant AR
   c. Biphasic contour of mitral inflow Doppler
   d. All of the above

30. Which of the following parameter is suggestive of severe aortic regurgitation on echocardiography of Doppler examination?
   a. Regurgitant volume of 60 mL or more
   b. EROA of 0.30 cm^2 or greater
   c. Vena contracta >6 mm
   d. All of the above

31. Which of the following is echocardiographic correlates to the clinical phenomenon of pulses paradoxus?
   a. Right atrial collapse
   b. Right ventricular diastolic collapse
   c. Exaggerated tricuspid inflow Doppler 'E' wave peak velocities with reciprocal decrease of mitral 'E' wave velocities
   d. Dilated IVC

32. The echocardiographic hallmark of pulmonary embolism is:
   a. Pulmonary artery dilatation
   b. Right ventricular dilatation
   c. Severe tricuspid regurgitation
   d. Presence of thrombus in pulmonary artery

33. What is *incorrect* regarding McConnell sign?
   a. The free RV mid wall becomes dyskinetic with relative sparing of apex and base
   b. It is due to abrupt increase in pulmonary vascular resistance
   c. It is seen in acute pulmonary embolism
   d. It is highly specific sign for diagnosis of pulmonary embolism

34. Vegetation which are large and dendritic in appearance is a feature of endocarditis due to which of the following organism?
   a. *Staphylococcus aureus*
   b. Streptococcus
   c. Fungal infection
   d. Noninfectious endocarditis

35. Which is the commonest cause of noninfective endocarditis?
   a. Antiphospholipid syndrome
   b. Systemic lupus erythematosus
   c. Advanced neoplasms
   d. Sepsis

36. Echocardiographic characteristic associated with a poor prognosis and embolization in infective endocarditis includes all of the following, *except*:
   a. Vegetation size >1 cm
   b. Increasing size of vegetation despite therapy
   c. Mobile vegetation
   d. All of the above

37. Which is not correct regarding vegetation and infective endocarditis treatment?
   a. Vegetation may persist after successful medical treatment
   b. Vegetation become more echodense over time
   c. The treatment of endocarditis should be guided by morphology of vegetation
   d. All are correct

38. Complete AV block or bundle branch block is a feature of infective endocarditis involving:
   a. Mitral valve
   b. Aortic valve
   c. Pulmonary valve
   d. Tricuspid valve

39. Involvement of which of the following in aortic valve infective endocarditis is likely to produce AV block?
   a. Right coronary cusp
   b. Left coronary cusp
   c. Noncoronary cusp
   d. It is equally seen with all the three cusps

40. Which of the following condition leads to poor atrial contractility and a high prevalence of atrial thrombi even in presence of sinus rhythm?
   a. Sarcoidosis
   b. Uremia
   c. Hypothyroidism
   d. Amyloidosis

41. Which of the following is more sensitive and earlier predictor of cardiotoxicity due to chemotherapeutic agent?
   a. Appearance of global hypokinesia
   b. >10% decrement in LVEF
   c. Presence of marantic endocarditis
   d. Decrease in peak systolic GLS

42. Plaque like deposit on the ventricular aspect of tricuspid valve and the arterial aspect of pulmonary valve is a characteristic feature of:
   a. Systemic lupus erythematosus
   b. Takayasu arteritis
   c. Behcet disease
   d. Carcinoid tumor

43. Which of the following is feature of acute pulmonary embolism?
   a. RV hypertrophy
   b. Elevation in pulmonary arterial pressure
   c. Flattening of interventricular septum in systole
   d. Regional RV dysfunction sparing the apex

44. Rope like vacillating masses in the right side of heart represents:
   a. Myxoma
   b. Fibroelastoma
   c. Melanoma
   d. Thromboemboli

45. Transesophagel echocardiography is required for diagnosis of which variety of atrial septal defect?
   a. Ostium secundum variety
   b. Ostium primum variety
   c. Sinus venosus ASD
   d. Coronary sinus variety

46. Which variety of atrial septal defect is frequently associated with persistent left superior vena cava?
   a. Secundum atrial septal defect (ASD)
   b. Primum ASD
   c. Sinus venosus ASD
   d. Coronary sinus ASD

47. The parallel orientation of great vessels on parasternal long axis or apical view is hallmark feature of:
   a. Tetralogy of Fallot
   b. Double outlet right ventricle
   c. Transposition of great arteries
   d. Truncus arteriosus

ANSWERS WITH EXPLANATIONS

1. Ans. d. All are correct

Braunwald 11th Ed; Page 177

Color flow Doppler is a pulse wave Doppler-based technique in which the velocities of a region of interest are encoded with colors that represent both mean velocities and directionality of the flow, which are superimposed on a 2D image in the region of interest. By convention, flow moving away from the transducer is encoded in blue, and flow toward the transducer is encoded in red. Because color flow Doppler is a form of pulse wave Doppler, it is subject to aliasing, such that high velocities (greater than the Nyquist limit) demonstrate "wraparound" in the color coding to the color of the opposite direction. Turbulent flow, in which a wide range of velocities exist, appears as a multicolored mosaic pattern. Color flow Doppler allows direct real-time visualization of the movement of blood in the heart and is particularly useful for identifying blood flow acceleration and turbulence. This technology is useful for delineating both regurgitant lesions, in which blood moves rapidly and opposite to the expected direction of flow, and discrete stenoses in which there is a flow acceleration. However, in contrast to PW and CW Doppler color Doppler only permits semiquantitative assessment of blood flow velocity.

2. Ans. a. Velocity

Braunwald 11th Ed; Page 178

Doppler echocardiography measures velocity. It does not measure pressure or flow directly. Pressure gradients are inferred from velocities based on the Bernoulli equation, but the absolute pressure within cardiac chambers cannot be directly measured as it is done in cardiac catheterization.

3. Ans. b. >1.5 m/sec

Braunwald 11th Ed; Page 176

The Nyquist limit refers to the maximum velocity that can be accurately quantified within a given sample volume during the Doppler imaging. It is directly related to the pulse repetition frequency. The pulse repetition frequency in turn is inversely related to the distance from the sample volume to the transducer. Pulse wave Doppler is primarily used to assess flow with relatively low velocity (typically ≤1.5 m/sec) present at a specific location, whereas continuous wave Doppler is used to assess higher velocities (typically ≥1.5 m/sec) along the transducer beam, but cannot specify at what location the highest velocity occurs.

4. Ans. d. LV aneurysm

Braunwald 11th Ed; Page 179

M-mode echocardiography provides greater temporal resolution than compared to standard 2D imaging and therefore it remains the method of choice for certain linear measurements, such as septal and posterior wall thickness and left ventricular (LV) chamber dimensions on a particular view. Because M-mode echocardiography is essentially a one dimensional imaging technique, for accurate measurements the cursor scan line must be oriented perpendicular to the long axis of the left ventricle or left atrium. M-mode-based estimates of LV volume, mass, and function can be inaccurate in patients with LV geometries that deviate substantially from normal, such as seen in patients with LV aneurysms or focal wall motion abnormalities. M-mode of valvular leaflets is of importance for diagnosis and still remains useful for demonstrating abnormalities in valvular motion, including rheumatic mitral stenosis, mitral valve prolapse, and systolic anterior motion of the mitral valve as occurs in obstructive hypertrophic cardiomyopathy.

5. Ans. d. 1540 m/sec

Braunwald 11th Ed; Page 176

The speed of ultrasound through body tissue averages 1540 m/sec, especially the speed of sound through the water, but varies minutely as ultrasound waves traverse various body constituents. These slight differences in ultrasound speed through different media (blood, muscle, fat, air) result in impedance mismatches at the tissue interfaces, which produces the specular reflections that mark the boundaries between different tissues.

6. Ans. c. >95 g/m² for women and >115 g/m² for men

Braunwald 11th Ed; Page 184

Left ventricular mass can be calculated by using wall thickness and chambers size with the help of M-mode or 2D measurements together with geometric modeling of the shape of LV myocardial shell. The measurements must be taken to measure the walls at end diastole. An LV mass index (derived from 2D measurements) of >95 g/m² for women or >115 g/m² for men is considered abnormally high. Pathologically, LV hypertrophy is defined as increased overall LV mass and is distinct from wall thickness per se.

7. Ans. d. Ejection fraction

Braunwald 11th Ed; Page 185

The myocardia performance index (MPI) also known as Tei index is defined as the sum of isovolumic relaxation time and isovolumic contraction time divided by ejection time. This method takes into account both systolic and diastolic performance. A higher index is associated with worse function. In adults, values of LV MPI >0.40 and RV MPI >0.43 are considered abnormal.

8. Ans. d. >1.7

Braunwald 11th Ed; Page 186

Regional wall motion can be assessed qualitative or semi-qualitatively using a scoring system. The popular current scoring system is based on a 17-segment model proposed by the American Society of Echocardiography (ASE) in which each segment is scored as normal (1 point), hypokinetic (2 points), akinetic (3 points), or dyskinetic (4 points). The wall motion score index (WMSI) is equal to the sum of these grades divided by the number of segments visualized. A normally contracting ventricle should have a score of 1.0. A WMSI of 1.7 or greater is usually associated with the physical examination findings of heart failure.

9. Ans. d. Invasively obtained pressure volume loop

Braunwald 11th Ed; Page 186

Diastolic function of left ventricle can be assessed by invasively obtained pressure volume loop in which diastolic function is assessed as the instantaneous relationship between pressure and volume of left ventricle and it is considered as gold standard for assessment of diastolic dysfunction. Noninvasively several echo based method can be used to assess cardiac diastolic performance and estimate LV end diastolic pressure. More commonly used variables are (a) mitral inflow Doppler pattern (b) Doppler tissue imaging of mitral annular motion and (c) pulmonary venous Doppler flow patterns.

10. Ans. c. M-mode imaging

Braunwald 11th Ed; Page 188

Tricuspid annular plane systolic excursion (TAPSE) is a measure of RV contractility, and it is usually measured with M-mode imaging. This longitudinal motion of the tricuspid annulus can be assessed similarly by pulsed or tissue Doppler as the peak velocity of the systolic wave, S'.

11. Ans. b. 5 to 10 mm

Braunwald 11th Ed; Page 191

Estimation of right atrial pressure on inferior vena cava (IVC) diameter and collapse

Variable	Normal [0–5 (3) mm Hg]	Intermediate [5–10 (8) mm Hg]		High (15 mm Hg)
IVC diameter	≤2.1 cm	≤2.1 cm	>2.1 cm	>2.1 cm
Collapse with sniff	>50%	<50%	>50%	<50%
Secondary indices				• Restrictive filling by tricuspid valve inflow tricuspid E/e' >6 • Diastolic flow predominance in hepatic veins (systolic filling <55%)

12. Ans. a. Mitral valve and mitral prostheses

Braunwald 11th Ed; Page 191

Advantages and disadvantages of TEE relative to transthoracic echocardiography (TTE)

Advantages	Disadvantages
Useful in percutaneous and surgical procedures, as well as at the bedside	Semi-invasive—usually requires sedation, hence associated risks with probe intubation (gastrointestinal and pulmonary implications) and sedation effects (hypotension). Long procedures may necessitate general anesthesia. Generally a minimum of two staff members required: one operator and one person to monitor the sedation needed
Higher resolution: Better to definitively detect vegetations, thrombi, masses, and intracardiac shunts. Superior imaging of valves, especially the mitral and aortic, left atrium and appendage, left ventricle, thoracic aorta and arch, and interatrial septum, as well as the pulmonary veins	May not view the LV apex or right-sided structures well (structures that are further from probe, particularly in large patients)
"Continuous" acoustic window when compared with TTE (no ribs to cause acoustic shadowing)	• "Blind spot" of acoustic shadowing where the trachea is interposed between the esophagus and heart • Much of the abdominal aorta is out of range

Continued

Continued

Advantages	Disadvantages
Superior imaging of the mitral valve and mitral prostheses in general, with the ability to precisely localize valvular and paravalvular defects	• Mechanical aortic prostheses can cause excessive shadowing • May be technically difficult to achieve the best angle of insonation (i.e., less reproducible and accurate) for assessing aortic stenosis gradients • Maneuvers to increase or decrease preload may be more difficult (e.g., Valsalva maneuver), although most patients can cooperate • Real-time 3D imaging and reconstruction dependent on a slow regular heart rate and "stable" window (i.e., still patient)

13. Ans. d. All of the above

Braunwald 11th Ed; Page 194

Stress echocardiography using either treadmill, bicycle, or pharmacologic (dobutamine or vasodilator) stress has proved to be more accurate than the exercise ECG alone for diagnosing flow-limiting CAD, particularly in women and in patients with left ventricular hypertrophy. Compared with nuclear imaging, stress echocardiography is equally sensitive and specific. However, the presence of previous infarcted segments, known multivessel CAD, and a left bundle branch block may decrease the sensitivity and specificity of stress echocardiography because of difficulty interpreting wall thickening in the presence of resting regional dysfunction and translational motion.

14. Ans. d. Echocardiography

Braunwald 11th Ed; Page 194

Echocardiography is helpful in diagnosing structural abnormalities of the myocardium, pericardium, valves, and vessels. Echocardiography can directly demonstrate the consequent physiologic and hemodynamic derangements, especially in pericardial disease like pericardial effusions. However, defining the thickness of the pericardium is a limitation with echocardiography. Cardiac ultrasound is poorly sensitive for pericardial thickening, and CT and CMR provide a more sensitive and comprehensive method of evaluation. However, echocardiography remains the first-line modality for detecting the characteristic respirophasic septal bounce and respiratory variations in cardiac output caused by constriction and continues to be the mainstay of follow-up regardless of treatment.

15. Ans. b. 20%

Braunwald 11th Ed; Page 195

Echocardiography plays an essential diagnostic and prognostic role in assessing patients during and after acute MI. Normal wall contractility (normokinesis) is seen as wall thickening caused by the contraction of individual myocardial fibers during systole. On echocardiography the radial distance between the epicardial and endocardial borders normally increases by at least 20% during systole.

16. Ans. d. All of the above

Braunwald 11th Ed; Page 195

Myocardial ischemia affects LV systolic function both focally and globally. Focal hypokinesis—decreased systolic thickening occurs within seconds of the onset of myocardial ischemia. Ischemia may also manifest as delayed contractility of a segment. Persistence or increasing severity of the wall motion abnormality after the initial insult implies that the tissue is becoming nonfunctional (not metabolically active or hibernating) or nonviable (infarcted). Akinetic myocardial segments do not thicken at all, and dyskinetic segments bulge paradoxically outward in systole, thus implying that no functioning myocardium is present. Thinning of the walls to <6 mm, echo brightness, and dyskinesis usually indicate scar.

17. Ans. c. Inferior infarct

Braunwald 11th Ed; Page 196

A pseudoaneurysm is a ventricular free wall perforation that is locally contained by adjacent pericardium and adhesions. Pseudoaneurysms appear more often after inferior MI, although they may arise in the lateral and apical regions.

18. Ans. c. Free wall rupture

Braunwald 11th Ed; Page 196

Free wall rupture following acute MI is often lethal. The Echocardiographic findings consist of a sudden new pericardial effusion in a patient with marked thinning and akinesis at the terminal myocardial territory of the occluded artery. Echocardiographic features of tamponade are usually present. The pericardial effusion may contain spontaneous echocardiographic contrast or organized clot. Demonstration of low-velocity color Doppler flow or extravasation of intravenous echocardiographic contrast from the LV cavity into the effusion confirm the diagnosis of free wall rupture.

19. Ans. b. Hemopericardium

Braunwald 11th Ed; Page 197

Hemopericardium is associated with a distinctive gel-like appearance of pericardial fluid on echocardiography.

20. Ans. d. Sphericity index

Braunwald 11th Ed; Page 198

Left ventricle can continue to expand in size and mass and display hypokinesis in noninfarcted areas, even after the initial insult has ended. This process is called as left ventricular remodeling. Remodeling is defined as an increase in LV volume, but concomitant changes in the geometry of the ventricle is also frequently observed. An increase in the globular shape of the heart is quantified by the sphericity index. On 2D echocardiography, this is the ratio of the long-axis dimension to the short-axis dimension. Sphericity index is 1.5 or higher in normal hearts but approaches 1.0 in globular hearts.

21. Ans. d. Sarcoidosis

Braunwald 11th Ed; Page 199

Dilated cardiomyopathy is characterized by increase in the left ventricular end diastolic volumes as well as LVED dimensions and overall LV mass along with subnormal overall LVEF. Dilated cardiomyopathies caused by processes such as viral, postpartum, genetic, chemotherapy, tachycardia, and toxic-metabolic causes typically display diffuse LV hypokinesis. Those caused by more focal processes such as sarcoidosis are more likely to have discrete areas of hypokinesis or akinesis.

22. Ans. c. Discrete inflammatory process

Braunwald 11th Ed; Page 200

The clue to the presence of focal inflammatory processes is wall motion abnormalities that do not follow a coronary distribution and associated thickening secondary to edema.

23. Ans. c. Left ventricular noncompaction

Braunwald 11th Ed; Page 201

Left ventricular noncompaction is a genetic abnormality and is characterized by abundant trabeculations and deep endothelial-lined recesses extending into the myocardial layer that have failed to compact. On echocardiography this confers a "spongy" appearance to the inner layer of the myocardium, whereas the outer layer has the normal "compacted" morphology.

24. Ans. a. RVOT long axis dimension of >30 mm

Braunwald 11th Ed; Page 201

Arrhythmogenic right ventricular dysplasia or arrhythmogenic cardiomyopathy affects primarily right ventricle. In the most classic form, RV dilatation (RVOT long axis dimension >30 mm) is the most commonly associated abnormality, and RV global hypokinesis (FAC <32%) is present in most of the cases. Segmental wall motion abnormalities, including thinning and aneurysms, may be present and are caused by fibrofatty infiltration. The inferoposterior wall of the RV inflow tract is the most frequent segment affected.

25. Ans. c. Cardiac amyloidosis

Braunwald 11th Ed; Page 201

The most common condition leading to restrictive myocarditis is amyloidosis. Deposition of amyloid proteins in the heart causes a very distinct appearance on echocardiography, including increased LV and RV wall thickness in association with a very finely granular or "scintillating" echo bright appearance of the myocardium and initially a preserved LVEF.

26. Ans. c. Endomyocardial fibrosis

Braunwald 11th Page 202

Endomyocardial fibrosis, also termed as Löffler endocarditis, is a rare variety of restrictive cardiomyopathy frequently accompanied by peripheral eosinophilia. Eosinophilic endocarditis and infiltration of the myocardium lead to changes that can be striking on echocardiography. LV size and systolic function may be preserved, but a hallmark of this condition is the formation of prominent diffuse thrombi along the endocardium in one or both LV apices that may embolize and can grow large enough to actually obliterate the cavities.

27. Ans. d. Left main and triple vessel coronary artery disease

Braunwald 11th Ed; Page 204

The sensitivity of stress echocardiography for significant coronary artery disease averages approximately 88%, and its specificity is 83%. The specificity of stress echocardiography appears to be higher than that of nuclear imaging for left main and triple-vessel CAD.

28. Ans. d. 20%

Braunwald 11th Ed; Page 205

In patients with low gradient, low output aortic stenosis and LV dysfunction (defined classically as a calculated aortic valve area by Doppler <1.0 cm^2, mean transaortic gradient <30–40 mm Hg, and LVEF ≤ 40%), DSE can be used to assess both the true severity of AS and the amount of LV contractile reserve. During the test dobutamine is infused in graded doses from 5 to 20 µg/kg/min, for longer stages than used for conventional ischemia testing, to allow for steady-state measurements of spectral Doppler of the LVOT and CW Doppler across the aortic valve. Stroke volume is calculated from VTI of LVOT. An increase of 20% or higher in stroke volume is indicative of significant contractile reserve.

29. Ans. d. All of the above

Braunwald 11th Ed; Page 207

Pressure half-time is most widely used approach to determine mitral valve area. This method relies on the rate at which LA and LV pressures equalize. MVA is calculated as 220 divided by pressure half-time, with 220 being an empirically derived constant. Pressure half time is the time that it takes the initial transvalvular gradient to fall to half of its initial value. The pressure half-time method should not be used in the immediate postvalvuloplasty setting because acute changes in the LA-LV compliance relationship and in the initial transmitral gradient which occurs may give error. This method is also invalid in the setting of significant aortic regurgitation and reduced LV compliance, both of which will result in overestimation of mitral valve area. Pressure half-time may be indeterminate when the mitral inflow Doppler spectrum has a biphasic contour. This method has also not been validated for other causes of mitral stenosis, such as mitral annular calcification, or for prosthetic valves.

30. Ans. d. All of the above

Braunwald 11th Ed; Page 213

The diagnosis of aortic regurgitation is by several parameters including evidence of LV enlargement, color jet dimensions, spectral Doppler signal intensity, pressure half-time, vena contracta, and diastolic flow reversal in the descending thoracic or abdominal aorta. Regurgitant volume and fraction can be calculated using a continuity-based approach, or by PISA approach. A regurgitant volume of 60 mL or more and EROA of 0.30 cm^2 or greater are consistent with severe aortic regurgitation. The vena contracta is the waist (smallest diameter) of the regurgitant flow jet at the level of the valve. A measurement >6 mm generally correlates with severe aortic regurgitation. Holo-diastolic flow reversal in the descending thoracic aorta as detected by pulsed Doppler is a marker of at least moderate aortic regurgitation.

31. Ans. c. Exaggerated tricuspid inflow Doppler 'E' wave peak velocities with reciprocal decrease of mitral 'E' wave velocities

Braunwald 11th Ed; Page 219

Echocardiographic markers of cardiac tamponade fall into two categories: (1) cardiac chamber invagination reflecting elevated intrapericardial pressure and the resultant pressure gradients across the chamber walls and (2) echocardiographic markers of pulsus paradoxus. Echocardiographic correlate to the clinical phenomenon of pulsus paradoxus is change in the flow pattern of atrioventricular valve. In the normal state, a slight increase (up to 17%) in flow velocities through the right heart occurs on inspiration, and a reciprocal but smaller decrease (up to 10%) in flow velocities through the left heart occurs during expiration. These tendencies are exaggerated when a tense, fluid-filled pericardium constrains the overall heart size and increases interdependence between the right and left ventricles. The most widely used signs are an exaggerated (>25%, and often >60% in frank tamponade) increase in the tricuspid inflow Doppler E wave peak velocities with a reciprocal decrease (of >30%) in the mitral E wave velocities, as well as corresponding changes in the pulmonic and aortic systolic Doppler spectra. Additional signs of tamponade include the characteristic appearance of the heart oscillating or "swimming" in the pericardial fluid.

32. Ans. b. Right ventricular dilatation

Braunwald 11th Ed; Page 226

The right ventricular dilation is the echocardiographic hallmark of pulmonary embolism. It is best visualized on the apical four-chamber view, where classic findings include RV diameter greater than LV diameter (ratio >1.0) and a small, underfilled, but normally functioning left ventricle. This is due to sudden rise in the pulmonary artery pressure.

33. Ans. d. It is highly specific sign for diagnosis of pulmonary embolism

Braunwald 11th Ed; Page 226

Acute pulmonary embolism is characterized by a distinctive regional wall motion abnormality in which the free RV mid wall becomes dyskinetic, with relative sparing of the apex and base. This pattern, known as the McConnell sign, it is highly specific for conditions in which PVR increases rapidly.

34. Ans. c. Fungal infection

Braunwald 11th Ed; Page 228

There are no distinguishing characteristics that are organism specific in infective endocarditis, although staphylococcal infections (particularly methicillin-resistant *Staphylococcus aureus* and *S. lugdunensis*) tend to be more destructive and form abscesses, and fungal infections are often large and dendritic in appearance.

35. Ans. b. Systemic lupus erythematosus

Braunwald 11th Ed; Page 228

Vegetations devoid of microorganisms are the hallmark of noninfectious endocarditis or "nonbacterial marantic" endocarditis. In this condition, the typical vegetation are small, verrucous, nondestructive nodules that are seen in upstream side of the valve (typically mitral or aortic) along the line of closure and contain only cellular and fibrin elements. These aseptic lesions are seen in up to 43% of patients with systemic lupus erythematosus (SLE) and 29% of those with antiphospholipid syndrome (APS), in whom they can cause cerebral embolization. These lesions are also seen in patients with advanced neoplasms, sepsis, and condition associated with prothrombotic tendencies.

36. Ans. d. All of the above

Braunwald 11th Ed; Page 228

Echocardiographic characteristics associated with a poorer prognosis and embolization include vegetation size >1.0 cm, increasing size of the vegetation over time despite therapy, very mobile vegetation, and paravalvular abscess.

37. Ans. c. The treatment of endocarditis should be guided by morphology of vegetation

Braunwald 11th Ed; Page 228

Following the medical therapy most of the vegetation will be apparent on follow-up echocardiography for 1 to 2 months, even after successful medical treatment. More than half of the vegetation become more echodense over time. This is due to the presence of varied components of the vegetation, which include not only bacteria but also inflammatory cells, fibroblasts, and extracellular matrix. Growth of a vegetation over time and increasing valvular regurgitation are poor prognostic signs. The mere persistence of vegetations in the absence of symptoms or positive blood cultures is not associated with increased clinical complications. The treatment of endocarditis should not be guided by the echocardiographic morphology of the vegetation over time but by clinical response to therapy.

38. Ans. b. Aortic valve

Braunwald 11th Ed; Page 228

Echocardiography is helpful in assessment of paravalvular extension of infection. On the aortic valve, involvement of right cusp can lead to necrosis of membranous interventricular septum, aneurysm of the right sinus of Valsalva, and valve dehiscence. Embolization into the right coronary artery can occur and cause MI. Involvement of the left cusp can affect the intervalvular fibrosa and extend to infect the base of the anterior mitral valve leaflet. There is also the potential to form an aortic-to-LVOT fistula, or paravalvular leak. Involvement of the noncoronary cusp can extend to the posterior interventricular septum, where the HIS conduction fibers are located, can lead to the development of an intra- or infrahisian block (third-degree atrioventricular block) or bundle branch block. Severe infection of the mitral valve less frequently leads to conduction disturbances.

39. Ans. c. Noncoronary cusp

Refer to explanation for Q. No 38.

Braunwald 11th Ed; Page 228

40. Ans. d. Amyloidosis

Braunwald 11th Ed; Page 229

Amyloidosis is an infiltrative disorder and is known to cause restrictive cardiomyopathy. It also causes valvular thickening and pericardial effusions. Infiltration of amyloid into the atrial walls leads to poor atrial contractility and a high prevalence of atrial thrombi, even when sinus rhythm is still present.

41. Ans. d. Decrease in peak systolic GLS

Braunwald 11th Ed; Page 230

Chemotherapeutic drugs and radiation have adverse effect on cardiac tissue. Early detection of cardiomyopathy especially with anthracyclines group of drugs helps in modification of protocol before irreversible damage occurs. Screening for LVEF is the most widely used strategy. A decrease in peak systolic GLS (>15% change from baseline) is a more sensitive and earlier predictor of cardiotoxicity.

42. Ans. d. Carcinoid tumor

Braunwald 11th Ed; Page 230

More than 50% of patients with carcinoid tumors have cardiac involvement in which plaque like deposits build up on the right-sided heart valves (typically the ventricular aspect of the tricuspid valve and the arterial aspect of the pulmonic valve). This causes a retracted and fixed appearance of the tricuspid and pulmonary leaflets and a combination of valvular stenosis and regurgitation. Cardiac involvement portends a worse prognosis in carcinoid syndrome.

43. Ans. d. Regional RV dysfunction sparing the apex

Braunwald 11th Ed; Page 230-31

Acute pulmonary embolism and pulmonary hypertension can be differentiated by several echocardiographic features. Acute pulmonary embolism is not usually associated with right ventricular hypertrophy, elevation in pulmonary arterial pressure or flattening of interventricular septum in systole unless the pulmonary embolism is chronic or longstanding thromboembolic disease has resulted in pulmonary hypertension. Beside this, the regional RV dysfunction in acute pulmonary embolism spares the apex, whereas there is global RV hypokinesis in pulmonary hypertension.

44. Ans. d. Thromboemboli

Braunwald 11th Ed; Page 233-234

Echocardiography is a versatile tool to diagnose nature of mass in cardiac chamber. Clues that a mass is actually a thrombus include residence in areas of stasis (tip of LA appendage or within LV aneurysm), "wisps" of spontaneous echocardiographic contrast, and associated predisposing cardiac conditions like mitral stenosis, prosthetic valves and cardiomyopathy. Ropelike vacillating masses in the right side of the heart often represent thromboemboli from the deep venous system and finding of such thing calls for assessment of IVC, as well as the pulmonary arteries for presence of similar clot. With anticoagulation, intracardiac thrombi frequently regress.

45. Ans. c. Sinus venosus ASD

Braunwald 11th Ed; Page 236

Sinus venosus ASDs occurs in 2 to 10% of all ASDs and occur in two locations. The Sinus venosus ASD can be SVC type or IVC type. Typically, transesophageal echocardiography is required to make the diagnosis, although SVC-type defects may be demonstrated with subcostal transthoracic echocardiography TTE. The SVC type creates a confluence among the left atrium, right atrium, and SVC as it enters the right atrium. It is frequently accompanied by partial anomalous drainage of the right upper pulmonary vein. IVC-type defects are less common and create a confluence among the left atrium, right atrium, and IVC as it enters the right atrium. This may be accompanied by partial anomalous drainage of the right lower pulmonary vein.

46. Ans. d. Coronary sinus ASD

Braunwald 11th Ed; Page 236

Coronary sinus ASDs are rare and are associated with fenestrations or complete unroofing of the coronary sinus into the left atrium. This variety is also associated frequently with a persistent left superior vena cava (SVC).

47. Ans. c. Transposition of great arteries

Braunwald 11th Ed; Page 238

Transposition of the great arteries (TGA) arises from failure of the aorticopulmonary septum to take its normal spiraling course. The echocardiographic hallmark of transposition is parallel orientation of the great vessels, best appreciated on parasternal long-axis or apical views.

Chapter 5: Cardiac Radiology

1. Reversible defect indicates:
   a. Normal myocardium
   b. Myocardial ischemia
   c. Myocardial necrosis
   d. Myocardial scarring

2. Reverse redistribution occurs only with:
   a. Thallium imaging
   b. Technetium pyrophosphate imaging
   c. PET
   d. Sestamibi imaging

3. The most informative imaging in emergency department in patient with acute chest pain is:
   a. Thallium imaging
   b. Tc 99m imaging
   c. SPECT sestamibi imaging
   d. None of the above

4. To assess the success of thrombolytic therapy which is the imaging of choice:
   a. Thallium perfusion scan
   b. Tc-sestamibi imaging
   c. Tc-pyrophosphate imaging
   d. None of the above

5. Frequently the disease in which of the following vascular territory is *not* detected by planar stress myocardial perfusion images:
   a. Left anterior descending artery
   b. Left circumflex artery
   c. Left main disease
   d. Right coronary artery

6. Which of the following is *not* a high risk myocardial perfusion image?
   a. Multiple reversible defect in a coronary territory
   b. Quantitatively large myocardial perfusion defects
   c. Increased pulmonary radiotracer uptake after exercise
   d. Transient dilatation of left ventricle immediately after exercise

7. Doxorubicin therapy should *not* be initiated in patients with EF below:
   a. 60%   b. 50%
   c. 40%   d. 30%

8. Doxorubicin therapy should be discontinued if the serial estimation of cardiac function reveals fall of EF by:
   a. > 30%   b. > 20%
   c. > 10%   d. > 50%

9. Which of the following is *not* a projection imaging method?
   a. Roentgenography   b. Fluoroscopy
   c. Angiography   d. Ultrasonography

10. Which of the following is *not* a tomographic imaging method?
    a. X-ray CT
    b. MRI
    c. Two-D Echocardiography
    d. Angiography

11. Which of the following imaging technique is precise and accurate in the derivation of right ventricular volume?
    a. Fast CT
    b. MRI
    c. First pass radionuclide ventriculography
    d. Echocardiography

12. The accurate and absolute measurement of regional myocardial perfusion at rest and with stress can be achieved by:
    a. 2 D-echocardiography   b. MRI
    c. PET   d. Angiography

13. The presence and extent of coronary atherosclerosis is most accurately defined by:
    a. Coronary angiography
    b. Intravascular ultrasound
    c. Computerized tomography
    d. MRI

14. The only imaging method capable of directly identifying acutely necrosed myocardium is:
   a. 99mTc-Pyrophosphate scintigraphy
   b. Labeled monoclonal antimyosin specific antibody scintigraphy
   c. Both a and b
   d. None of the above

15. The most direct method to assess the myocardial viability is:
   a. CT
   b. MRI
   c. Thallium scintigraphy
   d. PET

16. In a regurgitant valvular lesion, the regurgitant volume can be determined accurately by:
   a. MRI
   b. CT
   c. Two D-echocardiography
   d. First pass RVG

17. Which of the following catheter is used for measurement of suspected intraventricular pressure gradient?
   a. Pigtail catheter
   b. Cournard catheter
   c. Endhole multipurpose catheter
   d. Sidehole multipurpose catheter

18. The only indication for direct left ventricular puncture is in patient with:
   a. Tricuspid atresia
   b. Severe aortic stenosis
   c. Coarctation of aorta
   d. Mechanical prosthetic valves in both aortic and mitral position

19. Which of the following is a contraindication for intra-aortic balloon counterpulsation?
   a. Acute MI with cardiogenic shock
   b. Acute MI with ventricular septal rupture
   c. Acute MI with mitral regurgitation
   d. Acute MI with moderate-to-severe regurgitation

20. Intra-aortic balloon counterpulsation is indicated in which of the following condition:
   a. Aortic dissection
   b. Moderate-to-severe aortic regurgitation
   c. Aortic aneurysm
   d. Acute MI with cardiogenic shock

21. Which of the following is a contraindication for IABP insertion?
   a. Aortic aneurysm or dissection
   b. Moderate-to-severe aortic regurgitation
   c. Patent ductus arteriosus
   d. All of the above

22. Which of the following is a source of error during pressure recording from a cardiac chamber?
   a. Catheter whip artifact
   b. End pressure artifact
   c. Catheter impact artifact
   d. All of the above

23. Which is the normal range of pulmonary capillary wedge pressure?
   a. 2–7 mm Hg
   b. 4–12 mm Hg
   c. 6–21 mm Hg
   d. 15–30 mm Hg

24. In which of the following condition pulmonary capillary wedge overestimates the true left atrial pressure?
   a. Hypoxemia
   b. Pulmonary embolism
   c. Chronic pulmonary hypertension
   d. All of the above

25. Canon 'A' wave in right atrial pressure waveform indicates:
   a. Decreased ventricular compliance
   b. Atrioventricular asynchrony
   c. Atrial fibrillation
   d. None of the above

26. Canon 'A' wave in right atrial waveform is seen in all *except*:
   a. Complete heart block
   b. Premature ventricular contractions
   c. Ventricular tachycardia
   d. Atrial fibrillation

27. Elevated 'V' wave in right atrial waveform is seen in all *except*:
   a. Tricuspid regurgitation
   b. Right ventricular failure
   c. Restrictive cardiomyopathy
   d. Hypovolemia

28. 'A' wave equal to 'V' wave in right atrial pressure waveform is seen in all conditions *except*:
   a. Cardiac tamponade
   b. Tricuspid regurgitation
   c. Constrictive pericardial disease
   d. Hypervolemia

29. Prominent 'Y' descent in right atrial waveform is seen in all *except*:
   a. Constrictive pericarditis
   b. Restrictive cardiomyopathy
   c. Tricuspid regurgitation
   d. Right atrial ischemia

30. Kussmaul's sign (inspiratory rise or lack of decline in right atrial pressure) is seen in:
   a. Cardiac tamponade
   b. Restrictive cardiomyopathy
   c. Tricuspid regurgitation
   d. Right ventricular ischemia

31. Ventricularization of right atrial pressure is seen in:
   a. Ebstein's anomaly
   b. Severe tricuspid regurgitation
   c. Cardiac tamponade
   d. Right heart failure

32. Equalization (<5 mm Hg) of mean right atrial, right ventricular diastolic, pulmonary artery diastolic, pulmonary capillary wedge and pericardial pressure is suggestive of:
   a. Cardiac tamponade
   b. Constrictive pericarditis
   c. Chronic obstructive lung disease
   d. Effusive constrictive pericarditis

33. Dissociation between pressure recording and intracardiac ECG suggest diagnosis of:
   a. Single atrium   b. Single ventricle
   c. Ebstein's anomaly   d. Ulhs anomaly

34. Pulmonary capillary wedge pressure not equal to left ventricular end diastolic pressure, is found in all *except*:
   a. Left atrial myxoma
   b. Cor triatriatum
   c. Pulmonary venous obstruction
   d. Hypertrophic obstructive cardiomyopathy

35. Bifid pulmonary artery waveform is seen in:
   a. Severe tricuspid regurgitation
   b. Severe mitral regurgitation
   c. Severe mitral stenosis
   d. Severe mitral stenosis and regurgitation

36. Dip and plateau in diastolic pressure wave is found in all *except*:
   a. Constrictive pericarditis
   b. Restrictive cardiomyopathies
   c. Right ventricular ischemia
   d. Cardiac tamponade

37. Pulsus bisferiens is found in:
   a. Aortic stenosis   b. Aortic regurgitation
   c. Cardiac tamponade   d. Mitral regurgitation

38. Pulsus paradoxus is seen in all *except*:
   a. Cardiac tamponade
   b. Pulmonary embolism
   c. Chronic obstructive airway disease
   d. Hypertrophic obstructive cardiomyopathy

39. Spike and dome configuration in aortic pressure waveform is found in:
   a. Aortic stenosis with regurgitation
   b. Hypertrophic obstructive cardiomyopathy
   c. Coarctation of aorta
   d. Dilated cardiomyopathy

40. Pulsus parvus et tardus is found in:
   a. Aortic regurgitation
   b. Aortic stenosis
   c. Hypertrophic obstructive cardiomyopathy
   d. Pulmonic stenosis

41. What is the normal exercise index (actual cardiac index divided by the predicted cardiac index)?
   a. 0.4   b. 0.8
   c. 0.6   d. 0.1

42. Normally for every 100 mL/min increase in oxygen consumption with exercise, the cardiac output should increase by at least:
   a. 100%   b. 200%
   c. 400%   d. 600%

43. Which of the following agent is used to provoke coronary spasm?
   a. Phenylephrine   b. Isoproterenol
   c. Ergonovine   d. Sodium nitroprusside

44. Most widely applied technique for measurement of coronary blood flow in humans is:
   a. Thermodilution
   b. Digital substraction angiography
   c. Electromagnetic flow meter
   d. Doppler velocity probes

45. A positive inotropic effect following an abrupt elevation in aortic pressure is:
   a. Frank–Starling effect   b. Anrep effect
   c. Bowditch effect   d. Concertina effect

46. An increased heart rate progressively increases the force of ventricular contraction is:
   a. Frank–Starling phenomenon
   b. Bowditch phenomenon
   c. Anrep effect
   d. Ashman phenomenon

47. Bernheim effect is a:
   a. Diastolic dysfunction in hypertrophic myocardium
   b. Aortic-ventricular coupling
   c. Systolic-ventricular interaction
   d. Diastolic-ventricular interaction

48. Ischemic preconditioning is mediated by:
   a. Inhibitory G protein
   b. B receptors
   c. Potassium efflux
   d. Calcium influx

49. The term smart heart is applied for:
   a. Ischemic contraction
   b. Ischemic preconditioning
   c. Hibernating heart
   d. Myocardial stunning

ANSWERS WITH EXPLANATIONS

1. Ans. a. Normal myocardium

Braunwald 5th Ed; Page 281

Planar and Spect images are interpreted qualitatively by visual analysis often added by computer quantification. Image interpretation can be described as follows:
A. Normal—homogenous uptake of radiopharmaceutical throughout the myocardium.
B. Defect—a localized myocardial area with a relative decrease in radiotracer uptake. Defects may vary in intensity, from slightly reduced activity to almost absent activity.
C. Reversible defect—a defect present on initial stress images is no longer present or is present to a lesser degree on the resting or delayed images. This pattern indicates myocardial ischemia. Improvement overtime on Thallium-201 imaging is referred to as redistribution. It is not appropriate to use this terminology for 99mTc – labeled agents.
D. Fixed defect—a defect is unchanged and present on both exercise and rest (delayed images); this pattern generally indicates an infarction of heart issue. However, in some patient with fixed Thallium 201 defect, on 24 hour delayed imaging, improved uptake can be noted on 24 hours redistribution imaging or after a new resting injection.
E. Reverse distribution—this pattern occurs only with Thallium-201 (TI-201) imaging. The initial stress images either are normal or show a defect, whereas the delayed image shows a new or more severe defect. This pattern is frequently observed in patients with infarction who have undergone thrombolytic therapy or percutaneous coronary angioplasty. The phenomenon is thought to be caused by initial access of tracer uptake in a reperfused area with a mixture of scar tissue and viable myocytes. Initial accumulation is followed by rapid clearance from scar tissue. Although the significance of these finding is controversial, it does not represent evidence of exercise induced ischemia.

With positron emission tomography with (F^{18}) Fluoro—2—deoxyglucose (PET + DG), the presence of residual viable myocardium has been demonstrated within areas with reverse distribution.

2. Ans. a. Thallium imaging

Braunwald 5th Ed; Page 281

Refer to explanation for Q. No 1.

3. Ans. c. SPECT sestamibi imaging

Braunwald 5th Ed; Page 286

Because acute regional myocardial hypoperfusion can be visualized almost instantaneously in myocardial perfusion imaging, its potential use as means to triage patient in emergency department has been evaluated. A substantial number of patients seen in emergency department with complaint of acute chest pain have a nondiagnostic electrocardiogram. These patients are often admitted to rule out acute myocardial infarction. However, only a small proportion of these patients (15–20%), acute coronary disease is found. The majority of patients have hospital admission without having a true cardiac cause for their symptom. In one of the study, none of these patients with normal acute TI-201 images "had either acute infarction or unstable angina after further clinical evaluation". In contrast, more than 80% of patients who later were proven to have either acute infarction or unstable angina had abnormal TI-201 perfusion images on admission in emergency room. The new 99mTc labeled myocardial perfusion imaging agents are better suited than TI-201 for imaging patients with chest pain in emergency department. Because these agents do not redistribute significantly, imaging does not have to be performed immediately and myocardial perfusion during chest pain can be imaged at a convenient time. Moreover, Spect imaging can be performed which allows detailed evaluation of various coronary vascular territories. Patient with abnormal Spect images had a higher incidence of coronary event (death, acute infarction or revascularization) during follow-up whereas patient with normal acute myocardial perfusion images in general had a favorable outcome.

4. Ans. b. Tc-sestamibi imaging

Braunwald 5th Ed; Page 286

During the early hours of acute myocardial infarction, evaluation of myocardial perfusion is of interest in patients who have thrombolytic therapy. Serial myocardial perfusion imaging can demonstrate a decrease in the myocardial perfusion defects size overtime in patient who had successful reperfusion. Imaging with TI-201 is not practical in this setting because of TI-201 redistribution myocardial imaging has to be performed before initiation of therapy. This would cause a clinically unacceptable delay in the treatment. A more practical approach is the use of 99mTc—Sestamibi. Because of the lack of significant redistribution, this imaging agent can be injected before initiation of thrombolytic therapy and imaging of myocardial perfusion can be performed later using either planar imaging at the bed side or Spect imaging in the nuclear laboratory. Successful thrombolysis of the infarct artery can be predicted by a decrease of the size of myocardial perfusion defect on serial 99mTc— Sestamibi imaging.

5. Ans. b. Left circumflex artery

Braunwald 5th Ed; Page 291

Detection of high-risk coronary artery disease: The greater the functional severity of coronary artery disease, the more abnormal exercise myocardial perfusion images are likely to be. Most patients (~95%) with left main coronary artery disease have abnormal stress myocardial perfusion images. However, the expected typical left main pattern, i.e., defects in anteroseptal and posterolateral walls is found in only a minority (~14%) of patient with left main coronary artery disease. The majority (~75%) of patients have multiple perfusion defects and frequently abnormal increase uptake of TI-201. Although most patients with triple vessel disease have abnormal stress images, approximately 60% have multiple defects in two or more vascular reasons. Most frequently, disease in the left circumflex artery is not detected on planar stress myocardial perfusion images. High-risk myocardial perfusion images can be characterized by: (1) multiple reversible defects in two or more coronary artery territories; (2) quantitatively large myocardial perfusion defects; (3) increase pulmonary radiotracer uptake after exercise; (4) transient dilatation of the left ventricle immediately after exercise. These high risk pattern is highly specific (~95%) for multivessel coronary artery disease. However, the sensitivity is only about 70%. Therefore, in the absence of the above mentioned scintigraphic characteristics, the presence of multi vessel disease cannot be ruled out.

6. Ans. a. Multiple reversible defect in a coronary territory

Braunwald 5th Ed; Page 291

Refer to explanation for Q. No 5.

7. Ans. d. 30%

Braunwald 5th Ed; Page 303

Guidelines for monitoring patients receiving doxorubicin: Perform baseline radionuclide angio-cardiography at rest for LVEF prior to administration of 100 mg/m^2 doxorubicin. Subsequent studies at least 3 weeks after the indicated total cumulative doses have been given, but before next dose.

Patients with normal baseline LVEF (≥ 50%)
- Perform the second study after 250 to 300 mg/m^2
- Repeat study after 400 mg/m^2 in patients with known heart disease, radiation exposure, abnormal electrocardiogram, or cyclophosphamide therapy; or after 450 mg/m^2 in the absence of any of these risk factors.
- Perform sequential studies thereafter before each dose.
- Discontinue doxorubicin if absolute decrease in LVEF ≥ 10% (EF units) with a decline to a level ≤ 50% (EF units).

Patients with abnormal baseline LVEF (<50%)
- Doxorubicin therapy should not be initiated with baseline LVEF ≤ 30%
- In patients with LVEF > 30% and < 50% sequential studies should be obtained before each dose.
- Discontinue doxorubicin if absolute decrease in LVEF > 10% (EF units) and/or final LVEF < 30%.

8. Ans. c. >10%

Braunwald 5th Ed; Page 303

Refer to explanation for Q. No 7.

9. Ans. d. Ultrasonography

Braunwald 5th Ed; Page 349

Projection versus tomographic imaging: The distinction between projection and tomographic imaging is of theoretical and practical importance. The standard chest X-ray is a good example of projection imaging method. The patient is placed between X-ray source and an X-ray detector (a film is screen system). The X-rays are launched, then pass through the patient and/or then received and detected on film. Thus, the imaging energy is projected through the patient, so that attenuation of X-ray occurs not only due to the structure of interest (e.g., the heart) but also due to other structures interposed along the path taken by X-rays (such as chest-wall and lung). Because of this projection phenomena, X-ray shadows in the resulting roentgenogram represents a superimposition of wanted and unwanted information. Plain film Roentgenography, fluoroscopy and angiography are all example of projection imaging method.

The other basic approach to imaging is selective depiction of a slice or tomogram through the patient. For example, in case of X-ray computed tomography (CT) the production of a tomogram is accomplished by acquiring X-ray attenuation measurement from many different angle around the patient within a selected plane. At each angle, X-rays are sent from an X-ray source through the patient and or then received by a detector on the opposite side of the patient. This process is repeated for many angles around the patient yielding a set of X-ray attenuation profile. By computer reconstruction methods, these many X-ray attenuation profiles are combined to produce an image depicting the two dimensional distribution of X-ray attenuation data or a slice or tomogram through the patient. Since the resulting data selectively represent X-ray attenuation only in the slice under the study, the problem of superimposition found in projection image and projection method does not occur.

Thus, the tomographic imaging technique permits clear delineation of physical characteristics and anatomical features of selected body region, which is not possible with non-tomographic projection methods. Two dimensional echocardiography, single photon emission radionuclide CT, X-ray CT, and magnetic resonance imaging (MRI) are all examples of tomographic imaging methods. Tomographic imaging method virtually all depend on digital computer image processing method for image generation, display and analysis.

10. Ans. a. X-ray CT

Braunwald 5th Ed; Page 349

Refer to explanation for Q. No 9.

11. Ans. a. Fast CT

Braunwald 5th Ed; Page 352

Assessment of the function of the right ventricle is more difficult than of left ventricle because of the complex shape of right ventricle, which defies easy representation by simple geometrical models. Although echocardiographic methods of quantitatively assessing right ventricular function have been developed, there has not been widespread use of this technique. Fast CT is extremely precise and accurate in derivation of right ventricular volumes and stroke volume and MRI methods also appear to have impressive accuracy for assessment of right ventricular function and mass. First pass radionuclide ventriculography is a relatively inexpensive and simple method that can determine right ventricular ejection fraction accurately on the bedside or in the clinical imaging area.

12. Ans. c. PET

Braunwald 5th Ed; Page 353

The most promising radionuclide approach to quantitative myocardial perfusion imaging is PET. The combination of high energy photons released during positron annihilation (511 keV) and the method of coincidence detection for image formation permits high resolution depiction of the distribution of a perfusion tracer. The high temporal resolution, together with a quantitative imaging capability combined with a use of multicompartment tracer kinetic module, permits accurate estimate of absolute level of myocardial perfusion. PET and fast CT appears to be the method most capable of accurate, absolute measurement of regional myocardial perfusion at rest and with stress.

13. Ans. b. Intravascular ultrasound

Braunwald 5th Ed; Page 354

The presence and extent of coronary atherosclerosis can be characterized most definitively utilizing selective coronary angiography. The intravascular ultrasound permits extremely high-resolution imaging of coronary lumen and adjacent wall thickness and composition (e.g., the presence of calcified plaque). Intravascular ultrasound can demonstrate atherosclerosis in the region of coronary arteries judged normal on angiography. CT can also contribute to the diagnosis of coronary atherosclerosis by the identification of coronary calcification.

14. Ans. c. a+b

Braunwald 5th Ed; Page 355

The only clinically available imaging methods capable of directly identifying acutely necrotic myocardium are 99mTc-Pyrophosphate scintigraphy and labeled monoclonal antimyosin-specific-antibody scintigraphy. Although these methods permit the identification of acute necrosis, their clinical applicability is somewhat limited by their poor spatial resolution, which precludes detail assessment of the size of myocardial infarction. Nonetheless, infarct avid scintigraphy in selected patient is a useful method of infarct identification. Metabolic imaging with PET shows great promise in the identification and quantification of acute myocardial infarction. MR spectroscopy using ^{31}P also may prove to be useful in identifying infarction.

15. Ans. d. PET

Braunwald 5th Ed; Page 355

The most direct method available to help Clinician to negotiate the quandary of assessing myocardial viability is metabolic imaging with PET.

16. Ans. b. CT

Braunwald 5th Ed; Page 355

Echocardiography remains the procedure of choice for the initial assessment of patients with valvular heart disease. Frequently decisions regarding medical and surgical management are based on echocardiography without the need for invasive evaluation. In selected patients, angiography and cardiac catheterization are still quite useful particularly in the identification of concomitant coronary artery disease and when ultrasound examination yield equivocal results. CT and MRI methods have the ability to determine left ventricular mass more precisely than does echocardiography. Regurgitant volume can be determined accurately with CT. This may prove useful in selected patients with valvular heart disease.

17. Ans. c. Endhole multipurpose catheter

Braunwald 5th Ed; Page 184

For measurement of suspected intraventricular gradients, a multipurpose catheter with end hole is desirable to localize the gradient in the left ventricle. Pigtail catheters contain side holes which will up augment the capacity to define whether the gradient is intraventricular or transvalvular.

18. Ans. d. Mechanical prosthetic valves in both aortic and mitral position

Braunwald 5th Ed; Page 186

The sole indication for direct left ventricular puncture is to measure left ventricular pressure and to perform ventriculography in patients with mechanical prosthetic valves in both mitral and aortic positions thus preventing retrograde arterial and transseptal catheterization. Crossing mechanical prosthesis with catheter should be avoided as this may result in catheter entrapment, occlusion of the valve and possible dislodgement of the disk with embolization. The risk of this procedure includes cardiac tamponade, hemothorax, pneumothorax, laceration of left anterior descending artery, embolism of left ventricular thrombus, vagal reaction and ventricular arrhythmias. With the advent of transesophageal echocardiography, this procedure is now infrequently performed.

19. Ans. d. Acute MI with moderate-to-severe regurgitation

Braunwald 5th Ed; Page 187

Intra-aortic balloon insertion is indicated for patient with:
1. Angina refractory to medical therapy,
2. Cardiogenic shock,
3. Mechanical complication of myocardial infarction (including severe mitral regurgitation, ventricular septal defect;
4. Patients with severe left main coronary artery stenosis who is to undergo bypass surgery;
5. High-risk angioplasty and after primary angioplasty in setting of acute myocardial infarction.

IABP is contraindicated in patient with:
1. Moderate-to-severe insufficiency;
2. Aortic dissection;
3. Aortic aneurysm;
4. Patent ductus arteriosus;
5. Severe peripheral vascular disease;
6. Bleeding disorders or sepsis.

20. Ans. d. Acute MI with cardiogenic shock

Braunwald 5th Ed; Page 187

Refer to explanation for Q. No 19.

21. Ans. d. All of the above

Braunwald 5th Ed; Page 187

Refer to explanation for Q. No 19.

22. Ans. d. All of the above

Braunwald 5th Ed; Page 188

Intravascular pressures are typically measured using a fluid filled catheter, i.e., attached to a pressure transducer. The pressure wave is transmitted from the catheter tip to the transducer by the fluid column within the catheter. The majority of pressure transducers used currently are disposable electrical strain-gauges. The pressure wave distort the diaphragm are wire within the transducer. This energy is then converted to an electric signal proportional to the pressure being applied using the principal of wheat stone bridge. This signal is then amplified and recorded as an analog signal. There are a number of sources of error when pressure are measured using a fluid filled catheter/transducer system:
1. Distortion of output signal due to the frequency response characteristic and damping characteristic of the system;
2. Improper calibration of zero reference;
3. Catheter whip artifact, i.e., motion of the tip of the catheter within the measured chamber;
4. End pressure artefact, i.e., an end hole catheter measures an artificially elevated pressure on account of strumming or high velocity of the pressure wave;
5. Catheter impact artifact, i.e., when the catheter is impacted by the walls or valves of the cardiac chambers;
6. Catheter tip obstruction within a small vessels or valvular orifice occurring because of the size of catheter itself.

23. Ans. b. 4–12 mm Hg

Braunwald 5th Ed; Page 188

Normal pressures and vascular resistances

Pressures	Average (mm Hg)	Range (mm Hg)
Right atrium		
'A' wave	6	2–7
'V' wave	5	2–7
Mean	3	1–5
Right ventricle		
Peak systolic	25	15–30
End-diastolic	4	1–7
Pulmonary artery		
Peak systolic	25	15–30
End-diastolic	9	4–12
Mean	15	9–19
Pulmonary capillary wedge		
Mean	9	4–12
Left atrium		
A wave	10	4–16
V wave	12	6–21
Mean	8	2–12
Left ventricle		
Peak systolic	130	90–140
End-diastolic	8	5–12
Central aorta		
Peak systolic	130	90–140
End-diastolic	70	60–90
Mean	85	70–105

Continued

Continued

Pressures	Average (mm Hg)	Range (mm Hg)
Vascular resistances	Mean (dyne/sec/cm^{-5})	Range (dyne/sec/cm^{-5})
Systemic vascular resistance	100	700–1600
Total pulmonary resistance	200	100–300
Pulmonary vascular resistance	70	20–130

24. Ans. d. All of the above

Braunwald 5th Ed; Page 189

The pulmonary capillary wedge pressure wave forms is similar to the left atrial pressure wave form but is slightly damped and delayed as a result of transmission through the lungs. The 'A' and 'V' waves with both 'X' and 'Y' descents are visible but 'C' wave may not be seen. In the normal state, the pulmonary artery diastolic pressure is similar to the mean pulmonary capillary wedge pressure because the pulmonary circulation has low resistance. In certain disease states that are associated with an elevated pulmonary vascular resistance like hypoxia, pulmonary embolism and chronic pulmonary hypertension and occasionally after mitral valve surgery, the pulmonary capillary wedge pressure may not accurately reflect left atrial pressure. Pulmonary capillary wedge may over estimate true left atrial pressure in this circumstance and therefore accurate measurement of mitral valve gradient may require obtaining direct left atrial pressure.

25. Ans. b. Atrioventricular asynchrony

Braunwald 5th Ed; Page 190

Pathological Waveforms

I. *Right atrial pressure waveforms*
   A. Low mean atrial pressure
      1. Hypovolemia.
      2. Improper zeroing of the transducer.
   B. Elevated mean atrial pressure
      1. Intravascular volume overload states.
      2. Right ventricular failure due to valvular disease (tricuspid or pulmonic stenosis or regurgitation).
      3. Right ventricular failure due to myocardial disease (right ventricular ischemia, cardiomyopathy).
      4. Right ventricular failure due to left heart failure (mitral stenosis/regurgitation, aortic stenosis/regurgitation, cardiomyopathy, ischemia).
      5. Right ventricular failure due to increased pulmonary vascular resistance (pulmonary embolism, chronic obstructive pulmonary disease, primary pulmonary hypertension).
      6. Pericardial effusion with tamponade physiology.
      7. Obstructive atrial myxoma.
   C. Elevated 'A' wave (any increase to ventricular filling)
      1. Tricuspid stenosis.
      2. Decreased ventricular compliance due to ventricular failure, pulmonic valve stenosis, or pulmonary hypertension.
   D. Cannon 'A' wave
      1. Atrial-ventricular asynchrony (atria contract against a closed tricuspid valve, as during complete heart block, following premature ventricular contraction, during ventricular tachycardia, with ventricular pacemaker).
   E. Absent 'A' wave
      1. Atrial fibrillation or atrial standstill.
      2. Atrial flutter.
   F. Elevated 'V' wave
      1. Tricuspid regurgitation.
      2. Right ventricular heart failure.
      3. Reduced atrial compliance (restrictive myopathy).
   G. 'A' wave equal to 'V' wave
      1. Tamponade.
      2. Constrictive pericardial disease.
      3. Hypervolemia.
   H. Prominent 'X' descent
      1. Tamponade.
      2. Subacute constriction and possibly chronic constriction.
      3. Right ventricular ischemia with preservation of atrial contractility
   I. Prominent 'Y' descent
      1. Constrictive pericarditis.
      2. Restrictive myopathies.
      3. Tricuspid regurgitation.
   J. Blunted 'X' descent
      1. Atrial fibrillation.
      2. Right atrial ischemia.
   K. Blunted 'Y' descent
      1. Tamponade.
      2. Right ventricular ischemia.
      3. Tricuspid stenosis.
   L. Miscellaneous abnormalities
      1. Kussmaul's sign (inspiratory rise or lack of decline in right atrial pressure): Constrictive pericarditis, right ventricular ischemia.
      2. Equalization (≤ 5 mm Hg) of mean right atrial, right ventricular diastolic, pulmonary artery diastolic, pulmonary capillary wedge, and pericardial pressures in tamponade.
      3. M or W patterns: Right ventricular ischemia, pericardial constriction, congestive heart failure.
      4. Ventricularization of the right atrial pressure: Severe tricuspid regurgitation.

5. Saw tooth pattern: Atrial flutter.
6. Dissociation between pressure recording and intracardiac ECG: Ebstein's anomaly.

II. **Left atrial pressure/pulmonary capillary wedge pressure waveforms**
   A. Low mean pressure
      1. Hypovolemia.
      2. Improper zeroing of the transducer.
   B. Elevated mean pressure
      1. Intravascular volume overload states.
      2. Left ventricular failure due to valvular disease (mitral or aortic stenosis or regurgitation).
      3. Left ventricular failure due to myocardial disease (ischemia or cardiomyopathy).
      4. Left ventricular failure due to systemic hypertension.
      5. Pericardial effusion with tamponade physiology.
      6. Obstructive atrial myxoma.
   C. Elevated 'A' wave (any increase to ventricular filling)
      1. Mitral stenosis.
      2. Decreased ventricular compliance due to ventricular failure, aortic valve stenosis, or systemic hypertension.
   D. Cannon 'A' wave
      1. Atrial-ventricular asynchrony (atria contract against a closed mitral valve, as during complete heart block following premature ventricular contraction, during ventricular tachycardia with ventricular pacemaker).
   E. Absent 'A' wave
      1. Atrial fibrillation or atrial standstill.
      2. Atrial flutter.
   F. Elevated 'V' wave
      1. Mitral regurgitation.
      2. Left ventricular heart failure.
      3. Ventricular septal defect.
   G. A wave equal to 'V' wave
      1. Tamponade.
      2. Constrictive pericardial disease.
      3. Hypervolemia.
   H. Prominent 'X' descent
      1. Tamponade.
      2. Subacute constriction and possibly chronic constriction.
   I. Prominent 'Y' descent
      1. Constrictive pericarditis.
      2. Restrictive myopathies.
      3. Mitral regurgitation.
   J. Blunted 'Y' descent
      1. Atrial fibrillation.
      2. Atrial ischemia.
   K. Blunted 'Y' descent
      1. Tamponade.
      2. Ventricular ischemia.
      3. Mitral stenosis.
   L. Pulmonary capillary wedge pressure not equal to left ventricular end diastolic pressure
      1. Mitral stenosis.
      2. Left atrial myxoma.
      3. Cor triatriatum.
      4. Pulmonary venous obstruction.
      5. Decreased ventricular compliance.
      6. Increased pleural pressure.
      7. Placement of catheter in a nondependent zone of lung.

III. **Pulmonary artery pressure waveforms**
   A. Elevated systolic pressure
      1. Primary pulmonary hypertension.
      2. Mitral stenosis or regurgitation.
      3. Congestive heart failure.
      4. Restrictive myopathies.
      5. Significant left to right shunt.
      6. Pulmonary disease (pulmonary embolism, hypoxemia, chronic obstructive pulmonary disease).
   B. Reduced systolic pressure
      1. Hypovolemia.
      2. Pulmonary artery stenosis.
      3. Sub- or supravalvular stenosis.
      4. Ebstein's anomaly.
      5. Tricuspid stenosis.
      6. Tricuspid atresia.
   C. Reduced pulse pressure
      1. Right heart ischemia.
      2. Right ventricular infarction.
      3. Pulmonary embolism.
      4. Tamponade.
   D. Bifid pulmonary artery waveform
      1. Large left atrial v wave transmitted backward (i.e., MR).
   E. Pulmonary artery diastolic pressure greater than pulmonary capillary wedge pressure
      1. Pulmonary disease.
      2. Pulmonary embolus.
      3. Tachycardia.

IV. **Ventricular pressure waveforms**
   A. Systolic pressure elevated
      1. Pulmonary or systemic hypertension.
      2. Pulmonary valve or aortic valve stenosis.
      3. Ventricular outflow tract obstruction.
      4. Supravalvular obstruction.
      5. Right ventricular pressure elevation with significant:
         a. Atrial septal defect
         b. Ventricular septal defect

6. Right ventricular pressure elevation due to factors that increase pulmonary vascular resistance (see factors that increase right atrial pressure).
B. Systolic pressure reduced
 1. Hypovolemia.
 2. Cardiogenic shock.
 3. Tamponade.
C. End-diastolic pressure elevated
 1. Hypervolemia.
 2. Congestive heart failure.
 3. Diminished compliance.
 4. Hypertrophy.
 5. Tamponade.
 6. Regurgitant valvular disease.
 7. Pericardial constriction.
D. End-diastolic pressure reduced
 1. Hypovolemia.
 2. Tricuspid or mitral stenosis.
E. Diminished or absent 'A' wave
 1. Atrial fibrillation or flutter.
 2. Tricuspid or mitral stenosis.
 3. Tricuspid or mitral regurgitation when ventricular compliance is increased.
F. Dip and plateau in diastolic pressure wave
 1. Constrictive pericarditis.
 2. Restrictive myopathies.
 3. Right ventricular ischemia.
 4. Acute dilatation associated with:
  a. Tricuspid regurgitation
  b. Mitral regurgitation
G. Left ventricular end-diastolic pressure > right ventricular end-diastolic pressure
 1. Restrictive cardiomyopathies.

V. **Aortic pressure waveforms**
A. Systolic pressure elevated
 1. Systemic hypertension.
 2. Arteriosclerosis.
 3. Aortic insufficiency.
B. Systolic pressure reduced
 1. Aortic stenosis.
 2. Heart failure.
 3. Hypovolemia.
C. Widened pulse pressure
 1. Systemic hypertension.
 2. Aortic insufficiency.
 3. Significant patent ductus arteriosus.
 4. Significant ruptures sinus of Valsalva aneurysm.
D. Reduced pulse pressure
 1. Tamponade.
 2. Congestive heart failure.
 3. Cardiogenic shock.
 4. Aortic stenosis.
E. Pulse bisferiens
 1. Aortic insufficiency.
 2. Obstructive hypertrophic cardiomyopathy.
F. Pulsus paradoxus
 1. Tamponade.
 2. Chronic obstructive airway disease.
 3. Pulmonary embolism.
G. Pulsus alternans
 1. Congestive heart failure.
 2. Cardiomyopathy.
H. Pulsus parvus et tardus
 1. Aortic stenosis.
I. Spike and dome configuration
 1. Obstructive hypertrophic cardiomyopathy.

26. Ans. d. Atrial fibrillation

Braunwald 5th Ed; Page 190

Refer to explanation for Q. No 25.

27. Ans. d. Hypovolemia

Braunwald 5th Ed; Page 190

Refer to explanation for Q. No 25.

28. Ans. b. Tricuspid regurgitation

Braunwald 5th Ed; Page 190

Refer to explanation for Q. No 25.

29. Ans. d. Right atrial ischemia

Braunwald 5th Ed; Page 190

Refer to explanation for Q. No 25.

30. Ans. c. Tricuspid regurgitation

Braunwald 5th Ed; Page 190

Refer to explanation for Q. No 25.

31. Ans. b. Severe tricuspid regurgitation

Braunwald 5th Ed; Page 190

Refer to explanation for Q. No 25.

32. Ans. a. Cardiac tamponade

Braunwald 5th Ed; Page 190

Refer to explanation for Q. No 25.

33. Ans. c. Ebstein's anomaly

Braunwald 5th Ed; Page 190

Refer to explanation for Q. No 25.

34. Ans. d. Hypertrophic obstructive cardiomyopathy

Braunwald 5th Ed; Page 190

Refer to explanation for Q. No 25.

35. Ans. b. Severe mitral regurgitation

Braunwald 5th Ed; Page 190

Refer to explanation for Q. No 25.

36. Ans. d. Cardiac tamponade

Braunwald 5th Ed; Page 190

Refer to explanation for Q. No 25.

37. Ans. b. Aortic regurgitation

Braunwald 5th Ed; Page 190

Refer to explanation for Q. No 25.

38. Ans. d. Hypertrophic obstructive cardiomyopathy

Braunwald 5th Ed; Page 190

Refer to explanation for Q. No 25.

39. Ans. b. Hypertrophic obstructive cardiomyopathy

Braunwald 5th Ed; Page 190

Refer to explanation for Q. No 25.

40. Ans. b. Aortic stenosis

Braunwald 5th Ed; Page 190

Refer to explanation for Q. No 25.

41. Ans. b. 0.8

Braunwald 5th Ed; Page 190

Refer to explanation for Q. No 25.

42. Ans. d. 600%

Braunwald 5th Ed; Page 198

Normally the increased oxygen requirements of exercise are made by an increase in the cardiac output and an increase in the oxygen extraction from arterial blood. Patient with cardiac dysfunction are unable to increase their cardiac output appropriately in response to exercise to meet the demands of exercising muscles grouped with increasing the extraction of oxygen from arterial blood and therefore there is increase in arteriovenous oxygen difference. The relationship between the cardiac output and oxygen consumption is linear and that a regression formula may be used to calculate the predicted cardiac index at a given level of oxygen consumption. The actual cardiac index divided by the predicted cardiac index is defined as exercise index. A value of 0.8 or more indicates a normal cardiac output response to exercise. The exercise factor is another method of describing the same relationship between the cardiac output and oxygen consumption. The exercise factor is the increase in the cardiac output divided by increase in the oxygen consumption. Normally for every 100 mL/min increase in the oxygen consumption with exercise the cardiac output should increase by at least 600 mL/min. Therefore, a normal exercise factor should be 0.6 or more.

43. Ans. c. Ergonovine

Braunwald 5th Ed; Page 198

Ergonovine is used for provocation of coronary spasm, however its use as a diagnostic tool is limited by its lack of specificity.

44. Ans. d. Doppler velocity probes

Braunwald 5th Ed; Page 199

Four methods are generally used to measure human coronary blood flow in the cardiac catheterization laboratory: (1) thermodilution, (2) digital subtraction angiography; (3) use of electromagnetic flow meters; (4) Doppler velocity probe. The Doppler flow meter is based on principal of Doppler effects and it is the most widely applied technique for measurement of coronary flow in humans. High frequency sound waves are reflected from moving red blood cells and undergo a shift sound frequency, i.e., proportional to the velocity of blood flow.

45. Ans. b. Anrep effect

Braunwald 5th Ed; Page 379

In experimental preparations and in normal humans, a sudden increase in blood pressure is compensated by an increased force of contraction and by a reflex decrease of peripheral vascular resistance mediated by baroreflexes and is called as Anrep effect.

46. Ans. b. Bowditch phenomenon

Braunwald 5th Ed; Page 380

Treppe or Bowditch effect: An increase heart rate progressively increases the force of ventricular contraction even in isolated papillary muscle preparation. Conversely, a decreased heart rate has a negative staircase effect. When stimulation becomes too rapid force decreases. The mechanism is that during rapid stimulation more sodium and calcium ions enter the myocardial cells that can be handled by the sodium pump and the mechanism for calcium exit. Opposing the force frequency effect is the negative contractile influence of the decreased duration of ventricular filling at high heart rate. The longer the filling interval the better the ventricular filling and stronger the subsequent contraction. This phenomena can be shown in patient with mitral stenosis and atrial fibrillation with a variable filling interval.

47. **Ans. d. Diastolic-ventricular interaction**

Braunwald 5th Ed; Page 385

Anatomically, the two ventricles are interlinked. They share a common septum. That septum constitutes part of the load against which each ventricle must work. In left ventricular hypertrophy, which includes the septum the right ventricle must therefore work harder and tend to become hypertrophied. This is called as systolic ventricular interaction. Bernheim effect is a type of diastolic ventricular interaction whereby a large left ventricle compress the right ventricle, the volume on the left side is so great that the right side is unable to fill properly. A converse ventricular interaction can occur in severe heart failure when dilated left ventricle may bulge on the left. When the right ventricle is unloaded by venodilator agents like nitroglycerine it can decrease in the size and allow the LV function to improve similarly following surgical thromboendarterectomy for chronic thromboembolic pulmonary hypertension, left ventricular diastolic function improve as the interventricular septum change position.

48. **Ans. a. Inhibitory G protein**

Braunwald 5th Ed; Page 387

Ischemic preconditioning: Whereas many repetitive episode of ischemia should produce cumulative damage, relatively few episodes or even one burst of short leaved severe ischemia followed by complete reperfusion causes preconditioning. The preconditioning is a condition in which the myocardium is protected against a greater subsequent ischemic insult with less threat of infarction. The mechanism of the productive effect of preconditioning is still speculative and one of the proposed mechanism is the upregulation of protein G1 which leads to the activation of receptor coupled to it such as adenosine (A1), and muscarinic (M2) receptors which leads to greater inhibition of adenylyl cyclase and hence to an indirect antiadrenergic effect.

In addition, GI may mediate other potentially protective mechanism such as direct inhibition of L calcium channel and activation of the ATP sensitive potassium channels in the ventricle. An alternate hypothesis is that the adenosine formed during the preconditioning ischemic period activates protein kinase C which mediates the subsequent protection by an unknown mechanism. Preconditioning is an important phenomenon probably with clinical implications because repetitive anginal episodes in patients may develop into full-fledged infarction. Patient with pre infarction angina may suffer from a less severe infarct than those thought to undergo sudden coronary occlusion without the opportunity for preconditioning. In contrast, patient with multiple short lived attacks of ischemia might become tolerant to development of protective preconditioning according to animal data.

49. **Ans. c. Hibernating heart**

Braunwald 5th Ed; Page 388

The hibernating myocardium like the hibernating animal temporarily sleeps and can wake up to function when the blood supply is fully restored. It is proposed that the fall of myocardial function to a lower level copes with the reduced myocardial oxygen supply and leads to self preservation and therefore it is called as 'smart heart'. However, a greater flow reduction may lead to the true ischemia. Hibernation is a complex clinical situation without a good animal model. When ischemia in patient is delineated echocardiographically, as depressed regional wall motion, the hypocontractile segment that still have a sustained glucose extraction as shown by positron emission tomography (PET) have a high chance of recovery after coronary artery bypass surgery, in contrast those segment with a decreased glucose extraction almost uniformly, fails to recover.

CHAPTER 6: Echocardiography and Doppler

1. In echocardiographic imaging of adults the frequency of ultrasound used is:
   a. 1–10 MHz
   b. 2–5 MHz
   c. 3–7 MHz
   d. 3.5–10 MHz

2. In echocardiographic imaging of children the frequency of ultrasound used is:
   a. 1–10 MHz
   b. 2–5 MHz
   c. 3–7 MHz
   d. 3.5–10 MHz

3. Which of the following demonstrates both systolic and diastolic components during Doppler echocardiography?
   a. Venous flow
   b. Ventricular inflow
   c. Ventricular outflow
   d. All

4. The upper limit of normal of the mitral E point-septal separation (EPSS) is approximately:
   a. 4 mm
   b. 6 mm
   c. 8 mm
   d. 10 mm

5. In Doppler echocardiography, a markedly increase in E velocity with reduced atrial velocity (A) and an elevated 'V' wave in left atrial pressure is found in which of the following condition:
   a. Mitral regurgitation
   b. Constrictive pericarditis
   c. Restrictive cardiomyopathy
   d. All of the above

6. During echocardiography assessment the opening of pulmonary valve prior to the onset of right ventricular systole is often found in:
   a. Pulmonic stenosis
   b. Tricuspid regurgitation
   c. Constrictive pericarditis
   d. Communication between aorta and RV

7. The M mode echocardiographic hallmark of mitral stenosis is:
   a. Reduced diastolic (E-F slope)
   b. Diastolic doming
   c. Calcification with restricted movement of mitral leaflets
   d. Absence of valve closure in mid diastole and of reopening in late diastole

8. Doming of any valve on two-dimensional echocardiography is a characteristic sign of:
   a. Stenosis
   b. Regurgitation
   c. Calcification
   d. Rheumatic activity

9. The presence and severity of mitral regurgitation is best assessed by:
   a. M mode echocardiography
   b. Two-dimensional echocardiography
   c. Color flow Doppler imaging
   d. Transesophageal echocardiography

10. Premature closure of mitral valve during echocardiography is seen in:
    a. Severe mitral stenosis
    b. Severe chronic mitral regurgitation
    c. Severe acute mitral regurgitation
    d. Severe acute aortic regurgitation

11. A stiff immobile tricuspid leaflets that are continuously open is a echocardiographic finding of:
    a. Rheumatic tricuspid regurgitation
    b. Ebstein's anomaly
    c. Rheumatic tricuspid stenosis and regurgitation
    d. Tricuspid carcinoid disease

12. Which of the following view best demonstrates the MVP on Two-dimensional echocardiographic?
    a. Subcostal view
    b. Apical 4 chamber view
    c. Right parasternal view
    d. Suprasternal view

13. Which of the following waveform of normal ECG represents ventricular recovery?
    a. P wave
    b. PR interval
    c. QRS complex
    d. ST-T wave

14. Normal mean frontal plane P wave axis is approximately:
    a. 40°
    b. 60°
    c. 80°
    d. 90°

15. What is the normal P wave duration?
    a. 40 msec
    b. 80 msec
    c. 120 msec
    d. 140 msec

CHAPTER 6 | Echocardiography and Doppler

16. When all six extremity lead of ECG shows biphasic (QR or RS) pattern, it indicates:
 a. Normal axis
 b. Right axis deviation
 c. Left axis deviation
 d. Indeterminate axis

17. J wave is seen in which of the following condition?
 a. Hypothermia
 b. Brugada syndrome
 c. Early repolarization
 d. All

18. Which of the following is *correct* regarding the QT interval?
 a. QT interval duration varies from lead to lead
 b. QT interval is a rate dependent
 c. Bazett formula overcorrects the QT interval at high heart rate and under correct it at low heart rate
 d. All of the above

19. Wide and biphasic P wave (an initial positive wave followed by a negative deflection) in the inferior lead suggests:
 a. Left atrial activation site
 b. Posterior atrial activation site
 c. Inferior atrial activation site
 d. Interatrial block

20. The ECG features of left atrial abnormality is associated with which of the following?
 a. More severe LV dysfunction
 b. Higher incidence of atrial tachyarrhythmia including AF
 c. Higher incidence of left atrial thrombi and systemic embolism
 d. All of the above

ANSWERS WITH EXPLANATIONS

1. Ans. b. 2–5 MHz

Braunwald 5th Ed; Page 53

Echocardiography utilizes the ultrasound to examine the heart and record information in the form of echoes, i.e., reflected sonic waves. The sonic frequency used for echocardiography ranges from 1 to 10 Mega Hertz (MHz). In adults the frequencies commonly employed are 2.0 to 5.0 MHz while in children they are usually higher ranging from 3.5 to 10.0 MHz. The resolution of the recording which is the ability to distinguish two objects that are spatially closer together varies directly with the frequency and inversely with the wavelength. High frequency (short wavelength) ultrasound can identify separate objects that are less than 1 mm apart. Beams having lower frequency and longer wavelength have poorer resolution. However, the degree of penetration which is the ability to transmit sufficient ultrasonic energy into chest to provide a satisfactory recording is inversely proportional to the frequency of the signal. Since a high frequency ultrasonic beam (i.e., 5 or 10 MHz) is unable to penetrate a thick chest wall, lower frequency ultrasonic beams are used in adults.

2. Ans. d. 3.5–10 MHz

Braunwald 5th Ed; Page 53

Refer to explanation for Q. No 1.

3. Ans. a. Venous flow

Braunwald 5th Ed; Page 63

Spectral Doppler echocardiographic recordings are basically of three types. There is the venous ventricular inflow and ventricular outflow pattern of Doppler flow. Venous flow has both systolic and diastolic components. There will be some slight variation whether the recording is from systemic or pulmonary veins. There is frequently reverse flow that moves downward or away from transducer following atrial contraction. Ventricular inflow is totally diastolic. There is an early component that peaks at the 'E' wave and a late component following atrial contraction that peaks with an 'A' wave. Ventricular outflow is entirely systolic in nature.

4. Ans. c. 8 mm

Braunwald 5th Ed; Page 65

In the M-mode echocardiographic technique to assess ventricular size, the distance between the E point of mitral valve and the left side of interventricular septum is measured. Normally the mitral E point and the left side of the septum are within a few millimeters of each other. Upper limit of normal of mitral E points septal separation (EPSS) is approximately 8 mm. As the left ventricular ejection fraction decreases the EPSS increases. The left ventricle dilates the septum moves anteriorly. The opening of mitral valve is largely dependent upon the volume of blood passing through the orifice. As the mitral valve flow or left ventricular stroke volume decreases the amplitude of E point is decreased. Thus with a decrease stroke volume and/or left ventricular dilatation the septum and anterior mitral leaflet would move in opposite direction.

5. Ans. d. All of the above

Brauwald 5th Ed; Page 67

Doppler echocardiography is the primary technique used for evaluating left ventricular diastolic function. If the left ventricular filling pressure is markedly elevated as it occurs in patient with severe heart failure then the left ventricular inflow velocity pattern changes dramatically. There is a marked increase in the early diastolic velocity with an increase in the E velocity. The atrial velocity is reduced. A similar pattern may also occur if a patient has severe mitral regurgitation with an elevated V wave in the left atrial pressure. This type of mitral flow may also occur if there is a restrictive pattern of filling of the left ventricle as may occur with constrictive pericarditis or restrictive cardiomyopathy.

6. Ans. a. Pulmonic stenosis

Braunwald 5th Ed; Page 70

There is a direct relationship of the M mode pulmonary wall motion and right sided pressure. Normally, atrial systole produces a slight downward motion of the pulmonary valve. With pulmonary stenosis, the right ventricular systolic and diastolic pressure rises without any similar elevation in pulmonary artery pressure. As a result, atrial contribution to right ventricular pressure is exaggerated and is usually sufficient to open the pulmonary valve prior to ventricular systole. In patients with elevated right ventricular diastolic pressure due to right ventricular failure, tricuspid regurgitation, constrictive pericarditis or communication between aorta and left ventricle, the elevated pressure in the right ventricular in early diastole may cause opening of pulmonary valve even before the onset of atrial systole.

7. Ans. d. Absence of valve closure in mid diastole and of reopening in late diastole

Braunwald 5th Ed; Page 71

The detection of mitral stenosis was the first clinical application of echocardiography. The M-mode examination provides a sensitive assessment of the motion and thickness of the valve leaflet while the two-dimensional technique provides a spatial image of the valve and allows direct measurement of valve orifice. Doppler echocardiography provides hemodynamic assessment of the stenotic orifice. The motion of mitral valve is considerably altered from the normal pattern in patient with mitral stenosis, because of the presence of a holodiastolic atrioventricular pressure gradient, the rapid closure of valve in mid diastole is absent in patient with mitral stenosis. There is no reopening of the valve with atrial contraction and there is no 'A' wave noted in mitral stenosis. The M-mode echocardiographic hallmark of mitral stenosis is absence of valve closure in mid diastole and of reopening in late diastole. Although this decreased (flat) diastolic (E-F) slope is characteristic of mitral stenosis, it is not specific. Other condition such as decreased left ventricular compliance or low cardiac output may also reduce the diastolic slope of mitral valve motion.

8. Ans. a. Stenosis

Braunwald 5th Ed; Page 71

The diagnosis of mitral stenosis by two-dimensional echocardiograph is made by noting thickening, doming and restricted motion of the leaflet. Doming of any valve on two-dimensional echocardiography is a characteristic sign of stenosis. This distortion in shape with the opening of valve indicates that the tip of the leaflets are restricted in their ability to open, whereas the body of the leaflet still wish to accommodate more blood flow thus the leaflets are curved or domed. The presence of doming distinguishes a valve, i.e., truly stenotic from one that opens poorly because of low flow.

9. Ans. c. Color flow Doppler imaging

Braunwald 5th Ed; Page 72

Doppler echocardiography is the ultrasonic procedure of choice for detection of any valvular regurgitation. Color flow Doppler is the principal echocardiographic technique for assessing the presence and severity of mitral regurgitation. Transesophageal echocardiography is more sensitive in detecting mitral regurgitation than is transthoracic approach.

10. Ans. d. Severe acute aortic regurgitation

Braunwald 5th Ed; Page 76

As with all valvular regurgitation, Doppler echocardiography is the examination of choice for detecting the presence of aortic regurgitation. The accuracy of Doppler flow mapping for quantitating aortic regurgitation is at best semiquantitative. The width of aortic jet at the valve orifice as judged by color flow Doppler is used to judge the severity of aortic regurgitation and is clinically useful. The M-mode sign of aortic regurgitation that remain useful is premature closure of mitral valve in the presence of severe usually acute aortic regurgitation. This premature mitral closure can also be noted on Doppler recording. With an elevated left ventricular diastolic pressure there may even be early opening of aortic valve on M-mode recording. Both of these signs represent severe aortic regurgitation and markedly elevated left ventricular diastolic pressure.

11. Ans. d. Tricuspid carcinoid disease

Braunwald 5th Ed; Page 76

The tricuspid valve disease are best assessed by echocardiography and Doppler. Two-dimensional and Doppler echocardiography are procedure of choice for detecting tricuspid stenosis and tricuspid regurgitation. Tricuspid regurgitation is best determined by pulsed, continuous wave or color flow Doppler echocardiography. Two-dimensional echocardiography can help determining the etiology of tricuspid regurgitation. Rheumatic tricuspid regurgitation usually has an element of tricuspid stenosis and invariably exhibit mitral stenosis. Pulmonary hypertension can be detected by estimating the right ventricular systolic pressure. Tricuspid valve prolapse gives an appearance similar to that of mitral valve prolapse. A stiff tricuspid valve is indicated by the finding of parts of the tricuspid valve bulging into the right atrium in ventricular systole. Carcinoid valve disease produces steep mobile tricuspid leaflet that are continuously open. As with all valvular disease transesophageal echocardiography can provide higher quality image of tricuspid valve pathology.

12. Ans. c. Right parasternal view

Braunwald 5th Ed; Page 73

Echocardiography is particularly useful in the diagnosis of mitral valve prolapse. Several findings on two-dimensional echocardiography have been suggested for diagnosis of mitral valve prolapse including the recording of buckling of one or both mitral leaflets into left atrium during systole. Parasternal long axis and a four chamber examination can demonstrate mitral valve prolapse. The parasternal long axis view is more specific for the diagnosis of prolapse than is the four chamber view.

13. Ans. d. ST-T wave

Braunwald 11th Ed; Page 121

The waveforms and intervals that make up the standard ECG reflects activation of various chambers like atria and ventricular and their recovery. The P wave is generated by activation of the atria, the PR interval corresponds to the duration of atrioventricular conduction, the QRS complex is produced by the activation of the two ventricles, and the ST-T wave reflects ventricular recovery.

14. Ans. b. 60°

Braunwald 11th Ed; Page 122

The normal P wave reflects activation patterns of atria. P waves are positive in lead II and usually in leads I, aVL, and aVF, reflecting the leftward and inferior direction of activation during sinus rhythm. This corresponds to a mean frontal plane P wave axis of approximately 60°. The pattern in leads aVL and III may be upright or downward, depending on the exact orientation of the mean P wave axis.

15. Ans. c. 120 msec

Braunwald 11th Ed; Page 123

The upper limit for a normal P wave duration is 120 milliseconds, as measured in the lead with the widest P wave. The amplitude in the limb leads normally is less than 0.25 mV, and the terminal negative deflection in the right precordial leads normally is less than 0.1 mV in depth.

16. Ans. d. Indeterminate axis

Braunwald 11th Ed; Page 124

The normal mean QRS axis in adults lies between −30 to +90°. If the mean axis is near 90°, the QRS complex in leads II, III, and aVF will be predominantly upright, with qR complexes. Lead I will record an isoelectric RS pattern because the heart vector lies perpendicular to the lead axis. Mean QRS axes more positive than +90° (usually with an rS pattern in lead I) represent right axis deviation. Axes between +90 and +120° are referred to as moderate right axis deviation, and those between +120 and +180°, reflects marked right axis deviation. Axes more negative than −30° (with an rS pattern in lead II) represent left axis deviation, with axes between −30 and −45° called moderate and those between −45 and −90° called marked left axis deviation. Mean axes lying between −90 and −180° are referred to as extreme axis deviations or, alternatively, as right superior axis deviations. The term indeterminate axis is applied when all six extremity leads show biphasic (QR or RS) patterns, indicating a mean axis that is perpendicular to the frontal plane. This finding may be seen as a normal variant and also it is seen in a variety of pathologic conditions.

17. Ans. d. All

Braunwald 11th Ed; Page 125

A J wave is a dome or hump-shaped wave or notch that appears at the end of the QRS complex and it is of same polarity as the preceding QRS complex. It may be prominent as a normal variant and in certain pathological conditions, such as systemic hypothermia (referred as an Osborn wave) and in a set of conditions commonly referred to as the J wave syndromes which include Brugada pattern and the early repolarization pattern.

18. Ans. d. All of the above

Braunwald 11th Ed; Page 125

The QT interval extends from onset of the QRS complex to the end of T wave. Because the onset of the QRS and the end of the T wave do not occur simultaneously in every lead, the QT interval duration will vary from lead to lead by as much as 50 to 65 milliseconds (QT dispersion).

The normal QT interval is rate dependent, decreasing as heart rate increases. This corresponds to rate related changes in the duration of the normal ventricular action potential. Numerous formulas have been proposed to correct the QT interval for this rate effect, including one proposed by Bazett in 1920. The result is the corrected QT interval, or QTc, defined by a formula.

$$QTc = QT/\sqrt{RR}$$

The QT and RR intervals are measured in seconds. The Bazett formula has limited accuracy in correcting for the effects of heart rate on QT interval. Large database studies have shown that the QTc interval based on the Bazett formula remains significantly affected by heart rate. In general, Bazett formula overcorrects the QT interval at high heart rates and under corrects it at low rates.

19. Ans. d. Interatrial block

Braunwald 11th Ed; Page 127

P wave patterns may suggest the site of impulse formation and path of subsequent activation. A negative P wave in lead I suggests activation beginning in the left atrium, and an inverted P wave in the inferior leads generally corresponds to a posterior atrial activation site. Interatrial block, with conduction delay between the atria, alters the duration and pattern of P waves. When conduction from the right to the left atrium is delayed, the normal lag in left atrial activation relative to that of the right atrium increases. P wave duration is prolonged beyond 120 milliseconds, and P waves typically have two humps in lead II, with the first representing right atrial and the second reflecting left atrial activation. With more advanced block, the sinus node impulses reach the left atrium only after passing inferiorly toward the atrioventricular junction and then superiorly through the left atrium. In such cases, P waves are wide and biphasic (an initial positive wave followed by a negative deflection) in the inferior leads.

20. Ans. d. All of the above

Braunwald 11th Ed; Page 127

The ECG features of left atrial abnormality are associated with more severe left ventricular dysfunction in patients with ischemic heart disease and with more severe valve damage in patients with mitral or aortic valve disease. Patients with left atrial abnormalities also have a higher-than-normal incidence of atrial tachyarrhythmias, including atrial fibrillation, left atrial thrombi, cerebrovascular accident and all-cause and cardiovascular mortality.

Chapter 7: Ambulatory Blood Pressure Monitoring

1. All are correct regarding the definition of normal blood pressure in a ambulatory blood pressure monitoring *except*:
   a. 24 hours mean BP of 125/75 mm Hg
   b. Day time BP of 130/80 mm Hg or less
   c. Nighttime BP of 110/75 mm Hg or less with nocturnal dipping of 10–20%
   d. All of the above

2. Which of the following is *not* associated with higher cardiovascular risk than normal blood pressure?
   a. Masked hypertension
   b. White coat hypertension
   c. Non dippers
   d. All are associated with higher risk

ANSWERS WITH EXPLANATIONS

1. Ans. c. Nighttime BP of 110/75 mm Hg or less with nocturnal dipping of 10–20%

Camilo Pena Hernandez et al; Journal of Primary Care & Community Health 2020, Vol 11: 1–8

The most commonly utilized data for clinical purposes including diagnosis and treatment of blood pressure (BP) is 24 hours average BP, daytime BP, nighttime BP and nocturnal dipping patterns. The threshold for normality depends on the measurement used and the current definition of normal BP. In most instances, a 24 hour mean BP of 125/75 mm Hg or less, a daytime BP of 130/80 mm Hg or less or a nighttime BP of 110/65 mm Hg or less with nocturnal dipping of 10–20% are considered normal values for ABPM.

2. Ans. b. White coat hypertension

Camilo Pena Hernandez et al; Journal of Primary Care & Community Health 2020, Vol 11: 1–8

A diagnosis of white coat hypertension is based on an office blood pressure of 130/80 mm Hg or higher in individuals with normal ABPM measurement. The prevalence of office hypertension has been estimated to be approximately 10 to 30% of patients. This condition has been described more frequently in women and at this time no evidence to suggest that it is associated with higher cardiovascular risk than normal blood pressure. However, white coat hypertension does seem to be a risk factor for development of sustained hypertension and possibly stroke. Masked hypertension occurs when a patient has out of office hypertension i.e., not apparent in clinic BP reading, but is evident with ABPM. The prevalence of masked hypertension is approximately 10 to 25% in normotensive patients and is associated with increased cardiovascular risk. Masked hypertension occurs more frequently in elderly men, smokers, patients with high alcohol intake and patients with diabetes mellitus with or without chronic kidney disease. Masked hypertension patient should be treated with antihypertensive drugs to achieve normotension and decrease the risk for major cardiovascular events in the future.

Blood pressure homeostasis involves dynamic changes in the cardiovascular system based on physiological needs, which also involves neurohormonal changes occurring from internal day night clocks. Normal subjects have higher diurnal blood pressure with a nocturnal decrease in both systolic and diastolic BP while sleeping (dipping), of 10 to 20% and a rapid increase in the blood pressure in the morning related to waking up. The strongest correlation between cardiovascular risk and hypertension is related to 24 hours average BP and nighttime BP.

Cardiac Catheterization and Angiography

1. Which of the following is *not* a primary indication for coronary angiography?
   a. To establish the presence or absence of CAD
   b. To define the physiological significance of a given stenosis
   c. To define the therapeutic option
   d. To determine the prognosis

2. Coronary angiography is to be performed annually in absence of any symptoms in which of the following group of patients:
   a. Non Q infarction
   b. Unexplained CHF
   c. Intractable cardiac arrhythmia
   d. Cardiac transplantation

3. Each French number is equal to ___ mm in diameter:
   a. 0–22 mm
   b. 0–33 mm
   c. 0–34 mm
   d. 0–36 mm

4. A single catheter which can be used for selective left and right coronary angiography as well as left ventriculography and pressure study is:
   a. Judkins catheter
   b. Amplatz catheter
   c. Schoonmaker and king catheter
   d. Sones catheter

5. In which of the following approach Allen test should be performed prior to coronary arteriography?
   a. Femoral
   b. Radial
   c. Brachial
   d. Axillary

6. To evaluate possible left main coronary artery disease, which of the angiographic projection is most informative:
   a. RAO with shallow cranial angulation
   b. Anteroposterior view with shallow caudal angulation
   c. LAO with caudal angulation
   d. RAO with steep caudal angulation

7. Which of the following view is most informative to evaluate the possible disease in proximal left anterior descending artery?
   a. RAO with shallow cranial angulation
   b. LAO with cranial angulation
   c. RAO with caudal angulation
   d. Anteroposterior view with caudal angulation

8. The proximal segment of left circumflex artery is best visualized in:
   a. AP with caudal angulation
   b. Anteroposterior view
   c. RAO with cranial tilt
   d. LAO with caudal angulation

9. The left circumflex artery and its marginal branches in full profile can be obtained in:
   a. Anteroposterior with caudal angulation
   b. RAO with caudal angulation
   c. LAO with cranial angulation
   d. RAO with cranial angulation

10. Which of the following regarding dominance of coronary artery anatomy is *incorrect*?
    a. The dominant vessel is one that supplies the posterior diaphragmatic surface of the interventricular septum and of left ventricle
    b. The right coronary artery is dominant in about 85% of humans
    c. Dominance is most easily assessed in the LAO cranial view
    d. All are correct

11. Which of the following is *correct* regarding left main coronary artery (LMCA)?
    a. The diameter of LMCA ranges from 3 to 6 mm
    b. Diameter of LMCA is greater for patients with normal coronaries than in those with disease in left coronary artery
    c. The length of LMCA varies from 0–10 mm
    d. All are true

12. Which is the most densely vascularized area of the heart?
a. Left ventricular outflow tract
b. Left ventricular free wall
c. Right ventricular musculature
d. Interventricular septum

13. The lateral and posterior aspect of left atrium is supplied by branches from:
a. Left anterior descending artery
b. Left circumflex artery
c. Right coronary artery
d. Posterior descending artery

14. Catheterization of the right coronary artery is best performed in:
a. Anteroposterior view   b. LAO view
c. RAO view   d. Lateral view

15. The sinoatrial node artery arises most commonly from:
a. Right coronary artery
b. Left coronary artery
c. Both RCA and left circumflex artery
d. Left anterior descending artery

16. The development of symptoms in the immediate postoperative period after coronary artery bypass surgery is due to:
a. Incomplete revascularization
b. Spasm of left internal mammary artery
c. Early thrombotic graft occlusion of saphenous vein graft
d. Any of the above

17. The reappearance of symptoms in patient with prior coronary artery bypass surgery done within 2 years is due to:
a. Development of atherosclerosis in bypass graft
b. Progression of native vessel disease
c. Any of the two (a+b)
d. None of the above

18. The vessel most commonly affected by myocardial bridging is:
a. Left anterior descending artery
b. Left circumflex artery
c. Right coronary artery
d. Posterior descending artery

19. Which of the following is *not* correct regarding myocardial bridging?
a. It occurs in 5–10% of cases
b. It has no hemodynamic significance
c. It is almost always confined to LAD
d. It is amenable to balloon angioplasty

20. The most common site of origin of coronary fistula is:
a. Right coronary artery
b. Left circumflex artery
c. Left anterior descending artery
d. Obtuse marginal artery

21. Most common site of drainage of coronary fistula is:
a. Right ventricle   b. Right atrium
c. Left atrium   d. Pulmonary artery

22. Coronary artery fistula can drain into any of the following *except*:
a. Right ventricle   b. Pulmonary artery
c. Superior vena cava   d. Left atrium

23. Congenital coronary stenosis or atresia is seen with which of the following syndrome:
a. Friedreich's ataxia
b. Homocystinuria
c. Hunter syndrome
d. All of the above

24. Which of the following congenital coronary anomaly causes myocardial ischemia?
a. Origin of left circumflex artery from right aortic sinus
b. Origin of left coronary artery from pulmonary trunk
c. Single coronary artery
d. High anterior origin of RCA

25. TIMI grade 0 flow is:
a. No perfusion
b. Penetration without perfusion
c. Partial perfusion
d. Complete perfusion

26. Coronary collaterals are usually demonstrated when recipient coronary artery develops stenosis more than:
a. 50%   b. 75%
c. 90%   d. Total occlusion

27. Which of the following factor plays important role in collateral formation in coronary circulation?
a. Severity of obstruction in recipient vessel
b. Patency of feeding arteries
c. Size and vascular resistance of the postobstructive segment
d. All of the above

28. In Rentrop and Cohen system of grading coronary collaterals, grade 2 indicates when?
a. No collateral is present
b. Contrast medium passes through collateral channels but fails to opacify the epicardial vessel at any time

c. Contrast material enters but fails to opacify the target epicardial vessel completely
d. Contrast material enters and completely opacify the target epicardial vessel

29. First selective coronary angiography was performed by:
a. Grossmann
b. Sones
c. Judkins
d. Amplatz

30. First human cardiac catheterization was performed by:
a. Grossmann
b. Werner Forssmann
c. Judkins
d. Wales

31. The technique of percutaneous transluminal angioplasty was developed by:
a. Andreas Gruentzig
b. Dotter
c. Judkins
d. Dotter and Judkins

32. First percutaneous balloon coronary angioplasty in humans was performed by:
a. Dotter
b. Amplatz
c. Judkins
d. Andreas Gruentzig

33. Which of the following is most effective drug in preventing acute renal dysfunction due to contrast agents?
a. Saline
b. Mannitol
c. Frusemide
d. Spironolactone

34. The combination of right sided aortic arch and cyanosis suggests diagnosis of:
a. Tetralogy of Fallot
b. Double outlet right ventricle
c. Truncus arteriosus
d. All of the above

35. The normal pericardium is best defined by:
a. Lateral film projections of the chest as a thin linear opacity separating the anterior subxiphoid fat from subepicardial fat.
b. Frontal projections paralleling left border of heart
c. CT chest
d. MRI chest

36. Epicardial fat pad sign suggest diagnosis of:
a. Pericardial effusion
b. Constrictive pericarditis
c. Massive epicardial fat
d. Obesity

37. Which of the following statement is *not* correct regarding pericardial constriction?
a. Small to large pleural effusion are found in > 60% of cases with pericardial constriction
b. Enlargement of left atrium and azygos vein occurs in 20% of cases
c. Pericardial calcification is seen in fewer than 20% of cases with chronic pericardial constriction
d. Presence of pericardial calcification establishes the diagnosis of pericardial constriction

38. A straight or convex left supra-aortic border is found in patients with:
a. Left subclavian artery aneurysm
b. Persistent left azygos vein
c. Persistent left superior vena cava
d. Anomalous origin of left subclavian artery

39. Which of the following nonvascular pathology simulates the enlargement of left atrial appendage?
a. Pericardial fibroma
b. Mediastinal lymphoma
c. Congenital absence of pericardium
d. All of the above

40. Which of the following view in angiography best visualizes the anterior mitral leaflet?
a. RAO
b. LAO
c. Lateral
d. AP view

41. Which of the following view best visualizes the posterior mitral leaflet on angiogram?
a. RAO
b. LAO
c. PA view
d. Lateral view

42. Hourglass appearance due to indentation of anterior as well as inferior wall of LV in angiography in characteristic of:
a. MVP
b. IHSS
c. Tetralogy of Fallot's
d. TGA

43. Which of the following statement is *true* regarding the bronchial circulation?
a. It constitutes a physiological R-L shunt
b. It drains about 1% of total cardiac output
c. In cyanotic CHD the bronchial circulation participates in gas exchange and improve oxygenation
d. All are true

44. What is normal mean pulmonary artery pressure?
a. 12–16 mm Hg
b. 18–20 mm Hg
c. 10–15 mm Hg
d. 12–18 mm Hg

45. What is mean pulmonary venous pressure?
   a. 2–4 mm Hg
   b. 4–6 mm Hg
   c. 6–10 mm Hg
   d. 12 mm Hg

46. What is normal arteriovenous pressure difference across the pulmonary circulations?
   a. 2–10 mm Hg
   b. 6–12 mm Hg
   c. 8–14 mm Hg
   d. 12–16 mm Hg

47. What is the normal arteriovenous difference required for the movement of cardiac output through systemic circulation?
   a. 40 mm Hg
   b. 60 mm Hg
   c. 80 mm Hg
   d. 90 mm Hg

48. Normal pulmonary vascular resistance in adult is:
   a. 20–40 dynes-sec-cm^5
   b. 40–60 dynes-sec-cm^5
   c. 10–30 dynes-sec-cm^5
   d. 67–87 dynes-sec-cm^5

ANSWERS WITH EXPLANATIONS

1. Ans. b. To define the physiological significance of a given stenosis

Braunwald 5th Ed; Page 240

The primary indications for coronary angiography are to establish the presence or absence of coronary artery disease, define therapeutic options and determine prognosis. Coronary angiography is recommended for patients with history of stable angina, refractory to medical management, patient with history of angina and an exercise treadmill test showing high-risk features such as hypotension, more than 2 mm of ST segment depression associated with decrease exercise capacity, or myocardial perfusion scanning showing increase lung uptake or multiple perfusion defects, ordinarily should undergo coronary angiography. Coronary angiography is also recommended for middle aged and older patient scheduled to undergo surgery for valvular heart disease or congenital heart disease. Patients with a history of angina or provocable ischemia who are scheduled for vascular surgery should also undergo coronary angiography. Coronary angiography is important in certain patients who present with chest pain of unclear etiology. In patients with cardiac risk factor and chest pain atypical for angina, the findings of angiographically normal coronary arteries provide important information about therapy and prognosis. The diagnosis of coronary artery spasm relies on clinical presentation but coronary angiography remains useful in patient with clinical evidences of coronary spasm to exclude the presence of fixed atherosclerotic lesion.

2. Ans. d. Cardiac transplantation

Braunwald 5th Ed; Page 241

Coronary angiography is commonly performed annually in patients after cardiac transplantation in the absence of clinical symptoms because of the diffuse nature of graft atherosclerosis. Coronary angiography is useful in potential donors for cardiac transplantation whose age or cardiac risk profile increases the likelihood of coronary artery disease.

3. Ans. b. 0–33 mm

Braunwald 5th Ed; Page 241

The diagnostic catheters used for cardiac catheterization and angiography are constructed of polyethylene or polyurethane with a fine wire braided within the wall to allow advancement and directional control (torque ability) and yet prevent kinking. The size of the catheters ranges from No. 4 French (4F) to 8F. Each French number is equal to 0.33 mm in diameter. Commonly used catheters are 6F size. Diagnostic catheter dimension are given by the outer diameter. Most diagnostic catheters have 0.45 inch inner lumen diameter.

4. Ans. c. Schoonmaker and king catheter

Braunwald 5th Ed; Page 242

A single catheter that can be used for selective left and right coronary angiography as well as for left ventriculography via femoral approach was originally described by Schoonmaker and King. The catheter is similar to the Sones catheter and has a shorter tip. Some maneuver are required to hook the coronary artery with this multipurpose or Schoonmaker catheter.

5. Ans. b. Radial

Braunwald 5th Ed; Page 244

Coronary angiography can be performed through the radial artery with 5F and 6F catheters in adults. Before the procedure is performed the Allen test should be carried out to ensure that ulnar artery is patent.

6. Ans. b. Anteroposterior view with shallow caudal angulation

Braunwald 5th Ed; Page 247

The heart is oriented obliquely in the thoracic cavity and the direct frontal and lateral views are not commonly used during coronary angiography. Instead the coronary circulation is imaged in right anterior oblique (RAO) and left anterior oblique (LAO) views. The major coronary arteries traverse the atrioventricular and interventricular grooves, which in turn are align with the long and short axis of the heart. Thus, the best angiographic projection to visualize this vessel in profile are the oblique views. Because the straight RAO and LAO views of the heart have serious shortcomings caused by foreshortening and superimposition of branches, the rotation of X-ray beam around the patient in transverse plane for RAO and LAO projection is almost always accompanied by rotation of the X-ray beam around the patient in the sagittal plane for cranial or caudal angulations. General recommendations about routine views can be made for most patients and tailored views are required to accommodate possible variations. During coronary angiography, the anteroposterior (AP view) with shallow caudal angulation is performed first to evaluate the possibility of left main coronary artery disease.

Other important views include the LAO view with cranial angulation to evaluate left anterior descending artery. This view should have sufficient leftward positioning of the image intensifier to prevent overlap between the left anterior descending artery (LAD) and the spine. This is followed by LAO caudal view to evaluate the proximal segment of left circumflex artery (LCx) RAO view with caudal angulation to assess left circumflex and marginal branches in full profile and shallow RAO and AP cranial view to evaluate the mid portion of LAD. Although this sequence of viewing is recommended for minimal assessment of left coronary artery, a rigid sequence of view is not mandated. Instead, the views must be selected based on the rotation of the heart and presence of lesion that may be targeted for revascularization techniques.

7. Ans. b. LAO with cranial angulation

Braunwald 5th Ed; Page 247

Refer to explanation for Q. No 6.

8. Ans. d. LAO with caudal angulation

Braunwald 5th Ed; Page 247

Refer to explanation for Q. No 6.

9. Ans. b. RAO with caudal angulation

Braunwald 5th Ed; Page 247

Refer to explanation for Q. No 6.

10. Ans. d. All are correct

Braunwald 5th Ed; Page 249

The term 'dominance' is often used to describe coronary artery anatomy. The dominant vessel is the one that supplies the posterior diaphragmatic portion of the interventricular septum and diaphragmatic surface of the left ventricle. The right coronary artery is dominant in about 85% of humans. Because human coronary artery disease is primarily the result of interruption of blood supply to the left ventricular myocardium, a nondominant left coronary artery is almost always more important than dominant right coronary artery. Dominance is most easily assessed in the LAO cranial view.

11. Ans. d. All are true

Braunwald 5th Ed; Page 250

The left main coronary artery arise from the upper portion of left aortic sinus, just below the sinotubular ridge of the aorta, which defines the borders separating the left sinus of Valsalva from the smooth (tubular portion) of the aorta. The diameter of the left main coronary artery ranges from 3 to 6 mm. Quantitative analysis have shown that the diameter of left main coronary artery is greater for patients with entirely normal coronary arteries than in those with disease in the distal left coronary artery or disease in the adjacent segment of the left coronary artery. The left main coronary artery passes behind the right ventricular outflow tract and may extend for 0-10 mm. It usually than bifurcates into left anterior descending artery and left circumflex branches.

12. Ans. d. Interventricular septum

Braunwald 5th Ed; Page 250

The left anterior descending artery after arising from the left main passes down the anterior interventricular groove towards the cardiac apex. Its major branches are septal and diagonal branches. The septal branches emanate from the LAD at approximately 90 degree and pass into the interventricular septum. They vary in size, number and distribution. These septal branches interconnect with similar septal branches passing upward from posterior descending branch of right coronary artery to produce a network of potential collateral channel. The interventricular septum therefore is the most densely vascularized area of the heart and the first septal branch is its most important potential collateral channel.

13. Ans. b. Left circumflex artery

Braunwald 5th Ed; Page 251-252

The left circumflex artery originates at the bifurcation of left main coronary artery and passes on the left atrioventricular groove. The left circumflex artery give rise to obtuse marginal branches which vary in number from 1 to 3 and these are the principal branches of left circumflex artery since these branches supply the free wall of left ventricle along its lateral aspect. The left circumflex artery also give rise to one or two left atrial circumflex branches, these branches supply the lateral and posterior aspect of the left atrium.

14. Ans. b. LAO view

Braunwald 5th Ed; Page 252-253

Catheterization of right coronary artery is performed in LAO position but this requires different maneuver than catheterization of left main coronary artery. Whereas the left Judkin's catheter naturally seeks the ostium of the left main coronary artery (LMCA), the right coronary catheter must be rotated by the angiographer to engage the vessel. This is usually accomplished by first passing the catheter to a point just above the aortic valve in left sinus of Valsalva and then rotating the catheter clockwise which forces the catheter tip to move anteriorly from left sinus of Valsalva to right sinus of Valsalva. Entry into the right coronary ostium is signified by a sudden rightward and downward movement of the catheter tip. If the ostium of the right coronary artery is not easily located, most common reasons is that ostium has a higher and more anterior origin than anticipated.

15. Ans. a. Right coronary artery

Braunwald 5th Ed; Page 253

The right coronary artery originates from right aortic sinus. It passes down the right atrioventricular groove towards the crux (a point on the diaphragmatic surface of the heart where the right atrioventricular groove, the left atrioventricular groove and the posterior interventricular groove come together). The branches of right coronary artery are: (i) Conus artery—the primary importance of conus artery is to serve as a source of collateral circulation in patient with LAD occlusion; (ii) Second branch of right coronary artery is sinoatrial nodal artery. This vessel arise from right coronary artery in 59%, from left circumflex artery in 38% and from both arteries with dual blood supply in 3%. It sends branches to sinus node and usually also to the right atrium or both atrium; (iii) Mid portion of the right coronary artery usually gives rise to one or more medium size acute marginal branches which supplies the anterior wall of right ventricle; (iv) Posterior descending artery is the important branch of right coronary artery. When the right coronary artery is dominant as it is in about 85% of the patients, the posterior descending artery originate at or shortly before the crux and passes forward in the posterior interventricular groove; (v) A dominant right coronary artery continues beyond the crux and begin to pass upwards along the distal portion of left atrioventricular groove. There it gives rise to one or several posterior left ventricular branches which supply the diaphragmatic surface of the left ventricle.

16. Ans. d. Any of the above

Braunwald 5th Ed; Page 254

After coronary artery bypass surgery, several mechanisms leads to failure of bypass grafts. The development of symptoms in the immediate postoperative period after bypass surgery may be due to incomplete revascularization, spasm of internal mammary artery or early thrombotic graft occlusion of saphenous vein graft. The development of symptoms within one year of bypass surgery may be due to fibrointimal hyperplasia of saphenous venous graft. Symptom in patients more than 1 year after bypass surgery may be due to the development of atherosclerosis in the bypass graft or progression of native vessel disease.

17. Ans. c. Any of the two (a+b)

Braunwald 5th Ed; Page 254

Refer to explanation for Q. No 16.

18. Ans. a. Left anterior descending artery

Braunwald 5th Ed Page 258

Myocardial bridging: The major coronary arteries pass over the epicardial surface of the heart. In some cases, however short segment descends into the myocardium for the variable distance. This occurs in 5-12% of the humans and is almost always confined to left anterior descending artery (LAD). Because a bridge of myocardial fiber passes over the involved segment of LAD, early systolic contraction of these fibers can cause narrowing of the artery. Myocardial bridging has a characteristic appearance on cineangiography. The bridged segment is of normal caliber during diastole and abruptly narrows with each systole. Systolic narrowing caused by myocardial bridging should not be confused with atherosclerotic plaque. Although bridging is not thought to have any hemodynamic significance in most cases, some have suggested that when it produces severe systolic narrowing, ischemia or infarction may result. The presence of myocardial bridging has important implication for interventional cardiovascular therapy because myocardial bridges do not respond to angioplasty.

19. Ans. d. It is amenable to balloon angioplasty

Braunwald 5th Ed Page 258

Refer to explanation for Q. No 18.

20. Ans. a. Right coronary artery

Braunwald 5th Ed; Page 259-260

Coronary artery fistulas are the must common congenital anomalies of the coronary arteries. Although about half of the patients with large fistula remain asymptomatic, the other half develops congestive heart failure, infective endocarditis, myocardial ischemia or rupture of an aneurysmal fistula. About half of these fistula arise from right coronary artery or its branches, slightly fewer than half arise from LAD or LCx artery or their branches and in the remaining cases, there are multiple origins. Drainage occurs into right ventricle in 41%, into right atrium 26%, into the pulmonary artery in 17%, into the left ventricle in 3%, into the superior vena cava in 1%. A left to right shunt exist in more than 90% of the cases. Selective coronary arteriography is the only way to demonstrate the origin of this fistula.

21. **Ans. a. Right ventricle**

Braunwald 5th Ed; Page 259-260

Refer to explanation for Q. No 20.

22. **Ans. d. Left atrium**

Braunwald 5th Ed; Page 259-260

Refer to explanation for Q. No 20.

23. **Ans. d. All of the above**

Braunwald 5th Ed; Page 260

Congenital coronary stenosis or atresia: Congenital stenosis or atresia of coronary artery can occur as an isolated lesion or in association with other congenital diseases such as calcific coronary sclerosis, supravalvular aortic stenosis, homocystinuria, Friedreich's ataxia, Hurler's syndrome, progeria and rubella syndrome. In these cases, the atretic vessel usually fills by means of collateral circulation from the contralateral site.

24. **Ans. a. Origin of left circumflex artery from right aortic sinus**

Braunwald 5th Ed; Page 261

The abnormalities of coronary circulation can be classified into two categories: 1. **Congenital anomalies of coronary artery that causes myocardial ischemia** under this category are included, (i) coronary artery fistula; (ii) origin of the left coronary artery from the pulmonary artery, (iii) congenital coronary stenosis or atresia, and (iv) anomalous origin of either coronary artery from the contralateral sinus. 2. **Congenital coronary anomalies not causing myocardial ischemia**— in this category of anomalies the coronary artery originate from the aorta but their origins are in unusual location. Although myocardial perfusion is normal, but there may be difficulty in locating these arteries during angiography. These anomalies occurs in about 0.5 to 1.0% of the adult patients undergoing coronary angiography, in this category included are: (i) origin of the left circumflex artery from the right aortic sinus; (ii) single coronary artery; (iii) origin of all three coronary arteries from either the right or left aortic sinus via multiple separate ostia; (iv) high anterior origin of the right coronary artery.

25. **Ans. a. No perfusion**

Braunwald 5th Ed; Page 262

Angiographic evidence of coronary artery perfusion can be based on the flow grades first proposed by thrombolysis in myocardial infarction (TIMI) study group. With this scheme coronary perfusion is classified as follows:
Grade 0: No perfusion. No antegrade flow of contrast medium is detected beyond the point of occlusion.
Grade 1: Penetration without perfusion. Contrast medium passes through the point of obstruction but antegrade flow fail to opacify distal portion of vessel at any time.
Grade 2: Partial perfusion. Contrast material penetrates through the point of obstruction but enter the distal vessel at a rate slower than that of nonobstructed artery in the same patient.
Grade 3: Complete perfusion. Antegrade flow into the distal coronary bed is rapid and complete.

The rate of coronary flow as assessed by the TIMI flow grade is determined by two major factors i.e., 1. severity of stenosis in the vessel and 2. the status of microvasculature.

26. **Ans. c. 90%**

Braunwald 5th Ed; Page 262-263

Coronary collaterals circulation
In the normal heart, myriad tiny anastomotic branches interconnect the major coronary arteries. Most of these anatomical vessels are less than 200 mµ in diameter and they are precursors of the collateral circulation. In coronary arteriogram of patient with normal or mildly diseased coronary arteries, they cannot be visualized because they carry only minimal flow and there small caliber is well beyond the spatial resolution capability of the Cine imaging system. However when the obstruction of major coronary artery occur, a pressure gradient is created in the anastomotic vessels connecting the distal segment of the involved artery with either its proximal segment or the nearby segment of other vessels. With the creation of this gradient an increased volume of blood is propelled through the anastomotic vessel, which progressively dilate and eventually become visible angiographically as collateral channel. The most favorable clinical circumstances is gradual development of the obstruction, thereby allowing collateral channel to enlarge and becomes functional before the native vessel becomes totally occluded. Other factors that affect collateral development are patency of the feeding arteries, their size and vascular resistance of the postobstructive segment. Collaterals usually cannot be demonstrated at coronary angiography unless the recipient vessel has developed at least 90% diameter stenosis by visual estimate. A large number of collateral pathways exist in patient with severe coronary artery

disease. The advent of percutaneous transluminal coronary angioplasty (PTCA) has provided opportunity to study the hemodynamic aspects and angiographic pattern of the coronary collaterals circulation. Using bilateral coronary angiography, Rentrop and cohen developed a grading system of 0 to 3 for collateral filling classified as follows:
Grade 0: No collaterals present.
Grade 1: Barely detectable collateral flow. Contrast medium passes through collateral channel but fails to opacify the epicardial vessel at any time.
Grade 2: Partial collateral flow—Contrast materials enters but fail to opacify the target epicardial vessel completely.
Grade 3: Complete perfusion contrast material enters and completely opacifies the target epicardial vessel.

27. Ans. a. Severity of obstruction in recipient vessel

Braunwald 5th Ed; Page 262-263

Refer to explanation for Q. No 26.

28. Ans. c. Contrast material enters but fails to opacify the target epicardial vessel completely

Braunwald 5th Ed; Page 262-263

Refer to explanation for Q. No 26.

29. Ans. b. Sones

Braunwald 11th Ed; Page 374

Procedures in the cardiac catheterization laboratory have evolved from purely diagnostic and research technique to potentially life-saving interventional procedures. In 1929, it is Werner Forssmann who performed the first human cardiac catheterization by using fluoroscopic guidance to advance a urethral catheter through his own left antecubital vein into the right atrium. Zimmerman and Coworker undertook the first retrograde left heart catheterization in 1950 using a No. 6 F catheter. In 1958, it is Sones who performed the first selective coronary angiography. Dotter and Judkins developed the techniques of transluminal angioplasty in 1964. In 1977, Andreas Gruentzig performed the first percutaneous coronary balloon angioplasty in humans. Percutaneous revascularization strategies have evolved to include the use of intracoronary stents, various atherectomy methods and laser technology. Technology is advancing to the point that genetic manipulation may be feasible in the catheterization laboratory.

30. Ans. b. Werner forssmann

Braunwald 11th Ed; Page 374

Refer to explanation for Q. No 29.

31. Ans. d. Dotter and Judkins

Braunwald 11th Ed; Page 374

Refer to explanation for Q. No 29.

32. Ans. d. Andreas gruentzig

Braunwald 11th Ed; Page 374

Refer to explanation for Q. No 29.

33. Ans. a. Saline

Braunwald 5th Ed; Page 245

Radiographic contrast agents used during angiography can lead to worsening azotemia. Patients with preexisting renal impairment or diabetes mellitus are at increased risk for developing radiocontrast induced renal failure. Other risk factor for radiocontrast induced renal failure include advancing age, intravascular volume depletion, congestive heart failure and the volume of contrast media administered. In patients with renal insufficiency who undergo coronary angiography, hydration with intravenous saline provides better protection against radiocontrast induced renal failure than does mannitol or furosemide.

34. Ans. d. All of the above

Braunwald 5th Ed; Page 929

Tetralogy of Fallot (TOF) is the most common cyanotic congenital heart disease in adults as well as in the children. In X-ray of chest most adults with TOF demonstrates mild to moderate pulmonary hypovascularity. Those with mild infundibular pulmonary stenosis have normal pulmonary blood flow. A small tortuous bronchial arteries are found in both lungs when severe pulmonary outflow tract stenosis or atresia is present. There is a right aortic arch in 25% of the patients. The combination of right aortic arch and cyanosis should always suggest the diagnosis of TOF, although the same combination of finding can also be seen in the rare examples of truncus arteriosus or double outlet right ventricle in the adult patients. Echocardiography and MRI can demonstrate this defects with better clarity.

35. Ans. a. Lateral film projections of the chest as a thin linear opacity separating the anterior subxiphoid fat from subepicardial fat

Braunwald 11th Ed; Page 1674

The normal pericardium is frequently identified on lateral plane film projection of the chest as a thin linear opacity separating the anterior subxiphoid mediastinal fat from the subepicardial fat. The pericardium may also be visualized in the frontal projection paralleling the left heart border. The extent of the normal and abnormal pericardium is best appreciated with CT and MRI in most patients because of the superior contrast resolution of both techniques.

36. Ans. a. Pericardial effusion

Braunwald 11th Ed; Page 258

The pericardial effusion can be diagnosed by X-ray of chest. When fluid accumulates in pericardial space the cardiac silhouette develops a flask like, triangular or globular silhouette. The normal indentation and prominences along both the left and right heart border are effaced so that the shape of the cardiac silhouette becomes smooth and featureless. In the lateral chest radiography in the patient with pericardial effusion, the retrosternal space is typically narrowed or obliterated by the expanding cardiac silhouette. Normally the low density subepicardial fat merges imperceptibly with the mediastinal fat since the two fat planes are separated only by the 2 mm thick strip of pericardium. When pericardial effusion is present, the subepicardial fat is displaced posteriorly by the high density fluid which may be visible as a wide opaque vertical band between the anterior border of the heart and the mediastinum. This 'epicardial fat pad sign' is visualized best on the lateral projection and is highly specific for pericardial effusion.

37. Ans. d. Presence of pericardial calcification establishes the diagnosis of pericardial constriction

Braunwald 5th Ed; Page 373

Pericardial constriction may complicate viral or tubercular pericarditis, hemopericardium, pericarditis associated with radiation and postpericardiotomy syndrome. In patients with chronic pericardial constriction, the overall heart size is large when the pericardium is thickened to 2 cm or more. Otherwise the cardiac silhouette remains normal or small. The atrial border is flattened and there may be pulmonary vascular redistribution. A small to large pleural effusion are found in 60% of patients with pericardial constriction and enlargement of the azygos vein and left atrium occurs in 20% of the patient. Tubercular pericarditis is a frequent cause of pericardial calcification and constriction. Pericardial calcification occurs in fewer than 20% of patients with chronic pericardial constriction. Pericardial calcification is best appreciated along the anterior and inferior cardiac border and in the atrioventricular groove. Pericardial constriction is often confused with restrictive cardiomyopathy and MRI and CT are helpful in differentiating between these two entities. While it is important to appreciate that the presence of pericardial calcification indicates chronic pericarditis it does not in itself establish a diagnosis of pericardial constriction.

38. Ans. c. Persistent left superior vena cava

Braunwald 5th Ed; Page 262

The left subclavian artery is the border forming structure along the upper left mediastinum above the aortic arch. Although the left innominate vein is actually lateral in position to the left subclavian artery, the left subclavian artery usually forms a concave border with the lungs extending from clavicle to the aortic arch. The left subclavian artery may bulge laterally when there is increased blood flow through the vessel as in postductal coarctation of the aorta or when the vessel is tortuous due to atherosclerosis or hypertension. A straight or a convex left supra, aortic border is found in patient with persistent left superior vena cava.

39. Ans. d. All of the above

Braunwald 5th Ed; Page 207

The left atrial appendage lies immediately below the left mainstem bronchus in the frontal projection. The left atrial appendage normally forms a smooth and slightly concave segment of the left heart border. When the left atrial border is straightened or bulges laterally, atrial enlargement should be suspected. Nonvascular pathology may simulate enlargement of the left atrial appendages, e.g., a pericardial fibroma or cyst, lymphoma or other mediastinal or pleural neoplasms may present as a convexity of the left upper mediastinal border. Congenital absence of the pericardium also causes bulging of left atrial appendages. An important sign of left atrial enlargement in the frontal projection is elevation of the mainstem bronchus so that carinal angle is greater than normal value of up to 75°.

40. Ans. b. LAO

Braunwald 5th Ed; Page 422-429

The left ventriculography is a confirmed way to diagnosed mitral valve prolapse. The configuration of the left ventriculogram during systole is helpful in the diagnosis of mitral valve prolapse. The right anterior projection (RAO) is most useful for defining the posterior leaflet of the mitral valve and the left anterior projection (LAO) for studying the anterior leaflet. The most helpful sign is extension of the mitral leaflet tissue inferiorly and posteriorly to the point of attachment of the mitral leaflets to the mitral annulus. Angiography may also reveal scalloped edges of the leaflet reflecting redundancy of the tissue. Other abnormality noted on angiography of some patients with mitral valve prolapse include dilatation, decrease systolic contraction and calcification of mitral annulus and poor contraction of the basal portion of the left ventricle. There may be an indentation at the base of the posteromedial papillary muscle associated with prolapse of the posterior leaflet resulting from abnormal traction of on this muscle. With the involvement of both papillary muscles, there may be an indentation of the anterior as well as inferior wall of the left ventricle giving the cardiac silhouette an hourglass appearance. These left ventricular contraction abnormalities are secondary to the redundancy of mitral valve leaflets and transmission of the abnormal tension on these leaflets to the papillary muscles and underlying left ventricle.

41. Ans. a. RAO

Braunwald 5th Ed; Page 422–429

Refer to explanation for Q. No 40.

42. Ans. a. MVP

Braunwald 5th Ed; Page 422–429

Refer to explanation for Q. No 40.

43. Ans. d. All are true

Braunwald 5th Ed; Page 780

Pulmonary circulation in the normal adults: Pulmonary blood flow refers to the volume of blood per unit of time that passes from the pulmonary artery through the capillary bed into the pulmonary veins. Lungs have a dual circulation and it receives both systemic venous blood (the pulmonary blood flow) through the pulmonary artery and arterial blood through the bronchial circulation. The bronchial arteries ramifies normally into a capillary network drained by bronchial veins, some of which empty into the pulmonary veins whereas reminder empty into the systemic venous bed. Therefore, the bronchial circulation constitutes a physiological right to left shunt. Function of the bronchial circulation is to provide nutrition to the airways. Normally blood flow through this system is quite low, amounting to approximately 1% of cardiac output, the resulting desaturation of left atrial blood is usually trivial. However, in some forms of pulmonary disease, e.g., severe bronchiectasis and in presence of many congenital cardiovascular malformation that cause cyanosis, the blood flow through bronchial circulation can increase significantly account for nearly 30% of left ventricular output and produces a significant right to left shunt. In pulmonary disease, significant right to left shunting through the bronchial circulation may also result in arterial desaturation. The normal pulmonary artery pressure in a person living at sea level has a peak systolic value of 18 to 25 mm Hg and end diastolic value of 6 to 10 mm Hg and mean value ranging from 12 to 16 mm Hg. Definite pulmonary hypertension is present when pulmonary artery systolic and mean pressure exceeds 30 and 20 mm Hg respectively. The normal mean pulmonary venous pressure is 6 to 10 mm Hg. Therefore, the normal arteriovenous pressure difference which moves the entire cardiac output across the pulmonary vascular bed ranges from 2 to 10 mm Hg. This small pressure gradient is all the more remarkable when one consider that to move the same amount of blood per minute through the systemic vascular bed a pressure difference of approximately 90 mm is required. Normal pulmonary vascular bed offers less than one-tenth of the resistance to flow offered by systemic bed. The normal pulmonary vascular resistance in adult is 67 ± 23 (SD) dynes-sec-cm^5 or 1 wood unit.

44. Ans. a. 12–16 mm Hg

Braunwald 5th Ed; Page 780

Refer to explanation for Q. No 43.

45. Ans. c. 6–10 mm Hg

Braunwald 5th Ed; Page 780

Refer to explanation for Q. No 43.

46. Ans. a. 2–10 mm Hg

Braunwald 5th Ed; Page 780

Refer to explanation for Q. No 43.

47. Ans. d. 90 mm Hg

Braunwald 5th Ed; Page 780

Refer to explanation for Q. No 43.

48. Ans. d. 67–87 dynes-sec-cm^5

Braunwald 5th Ed; Page 780

Refer to explanation for Q. No 43.

CHAPTER 9

Hypertension

1. **Common cause of renovascular hypertension in younger patient is:**
   a. Atherosclerotic renal artery stenosis
   b. Fibromuscular dysplasia
   c. Single kidney
   d. Horse kidney

2. **Acute renal failure precipitated by antihypertensive therapy, particularly ACE inhibitors, points to the diagnosis of:**
   a. Renovascular hypertension
   b. Renal parenchymal disease
   c. Salt sensitive hypertension
   d. Primary hyperaldosteronism

3. **Which is *incorrect* regarding obstructive sleep apnea and hypertension?**
   a. Obstructive sleep apnea may occur in up to 50% of patients with hypertension
   b. Aldosterone antagonist is more effective in treating this subset of patients
   c. Vasodilators are more effective in this subset of patients
   d. CPAP effectively reduces nocturnal blood pressure in OSA than day time blood pressure

4. **Coombs-positive hemolytic anemia is found with use of:**
   a. α-blockers
   b. β-blockers
   c. Vasodilators
   d. Methyldopa

5. **Resistant hypertension in defined as failure to reach goal blood pressure in patients who are taking:**
   a. Full dose of appropriate three drug regime
   b. Full dose of three drugs regime that includes a diuretic
   c. Full dose of three drugs regime that includes beta blocker
   d. Full dose of three drugs regime that includes vasodilators

6. **Which is the most dramatic and most rapidly fatal complication of severe hypertension?**
   a. Acute heart failure
   b. Stroke
   c. Aortic dissection
   d. Symptomatic CAD

7. **Most end-organ damage is noted with:**
   a. SBP exceeding 220 mm Hg or DBP exceeding 120 mm Hg
   b. SBP ≥ 200 mm Hg or DBP ≥ 120 mm Hg
   c. SBP ≥ 220 mm Hg and DBP ≥ 120 mm Hg
   d. SBP ≥ 200 mm Hg and DBP ≥ 100 mm Hg

8. **The drug of choice for most hypertensive emergencies is:**
   a. Sodium nitroprusside
   b. Parenteral labetalol
   c. Nicardipine
   d. Esmolol

9. **Gestational hypertension is defined as elevated BP detected:**
   a. After 20 weeks of gestation without proteinuria
   b. Before 20 weeks of gestation without proteinuria
   c. After 20 weeks of gestation with proteinuria
   d. Before 20 weeks of gestation with proteinuria

10. **Which of the following adverse effects of hypertension is due to direct effects of blood pressure?**
    a. Coronary heart disease
    b. Heart failure
    c. Stroke
    d. Chronic kidney disease

11. **Which measures of blood pressure is most closely related to risk?**
    a. Systolic BP for all age groups
    b. Diastolic BP for all age groups
    c. Mean blood pressure for all age groups
    d. Diastolic BP for subjects younger than age 50 years and systolic BP for subjects older than 60 years

12. **Secondary aldosteronism is seen in all, *except*:**
    a. CHF
    b. Renal artery stenosis
    c. Hyperinsulinemia
    d. Sleep apnea syndrome

13. **Which of the following does *not* cause hypertension in humans:**
    a. Hyperinsulinemia
    b. Hyperaldosteronism
    c. Glucocorticoids excess
    d. Pheochromocytoma

14. **The J curve hypothesis is applicable to the hypertensive patient with:**
    a. CAD
    b. CHF
    c. Stroke
    d. Chronic kidney disease

15. Which of the following is a better predictor for stroke?
   a. Systolic BP
   b. Diastolic BP
   c. Mean pressure
   d. Pulse pressure

16. Which is *correct* regarding J curve phenomenon in patients with hypertension and myocardial infarction?
   a. It is applicable for first 2 years after MI
   b. With longer follow-up there is positive relationship
   c. It is applicable only in presence of a high SBP and low DBP
   d. All of the above

17. Efficacy of which of the following class of antihypertensive drugs diminishes with time when given as monotherapy:
   a. α-blockers
   b. α-agonists
   c. β-blockers
   d. Calcium channel blockers

18. Incorrect regarding α-2 agonists (clonidine, methyldopa) is?
   a. The antihypertensive efficacy of these drugs diminishes with time when given as monotherapy
   b. Their effect is enhanced by concomitant use of diuretics, vasodilators or calcium channel blockers
   c. They are less effective when prescribed with ACE inhibitors
   d. These drugs are not useful in treating hypertensive emergencies

19. Which of the following statement is *not* correct regarding hypertension?
   a. There is a continuous positive relationship between the risk of CAD and stroke death with systolic or diastolic BP down to values as low as 115 or 75 mm Hg respectively
   b. There is continuous positive relationship between the risk of CAD and stroke death with systolic or diastolic blood pressure values of 140/90 mm Hg
   c. Before the age of 50 years, women have lower prevalence of hypertension than men
   d. After menopause, prevalence of hypertension increases rapidly in women and surpasses that in men

20. All the following statements about hypertension are correct, *except*:
   a. Teetotaller has less hypertension
   b. Moderate alcohol drinkers (1 or 2 drinks per day) have less hypertension than teetotaller
   c. The heavy drinker (3 or more drinks per day) has higher prevalence of hypertension
   d. Risk for hypertension increases steeply when caffeine is consumed in diet sodas

21. Risk of developing hypertension increases with all, *except*:
   a. Increasing average body mass index (BMI)
   b. Dietary sodium intake
   c. Dietary potassium intake
   d. Caffeine consumption with sodas

22. Progressive fall in diastolic blood pressure and resultant widening of pulse pressure starts around age of:
   a. 45 years
   b. 55 years
   c. 65 years
   d. 75 years

23. Which of the following statement is *correct* regarding isolated systolic hypertension?
   a. Systolic BP and pulse pressure do not rise with age in absence of urbanization
   b. Isolated systolic hypertension is more common in women
   c. It is more often associated with heart failure with preserved systolic function
   d. All of the above

24. Which of the following is *not* a strong risk factor for developing hypertension?
   a. Coffee consumption
   b. Obesity
   c. Obstructive sleep apnea
   d. Low birth weight

25. Which of the following may be an unrecognized symptom of uncontrolled primary hypertension?
   a. Insomnia
   b. Excessive day time fatigue
   c. Nocturia
   d. Anorexia

26. Which of the following is the gold standard for diagnosis of hypertension?
   a. Conventional office blood pressure measurement
   b. Automated office blood pressure measurement
   c. Home blood pressure monitoring
   d. Ambulatory blood pressure monitoring

27. Which of the following is correct regarding white coat hypertension, *except*:
   a. Patient with white coat hypertension have no target organ damage despite consistently elevated office readings
   b. Patient with white coat hypertension typically show exaggerated pressor reactions to stressful stimuli in their daily lives
   c. Prevalence and severity of white coat hypertension increases sharply with age
   d. All are correct

28. Masked hypertension is more common in all, *except*:
a. Elderly
b. Patient with diabetes
c. Patient with CKD
d. Patient treated with BP medication

29. Noninvasive measurement of aortic stiffness and central aortic pressure can be obtained by:
a. Plethysmography
b. Polysomnography
c. Ambulatory blood pressure monitoring
d. Pulse tonometry

30. Hypertensive heart disease can present as:
a. Symptomatic or asymptomatic diastolic dysfunction
b. Heart failure with preserved ejection fraction
c. Heart failure with reduced ejection fraction
d. All of the above

31. Which of the following renal parameter closely relates with target organ damage in hypertension?
a. Serum creatinine level
b. Blood BUN level
c. Microalbuminuria of 30–300 mg/day
d. Serum cystatin C

32. Nonsteroidal anti-inflammatory drugs (NSAIDs) can precipitate acute kidney injury (AKI) in patients with pre-existing CKD by which of the following mechanism?
a. RAAS inhibition
b. Blocking the synthesis of prostaglandin
c. Accumulation of endogenous inhibitors of NOS
d. Sympathetic overactivity

33. Which of the following is *true* regarding hypertension in hemodialysis patient?
a. Blood pressure is often labile
b. Blood pressure is sensitive to change in fluid volume
c. Blood pressure tends to fall progressively after dialysis
d. All of the above

34. Which is the cause of hypertension in patients with renal transplant?
a. Stenosis of renal artery at the site of anastomosis
b. Rejection
c. Excess renin derived from the retained diseased kidney
d. All of the above

35. Which is *correct* regarding hypertension in patient with renal transplantation?
a. Successful renal transplantation may cure hypertension
b. 50% of the renal transplant patients become hypertensive within one year
c. Hypertension occurs more frequently when donors have a family history of hypertension
d. All of the above

36. Which of the following is *not* correct regarding the renovascular hypertension due to fibromuscular disease?
a. It affects elderly people
b. It is more common in women
c. It affects distal two third and branches of renal artery
d. Carotid FMD often accompanied renal artery FMD

37. Progressive renal failure developing after the start of ACEI or ARB therapy points to diagnosis of:
a. Atherosclerotic renal artery stenosis
b. Renal parenchymal disease
c. Bilateral renal artery stenosis
d. Unilateral nonfunctioning kidney

38. Which of the following is a strong clinical clue for renovascular hypertension?
a. Acceleration of treated primary hypertension
b. Deterioration in renal function in treated primary hypertension
c. Acute kidney injury during treatment of hypertension
d. All of the above

39. Which of the following is the best candidate for renal artery stenting for treatment of renovascular hypertension?
a. Intractable hypertension
b. AKI induced by ACEI or ARB treatment of hypertension
c. Recurrent, episodic flash pulmonary edema
d. All of the above

40. Excessive hypokalemia on diuretic therapy for hypertension often points to the diagnosis of:
a. Primary aldosteronism
b. Adrenaloma
c. Pheochromocytoma
d. Renovascular hypertension

41. In dietary intervention for blood pressure control, which of the following has high strength of evidence?
a. Mediterranean diet pattern
b. DASH diet pattern and low sodium consumption
c. DASH diet pattern and high potassium consumption
d. Mediterranean diet pattern and low sodium consumption

42. In the current practice guidelines for management of hypertension which of the following is *not* included as first line drug for treatment of hypertension?
   a. Calcium channel blockers
   b. Renin angiotensin system inhibitors
   c. Thiazide type of diuretic
   d. Beta blockers

43. In ALLHAT (Antihypertensive Lowering to Prevent Heart Attack Trial) which was the representative drug among the calcium channel blockers?
   a. Nifedipine   b. Benidipine
   c. Cilnidipine   d. Amlodipine

44. As antihypertensive what is the rank order of potency among the calcium channel blockers?
   a. Dihydropyridines > Diltiazem > Verapamil
   b. Diltiazem > Dihydropyridines, i.e., > Verapamil
   c. Verapamil > Diltiazem, i.e., > Dihydropyridines
   d. All are equally efficacious

45. A high salt diet or concurrent nonsteroidal anti-inflammatory drug therapy does not compromise the effectiveness of which of the following antihypertensive drugs?
   a. ACE inhibitors   b. Diuretics
   c. Beta blockers   d. Dihydropyridine CCBs

46. Which of the following statement is *correct* regarding dihydropyridine CCBs?
   a. High salt diet or concurrent NSAID therapy does not compromise its effectiveness
   b. It has diuretic action
   c. Dihydropyridine CCBs are less renoprotective than ACEI or ARBs in patients with proteinuric CKD
   d. All of the above

47. Gingival hyperplasia is a serious side effect associated with which class of antihypertensive drugs?
   a. Beta blockers
   b. ACE inhibitors
   c. ARBs
   d. Calcium channel blockers

48. Which of the following is *correct* regarding Amlodipine induced ankle edema?
   a. It is more common with 10 mg dose than with 2.5 or 5 mg doses
   b. It can be improved by concomitant therapy with ACEI or ARB
   c. Only (a)
   d. Both a and b

49. Which of the following ARB has shorter half-life?
   a. Olmesartan   b. Irbesartan
   c. Telmisartan   d. Valsartan

50. Which of the following is the most potent ARBs?
   a. Olmesartan   b. Azilsartan
   c. Irbesartan   d. Telmisartan

51. Maximum regression of left ventricular hypertrophy is seen in which of the following antihypertensive drug?
   a. Calcium channel blockers
   b. Beta blockers
   c. ACEIs
   d. ARBs

52. Which of the following statement is *correct* regarding RAS inhibitors?
   a. RAS inhibitors provides superior renal protection than other antihypertensive agents mainly for non-diabetic proteinuric CKD
   b. RAS inhibitors provides superior renal protection than other antihypertensive drug mainly for diabetic proteinuric CKD
   c. RAS blockers slows progression from glucose intolerance to type 2 diabetes mellitus (T2DM)
   d. ACEIs and ARBs are superior to other antihypertensive agents for hypertensive patients with diabetes

53. Which of the following side effects are seen with spironolactone?
   a. Painful gynecomastia
   b. Erectile dysfunction
   c. Nonmenstrual uterine bleeding
   d. All of the above

54. Which of the following is *not* a vasodilating beta blockers?
   a. Labetalol   b. Carvedilol
   c. Nebivolol   d. Metoprolol

55. Beta blockers are known to increase the risk of diabetes especially when combined with:
   a. Calcium channel blockers   b. ACE inhibitors
   c. ARBs   d. Diuretics

56. Which of the following is the drug of choice for preoperative management of pheochromocytoma?
   a. Labetalol   b. Central sympatholytic
   c. Phenoxybenzamine   d. Prazosin

57. Which of the following is drug of choice for short time oral treatment of hypertensive urgency when beta blockers (Labetalol) are contraindicated?
   a. Alpha adrenergic blockers
   b. Central sympatholytic such as clonidine
   c. Direct vasodilators
   d. All can be used

CHAPTER 9 | Hypertension

58. Which of the following antihypertensive drug has been proved to be useful for treating prehypertension?
   a. Thiazide diuretic
   b. Beta blockers
   c. ARB
   d. Calcium channel blockers

59. Which of the following is *incorrect*?
   a. Beta blockers provides less stroke protection
   b. Calcium channel blocker provide more stroke protection than any other class of drug
   c. Combination of ACEI/ARB and CCB prevents more CV event than beta blocker/thiazide diuretic combination
   d. Dual RAS blockade with ACEI and ARB provides better cardiovascular outcome over monotherapy with either drug

60. Postprandial hypotension is seen in which group of hypertensive patients?
   a. Pregnant woman
   b. Elderly people
   c. Patients with CKD
   d. Patient hypertension with Parkinsonism

61. Pre-eclampsia is a risk factor for:
   a. Maternal death
   b. Chronic hypertension
   c. Peripartum cardiomyopathy
   d. All of the above

62. Which is a drug of choice for treating severe pre-eclampsia/eclampsia?
   a. IV Sodium nitroprusside
   b. Hydralazine
   c. Labetalol
   d. IV Magnesium

63. Which of the following antihypertensive drug used during pregnancy can lead to postpartum depression?
   a. Nifedipine
   b. Labetalol
   c. Methyldopa
   d. Calcium channel blockers

64. Which of the following antihypertensive drug do *not* enter into human breast milk?
   a. Calcium channel blocker
   b. Beta blocker
   c. Methyldopa
   d. All BP drug enters into human breast milk

65. Which of the following is a cause of true resistant hypertension?
   a. Inadequate blood pressure regime
   b. Medication nonadherence
   c. White coat reaction
   d. Chronic kidney disease

66. Which of the following drug should be avoided for lowering blood pressure in patients with ischemic or hemorrhagic stroke?
   a. Urapidil   b. Nicardipine
   c. Labetalol   d. Nitroprusside

67. Which of the following drug should be avoided to lower blood pressure in hypertensive patients with acute coronary syndrome?
   a. IV Nitroglycerin   b. IV Esmolol
   c. IV Nitroprusside   d. All can be used

68. Which of the following is a drug of choice to treat hypertensive crisis with acute heart failure?
   a. IV Esmolol   b. IV Nitroglycerin
   c. IV Labetalol   d. IV Nitroprusside

ANSWERS WITH EXPLANATIONS

1. Ans. b. Fibromuscular dysplasia

Hurst's 10th Ed; Page 1612

Renovascular hypertension occurs in 1 to 2% of the overall hypertensive population, but the prevalence may be as high as 10% in patients with resistant hypertension, and even higher in patients with accelerated or malignant hypertension. Clinical clues to renovascular disease include: (1) onset of hypertension before age 30 years (especially without a family history) or recent onset of significant hypertension after age 55 years; (2) an abdominal bruit, particularly if it continues into diastolic and is lateralized; (3) accelerated or resistant hypertension; (4) recurrent (flash) pulmonary edema; (5) renal failure of uncertain etiology, especially with a normal urinary sediment; (6) coexistent diffuse atherosclerotic vascular disease, especially in heavy smokers; or (7) acute renal failure precipitated by antihypertensive therapy, particularly angiotensin-converting enzyme (ACE) inhibitors or angiotensin receptor blockers (ARBs). Fibromuscular dysplasia is a common cause of renovascular hypertension in younger patients, especially women between 15 and 50 years of age. On the other hand, atherosclerotic renal artery stenosis occurs in older persons, is bilateral in 35 to 50% of cases, and is associated with atherosclerosis of the coronary, carotid, and lower-extremity vessels. Hypertension in this setting is often resistant to standard therapy.

2. Ans. a. Renovascular hypertension

Hurst's 10th Ed; Page 1612

Refer to explanation for Q. No 1.

3. Ans. c. Vasodilators are more effective in this subset of patients

Hurst's 10th Ed; Page 1613

Obstructive sleep apnea is a common medical condition characterized by abnormal collapse of the pharyngeal airway during sleep, causing repetitive arousals from sleep. It affects 4% of middle aged men and 2% of middle aged women. Obstructive sleep apnea may occur in up to 50% of patients with hypertension. A formal sleep study usually is needed for diagnosis of obstructive sleep apnea and the determination of corrective interventions. Continuous positive airway pressure treatment can reduce nocturnal blood pressure in patients with obstructive sleep apnea, the effect on daytime blood pressure is less clear. Sleep apnea is associated with elevated aldosterone levels, and aldosterone antagonists have been used to treat sleep apnea related hypertension.

4. Ans. d. Methyldopa

Hurst's 10th Ed; Page 1619

Central alpha to agonists include methyldopa, clonidine, guanabenz and guanfacine, and stimulate central nervous system α-2 receptors to reduce central nervous system sympathetic outflow. The antihypertensive efficacy of these agents diminish with time when given as monotherapy. Their effect is enhanced by concomitant diuretic, vasodilator, or CCB administration. They are less effective when prescribed with other sympatholytics or with inhibitors of the rennin-angiotensin system. Clonidine is useful in treating hypertensive urgencies and emergencies. The most common side effects include sedation, dry mouth, and fatigue. Liver dysfunction and a Coombs-positive hemolytic anemia can be seen with methyldopa.

5. Ans. b. Full dose of three drugs regime that includes a diuretic

Hurst's 10th Ed; Page 1626

Resistance hypertension is the failure to reach goal blood pressure in patients who are adhering to full doses of an appropriate three drugs regime that includes the diuretics.

6. Ans. c. Aortic dissection

Hurst's 10th Ed; Page 1626

Aortic dissection is the most dramatic and most rapidly fatal complication of severe hypertension. Mortality rates from aortic dissection remain high. Systolic blood pressure should be decreased as rapidly as possible to 100–110 mm Hg or lower. This reduction is best achieved with a combination of β-blockers and intravenous vasodilators such as sodium nitroprusside. Therapy for acute aortic dissection aims to reduce stress on the aortic wall by lowering both blood pressure and heart rate and consequently the change in blood pressure versus time (dP/dt). Because sodium nitroprusside can cause reflex tachycardia, therapy with β-blocking agents should be started before hand.

7. Ans. a. SBP exceeding 220 mm Hg or DBP exceeding 120 mm Hg

Hurst's 10th Ed; Page 1624–1625

Hypertensive emergency is defined by acute and rapidly evolving end organ damage, such as aortic dissection, heart failure, symptomatic coronary heart disease, progressive renal disease, stroke or cerebral dysfunction associated with significant hypertension. Although there is no blood pressure threshold for the diagnosis of hypertensive emergency, most end organ damage is noted with systolic blood pressure exceeding 220 mm Hg or diastolic blood pressures exceeding 120 mm Hg. Hypertensive urgency is defined by a markedly elevated blood pressure, usually in the same range seen in a hypertension emergency, but without the rapid progression of target-organ damage. If the patient is asymptomatic or clinically stable, the patient can be managed as an outpatient with close follow-up within days. Blood pressure lowering is essential, but the reduction can be achieved over a period of days without an intensive monitoring setting usually with oral medications. Multiple medications are available for the treatment of hypertension crisis. Sodium nitroprusside is the drug of choice for most hypertensive emergencies because it has an immediate onset of action and can be titrated quickly and accurately. The duration of effect is 1 to 2 minutes. Parenteral labetalol is another first line agent for hypertensive emergency. Its onset of action is within 5 to 10 minutes, and the duration of action is about 3 to 6 hours. Nicardipine is a calcium-channel blocker administered parenterally by continuous infusion for hypertensive crises. The onset of action of this drug is 5 to 10 minutes, and the duration of action is 1 to 4 hours. Esmolol is a cardioselective β-blocker with a short duration of action. It reduces systolic blood pressure and mean arterial pressure, as well as heart rate, cardiac output, and stroke volume.

8. Ans. a. Sodium nitroprusside

Hurst's 10th Ed; Page 1624-1625

Refer to explanation for Q. No 7.

9. Ans. a. After 20 weeks of gestation without proteinuria

Hurst's 14th Ed; Page 2349

Gestational hypertension (also called transient hypertension) refers to elevated blood pressure first detected after 20 weeks of gestation without proteinuria.

10. Ans. c. Stroke

Hurst's 10th Ed; Page 1542

Hypertension leads to adverse events in the brain, heart, and kidneys through two related mechanisms, both of which involve the effects of increased pressure on the arteries. The first is the effect on the structure and function of the heart and arteries, and the second is the acceleration of the development of atherosclerosis. The former is directly the result of the blood pressure, whereas the latter requires an interaction with other risk factors for cardiovascular disease, most importantly cholesterol. Thus strokes are closely related to the direct effects of blood pressure, whereas coronary heart disease is related to atherosclerosis, and the relationship between blood pressure and events is steeper for stroke than for coronary heart disease events.

11. Ans. d. Diastolic BP for subjects younger than age 50 years and systolic BP for subjects older than 60 years

Hurst's 10th Ed; Page 1537

A continuing debate in the field of hypertension is the relative importance of the different components of the arterial pressure wave in determining cardiovascular risk. There are four candidates: systolic, diastolic, pulse, and mean pressure. For many years, the diastolic pressure reigned supreme, and most the early hypertension treatment trials used a high diastolic pressure as an entry criterion. Although the importance of systolic pressure was never in doubt, it gained precedence over diastolic pressure with the publication of a series of epidemiologic studies showing not only that high-systolic pressure was the best predictor of risk in the elderly, but also that a low-diastolic pressure was associated with increased risk. The Framingham Heart Study data provided an elegant solution to this apparent paradox. In subjects younger than age 50 years the best predictor of risk was a high diastolic pressure, but in those older than age 60 years systolic pressure was the best predictor, and the relationship between diastolic pressure and risk was now negative, so that a low diastolic pressure was related to higher risk.

12. Ans. c. Hyperinsulinemia

Hurst's 10th Ed; Page 1570

Secondary aldosteronism refers to increased aldosterone secretion that occurs secondary to know stimulus, such as activation of the RAS. This is the most common form of aldosteronism seen in clinical practice and occurs in various conditions associated with stimulation of rennin secretion, such as congestive heart failure, sodium depletion, or renal artery stenosis and obstructive sleep apnea.

13. Ans. a. Hyperinsulinemia

Hurst's 10th Ed; Page 1579

Hyperinsulinemia, which occurs as a compensation for insulin resistance, is postulated to mediate increased blood pressure in essential hypertensional via multiple mechanisms, such as stimulation of SNS activity and renal tubular sodium reabsorption. Chronic hyperinsulinemia, in the absence of obesity does not raise blood pressure in either dogs or humans.

14. Ans. a. CAD

Hurst's 10th Ed; Page 1541

The official; recommendation for the treatment of hypertensive patients with coronary heart disease is that the target blood pressure should be 140/90 mm Hg; whether further reduction is beneficial or harmful is controversial. The J-curve hypothesis was postulated on the basis of observations suggesting that if diastolic pressure was lowered below a certain level (about 85 mm Hg) there was a paradoxical increase of events. The proposed explanation was that because coronary artery perfusion occurs during diastole, excessive reduction in combination with diseased coronary arteries would result in ischemia. Subsequent work supported this idea, because the J-curve was seen for myocardial infarction but not with stroke, where the adage that the lower the blood pressure, the better still holds.

The relationship between risk and blood pressure in individuals who have already had a myocardial infarction is different, and has been reported to be J-shaped for the first 2 years after the MI (i.e., there is a paradoxical increase of risk in those with the lowest blood pressure, e.g., below 110/70 mm Hg) but with longer follow-up there is a positive relationship. The increased mortality at lower levels of pressure may be an example of reverse causality; that is the pressure is low because of extensive damage to the heart.

15. Ans. c. Mean pressure

Hurst's 10th Ed; Page 1540

Mean pressure is a potential candidate as a risk marker. It is defined as diastolic pressure plus 1/3rd of pulse pressure.

In the major intervention studies in elderly patients, it has been found that pulse pressure but not mean pressure predicts the cardiovascular outcome. However, in young patients, mean pressure is more important. In major studies of younger patients, pulse pressure was strongest predictor of coronary event whereas mean pressure was best predictor of stroke. The reason while mean pressure is a better predictor of stroke may be that it is closer to diastolic than to systolic pressure and many studies have shown that the relationship between diastolic pressure and stroke is steeper than for coronary event.

16. Ans. d. All of the above

Hurst's 10th Ed; Page 1541

Refer to explanation for Q. No 14.

17. Ans. b. α-agonists

Hurst's 10th Ed; Page 1619

Refer to explanation for Q. No 4.

18. Ans. d. These drugs are not useful in treating hypertensive emergencies

Hurst's 10th Ed; Page 1619

Refer to explanation for Q. No 4.

19. Ans. b. There is continuous positive relationship between the risk of CAD and stroke death with systolic or diastolic blood pressure values of 140/90 mm Hg

Braunwald 11th Ed; Page 910

Hypertension is defined as usual BP of 140/90 mm Hg or higher. Epidemiological data shows continuous positive relationship between the risk of CAD and stroke death with systolic or diastolic BP down to values as low as 115 or 75 mm Hg respectively. Before 50 years of age, women have a somewhat lower prevalence of hypertension than men. After menopause, the prevalence of hypertension increases rapidly in women and surpasses that in men.

20. Ans. a. Teetotaller has less hypertension

Braunwald 11th Ed; Page 912

Among the various behavioural determinants of hypertension commonly identifiable are nicotine, alcohol and caffeine consumption, physical inactivity, and dietary habits. The nicotine in cigarette smoke transiently increases BP by 10 to 20 mm Hg. Moderate alcohol drinkers (1 or 2 drinks per day) generally have less hypertension than teetotallers, but the risk for development of hypertension increases in heavy drinkers (3 or more drinks per day). Caffeine consumption typically causes only a small transient rise in BP, which in some individuals habituates after the first cup of coffee. The risk for development of hypertension does not vary with the coffee consumption but increases steeply when caffeine is consumed in diet sodas. Coffee contains protective polyphenols not present in sodas.

21. Ans. c. Dietary potassium intake

Braunwald 11th Ed; Page 912

Dietary habits influence the risk for developing hypertension. Hypertension prevalence increases linearly with average body mass index (BMI). Risk of developing hypertension also increases with dietary sodium intake and decreases with dietary potassium intake.

22. Ans. b. 55 years

Braunwald 11th Ed; Page 915

Systolic blood pressure rises steadily with age. Diastolic blood pressure rises until about 55 years of age, then falls progressively thereafter. The resultant widening of pulse pressure is indicative of stiffening of the central aorta and a more rapid return of reflected pulse waves from the periphery, augmenting systolic aortic pressure.

23. Ans. d. All of the above

Braunwald 11th Ed; Page 916

After 55 years of age, ISH (systolic BP >140 mm Hg and diastolic BP <90 mm Hg) predominates. ISH represent an exaggeration of this age-dependent stiffening process. Systolic BP and pulse pressure do not rise with age in the absence of urbanization. ISH is more common in women and is associated prominently with heart failure with preserved systolic function. Many neurohormonal, renal, and vascular mechanisms interact to varying degrees to the pathogenesis and progression of this forms of hypertension.

24. Ans. a. Coffee consumption

Braunwald 11th Ed; Page 914

The risk for development of hypertension does not vary with coffee consumption but increases steeply when caffeine is consumed in diet sodas. Coffee may contain protective antioxidant polyphenols not present in sodas. With weight gain, reflex sympathetic activation is important compensatory mechanism to burn fat, but at the expense of sympathetic overactivity in target tissues such as vascular smooth muscle and kidney that produces hypertension.

Obstructive sleep apnea (OSA) is an important cause of hypertension. In OSA repeated arterial desaturation during apneas, activation of carotid body chemoreceptors triggers BP surges throughout the night and resets the chemoreceptor reflex. Daytime normoxia is misinterpreted as hypoxia, producing sustained reflex sympathetic activation and hypertension even during waking hours. The OSA accelerates the emergence of hypertensive complications such as atrial fibrillation and stroke.

Because of fetal undernutrition, low birth weight with reduced nephrogenesis increases the risk for development of adult salt-dependent hypertension. Hypertensive adults have fewer glomeruli per kidney but very few obsolescent glomeruli with decreased total filtration surface area leading to the hypertension. When low-birth-weight children consume a fast-food diet, they are susceptible to rapid postnatal weight gain, leading to adolescent obesity and hypertension.

25. Ans. c. Nocturia

Braunwald 11th Ed; Page 914

In normotensive individual blood pressure elevation stimulate an immediate increase in renal sodium excretion to shrink plasma volume and to return BP to normal. In hypertension, this pressure-natriuresis curve is shifted to the right, and in salt-sensitive hypertension, the slope is reduced. Resetting of pressure natriuresis prevents the return of BP to normal so that fluid balance is maintained, but at the expense of high BP. Pressure-natriuresis causes profound nocturia due to autonomic failure in patients who have supine nocturnal hypertension and therefore nocturia may be an unrecognized symptom of uncontrolled primary hypertension.

26. Ans. d. Ambulatory blood pressure monitoring

Braunwald 11th Ed; Page 917

Conventional blood pressure monitoring by clinician in the clinic is known to both overestimate and underestimate a person's blood pressure. Home blood pressure is often lower than the blood pressure measured at clinician's office. Automated office blood pressure is a method (which was used in the SPRINT trial), where Oslo metric monitor is set to take 3 readings at one minute interval after the patient was unattended by medical staff and unaccompanied by family member in an examination room for 5 minutes. Automated office blood pressure measure is a preferred method over conventional office blood pressure because it minimizes white coat reaction, it correlates better with home or awake ambulatory blood pressure and it eliminates digital preference. Ambulatory blood pressure monitoring is the gold standard, it provides automated measurement of blood pressure during 24 hours or 48 hours periods while patients are engaged in their usual activity including sleep. Prospective studies have shown that ABPM predicts fatal and nonfatal MI and stroke better than standard office measurements.

27. Ans. b. Patient with white coat hypertension typically show exaggerated pressor reactions to stressful stimuli in their daily lives

Braunwald 11th Ed; Page 918

Patients with elevated office BP can have normal home and ambulatory BP and they are labelled as white coat hypertension. If the daytime BP is less than 135/85 mm Hg and there is no target-organ damage despite consistently elevated office readings, the patient is labelled as white coat hypertension, caused by a transient adrenergic response to the measurement of BP in the physician's office. Patients with white coat hypertension typically do not show exaggerated pressor reactions to stressful stimuli in their daily lives. White coat hypertension is usually a benign phenomenon. Prevalence and severity of white coat hypertension sharply increases with the age.

28. Ans. a. Elderly

Braunwald 11th Ed; Page 918

Masked hypertension is a situation when the out-of-office BP measured is higher compared to measure in Clinician's chamber. It is because of the sympathetic overactivity daily life caused by different stresses like job or home stress, tobacco abuse, or other adrenergic stimulation (OSA) that dissipates when they come to the clinician's office. Masked hypertension increases CVD risk despite normal office blood pressure readings. Masked hypertension is particularly common in African American patients and in patients with diabetes or those with CKD. Masked hypertension is more common in patients being treated with BP medication than in untreated patients. It is because of the fact that patients are more likely to take their BP medication in the morning before coming to the doctor. Sometime, short-acting drugs like hydrochlorothiazide (HCTZ), when dosed in the morning, causes a sizable decrease in BP for the clinic visit but their effect wears off before bedtime, providing no protection against nocturnal hypertension.

29. Ans. d. Pulse tonometry

Braunwald 11th Ed; Page 920

Aortic stiffness is both the cause and consequence of isolated systolic hypertension. It can be measured non-invasively. Sphygmocor is a commercial device, that uses brachial artery BP and a generalized transfer function (by software) to convert the radial waveform, measured by applanation tomography, to a derived central aortic BP waveform. Pulse tonometry provides two principal measures of aortic stiffness that are typically increased in hypertension—pulse wave velocity and augmentation index.

30. Ans. d. All of the above

Braunwald 11th Ed; Page 920

Hypertensive heart disease is classified by severity of the complication. These ranges from mild asymptomatic diastolic dysfunction to heart failure with preserved (HFpEF) or reduced (HFrEF) ejection fraction.

Classification of Hypertensive Heart Disease

Class I: Subclinical diastolic dysfunction by echocardiography without left ventricular hypertrophy. Asymptomatic patients with abnormal left ventricular relaxation/stiffness by Doppler echocardiography, a common finding in hypertensive individuals >65 years

Class II: Left ventricular hypertrophy

Class IIA: With normal functional capacity (NYHA Class I)

IIB: With abnormal functional capacity (NYHA Class >II)

Class III: Heart failure with preserved ejection fraction (HFpEF)

Class IV: Heart failure with reduced ejection fraction (HFrEF)

31. Ans. c. Microalbuminuria of 30–300 mg/day

Braunwald 11th Ed; Page 921

Renal parenchymal disease is the most common cause of secondary hypertension. Diabetes and hypertension are the most common risk factors for CKD as the cases of chronic glomerulonephritis has become less common. Microalbuminuria of 30 to 300 mg/day closely relates to target-organ damage and it should be determined in every new hypertensive patient by testing of a single-voided urine specimen. Serum creatinine level measurement is an inadequate screening test for significant renal damage, especially in elderly patients. Ideally, creatinine clearance should be calculated. Serum cystatin C, is an endogenous 13-kDa protein filtered by the glomeruli and reabsorbed and metabolized by the proximal tubular epithelium, with very little being excreted in urine, has promise as a replacement for serum creatinine because it is less affected by muscle mass.

32. Ans. b. Blocking the synthesis of prostaglandin

Braunwald 11th Ed; Page 922

The kidney is both the culprit and victim in hypertension. In patients with CKD, aggressive antihypertensive regimen including a potent RAAS inhibitor and potent diuretic, can precipitate acute kidney injury (AKI). Another class of drug nonsteroidal anti-inflammatory drugs, i.e., NSAIDs can precipitate acute injury in patients with pre-existing CKD. NSAIDs block the synthesis of prostaglandin, which acts as vasodilator within the kidney. Renin-angiotensin inhibitors, including ACE inhibitors (ACEIs) and angiotensin receptor blockers may precipitate acute renal failure in patients with bilateral renovascular disease whose renal perfusion depends on high levels of A II. The accumulation of endogenous inhibitors of NOS and sympathetic overactivity are responsible for accentuate hypertension in hemodialysis patients.

33. Ans. d. All of the above

Braunwald 11th Ed; Page 922

In patients on dialysis, hypertension is a risk factors for mortality. The common cause of accentuation of hypertension in patients with hemodialysis are excess fluid volume and accumulation of endogenous inhibitors of NOS. The blood pressure may be particularly labile and sensitive to change in fluid volume. In patients receiving maintenance hemodialysis every 48 hours, elevated BPs tend to fall progressively after dialysis, remain low during the first 24 hours, and rise again during the second day due to fluid retention. Gradually achieving and maintaining dry weight, as with 8-hour nocturnal hemodialysis, can greatly improve BP control in hemodialysis patients.

34. Ans. d. All of the above

Braunwald 11th Ed; Page 922

Successful renal transplantation may cure primary hypertension. But due to various reasons about 50% of recipients becomes hypertensive within 1 year. The usual causes are stenosis of the renal artery at the site of anastomosis, rejection episodes, high doses of glucocorticoids and cyclosporine or tacrolimus, and excess renin derived from the retained diseased kidneys. ACEI or ARB therapy may obviate the need to remove the native diseased kidneys to relieve hypertension caused by their persistent secretion of renin. The source of the donor kidney may also play a role in subsequent development of hypertension in the recipient. Hypertension occurs more frequently when donors have a family history of hypertension or when donors have died of subarachnoid hemorrhage and had high BP.

35. Ans. d. All of the above

Braunwald 11th Ed; Page 922

Refer to explanation for Q. No 34.

36. Ans. a. It affects elderly people

Braunwald 11th Ed; Page 922

Atherosclerotic renal artery stenosis causes more than 85% cases of renovascular disease affecting the origin of main renal artery. Atherosclerotic renal artery disease occurs more frequently in older patients with CVD risk factors. In contrast, fibromuscular disease (FMD) involving mainly the distal two third branches of renal artery and often seen in women between ages of 20 to 60 years. Carotid FMD and less often coronary FMD may accompanied renal artery FMD.

37. Ans. c. Bilateral renal artery stenosis

Braunwald 11th Ed; Page 922

Renovascular stenosis is often bilateral although usually one side predominates. Bilateral disease should be suspected in those with renal insufficiency, particularly if rapidly progressive oliguric renal failure develops without evidence of obstructive uropathy, and even more so if it develops after the start of ACEI or ARB therapy.

38. Ans. d. All of the above

Braunwald 11th Ed; Page 923

Clinical clues for renovascular hypertension include:
- Onset of hypertension before age 30 or after 50
- Acceleration of treated primary hypertension
- Deterioration in renal function in treated primary hypertension
- Acute kidney injury (AKI) during treatment of hypertension
- Flash pulmonary edema
- Progressive renal failure
- Refractory heart failure
- Unilateral small (atrophic) kidney size by ultrasound examination

39. Ans. d. All of the above

Braunwald 11th Ed; Page 923

Renal angioplasty without stenting is the treatment of choice for renal artery FMD. A conservative approach based on medical management of cardiovascular risk factors with ACEI- or ARB-based antihypertensive regime, including statins, antiplatelet therapy, and smoking cessation is the cornerstone for the treatment for atherosclerotic renal artery stenosis. In the randomized clinical trial, renal angioplasty has not shown benefits. Registry data strongly indicate that following category of patients are benefitted best with renal artery stenting: (1) intractable hypertension, (2) AKI induced by ACEI or ARB treatment of hypertension, and (3) recurrent, episodic (flash) pulmonary edema.

40. Ans. a. Primary aldosteronism

Braunwald 11th Ed; Page 924

Hyperaldosteronism is a common secondary cause of hypertension seen in about 20% of patients with resistant hypertension. The classic picture of primary aldosteronism is a young, adult with severe systolic/diastolic hypertension and hypokalemia. Aldosterone producing adenoma is suspected in patients who developed unprovoked hypokalemia or excessive hypokalemia on diuretic therapy, a family history of aldosteronism, resistant hypertension, or an adrenal incidentaloma.

41. Ans. b. DASH diet pattern and low sodium consumption

Braunwald 11th Ed; Page 929

Two dietary patterns have undergone contemporary and rigorous study in relation to BP control "the Mediterranean diet pattern and the Dietary Approaches to Stop Hypertension (DASH) diet" pattern. The PREDIMED (Prevención con Dieta Mediteránea) study has shown potential benefits of a Mediterranean diet in hypertension. This study showed an overall reduction in cardiovascular outcomes in the dietary intervention groups defined by a decrease in stroke, an endpoint closely associated with BP. Meta-analysis shows small overall reductions in BP associated with a Mediterranean diet. Consumption of a Mediterranean diet pattern correlated with improvement in numerous biomarkers associated with cardiovascular benefit, including anti-inflammatory effects, as assessed by reduced C-reactive protein. However, the most recent AHA/ACC guidelines on lifestyle management assessed the strength of evidence as "low" regarding consumption of a Mediterranean diet pattern versus a low-fat dietary pattern. DASH diet evolves from studies supported by National Heart Lung and Blood Institute (NHLBI). These randomized, controlled DASH feeding studies showed that this dietary pattern could lower systolic blood pressure (SBP) by more than 5 mm Hg in adults with hypertension compared with the control diet, findings which was supported by further meta-analyses. The 2013 AHA/ACC guidelines consider the strength of evidence "high" for adherence to the DASH diet in individuals with hypertension.

The effects of sodium intake on BP and the cardiovascular benefits of limiting sodium consumption is a controversial subject. The 2013 AHA/ACC lifestyle management guidelines concluded that in adults aged 25 to 80 years with SBP of 120 to 159 mm Hg, reducing sodium intake lowers BP. The guidelines further found the evidence "strong" that for adults aged 30 to 80 with or without hypertension, reduction of sodium intake by approximately 1 g daily lowers SBP by 3 to 4 mm Hg. The observational data supports and association between high potassium intake and lower BP. Increased consumption of potassium may lower BP, particularly in blacks compared with whites. Although the American Society of Hypertension (ASH) recommends an increase in potassium intake to 4.7 g daily, the 2013 AHA/ACC lifestyle guidelines find the strength of evidence insufficient to establish a relationship between increased dietary potassium and lower BP or altered risk for coronary heart disease (CHD), HF, or cardiovascular mortality.

42. Ans. d. Beta blockers

Braunwald 11th Ed; Page 933

The current practice guidelines recommend initiating treatment of hypertension with one or more of three classes of first-line BP-lowering agents, i.e., (1) calcium channel blockers (CCBs); (2) renin-angiotensin system (RAS) inhibitors, either angiotensin-converting enzyme inhibitors (ACEIs) or angiotensin receptor blockers (ARBs); (3) thiazide-type diuretics. These drugs have been found to reduce the risk for nonfatal and fatal cardiovascular events. They have additive effects when used in combination. Although beta-adrenergic blockers (beta blockers) are first-line drugs for angina and heart failure, there is disagreement whether they should be included among the first-line drugs for uncomplicated hypertension because of their inferior stroke protection and increased risk for incident diabetes.

43. Ans. d. Amlodipine

Braunwald 11th Ed; Page 933

All calcium channel blockers block the opening of L-type of calcium channels in the cardiac myocytes and vascular smooth muscle cells. They lower blood pressure by causing peripheral arterial dilation, with the rank order of potency being dihydropyridines > diltiazem > verapamil. Calcium channel blockers (CCB) have antianginal and some antiarrhythmic effects. They also provide more protection against cerebrovascular accident (stroke) than other antihypertensive agents. ALLHAT (Antihypertensive Lowering to Preventive Heart Attack Trial) and other RCT have shown that CCB represented by Amlodipine prevent coronary events as effectively as Diuretics and RAS blockers.

44. Ans. a. Dihydropyridines > Diltiazem > Verapamil

Braunwald 11th Ed; Page 933

Refer to explanation for Q. No 43.

45. Ans. d. Dihydropyridine CCBs

Braunwald 11th Ed; Page 934

Amlodipine is a best studied dihydropyridine calcium channel blockers (CCBs), and has undergone evaluation in multiple RCTs. Advantages of Amlodipine includes predictable dose dependent potency, once daily dosing because of its long half-life, tolerability. Unlike diuretics and RAS inhibitors, a high-salt diet or concurrent nonsteroidal anti-inflammatory drug (NSAID) therapy does not compromise the effectiveness of dihydropyridine CCBs. These drugs have some diuretic action (due to dilation of the afferent renal arteriole), which may reduce requirements for additional diuretic therapy for mild hypertension.

46. Ans. d. All of the above

Braunwald 11th Ed; Page 934

The principal side effect of dihydropyridines is dose-dependent ankle edema. With amlodipine, ankle edema is much more common with a 10-mg dose than with 2.5- or 5-mg doses. The edema is mainly vasogenic because of selective arterial dilation and can be improved by concomitant therapy with an ACEI or ARB that causes balanced arterial and venous dilation. Long acting dihydropyridine CCBs are rarely associated with flushing and headache. All CCBs can cause gingival hyperplasia, a rare but serious side effect that is reversible if detected early.

47. Ans. d. Calcium channel blockers

Braunwald 11th Ed; Page 934

Refer to explanation for Q. No 46.

48. Ans. d. Both a and b

Braunwald 11th Ed; Page 934

Refer to explanation for Q. No 46.

49. Ans. d. Valsartan

Braunwald 11th Ed; Page 934

Refer to explanation for Q. No 50.

50. Ans. b. Azilsartan

Braunwald 11th Ed; Page 934

ARBs are potent antihypertensive drugs. They offer same benefit as ACEIs in treating hypertension while avoiding the ACEI related cough. They have once daily doses with long-acting ARBs such as olmesartan, irbesartan, telmisartan, azilsartan. The shorter half-life of valsartan requires twice daily doses. Azilsartan is most potent among this class of drug.

51. Ans. d. ARBs

Braunwald 11th Ed; Page 935

ARBs produces somewhat more regression of left ventricular hypertrophy than do other antihypertensive drugs as demonstrated in mets-analysis.

52. Ans. a. RAS inhibitors provides superior renal protection than other antihypertensive agents mainly for nondiabetic proteinuric CKD

Braunwald 11th Ed; Page 934

ACEIs and ARBs have become standard first-line antihypertensive therapy for patients with diabetic and nondiabetic CKD, but evidence indicates that RAS inhibitors provide superior renal protection than do other antihypertensive agents, mainly for nondiabetic proteinuric CKD, as seen in AASK (African American Study of Kidney Disease). Head-to-head comparison in ONTARGET has indicated that ACEIs and ARBs have comparable effects on renal outcomes. A recent meta-analysis has indicated that diabetes should no longer be a compelling indication for RAS inhibitors. For hypertensive patients with diabetes, ACEIs and ARBs are not superior to other antihypertensive agents at reducing the risk of cardiovascular outcomes or end-stage renal disease. RCTs have also not demonstrated that RAS blockers slow progression from glucose intolerance to type 2 diabetes mellitus (T2DM).

53. Ans. d. All of the above

Braunwald 11th Ed; Page 936

Sexual side effects of spironolactone include painful gynecomastia, erectile dysfunction, nonmenstrual uterine bleeding.

54. Ans. d. Metoprolol

Braunwald 11th Ed; Page 936

Among the beta blockers, Labetalol and Carvedilol are vasodilators as they block alpha-adrenergic receptor. Similarly, Nebivolol also acts as a vasodilator by stimulating endogenous production of nitric oxide.

55. Ans. d. Diuretics

Braunwald 11th Ed; Page 936

Standard beta blockers are weak antihypertensive drugs compared to ACE inhibitors, ARBs, CCBs or diuretics. Standard beta blocker provides modest protection against CV events, but do not reduce all cause mortality. They also increase the risk for diabetes particularly when combined with a diuretic.

56. Ans. c. Phenoxybenzamine

Braunwald 11th Ed; Page 936

Phenoxybenzamine remains the drug of choice for preoperative management of pheochromocytoma. After alpha blockade is achieved, a beta blocker should be added to block excessive reflex tachycardia.

57. Ans. b. Central sympatholytic such as clonidine

Braunwald 11th Ed; Page 937

The central sympatholytic drug such as clonidine are reserved for short-term oral treatment of hypertensive urgency when beta blockers (i.e., labetalol) are contraindicated. The central sympatholytics are potent antihypertensive agents used as add on therapy for difficult hypertensive patients.

58. Ans. c. ARB

Braunwald 11th Ed; Page 941

Prehypertension may precede stage 1 hypertension and predicts augmented cardiovascular risk. The outcomes of TROPHY (Trial of Preventing Hypertension) suggest that pharmacologic treatment of prehypertension with an ARB together with lifestyle coaching can postpone stage 1 hypertension.

59. Ans. d. Dual RAS blockade with ACEI and ARB provides better cardiovascular outcome over monotherapy with either drug

Braunwald 11th Ed; Page 941

Based on the results of various randomized controlled trials, it was found that beta blockers provide less stroke protection and CCBs more stroke protection than in any other class drugs. Combination of an ACEI (or ARB) and a CCB is an excellent option to initiate medication management for hypertension, because it prevents more cardiovascular events than did the beta blocker/thiazide diuretic combination in ASCOT and the ACEI/HCTZ combination in the ACCOMPLISH trial. ONTARGET trial showed that "dual RAS blockade" is dangerous as combined treatment with both an ACEI and an ARB (ramipril plus telmisartan) has no advantage on cardiovascular outcomes over monotherapy with either drug alone, rather it results in more symptomatic hypotension and more renal impairment.

60. Ans. b. Elderly people

Braunwald 11th Ed; Page 942

Postprandial hypotension and orthostatic hypotension are common in hypertensive elderly patients. To diagnose it ambulatory blood pressure monitoring is a suitable option. Management of postprandial hypotension is challenging. Useful strategies include frequent small low-carbohydrate meals, caffeine with meals, and liberalized salt intake. If these non-drug-related strategies fails, fludrocortisone can be added but often causes or worsens supine hypertension, which can be managed by elevation of the head of the bed and a low-dose short-acting ARB (losartan, 25 to 50 mg) at bedtime.

61. Ans. d. All of the above

Braunwald 11th Ed; Page 948

Pre-eclampsia is a severe progressive multisystem disorder diagnosed by hypertension accompanied by one of the following features: proteinuria, BP more than of 160/110 mm Hg or higher despite bed rest, thrombocytopenia, impaired liver function, progressive renal insufficiency, pulmonary edema, or new-onset cerebral or visual disturbance. Pre-eclampsia causes 15% of maternal deaths. Risk factors for pre-eclampsia includes maternal age younger than 20 or older than 35, positive personal or family history, pre-existing hypertension, obesity, diabetes, and antiphospholipid antibodies. Pre-eclampsia is a risk factor for peripartum cardiomyopathy.

Definitive cure of pre-eclampsia is termination of pregnancy. The intravenous (IV) magnesium sulphate is not a reliable antihypertensive agent but is effective in treating or preventing the seizures in the setting of eclampsia or severe pre-eclampsia. IV labetalol has replaced hydralazine as the drug of choice for treating severe pre-eclampsia/eclampsia. Compared with hydralazine, labetalol carries a lower risk for overshoot hypotension, which can impair fetal blood flow, and also does not cause reflex tachycardia.

62. **Ans. c. Labetalol**

Braunwald 11th Ed; Page 948

Refer to explanation for Q. No 61.

63. **Ans. c. Methyldopa**

Braunwald 11th Ed; Page 948

Pregnant women with stage 2 hypertension but without severe pre-eclampsia/eclampsia, can be treated with one of the three preferred class of drugs: labetalol, nifedipine, or methyldopa. Methyldopa is a conventional drug of choice. However, it poorly tolerated and, if used after delivery, it may cause postpartum depression. All class of antihypertensive drugs enter into human milk.

64. **Ans. d. All BP drug enters into human breast milk**

Braunwald 11th Ed; Page 948

Refer to explanation for Q. No 63.

65. **Ans. d. Chronic kidney disease**

Braunwald 11th Ed; Page 949

Resistant hypertension, defined as high BP uncontrolled with three or controlled with at least four antihypertensive drugs (including a diuretic), is associated with a higher prevalence of secondary hypertension and worse cardiovascular and renal outcomes. The prevalence of resistant hypertension ranges between 13 to 20% of the adult population. More than half of these patients have pseudo-resistant hypertension from improper BP measurement technique, white coat reactions, medication noncompliance, use of pressor substances (NSAIDs, excessive alcohol, psychiatric drugs), or an inadequate BP regimen. Truly drug-resistant patients are at a special high-risk population. Patients should be screened for secondary hypertension, especially primary aldosteronism and CKD, as well as pheochromocytoma.

66. **Ans. d. Nitroprusside**

Braunwald 11th Ed; Page 951

For ischemic or hemorrhagic stroke, agents of choice to lower BP include urapidil, nicardipine, or labetalol. Nitroprusside and hydralazine should be avoided because they may increase intracranial pressure.

67. **Ans. c. IV Nitroprusside**

Braunwald 11th Ed; Page 951

In hypertensive patients with acute coronary syndrome (ACS), BP should be lowered with IV nitroglycerin after administration of a beta blocker such as IV metoprolol to prevent reflex tachycardia. IV esmolol lowers BP more than metoprolol, is rapidly reversible, and produces a more predictable dose-dependent reduction in BP than IV nitroglycerin (which alleviates angina more reliably than lowering BP). Nitroprusside should be avoided as it can cause coronary steal.

68. **Ans. d. IV Nitroprusside**

Braunwald 11th Ed; Page 951

IV nitroprusside is a drug of choice to treat hypertensive crisis with acute heart failure. Concomitant loop diuretics both decrease acute pulmonary edema and lower BP.

CHAPTER 10

Hyperlipidemia

1. **Predominant lipoprotein in Apoprotein(a) is:**
   a. HDL
   b. VLDL
   c. Lp(a)
   d. Chylomicron

   (c)

2. **ApoB-100 contains predominantly which lipoprotein?**
   a. Chylomicrons
   b. HDL
   c. Lp(a)
   d. LDL, VLDL

3. **Measurement of non-HDL-C is equivalent to measurement of which of the following lipoprotein in the determination of CV risk?**
   a. ApoA
   b. ApoB
   c. ApoD
   d. ApoE

4. **Which of the following is *correct* regarding lipoprotein(a) – Lp(a)?**
   a. Lp(a) has antifibrinolytic potential
   b. It has strong association with aortic calcification and have a causal role in aortic stenosis
   c. It has ability to bind with oxidase lipoprotein
   d. All of the above

5. **Effect of statins on atherosclerosis includes all the following *except*:**
   a. Decreases C-reactive protein
   b. Decreases the collagen content of atherosclerotic plaque
   c. Alter the endothelial function
   d. Decreases the inflammatory component of the plaque

6. **In management of hypercholesterolemia, every doubling of statin dose brings down LDL-C by:**
   a. Additional 6%
   b. Additional 25%
   c. Additional 30%
   d. Additional 50%

7. **Which of the following is *not* a risk factor for statin induced rhabdomyolysis?**
   a. Advanced age
   b. Concomitant use of antifungal and gemfibrozil
   c. Hypothyroidism
   d. Diabetes

8. **Which of the following is a cholesterol absorption inhibitor?**
   a. Fibrates
   b. Statins
   c. Fish oil
   d. Ezetimibe

9. **Which of the following drug can cause hypertriglyceridemia?**
   a. Fibric acid derivatives
   b. Ezetimibe
   c. Statins
   d. Bile-acid binding resins

10. **Fish oil have a therapeutic role in treatment of:**
    a. Hypercholesterolemia
    b. Hypertriglyceridemia
    c. To increase HDL-C
    d. None of them

11. **Evolocumab and alirocumab are:**
    a. Cholesterol absorption inhibitor
    b. Cholesterol ester transfer protein inhibitor
    c. PCSK9 inhibitor
    d. Bile-acids binding resins

12. **All the following are known to lower Lp(a) *except*:**
    a. Niacin
    b. PCSK9 inhibitors
    c. Antisense RNA directed against ApoA.
    d. Ezetimibe

13. **Which of the following drug inhibits ATP-citrate lyase (ACL), a key enzyme in the "cholesterol biosynthesis pathway?**
    a. Evolocumab
    b. Torcetrapib
    c. Bempedoic acid
    d. Inclisiran

14. **Which of the following is also named as β-lipoprotein?**
    a. Chylomicron
    b. High density lipoprotein (HDL)
    c. Very low-density lipoprotein
    d. Low density lipoprotein

15. **Which of the following is called as pre β-lipoprotein?**
    a. Low density lipoprotein
    b. Very low density lipoprotein
    c. High density lipoprotein
    d. Chylomicron

16. Which of the following is named as α-lipoprotein?
   a. HDL (high density lipoprotein)
   b. Chylomicron
   c. Low density lipoprotein (LDL)
   d. Very low density lipoprotein (VLDL)

17. Lipoprotein (a) – Lp (a) is a form of:
   a. HDL   b. LDL
   c. VLDL   d. IDL

18. Which of the following combination is called as atherogenic lipoproteins?
   a. Chylomicrons and triglycerides
   b. Chylomicrons and VLDL
   c. LDL and VLDL
   d. LDL + IDL

19. Which of the following is *not* atherogenic?
   a. Chylomicrons   b. Triglycerides
   c. LDL   d. HDL

20. Which of the following do *not* contains ApoB?
   a. Chylomicron   b. Triglycerides
   c. LDL   d. HDL

21. Excessively high level of which of the following signifies and increases the risk of acute pancreatitis?
   a. LDL   b. Triglycerides
   c. Chylomicrons   d. ApoB

22. Dysbetalipoproteinemia is primarily:
   a. Hypertriglyceridemia
   b. Hypercholesterolemia
   c. Elevation of VLDL triglycerides
   d. Excess of cholesterol enriched VLDL remnant

23. Characteristic lipid abnormality in patients with nephrotic syndrome is:
   a. Hypertriglyceridemia
   b. Hypercholesterolemia
   c. Combined hyperlipidemia
   d. Very low HDL level

24. Which statement is *correct*?
   a. Hypothyroidism raises serum LDL-C level
   b. Hypothyroidism predisposes to statin induced myopathy
   c. All dyslipidemia patients should be tested for hypothyroidism
   d. All are correct

25. The use of retinoids is known to be associated with:
   a. Hypertriglyceridemia
   b. Hypercholesterolemia
   c. Combined hyperlipidemia
   d. Increase in the VLDL remnants

26. Traditional mediterranean diet is rich in:
   a. Saturated fatty acids
   b. Monounsaturated fatty acids
   c. Polyunsaturated fatty acids
   d. Carbohydrate

27. Which of the following is the consequence of excess of ectopic fat deposition?
   a. Insulin resistance and type 2 diabetes mellitus
   b. Non-alcoholic fatty liver disease
   c. Diastolic heart failure
   d. All of the above

28. Which of the following statement is *incorrect*?
   a. Statin can cause new neuromuscular disorders
   b. Hypothyroid patients who are pharmacologically euthyroid have higher rates of statin associated myopathy
   c. 60–70% of individuals tolerate reinduction of statin on blinded rechallenge
   d. Adverse muscle event is lowest with simvastatin

29. The risk of adverse muscle event appears to be lowest with:
   a. Simvastatin   b. Rosuvastatin
   c. Lovastatin   d. Fluvastatin

30. Which of the following is risk factors for statin associated myopathy?
   a. Hypothyroidism
   b. Chronic renal failure
   c. Preexisting neuromuscular disorder
   d. All of the above

31. What is the optimal level of LDL for primary prevention of atherosclerotic cardiovascular disease?
   a. < 120 mg/dL   b. < 100 mg/dL
   c. < 70 mg/dL   d. < 50 mg/dL

32. Which of the following method is most appropriate for selection of patients for statin therapy in primary prevention of CHD?
   a. 10-year risk for ASCVD based on multiple risk factors algorithm (Global Risk Assessment)
   b. Lifetime risk based on a single major risk factor
   c. 10-year risk based on imaging for subclinical atherosclerosis
   d. Anyone can be used

33. What is the cholesterol goal in primary prevention for high-risk individuals?
   a. 50% reduction in LDL-C level
   b. Non HDL-C < 100 mg/dL
   c. LDL-C < 70 mg/dL
   d. Either

ANSWERS WITH EXPLANATIONS

1. Ans. c. Lp(a)

Braunwald 11th Ed; Page 963

Name	Predominant lipoprotein	Molecular weight (kDa)	Plasma concentration (mg/dL)	Role	Human disease
ApoA	Lp(a)	250–800	0.2–200	Unknown	Lp(a) excess
ApoA-I	HDL	28.3	90–160	ACAT activation, structural	HDL deficiency
ApoA-II	HDL	17	25–45	Structural	
ApoA-IV	HDL	45	10–20	Structural, absorption	
ApoA-V	VLDL, HDL			TRL metabolism	Hypertriglyceridemia
ApoB-100	LDL, VLDL	512	50–150	Structural, LDL-R binding	Hypobetalipoproteinemia
ApoB-48	Chylomicrons	214	0–100	Structural	
ApoC-I	Chylomicrons	6.63	5–6	TRL metabolism	
ApoC-II	Chylomicrons, VLDL	8.84	3–5	LPL activation	Hyperchylomicronemia
ApoC-III	Chylomicrons, VLDL	8.76	10–14	LPL inhibition	Hypertriglyceridemia
ApoD	HDL	33	4–7	LCAT	
ApoE	Chylomicrons remnant, IDL	34	2–8	LDL-R, ApoE receptor binding	Type III hyperlipoproteinemia
ApoH	Chylomicrons, VLDL, LDL, HDL	38–50	1.4–1.6	Beta$_2$-glycoprotein Platelet aggregation	Cardiolipin-binding defect
ApoJ	HDL	70	10	Complement system	
APOL1–6	HDL	43.9	—	Unknown	
ApoM	HDL	25	1μM	Unknown	

2. Ans. d. LDL, VLDL

Braunwald 11th Ed; Page 963

Refer to explanation for Q. No 1.

3. Ans. b. ApoB

Braunwald 11th Ed; Page 967

The measurement of ApoB level provides information on the number of potentially atherogenic particles and can be used as a goal of lipid lowering therapy. LDL particle size correlates highly with plasma HDL-C and TG levels. The Emerging Risk Factors Collaboration studies have shown that measurement of non–HDL-C is equivalent to measurement of ApoB in determination of CV risk. Measurement of non–HDL-C captures the cholesterol content in apo B–containing lipoproteins.

4. Ans. d. All of the above

Braunwald 11th Ed; Page 968

Lp(a) consist of LDL particle linked covalently with one molecule of ApoA. The ApoA moiety consists of a protein with a high degree of homology with plasminogen. The pathogenesis of Lp(a) may result from an antifibrinolytic potential and ability to bind oxidized lipoproteins. Lp(a) has been implicated as a causal CV risk factors. Genetic polymorphisms at the *LPA* gene have shown a strong association with aortic calcification and may have a causal role in aortic stenosis.

5. Ans. b. Decreases the collagen content of atherosclerotic plaque

Braunwald 11th Ed; Page 971

Atherosclerosis involves inflammation. Statins have known to decrease C-reactive protein (CRP), augment the collagen content of atherosclerotic plaque, alter the endothelial function, and decrease the inflammatory component of plaque.

6. Ans. a. Additional 6%

Braunwald 11th Ed; Page 972

Statin do not reduce LDL in a linear manner. For every doubling of statin dose LDL-C drops by about an additional 6%.

7. Ans. d. Diabetes

Braunwald 11th Ed; Page 972

Drugs like antibiotics, antifungal medications, certain antiviral drugs, grapefruit juice, cyclosporine, amiodarone, are known to affect cytochrome P-450 and therefore, interfere with metabolism of statin. The major side effects of statins is due to muscle symptoms ranging from diffuse myalgias [normal creatinine kinase (CK) levels], seen in up to 10% to 15% of statin users, to myositis, defined as diffuse muscle pain with evidence of muscle inflamation and elevated CK levels. A minority of statin user may develop rhabdomyolysis. This life-threatening situation is often related to predisposing factors like advanced age, frailty, renal failure, shock, concomitant use of antifungal agents, antibiotics and the fibric acid derivative gemfibrozil, and hypothyroidism.

8. Ans. d. Ezetimibe

Braunwald 11th Ed; Page 974

Ezetimibe limits selective uptake of cholesterol and other sterols by intestinal epithelial cells by interfering with NPC1L1. This agent is to be added in patients whose LDL levels does not reach to the target while receiving the maximally tolerated statin dose. Ezetimibe lowers LDL-C by about 18% and adds to the effect of statins.

9. Ans. d. Bile-acid binding resins

Braunwald 11th Ed; Page 975

Bile acid–binding resins interrupt the enterohepatic circulation of bile acids by inhibiting their reabsorption in the intestine. They are mainly indicated in patients with severe hypercholesterolemia secondary to increased LDL-C. The important side effects of this drugs are gastrointestinal constipation, a sensation of fullness, and GI discomfort. These drugs can cause hypertriglyceridemia.

10. Ans. b. Hypertriglyceridemia

Braunwald 11th Ed; Page 975

Fish oils are rich in polyunsaturated fatty acids such as eicosapentaenoic acid (EPA) or docosahexaenoic acid (DHA). These fatty acids lower plasma triglyceride levels and have antithrombotic properties. The use of fish oil is reserved for patients with severe hypertriglyceridemia refractory to conventional therapy. Fish oils decrease VLDL synthesis and decrease VLDL ApoB.

11. Ans. c. PCSK9 inhibitor

Braunwald 11th Ed; Page 976

Evolocumab and alirocumab are monoclonal antibody, which inhibits proprotein convertase subtilisin/kexin type 9 (PCSK9) drug. Both these drugs have shown to reduce the LDL significantly. Evolocumab is to be given in a dose of 140 mg subcutaneously every two weeks or 420 mg monthly and Alirocumab is to be given 75 mg or up-titrated to 150 mg subcutaneously every two weeks. It is indicated in patients with established clinical atherosclerotic vascular disease or familial hypercholesterolemia, whose LDL remain above target despite maximally tolerated statin dosing with or without ezetimibe.

12. Ans. d. Ezetimibe

Braunwald 11th Ed; Page 976

Patients with elevated Lp(a) represent a therapeutic challenge. Statins have little effect on Lp(a) levels. Niacin can lower Lp(a) level by 20% to 30%, but its use is accompanied by adverse events. PCSK9 inhibitors such as evolocumab and alirocumab lower Lp(a) significantly by 20% to 25%. Antisense RNA directed against apo(a) has been shown to decrease Lp(a) level markedly in humans in a proof-of-concept study, which need future trials.

13. Ans. c. Bempedoic acid

Braunwald 11th Ed; Page 976

14. Ans. d. Low density lipoprotein

Hurst's 14th Ed; Page 817

The major lipids of plasma, cholesterol and triglycerides are transported in molecular complexes called lipoprotein. The lipoprotein consists of a core of neutral lipid (triglycerides and cholesterol ester) that is surrounded by a polar core containing nonsterified cholesterol, phospholipids, and proteins (called apolipoprotein). The major category of lipoprotein consists of low density lipoprotein (LDL), very low density lipoprotein (VLDL), high density lipoprotein (HDL) and chylomicrons. These lipoproteins vary in size and density. Because lipoprotein can be separated by electrophoresis, they have also been labelled according to their migration relative to serum protein. LDL is called β-lipoprotein, VLDL is pre-β-lipoprotein and HDL is α-lipoprotein.

15. Ans. b. Very low density lipoprotein

Hurst's 14th Ed; Page 817

Refer to explanation for Q. No 14.

16. Ans. a. HDL (high density lipoprotein)

Hurst's 14th Ed; Page 817

Refer to explanation for Q. No 14.

17. Ans. b. LDL

Hurst's 14th Ed; Page 818

Apolipoprotein(a) is a unique form of LDL. It is a LDL particle in which apo-B is covalently linked to another protein named apolipoprotein(a). Evidence suggests that Lp(a) carries atherogenic potential equal to or even greater than LDL.

18. Ans. c. LDL and VLDL

Hurst's 14th Ed; Page 818

There is growing evident that VLDL, like LDL is atherogenic for this reason many investigators favour combining LDL and VLDL into a single fraction of atherogenic lipoproteins. Chylomicrons are not atherogenic. Native chylomicrons are too large to filter into the arterial wall. However, chylomicron remnants may promote atherosclerosis. Normally, chylomicron remnants are rapidly removed from circulation, consequently their plasma levels are very low. In some circumstances, however, concentrations of chylomicron remnants can be relatively high which may contribute to atherosclerosis.

19. Ans. a. Chylomicrons

Hurst's 14th Ed; Page 818

Refer to explanation for Q. No 18.

20. Ans. d. HDL

Hurst's 14th Ed; Page 818

HDL do not contain ApoB, instead HDL particles are held together by ApoA1 and ApoA-1L. HDL are considered antiatherogenic.

21. Ans. c. Chylomicrons

Hurst's 14th Ed; Page 818-819

The two main categories of hyperlipidemia are hypercholesterolemia and hypertriglyceridemia. Most people with high and high triglycerides have elevation of VLDL-triglycerides, dysbetalipoproteinemia signifies an excess of cholesterol enriched VLDL remnants. When fasting triglycerides occurs in high range chylomicrons are present. Excess chylomicrons signify an increased risk of acute pancreatitis.

22. Ans. d. Excess of cholesterol enriched VLDL remnant

Hurst's 14th Ed; Page 818-819

Refer to explanation for Q. No 21.

23. Ans. b. Hypercholesterolemia

Hurst's 14th Ed; Page 828

The characteristic lipid abnormality in patients with nephrotic syndrome is hypercholesterolemia. This is attributed to low level of serum albumin (or low oncotic pressure). In response to hypoalbuminemia, there is overproduction of ApoB–containing lipoproteins by the liver. On the other hand, there is reduced clearance of LDL from the circulation.

24. Ans. d. All are correct

Hurst's 14th Ed; Page 828

Hypothyroidism is known to raise serum LDL-C levels. It is most commonly due to decreased expression of LDL receptors. Clinical experience mandates that all patients with hypercholesterolemia or other dyslipidemia should be tested for hypothyroidism. Not only can hypothyroidism cause hypercholesterolemia, it can unmask other forms of latent dyslipidemia. Hypothyroidism is known to predisposes to severe myopathy when statins are used for treatment of hypercholesterolemia.

25. Ans. a. Hypertriglyceridemia

Hurst's 14th Ed; Page 829

Oral retinoids used for treatment of skin disorder such as acne, can induce hypertriglyceridemia and in some cases severe hypertriglyceridemia precipitates acute pancreatitis.

26. Ans. b. Monounsaturated fatty acids

Hurst's 14th Ed; Page 829

Dietary fats/cholesterol as well as saturated and trans fatty acids are LDL raising nutrients. In population with high intake of these saturated fatty acids, LDL-C levels are raised by 10% to 50%. In contrast, unsaturated fatty acid (monounsaturated and polyunsaturated) do not raise LDL-C level. Therefore, these fats can be used in place of saturated fatty acids. High carbohydrate diet caused mild to moderate increase in VLDL and reduced HDL-C levels. Because of these effects monounsaturated fatty acids may be preference for carbohydrates as a replacement of saturated fatty acids. A diet high in monounsaturated fatty acid is characteristic of the traditional Mediterranean diet.

27. Ans. d. All of the above

Hurst's 14th Ed; Page 829-830

Fat can be stored either in upper body or lower body adipose tissue pools. Lower body fat occurs predominantly in subcutaneous adipose tissue in the gluteofemoral region. This appears to be a preferable location for fat storage because the metabolic consequences of gluteofemoral obesity tend to be minimal. It is common storage site for triglyceride in women. In contrast, men usually store excess fat in the upper body (abdominal obesity). Here fat storage can occur in either subcutaneous or visceral pools. Upper body obesity is accompanied by greater nutrient overload in other issues, which is called as ectopic fat. Accumulation of ectopic fat may occur in skeletal muscle, liver, heart and pancreatic β-cells. In muscles, ectopic fat contributes to insulin resistance and type 2 diabetes mellitus. In the liver, it predisposes to non-alcoholic fatty liver as well as to atherogenic dyslipidemia. In β-cells of pancreas, ectopic fat may impair insulin secretion and in the heart it may lead to systolic or diastolic dysfunction.

28. Ans. d. Adverse muscle event is lowest with simvastatin

Hurst's 14th Ed; Page 831–832

Statin intolerance is the inability to tolerate statins at the recommended doses to reduce adverse cardiovascular events. Statin may cause adverse muscle complaints like myalgia, myopathy, myositis, myonecrosis or clinical rhabdomyolysis. The ability to cause muscle injury varies among statins. Myositis has been reported in less than 0.5%, but frequency increases with higher doses. In clinical trial, this effect was 0.02% at simvastatin 20 mg/day to 0.07% at 40 mg/day and 0.3% at 80 mg/day. The risk of adverse muscle event appears to be lowest with fluvastatin. Preexisting neuromuscular disorder may become clinically manifest after initiation of statin therapy. In some cases, statin may cause new neuromuscular disorder. Hypothyroidism may predispose to the development of statin induced myopathy. Hypothyroid patients who are pharmacologically euthyroid have higher rates of statin associated adverse muscle complaint. Other risk factors for developing statin induced myopathy are chronic renal failure and concurrent drug therapy, particularly those drugs that inhibits cytochrome P450 like gemfibrozil and PPAR-α agonists. Important component of assessment of statins intolerance is dechallenge and rechallenge of statin therapy at reduced doses or selection of an alternate statin with different pharmacodynamic and pharmacokinetic properties. 60-70% of individual tolerate reintroduction of statin on blinded rechallenge.

29. Ans. d. Fluvastatin

Hurst's 14th Ed; Page 831–832

Refer to explanation for Q. No 28.

30. Ans. d. All of the above

Hurst's 14th Ed; Page 831–832

Refer to explanation for Q. No 28.

31. Ans. b. < 100 mg/dL

Hurst's 14th Ed; Page 834–835

Several epidemiological studies have indicated that CHD risk is progressive lower for a total cholesterol down to 150 mg/dL. This level corresponds to an LDL-C of about 100 mg/dL. Genetic epidemiology have demonstrated that lifetime levels of LDL-C of approximately 100 mg/dL are accompanied by a low lifetime risk of CHD. RCT's with cholesterol lowering drugs show that reducing LDL-C concentrations to near 100 mg/dL or below produce significant reduction in ASCVD rates. Based on these evidences, the Adult Treatment Panel (ATP) III defined an LDL-C level of less than 100 mg/dL as being optimal, whereas 100 to 129 mg/dL was called near optimal.

32. Ans. c. 10-year risk based on imaging for subclinical atherosclerosis

Hurst's 14th Ed; Page 835

Three methods have been used for selection of patients for initiation of cholesterol-lowering drugs. These are (1) 10-year risk for ASCVD based on multiple-risk-factor algorithms (global risk assessment), (2) lifetime risk based on single major risk factors, and (3) 10-year risk based on imaging for subclinical atherosclerosis. 10-year risk estimates based on multiple risk factor algorithms are Framingham Risk Score and QRISK risk score developed in United Kingdom. The major limitation of this method is that risk in individual can vary substantially from population mean. This is particularly so in older patients who exhibit wide variability in atherosclerotic burden. Population-risk algorithms derived in the past tend to overestimate current risk and therefore, it may not be applicable to wide range of population.

Lifetime risk assessment based on algorithms and on individual high-risk conditions are not as reliable as 10-year risk estimates because long-term risk is not as well substantiated. The major drawback of global risk algorithms is that excessive weight has been given to the age as a risk factor. Age is used as a surrogate for progressive atherosclerosis. The impact of age on estimated risk is so powerful that most men over 60 and most women over 70 are recommended for statin therapy. Atherosclerotic burden increases with age in the population as a whole; yet many older individuals have little or no atherosclerosis. They will not benefit from taking statins. The way to improve identification of individuals without atherosclerotic burden is to measure subclinical atherosclerosis. The most readily available and intensively studied modality for atherosclerosis imaging is coronary artery calcium (CAC). Measurement of CAC in older individuals who are at relatively low risk by global risk assessment will uncover a substantial portion who are devoid of coronary athcrosclcrosis. Recent studies have shown that actual 10-year risk for clinical CHD when CAC is zero is very low. In the absence of CAC, statin treatment is not needed.

33. Ans. d. Either

Hurst's 14th Ed; Page 837

For high-risk individuals with hypercholesterolemia whose 10-year risk is equivalent to that of a patient with established atherosclerotic cardiovascular disease (ASCVD) (i.e. ≥ 20%), cholesterol lowering should be as intense as in ASCVD patients. Accordingly, the goal can be either a 50% reduction in LDL-C levels or alternatively, a target non-HDL-C of less than 100 mg/dL (LDL-C < 70 mg/dL). For most patients, a high intensity statin can be justified.

CHAPTER 11: Congestive Heart Failure

1. **Which is the most common cause of heart failure?**
   a. Massive pulmonary embolism
   b. Dilated cardiomyopathy
   c. Hypertrophic cardiomyopathy
   d. Coronary atherosclerosis

2. **Which of the following condition produces combined systolic and diastolic heart failure?**
   a. Dilated cardiomyopathy
   b. Hypertrophic cardiomyopathy
   c. Subendocardial fibrosis
   d. Coronary atherosclerosis

3. **Kussmaul's sign—A paradoxical rise in the height of the jugular venous pressure during inspiration is seen in all the following conditions *except*:**
   a. Chronic constrictive pericarditis
   b. Congestive heart failure
   c. Tricuspid stenosis
   d. Tricuspid regurgitation

4. **Hepatojugular reflux is helpful in differentiating:**
   a. Right heart failure from left heart failure
   b. Systolic and diastolic heart failure
   c. Hepatic enlargement caused by heart failure from that caused by other conditions
   d. Tricuspid stenosis tricuspid regurgitation

5. **Which is *correct* regarding pulsus alternans?**
   a. It can be elicited by assumption of erect posture or application of venous tourniquets
   b. It is reduced by assuming recumbent posture and exercise
   c. It is often initiated by a premature beat
   d. All are correct

6. **Which of the following is found to be elevated in patient with CHF and contributes in causing cardiac cachexia?**
   a. Interleukin-II
   b. Interleukin-6
   c. Tumor necrosis factor
   d. Angiotensin-II

7. **In chest roentgenogram in a patient with CHF, a butterfly pattern and pleural effusion develops when pulmonary capillary pressure is:**
   a. 13–17 mm Hg
   b. 28–20 mm Hg
   c. 20–25 mm Hg
   d. > 25 mm Hg

8. **In chest X-ray of patient with CHF Kerley's lines are seen when pulmonary capillary pressure is approximately:**
   a. 13–17 mm Hg
   b. 18–20 mm Hg
   c. 20–25 mm Hg
   d. > 25 mm Hg

9. **Nicoladoni-Branham sign is elicitable in:**
   a. Hypersensitive carotid sinus syndrome
   b. Femoral artery aneurysm
   c. Brachial artery aneurysm
   d. Systemic arteriovenous fistula

10. **High—Altitude pulmonary edema (HAPE) occurs in ascending quickly above the height of**
    a. 1,000 m
    b. 1,500 m
    c. 2,000 m
    d. 2,500 m

11. **Which of the following central nervous system disorder can be associated with acute pulmonary edema without detectable left ventricular disease?**
    a. Grand mal seizures
    b. Subarachnoid hemorrhage
    c. Intracranial neoplasm
    d. Acoustic neuroma

12. **Potentially life-threatening digoxin or digitoxin toxicity can be reversed by:**
    a. Dose adjustment of digoxin
    b. Potassium administration
    c. Magnesium administration
    d. Antidigoxin immunotherapy with purified fab fragment

13. Which is *true* regarding the management of digitalis toxicity?
   a. Digoxin is not removed effectively by peritonear or hemodialysis
   b. Intravenous magnesium is specially useful in patients with atrial fibrillation and an accessory pathway with fast ventricular response
   c. Electrical cardioversion can precipitate severe rhythm disturbances
   d. All are true

14. Patients with past or current symptoms of heart failure associated with underlying structural heart disease is categorized (according to ACC/AHA guideline) as:
   a. Stage A
   b. Stage B
   c. Stage C
   d. Stage D

15. Which of the following is "fibrosis biomarker" used in assessment of heart failure?
   a. BNP
   b. NT-proBNP
   c. Troponin
   d. Soluble ST2

16. Which of the following is *not* the component of reversal of left ventricular remodeling?
   a. Decrease in LV volume
   b. Increase in LV mass
   c. Decrease in LV mass
   d. Restoration to normal elliptical shape of the ventricle

17. In a patient of heart failure with the medical or device therapy if there is normalization of the molecular, cellular, myocardial and LV geometric changes leading to the freedom from future heart failure event is called as:
   a. Reverse remodeling
   b. Myocardial recovery
   c. Myocardial remission
   d. All the terms are interchangeable

18. Which of the following compensatory adaptive mechanism occurs early in the course of developing heart failure?
   a. Activation of renin-angiotensin system
   b. Activation of adrenergic nervous system
   c. Release of inflammatory mediators responsible for cardiac repair and remodelling
   d. Stimulation of zona glomerulosa of the adrenal cortex to produce aldosterone

19. Which of the following attenuates LV remodeling?
   a. Angiotensin II
   b. Angiotensin III
   c. Angiotensin IV
   d. Angiotensin I–VII

20. In patients with heart failure, which of the following agent contribute to the hyponatremia seen even after correction for plasma osmolality?
   a. Noradrenaline
   b. Aldosterone
   c. Arginine vasopressin
   d. Use of diuretic drugs

21. All the following counterregulatory neurohormones are activated in heart failure in order to offset the deleterious effect of the vasoconstricting neuro-mechanism *except*:
   a. Prostaglandin E2 (PGE2)
   b. Prostacyclin (PGI2)
   c. Atrial natriuretic peptide (ANP) and brain (B-type) natriuretic peptide (BNP)
   d. Arginine vasopressin

22. Which of the following statement is *correct* regarding natriuretic peptides?
   a. ANP is secreted in short burst in response to acute changes in atrial pressure while the BNP is secreted and response to chronic increase in atrial/ventricular pressure
   b. ANP has a short half-life of approximately 3 minutes whereas BNP has a plasma half-life of approximately 20 minutes
   c. All natriuretic peptides are degraded by neutral endopeptidase (NEP)
   d. All are correct

23. Which of the following is the beneficial effect of neprilysin inhibition (NEP inhibition)?
   a. Inhibition of degradation of natriuretic peptides
   b. Inhibition of degradation of angiotensin II, angiotensin I–VII and ET1.
   c. Inhibition of degradation of the amyloid β-peptides (AB)
   d. All are beneficial

24. Omapatrilat inhibits:
   a. Angiotensin converting enzyme
   b. Neprilysin neutral endopeptidase (NEP) or neprilysin
   c. Both of the above
   d. None of the above

25. Which of the following changes in the myocyte component of the myocardium in failing heart leads to the inflammatory reaction and formation of fibrotic scar?
   a. Necrosis
   b. Autophagy
   c. Apoptosis
   d. All leads to scarring

26. Which of the following is the most prevalent comorbid condition found in patients with acute heart failure?
    a. Coronary artery disease
    b. Hypertension
    c. Dyslipidemia
    d. Chronic renal failure

27. Which of the following is a feature of hemodynamic congestion in patients with acute heart failure?
    a. Presence of rales
    b. Elevated jugular venous pressure
    c. Edema
    d. High ventricular diastolic pressure without overt clinical signs

28. Which of the following event occur first in the chronological orders of development of acute heart failure?
    a. Increase in the body weight
    b. Increase in LV filling pressure
    c. Pedal edema and raised JVP
    d. Presence of rales

29. Which of the following mechanisms leads to the worsening of heart failure in patients with elevated left ventricular filling pressure or hemodynamic congestion in absence of clinical congestion?
    a. Decreased biological activity of counterregulatory hormone such natriuretic peptides
    b. Decreased in coronary perfusion pressure leading to subendocardial ischemia
    c. Acute change in ventricular architecture leading to worsening of mitral regurgitation
    d. All of the above

30. Which of the following statement is *incorrect*?
    a. Approximately half of patients with acute heart failure have relatively preserved systolic function
    b. Abnormality in diastolic function are presented in heart failure patients regardless of ejection fraction
    c. Diastolic dysfunction alone is insufficient to lead to acute heart failure
    d. All are correct

31. Strongest predictor of worsening renal function in heart failure patients relates to:
    a. Low cardiac output
    b. Diminished renal blood flow
    c. Elevated central venous pressure
    d. Decreased urine output

32. Which is *incorrect* regarding acute hypertensive heart failure?
    a. More likely to have preserved systolic function
    b. More likely in man
    c. Frank pulmonary edema with evident rale and florid congestion on chest X-ray is much more common
    d. These patients have lower in-hospital mortality

33. Which of this is a barometer of systemic venous hypertension?
    a. Pulmonary rales or inspiratory crackles
    b. Pulse pressure
    c. Jugular venous pressure
    d. Peripheral edema

34. What is approximate quantity of fluid to be accumulated to produce clinically detectable edema?
    a. Minimum of 2 L
    b. Minimum of 4 L
    c. Minimum of 8 L
    d. Minimum of 10 L

35. Which statement is *correct* regarding natriuretic peptide estimation in setting of heart failure?
    a. Negative predictive value of BNP is generally greater than positive predictive value in setting of heart failure
    b. False negative values are commonly seen in patients with obesity and heart failure.
    c. Natriuretic peptide level tends to be lower in patients with heart failure with preserved ejection fraction (HFpEF) than those with reduced systolic function
    d. All are correct

36. Value of which of the following parameter is approximately proportional to the neurohormonal activation in acute heart failure?
    a. BNP and NT-proBNP
    b. Cardiac troponin
    c. Serum creatinine
    d. Blood urea nitrogen

37. Which of the following variable is associated with favourable prognosis in patients with heart failure?
    a. Rising blood urea and nitrogen
    b. Rising NT-pro BNP and BNP
    c. Elevated/high blood pressure
    d. Nonadherence to medication and diet

38. Which of the following statement is *incorrect* regarding treatment of patients with left ventricular dysfunction who have not developed symptom?
    a. Angiotensin converting enzyme or ARBs are recommended for all patients with history of myocardial infarction regardless of ejection fraction
    b. ACE inhibitor or ARBs should be used only in patients with MI who have reduced ejection fraction (< 35%)

c. ACE inhibitor/ARBs are recommended for all patients with diminished EF regardless history of myocardial infarction
d. ICD is recommended for asymptomatic ischemic cardiomyopathy who had a recent (> 40 days) MI with EF of 30% or less

39. Use of which one of the following beta blocker has *not* been proven to reduce mortality in patients with current or prior symptom of heart failure with reduced ejection fraction?
a. Bisoprolol
b. Carvedilol
c. Sustained release metoprolol succinate
d. Nebivolol

40. According to new guideline (ACC 2017), ACE inhibitor/ARB should be replaced by ARNI.
a. In all patients who are tolerant to ACEI/ARB to further reduce morbidity and mortality in patients with NYHA class II–III heart failure
b. Should be replaced only if a patient remains symptomatic after an ACEI (equivalent to 10 mg twice daily of enalapril) or ARB along with beta blocker and MRA
c. Should be replaced only if there is repeated heart failure hospitalization with an elevated plasma level of BNP and ProBNP
d. All of the above

41. In heart failure with preserved ejection fraction, BNP levels are elevated in all the following *except*:
a. Women and elderly population
b. Patients with concomitant pulmonary disease
c. Renal dysfunction
d. Obese patients

42. Which of the following drug has *not* shown to improve mortality in heart failure?
a. ACE inhibitors/ARNIs
b. Aldosterone receptor antagonists
c. Hydralazine and isosorbide dinitrate
d. Digoxin

43. Which of the following is *not* the pillar of guideline directed medical therapy for heart failure with reduced ejection fraction?
a. ARNI (neprilysin inhibitor)
b. Beta blocker
c. SGLT-2i
d. Digoxin

44. Tafamidis is used for treatment of:
a. Cardiac sarcoidosis
b. Cardiac amyloidosis
c. Arrhythmogenic right ventricular dysplasia
d. Hypertrophic cardiac myopathy

45. Recovery of left ventricular systolic function is seen commonly in which of the following disorder:
a. Chronic tachycardia
b. Peripartum cardiomyopathy
c. Patients who have undergone revascularization or device therapy
d. All of the above

46. Recovery of left ventricular systolic function is seen commonly in which condition?
a. Peripartum cardiomyopathy
b. Acute myocarditis
c. Cardiomyopathy as a result of systemic inflammatory response
d. All of the above

47. Which of the following diuretic acts in collecting duct?
a. Bumetanide
b. Furosemide
c. Thiazide diuretics
d. Potassium sparing diuretic (spironolactone)

48. All the following diuretics acts at loop of Henle *except*:
a. Thiazide
b. Bumetanide
c. Furosemide
d. Torsemide

49. Which of the following diuretic acts in distal convoluting tubule?
a. Spironolactone
b. Bumetanide
c. Thiazide diuretic
d. Furosemide

50. All the following may lead to unresponsiveness to high doses of diuretic drug in patients with congestive heart failure *except*:
a. Hepatic failure
b. Significant impairment of renal function
c. Consumption of large amount of dietary sodium
d. Concomitant use of NSAIDs

51. Which of the following method is used to overcome diuretic resistance without producing adverse metabolic consequence and affecting survival?
a. Escalation of dose of loop diuretic
b. Intravenous administration of diuretic (bolus or continuous infusion)
c. Combination of different diuretic class
d. All are equal

52. Vaginal bleeding as a side effect is seen with which of the following drug?
a. ARNI
b. Omapatrilat
c. Spironolactone
d. Diuretic

53. Which of the following statement is *incorrect* regarding ACE inhibitors in patient with HFrEF?
a. Benefit of ACE inhibition is seen only in the patient with moderate-to-severe symptoms of heart failure
b. Benefit of ACE inhibition is seen in patients with mild, moderate or severe symptoms of heart failure
c. Benefit is seen in patient with CAD
d. Benefit is seen in patients with or without CAD

54. All the following drugs are of unproven value in treatment of heart failure *except*?
a. Class 1C antiarrhythmic drugs
b. Calcium channel blocker
c. Dipeptidyl peptidase 4 (DPP-4) inhibitors
d. Omega-3 PUFA

55. Which of the following agent has been used to lower potassium level and enable treatment with RAAS in patients with heart failure and hyperkalemia?
a. Patiromer
b. Sodium zirconium cyclosilicate
c. Both of the above
d. None of the above

56. Which of the following drug can cause sodium and water retention and blunt the effect of diuretics?
a. Verapamil
b. Diltiazem
c. Amlodipine
d. NSAIDs

57. Which of the following statement is *incorrect* about treatment GDMT of heart failure with ACEI, ARB, ARNI, beta blockers?
a. Up-titration of medication dose should be done over time to a specified target dose, unless not well tolerated
b. If symptom improved at lower doses, the medication dose need not be titrated to the trial defined target dose
c. The beta blockers provide dose dependent improvement in LVF, reduction in heart failure hospitalization and reduction in all causes mortality
d. ACEI or ARBs have shown lower risk of cardiovascular death or heart failure stabilization with higher doses

58. What should be the initiation and titration sequences of GDMT in treatment of heart failure?
a. ACEI/ARNI/ARB should be started first
b. Beta blockers should be started first followed by ACEI
c. SGLT-2 inhibitor should be started first
d. Simultaneous initiation and sequencing should be done based on patient's symptoms, vital signs, functional status, tolerance and renal function

59. Which of the following trial demonstrated that reducing heart rate in patients with heart failure improved cardiovascular outcomes?
a. V-HeFT
b. RALES trial
c. PIONEER-HF
d. SHIFT

60. Which of the following statement is *correct* regarding the use of ivabradine in heart failure?
a. The greatest benefit of ivabradine in heart failure was reduction in heart failure hospitalization
b. It should be used only in patients with resting heart rate of > 70 bpm.
c. Before initiating Ivabradine, beta blockers should be titrated to the highest tolerated dose before assessing the resting heart rate for consideration of ivabradine
d. All are correct

61. Which of the following drug used in heart failure has *not* shown mortality benefit?
a. ACE inhibitors
b. Beta blockers
c. Ivabradine
d. Digoxin

62. Recently concluded VICTORIA trial studied which of the following drug in heart failure?
a. SGLT-2 inhibitor
b. ARNI
c. Vericiguat
d. Ivabradine

63. Which of the following is *not* correct regarding the indication of ICD for primary prophylaxis?
a. Patient should have LVEF < 35% and NYHA Class II or III symptom on chronic GDMT
b. Should have expected meaningful survival of >1 year
c. Should have risk of SCD demonstrated by having frequent VPCs or non-sustained VT
d. Should be ischemic cardiomyopathy only

64. The maximum benefit of CRT implantation in patients with heart failure is obtained in which of the following subgroup?
   a. Patient with wider QRS duration (> 150 msec) and with LBBB
   b. Patient with non LBBB, prolonged PR
   c. Patient with LVEF < 35%, non-LBBB 120–140 msec and NYHA class I–II heart failure
   d. Patient with LVEF < 35% with LBBB and QRS duration of 120 msec

65. Which of the following statement is *incorrect* regarding CABG in heart failure?
   a. It improves outcome in patients with left main or left main equivalent disease and heart failure
   b. Long term survival benefit is greater in those with more advanced ischemic cardiomyopathy (lower EF or three vessel disease)
   c. Benefit enhances with increasing with age
   d. All are correct

66. Which of the following therapy has been shown to improves mitral regurgitation and left ventricular dimension in patients with heart failure with reduced ejection fraction (HFrEF) and secondary mitral regurgitation?
   a. RAAS inhibition
   b. Beta blockers
   c. Biventricular pacing
   d. All

67. Which of the following statement is *not* true regarding management of heart failure?
   a. The benefit of CRT is seen in patients with QRS duration of > 150 msec, LBBB morphology
   b. The one year survival is standard inclusion for ICD and CRT implantation indication
   c. CABG has shown to improve outcome in patients with left main or left main equivalent disease and heart failure
   d. Following remission in patients with HFrEF and HFmrEF, it is important to withdraw GDMT

68. Pathogenic variants in transthyretin gene leads to:
   a. Sarcoidosis
   b. Hypertrophic cardiomyopathy
   c. Dilated cardiomyopathy
   d. Amyloidosis

69. Transthyretin amyloidosis is prevalent in which of the following condition?
   a. Severe aortic stenosis
   b. HFpEF
   c. Carpal tunnel syndrome
   d. All of the above

70. Discordance between wall thickness on echocardiogram and QRS voltage on ECG is characteristics of:
   a. Hypertrophic cardiomyopathy
   b. Arrhythmogenic RV dysplasia
   c. Ebstein anomaly
   d. Cardiac amyloidosis

71. Which of the following statement is *correct* regarding cardiac amyloidosis?
   a. There is often discordance between wall thickness on echocardiogram and QRS voltage on ECG in patient with cardiac amyloidosis
   b. Intracardiac thrombosis in absence of diagnosed AF and regardless of CHA_2DS_2-VASc score is common
   c. Guideline directed medical therapy is often poorly tolerated in patients with cardiac amyloidosis
   d. All of the above

72. What is the cause of dyspnea in a suspected heart failure patients with absence of jugular venous distention and edema?
   a. Proportional elevation of right and left sided cardiac filling pressure
   b. Disproportionate elevation of right sided pressure particularly with tricuspid regurgitation
   c. Disproportionate elevation of left sided filling pressure
   d. All of the above

73. Which of the following hinders effective decongestion in decompensated chronic heart failure?
   a. Proportional elevation of right and left sided cardiac filling pressure
   b. Disproportionate elevation of right sided pressure especially in presence of TR
   c. Disproportionate elevation of left sided filling pressure
   d. Improper fluid restriction

74. Which of the following is recommended for treatment of anemia in patients with heart failure?
   a. Oral iron supplementation
   b. Weekly intravenous ferric carboxymaltose
   c. Erythropoietin stimulating agents like darbepoetin
   d. All can be used

75. In patients with heart failure and central sleep apnea which of the following is recommended?
   a. Continuous positive air pressure ventilation
   b. Adaptive servo ventilation
   c. Both can be used
   d. Both are of no use

76. According to American Diabetes Association guideline which of the following is first line agent for treatment of hyperglycemia in patients with diabetes with heart failure or at high risk of heart failure?
   a. Acarbose
   b. Long-acting insulin
   c. SGLT-2i
   d. GLP-1 antagonist

77. In patients with heart failure and atrial fibrillation if a rhythm-controlled strategy fails, then which is the treatment of choice?
   a. Addition of digoxin in medical treatment
   b. AV nodal ablation with implantation of a ventricular pacemaker
   c. AV nodal ablation with implantation of a CRT device
   d. Any one of above can be chosen

78. Which of the following is *not* correct regarding anticoagulation in patients with heart failure?
   a. Anticoagulation should be used among patients with heart failure and AF
   b. Anticoagulation should be used in all patients with heart failure with or without AF
   c. Paroxysmal and new onset AF are associated with greater risk for hospitalization caused by heart failure or stroke
   d. Risk of stroke is particularly higher in initial period after diagnosis of heart failure among patients with prevalent AF

79. Which of the following DOAC is direct thrombin inhibitor?
   a. Apixaban
   b. Rivaroxaban
   c. Dabigatran
   d. Edoxaban

80. Which of the following drug is known to be effective in improving LV dysfunction in patients with anthracycline trastuzumab induced cardiomyopathy?
   a. ARNI
   b. ACEI and beta blockers
   c. ACEI and diuretics
   d. Ivabradine

81. Which of the following statement is *correct* regarding cancer therapy related cardiomyopathy?
   a. Use of trastuzumab leads to irreversible cardiomyopathy
   b. Pre-emptive use of ACEI and beta blockers prevents cancer therapy related cardiomyopathy
   c. Serial biomarkers estimation (troponin) may be useful in risk stratification
   d. All are incorrect

82. Titan gene mutation is linked with development of:
   a. Hypertrophic cardiomyopathy
   b. Cancer therapy related cardiomyopathy
   c. Peripartum cardiomyopathy
   d. Takotsubo cardiomyopathy

83. Which of the following group of drugs is considered acceptable during pregnancy for treatment of HFrEF?
   a. ACEI and ARBs
   b. ACEI, ARB, and spironolactone
   c. Furosemide, beta blockers, hydralazine, and nitrates
   d. ARNI and ivabradine

ANSWERS WITH EXPLANATIONS

1. Ans. d. Coronary atherosclerosis

Braunwald 5th Ed; Page 447–448

Heart failure can be caused by an abnormality in systolic function leading to a defect in the expulsion of blood (i.e. systolic heart failure) or by an abnormality in diastolic function leading to a defect in ventricular filling (i.e. diastolic heart failure). The former is the more familiar, classic heart failure in which an impaired inotropic state is responsible. Less familiar, but perhaps just as important, is diastolic heart failure, in which the ability of the ventricle(s) to accept blood is impaired. This may be due to slowed or incomplete ventricular relaxation which may be transient, as occurs in acute ischemia, or sustained, as in concentric myocardial hypertrophy or restrictive cardiomyopathy secondary to infiltrative conditions such as amyloidosis.

There are many examples of pure systolic or diastolic heart failure. Examples of the former are patients with acute massive pulmonary embolism or dilated cardiomyopathy, while examples of the latter are patients with hypertrophic cardiomyopathy or subendocardial fibrosis. However, in many patients, systolic and diastolic heart failure coexists. The most common form of heart failure, that caused by coronary atherosclerosis, is an example of combined systolic and diastolic failure.

2. Ans. d. Coronary atherosclerosis

Braunwald 5th Ed; Page 447–448

Refer to explanation for Q. No 1.

3. Ans. d. Tricuspid regurgitation

Hurst's 11th Ed; Page 247

Refer the answer from Chapter of Clinical Cardiology Question number 20.

4. Ans. c. Hepatic enlargement caused by heart failure from that caused by other conditions

Braunwald 5th Ed; Page 19

Abdominal-jugular reflux: This can be tested by applying firm pressure to the periumbilical region for 10 to 30 seconds with the patient breathing quietly while the jugular veins are observed; increased respiratory excursions or straining should be avoided. In normal subjects, jugular venous pressure rises <3 cm H_2O and only transiently, while abdominal pressure is continued, whereas in right or left ventricular failure and/or tricuspid regurgitation the jugular venous pressure remains elevated. In the absence of these conditions a positive abdominal jugular reflux suggests an elevated pulmonary artery wedge or central venous pressure.

5. Ans. d. All are correct

Braunwald 5th Ed; Page 455

Pulsus alternans is characterized by a regular rhythm with alternating strong and weak ventricular contraction. It is to be distinguished from the alternation of strong and weak beat that occurs in pulsus bigeminus in which the weak beat follows the strong beat by a shorter time interval than the strong beat follows the weak. Where is in pulsus alternans they are equally fixed or the weak beat is slightly closer to the succeeding than to the preceding beat. Severe pulsus alternans can be detected either by palpation of peripheral pulse or by sphygmomanometry. Pulsus alternans may be accompanied by alternation in the intensity of heart sound and of existing heart murmur. Pulsus alternans occurs most commonly in heart failure secondary to increase resistance to left ventricular ejection has occurs in systemic hypertension and aortic stenosis as well as in coronary atherosclerosis and dilated cardiomyopathy. It is usually associated with ventricular protodiastolic gallop sounds (S3). It signifies advance myocardial disease and often disappears with treatment of heart failure. In patient with heart failure, pulsus alternans often can be elicited by reduction in systemic venous return as occur with assumption of the erect posture or application of venous tourniquets and it is reduced by an increase in venous return as in recumbency or with exercise. Pulsus alternans tends to be present during tachycardia and is often initiated by premature beat. Pulsus alternans is attributed to an alternation in the stroke volume ejected by the left ventricle and ultimately to a deletion in the number of contracting sales in every other cycle presumably owing to incomplete recovery. Alternans is almost always concordant in the two sides of circulation. Rarely pulsus alternans is accompanied by electrical alternans. However, the later condition is usually not due to mechanical alternans but to alternating position of the heart within the fluid filled pericardial sac.

6. Ans. c. Tumor necrosis factor

Braunwald 5th Ed; Page 455

Cardiac cachexia: Long standing severe congestive heart failure particularly in the right ventricle may lead to anorexia, owing to the hepatic and intestinal congestion and sometime to digitalis intoxication. Occasionally, there is impairment of intestinal absorption of fat and rarely protein losing enteropathy. Patient with heart failure also may exhibit increase total metabolism secondary to: (1) an augmentation of myocardial oxygen consumption as occurs in patient with aortic stenosis and hypertension; (2) excessive work of breathing; (3) low grade fever and (4) elevated level of circulating tumor necrosis factor. This cytokine is produced by monocytes and causes cachexia and anorexia. The combination of reduced calorie intake and increase caloric expenditure however, produce mali to reduction of tissue mass and in severe cases to cardiac cachexia.

7. Ans. d. >25 mm Hg

Braunwald 5th Ed; Page 456–457

In chest X-ray of the patient with congestive heart failure, there are two principle features which helps in making diagnosis: (1) the size and shape of the cardiac silhouette which provide important information regarding the precise nature of underlying heart disease. Both the cardiothoracic ratio and the heart volume determine on plain film or relatively specific but insensitive indicator of increased left ventricular end diastolic volume; (2) in the presence of normal pulmonary capillary and venous pressure in the erect position the lung bases are better profuses than apices, and the vessel supplying the lower lobes are significantly larger than or those supplying the upper lobes. With elevation of left atrial, pulmonary venous and capillary pressure, interstitial and perivascular edema develops and is most prominent in the lung bases because hydrostatic pressure greater there. When pulmonary capillary pressure is slightly elevated, i.e., approximately 13–17 mm Hg, the resultant compression of the pulmonary vessel in the lower lobes causes equalization in the size of the vessels at the apices and bases. With greater pressure elevation (approximately 18–23 mm Hg), actual pulmonary vascular redistribution occurs (i.e., further constriction of vessel leading to the lower lobes and dilatation of vessel leading to the upper lobes). When the pulmonary capillary pressure exceeds approximately 20–25 mm Hg interstitial pulmonary edema occurs. This may be of several varieties: (1) Septal—producing Kerley's line (sharp, linear density of interlobular interstitial edema); (2) Perivascular—producing loss of sharpness of central and peripheral vessel and (3) Subpleural—producing spindle shaped accumulation of fluid between the lung and adjacent pleural surface. When the pulmonary capillary pressure exceeds 25 mm Hg, alveolar edema with cloud like appearance and concentration of fluid around the hili in the butterfly pattern and large pleural effusion may occur.

8. Ans. c. 20–25 mm Hg

Braunwald 5th Ed; Page 456 – 457

Refer to explanation for Q. No 7.

9. Ans. d. Systemic arteriovenous fistula

Braunwald 5th Ed; Page 460

Systemic arteriovenous fistulas may be congenital or acquired. The acquired fistulas are either post traumatic and iatrogenic. Increased cardiac output associated with such fistula depends on the size of a communication and magnitude of resultant reduction in systemic vascular resistance. The physical finding in general includes a widen pulse pressure, brisk carotid and peripheral arterial pulsation and mild tachycardia. Nicoladoni-Branham sign consist of slowing of the heart after manual compression of the fistula is present in the majority of the cases. This maneuver also raises arterial and lower venous pressure. It appears to result from operation of cardio accelerator reflects with both afferent and efferent pathways in the vagus nerve.

10. Ans. d. 2,500 m

Braunwald 5th Ed; Page 465

High altitude pulmonary edema (HAPE): Victims of this disorder are usually persons most in their teens or early 20's who have quickly ascended to altitudes in excess of 2,500 m and who then engage in strenuous physical exercise at that altitude before they become acclimated. The gradual ascent, allowing time for acclimatization and limiting physical exertion upon more rapid ascent are thought to be preventive. Reversal of this syndrome is both rapid (<48 hours) and certain either by returning the patient to a lower altitude and or by administering a high inspiratory concentration of oxygen. Sleeping below 2,500 m, gradual acclimatization and widens of heavy exertion for first 2 or 3 days at high altitudes appears to be preventive.

11. Ans. d. Acoustic neuroma

Braunwald 5th Ed; Page 465

Neurogenic pulmonary edema: Central nervous disorders ranging from head trauma to grand mal seizures can be associated with acute pulmonary edema without detectable left ventricular disease. The sympathetic over activity produces shift of blood volume from the systemic to pulmonary circulation with secondary elevation of left atrial and pulmonary capillary pressure. Thus, an imbalance of starling forces may be the bases for this form of pulmonary edema although capillary pressure quickly returns to normal after the acute and transitory sympathetic discharge.

12. Ans. d. Antidigoxin immunotherapy with purified fab fragment

Braunwald 5th Ed; Page 482

The half-life of digoxin elimination is 36 to 48 hours and therefore, in patient with normal or near normal renal function once a day dosing is permitted. In the absence of loading doses nearly steady state blood levels are achieved in 4 to 5 half-life or about one week after the initiation of maintenance therapy if normal renal function is present. Digoxin is largely excreted unchanged with a clearance rate proportional to the GFR, resulting in the excretion of approximately one-third of body stored daily. In patient with heart failure and reduced cardiac reserved, increased cardiac output and renal blood flow in response to treatment with vasodilators or sympathomimetic agents may increase renal digoxin clearance necessitating doses adjustment. Digoxin is not removed effectively by peritoneal dialysis or hemodialysis because of its large volume of distribution. The principle body reservoir is skeletal muscle and not adipose tissue and therefore, dosing should be based on estimated lean body mass. Neonates and infants tolerate and may require higher doses of digoxin than older children or adults. The overt digitalis toxicity tends to emerge at 2-to 3-fold higher serum concentration than the target 1.8 nmol/dL. The blood sample for serum digoxin level measurement should be taken at least 6 to 8 hours following the last digoxin dose. Disturbance of cardiac impulse formation, conduction or both are hallmark of digitalis toxicity. Potassium administration in setting of digitalis toxicity is often useful for atrial, AV junctional or ventricular ectopic rhythm even when the serum potassium level is in the normal range, unless high grade atrioventricular block is also present. Magnesium may be useful in patient with atrial fibrillation and an accessory pathway in whom digoxin administration has facilitated a rapid accessory pathway mediated ventricular response. Lidocaine or phenytoin which in conventional dose have minimal effects on atrioventricular conduction are useful in management of worsening ventricular arrhythmias that threaten hemodynamic compromise. Electrical cardioversion can precipitates severe rhythm disturbance in patient with overt digitalis toxicity and should be used with particular caution.

Potentially life-threatening digoxin or digitoxin can be reversed by antidigoxin immunotherapy. Purified Fab fragments from digoxin specific antisera are available. The smaller (molecular weight of 50,000) Fab fragments have a larger volume of distribution, more rapid onset of action and more rapid clearance than does intact IgG. Antidigoxin Fab is very effective in treating life-threatening digitalis toxicity.

13. Ans. d. All are true

Braunwald 5th Ed; Page 482

Refer to explanation for Q. No 12.

14. Ans. c. Stage C

Braunwald 11th Ed; Page 404

The ACC/AHA guideline classified patients of heart failure according to the following four stages:
- *Stage A*: Patient at high risk for developing heart failure but without structural disorder of the heart
- *Stage B*: Patient with structural disorder of the heart but no symptom of heart failure
- *Stage C*: Patient with past or current symptoms of heart failure associated with underlying structural heart disease
- *Stage D*: Patient with end stage disease who requires specialized treatment strategies such as mechanical circulatory support, continuous inotropic infusion, cardiac transplantation, or hospital care

15. Ans. d. Soluble ST2

Braunwald 11th Ed; Page 409

The biomarkers which are used for assessment of heart failure include B-type Natriuretic peptide (BNP) and N-Terminal proBNP (NT proBNP). The other biomarkers which may be useful for prognosticating heart failure include troponin and 'fibrosis markers' such as soluble ST2. Soluble concentration of ST2, a member of interleukin receptor family have been shown to be strongly linked to progressive heart failure and death in patients across all the four stages of heart failure. ST2 plays a pivotal role in the formation of fibrosis in the heart; elevated concentrations of ST2 are thus associated with progressive cardiovascular dysfunction, remodeling, and risk of death. Soluble ST2 concentrations are additive to natriuretic peptides for prognostication, and are useful in both HFrEF and HFpEF.

16. Ans. b. Increase in LV mass

Braunwald 11th Ed; Page 459

In patients with heart failure, medical and device therapy that reduce heart failure morbidity and mortality also lead to decrease in LV volume and mass and there is restoration to normal elliptical shape to the ventricle. These changes represent the final pathway in a series of integrated biologic changes in the cardiac myocytes size and function as well as modification in LV structure and organization that are accompanied by shift of the LV end diastolic pressure volume relationships towards normal. All these changes are collectively called as 'reverse LV remodelling'.

17. Ans. b. Myocardial recovery

Braunwald 11th Ed; Page 459

Refer to explanation for Q. No 16.

18. Ans. b. Activation of adrenergic nervous system

Braunwald 11th Ed; Page 442

Heart failure progresses as result of the over expression of biologically active molecule that are capable of exerting deleterious effect on heart and circulation. The main compensatory mechanism involved in pathogenies of heart failure are activation of adrenergic nervous system and renin–angiotensin system, which are responsible for maintaining cardiac output through increase retention of salt and water, peripheral vasoconstriction and increased contractility, and inflammatory mediators are responsible for cardiac repair and remodeling. The decrease in cardiac output in heart failure activates adrenergic system quite early in the course of heart failure. Activation of sympathetic nervous system in heart failure is accompanied by a concomitant withdrawal of parasympathetic tone.

In contrast with sympathetic nervous system, the component of renin–angiotensin system (RAS) are activated comparatively later in heart failure. The RAS activation in heart failure leads to renal hypoperfusion, decreased filtered sodium reaching the macula densa of the distal tubule, and increased sympathetic stimulation of the kidney, leading to increased renin release from juxtaglomerular apparatus.

Angiotensin II has several important actions that are critical to maintaining short-term circulatory homeostasis. The sustained expression of angiotensin II is maladaptive, leading to fibrosis of the heart, kidneys, and other organs. Angiotensin II can also lead to worsening neurohormonal activation by enhancing the release of noradrenaline from sympathetic nerve endings, as well as stimulating the zona glomerulosa of the adrenal cortex to produce aldosterone. Similar to angiotensin II, aldosterone provides short-term support to the circulation by promoting the reabsorption of sodium in exchange for potassium, in the distal segments of the nephron. However, the sustained expression of aldosterone may exert harmful effects by provoking hypertrophy and fibrosis within the vasculature and myocardium, contributing to reduced vascular compliance and increased ventricular stiffness. In addition, aldosterone also provokes endothelial cell dysfunction, baroreceptor dysfunction, and inhibition of noradrenaline uptake. All these leads to further worsening of heart failure. The mechanism of action of aldosterone in the cardiovascular system appears to involve oxidative stress, with resultant inflammation in target tissue.

19. Ans. d. Angiotensin I-VII

Braunwald 11th Ed; Page 444

The exact role of angiotensin III, angiotensin IV and angiotensin I-VII in heart failure are not known. However, experimental studies suggest that angiotensin I-VII counteracts the effects of angiotensin II, and attenuates LV remodeling. In contrast, angiotensin III directly stimulates the zona glomerulosa of the adrenal glands to produce aldosterone, which promotes sodium resorption in the distal collecting duct of the kidney. Angiotensin III also has an important role in vasopressin release in the brain, which controls water retention in distal collecting duct of the kidney. Angiotensin III in the brain can also modulate cardiac nervous sympathetic hyperactivity, as well as LV remodeling after myocardial infarction.

20. Ans. c. Arginine vasopressin

Braunwald 11th Ed; Page 446

Arginine vasopressin (AVP) is a pituitary hormone that plays important role in regulation of free water clearance and plasma osmolality. Under normal circumstances, AVP is released in response to an increase in plasma osmolality, leading to increased retention of water from the collecting duct. Circulating AVP is elevated in many patients with heart failure, even after correction for plasma osmolality and may contribute to the hyponatremia that occurs in heart failure.

21. Ans. d. Arginine vasopressin

Braunwald 11th Ed; Page 446

A number of counterregulatory neurohormonal systems is activated in heart failure in order to offset the deleterious effects of the vasoconstricting neurohormones. Prominent among these are the prostaglandin E2 and prostacyclin. In addition to being a vasodilator, PGE2 enhances renal sodium excretion and modulates the antidiuretic action of arginine vasopressin. Atrial natriuretic peptide and brain natriuretic peptide (BNP) function as natriuretic hormones that are released in response to increases in atrial and myocardial stretch, often secondary to excessive sodium intake. These peptides act on the kidney and peripheral circulation to unload the heart, through increased excretion of sodium and water, while inhibiting the release of renin and aldosterone.

22. Ans. d. All are correct

Braunwald 11th Ed; Page 447

The natriuretic peptide system consists of five structurally similar peptides: ANP, urodilatin, BNP, C-type natriuretic peptide (CNP), and dendroaspis natriuretic peptide (DNP). ANP is secreted in short bursts in response to acute changes in atrial pressure, while the activation of BNP is regulated transcriptionally in response to chronic increases in atrial/ventricular pressure. ANP and BNP initially are synthesized as prohormones that are subsequently proteolytically cleaved, respectively, to yield large, biologically inactive N-terminal fragments (NT-ANP and NT-BNP) and smaller, biologically active peptides (i.e., ANP and BNP). ANP has a relatively short half-life of approximately 3 minutes, whereas BNP has a plasma half-life of approximately 20 minutes. CNP, which is located primarily in the vasculature, is released as a prohormone that is cleaved into biologically inactive form (NT-CNP). All the three natriuretic peptides are degraded by two mechanisms: NPR-C–mediated internalization, followed by lysosomal degradation and enzymatic degradation by neutral endopeptidase (NEP) or neprilysin, which is widely expressed in multiple tissues, where it often is colocalized with angiotensin converting enzyme (ACE).

23. Ans. a. Inhibition of degradation of natriuretic peptides

Braunwald 11th Ed; Page 447

All the natriuretic peptides are degraded by two major mechanisms: NPR-C–mediated internalization, followed by lysosomal degradation and enzymatic degradation by neutral endopeptidase (NEP) neprilysin. Neprilysin is widely expressed in multiple tissues, where it often is colocalized with ACE. NEP or neprilysin degrades multiple peptides, including natriuretic peptides, angiotensin I, angiotensin II, ET-I, adrenomedullin, opioids, bradykinin, chemotactic peptides, enkephalins, and amyloid-β peptide (Aβ). NEP inhibition of degradation of natriuretic peptides results in vasorelaxation, natriuresis, inhibition of hypertrophy, and fibrosis. On the other hand, inhibition of degradation of other vasoactive peptides, such as angiotensin II, angiotensin I–VII, and ET, opposes the vasodilatory effects of natriuretic peptides. NEP inhibition increases urinary kinin levels, which may contribute to its natriuretic effects. NEP plays an important role in clearance of amyloid peptides in the brain. In particular, NEP or neprilysin is of major importance for degrading the amyloid-beta peptides (Aβ), which play a significant role in neurotoxicity, and formation of amyloid plaques from Aβ aggregates in complex with other proteins is a hallmark of Alzheimer disease. Overexpression of neprilysin ameliorated the development of Alzheimer disease, and disruption of the neprilysin gene induces cognitive dysfunction in a mouse model of Alzheimer disease. Because of the potentially beneficial effects of natriuretic peptides in heart failure, neprilysin is used as an important agent in the treatment of heart failure. The use of a combined AT1 receptor antagonist and a neprilysin inhibitor (valsartan/sacubitril) has been shown to have a favorable impact on heart failure outcome, including quality of life, exercise capacity, and more importantly, heart failure hospitalization and total mortality.

24. Ans. c. Both of the above

Braunwald 11th Ed; Page 447

The drug omapatrilat, is a dual vasopeptidase inhibitor that inhibits both ACE and NEP. However, it has not shown to be more effective than angiotensin converting enzyme inhibition alone in heart failure patients.

25. Ans. a. Necrosis

Braunwald 11th Ed; Page 454

In failing heart, there is a progressive myocytes loss, through necrotic, apoptotic, autophagic cell death pathway, which eventually contribute to progressive cardiac dysfunction and LV remodeling. Necrosis is a cell death which is a very important component of myocardial infarction, heart failure and cerebrovascular accident. The hallmark features of necrosis are loss of plasma membrane integrity and depletion of cellular adenosine triphosphate (ATP). Dysfunction of the plasma membrane in necrotic cells leads to cell swelling and rupture. In the heart, increased plasma membrane permeability allows Ca^{2+} to leak into the cell, exposing the contractile proteins to very high concentrations of this activator, which in turn initiates extreme interactions between the myofilaments, further contributing to disruption of the cellular membrane. Necrotic myocyte death occurs in ischemic heart disease, myocardial injury, toxin exposure (e.g., daunorubicin), infection, and inflammation. Neurohormonal activation can also lead to necrotic cell death. The rupture of cell membranes with cell necrosis releases intracellular contents, so-called danger-associated molecular patterns (DAMPS), which evoke an intense inflammatory reaction, leading to the influx of granulocytes, macrophages, and collagen-secreting fibroblasts into the area of injury. The final result is a fibrotic scar, which may alter the structural and functional properties of the myocardium.

Apoptosis, or programmed cell death, is an evolutionarily process. It is a mechanism by which selectively cells are removed through a highly regulated program of cell suicide. Apoptosis plays an important role in the development in postnatal life and it is critical for tissue homeostasis and surveillance of damaged or transformed cells. However, under certain pathological circumstances, such as acute ischemia and in dilated cardiomyopathy, the apoptotic program can be triggered inappropriately, resulting in inadvertent cell death that can lead to organ failure. In contrast with the cell swelling that characterizes necrosis, during apoptosis the cell shrinks and eventually breaks up into small, membrane-surrounded fragments. These are called as "*apoptotic bodies*". Maintenance of plasma membrane integrity until late in the apoptotic process allows the dying cell to be engulfed by macrophages, which prevents the release of the reactive intracellular contents and therefore preventing an inflammatory reaction.

Autophagy is the homeostatic cellular process of sequestering organelles, proteins, and lipids in a double-membrane vesicle inside the cell (*autophagosome*), where the contents are subsequently delivered to the lysosome for degradation. Unlike necrosis and apoptosis, autophagy is primarily a survival mechanism that regulates the quality and abundance of intracellular proteins and organelles. Autophagy has been shown to play a variety of physiologic roles in the heart, and impaired clearance of autophagosomes may be deleterious, rather than the process of autophagy per se. Autophagic cell death is seen in hypertrophied, failing and hibernating myocardium.

26. Ans. b. Hypertension

Braunwald 11th Ed; Page 463

Concomitant diseases are common in patients with acute heart failure. Hypertension is the most prevalent of the concurrent conditions, present in approximately two-thirds of acute heart failure patients followed by coronary artery disease (CAD) in about half of the patient and dyslipidemia in more than one-third. Other conditions resulting from the vascular injury produced by these diseases, such as CVA (stroke), peripheral vascular disease, and chronic renal insufficiency, are also common in patients with acute heart failure. Diabetes mellitus is present in around 40% of patients with acute heart failure.

27. Ans. d. High ventricular diastolic pressure without overt clinical signs

Braunwald 11th Ed; Page 465

In patients with acute heart failure, distinction is to be made between "clinical congestion" and "hemodynamic congestion." Although patients present with signs and symptoms of systemic congestion such as dyspnea, rales, elevated jugular venous pressure, and edema, this state is often preceded by *hemodynamic congestion,* defined as high ventricular diastolic pressures without overt clinical signs. The clinical congestion may resolve with treatment, but hemodynamic congestion may persist, leading to a high risk of rehospitalization. Hemodynamic congestion may contribute to the progression of heart failure because it may result in increased wall stress as well as in activation of renin–angiotensin–aldosterone system (RAAS) and sympathetic nervous system (SNS).

28. Ans. b. Increase in LV filling pressure

Braunwald 11th Ed; Page 464

Congestion is the common pathway producing clinical symptoms in patients with heart failure. Acute heart failure pathology involves gradual increase in intravascular volume leading to the symptom of congestion and clinical presentation. The studies using implantable hemodynamic monitors suggest that increase in the invasively measured LV filling pressure can occur without substantial changes in the body weight. However, some data suggests that increase in the body weight often precedes decompensation and hospitalization for heart failure. This phenomenon is mainly due to the volume redistribution and dynamic role of vasculature.

29. Ans. d. All of the above

Braunwald 11th Ed; Page 465

Hemodynamic congestion in absence of clinical congestion may contribute to the progression of heart failure, because it may result in increased wall stress as well as in activation of renin–angiotensin–aldosterone system (RAAS) and sympathetic nervous system (SNS). In presence of hemodynamic congestion, the natriuretic peptides which are the main intrinsic counter regulatory hormone in heart failure may undergo abnormal processing that leads to diminished biological activity. Elevated diastolic filling pressure may decrease coronary perfusion pressure resulting in subendocardial ischemia that may further exacerbate cardiac dysfunction. Increased LV filling pressures can also lead to acute changes in ventricular architecture (more spherical shape), contributing to the worsening mitral regurgitation.

30. Ans. d. All are correct

Braunwald 11th Ed; Page 465

Impairment of cardiac function (systolic, diastolic or both) is central to the pathogenesis of heart failure. Although decrease in systolic function plays a role in pathophysiology of acute heart failure, epidemiologically approximately half of patients with acute heart failure have relatively preserved systolic function. Abnormalities in diastolic function are present in heart failure patients regardless of ejection fraction. The impairment of the diastolic function may be related to passive stiffness, abnormal active relaxation of the left ventricle, or both. Hypertension, tachycardia, and myocardial ischemia (even in the absence of CAD) can further impair diastolic filling. All these mechanisms contribute to higher left ventricular end-diastolic pressure, which is reflected back to the pulmonary capillary circulation leading to the pulmonary congestion. Diastolic dysfunction alone may be insufficient to lead to acute heart failure, but it serves as a substrate on which other precipitating factors like atrial fibrillation, coronary artery disease, hypertension can lead to decompensation.

31. Ans. c. Elevated central venous pressure

Braunwald 11th Ed; Page 466

The term 'cardiorenal syndrome' is used to describe pathological interaction between the cardiac and renal axis in the setting of heart failure. Cardiorenal syndrome describes the clinical situation of worsening measures of renal function in the setting of persistent congestion. This clinical scenario has been associated with poor outcomes. Although often assumed to be related to low cardiac output and renal blood flow, hemodynamic studies have confirmed that strongest predictor of worsening renal function in heart failure patients relates to elevated central venous pressure, which is reflected back to the renal veins and leads directly to changes in GFR. There is importance of evaluating changes in renal function in the context of the overall clinical picture. Worsening renal function in the setting of ongoing clinical improvement is generally reflective of successful decongestion and does not portend a poor prognosis.

32. Ans. b. More likely in man

Braunwald 11th Ed; Page 467

Hypertension is seen in >50% of patients with acute heart failure with systolic blood pressure >140 mm Hg and 25% patients with >160 mm Hg. Hypertension is triggered by a high sympathetic tone related to dyspnea and accompanying anxiety or acute hypertension with accompanying changes in afterload may be triggered for decompensation. Acute hypertensive heart failure are more likely to have preserved systolic function, they more likely to be women patients and more likely to have sudden onset of symptom. Frank pulmonary edema with evident rales and florid congestion on chest X-ray is much more common in this group of patients than in those with more gradual onset of symptoms, likely related to the difference in LV compliance, acuity of pressure changes, and pulmonary lymphatic capacity. Although these patients are severely ill at the initial presentation with hypoxemia and possible need for non-invasive ventilation or even intubation, this group of patients tends to respond well to therapy and have lower in-hospital mortality.

33. Ans. c. Jugular venous pressure

Braunwald 11th Ed; Page 469

Although the blood pressure is generally related to the cardiac output and state of the organ perfusion, systemic hypoperfusion may present with normal blood pressure, and likewise, patients with advanced forms of heart failure may have chronically low blood pressure not associated with acute hypoperfusion. Pulse pressure (the difference between systolic and diastolic blood pressure) is a useful measure that is an indirect marker of cardiac output. A low pulse pressure is a marker of a low cardiac output and confers an increased risk in patients admitted with acute heart failure. The *jugular venous pressure* (JVP) is a barometer of systemic venous hypertension. The JVP reflects the right atrial pressure which typically is an indirect measure of LV filling pressures. *Rales* or inspiratory crackles are the most common physical examination finding in heart failure. However, rales are often not heard in patients with a background of chronic heart failure and pulmonary venous hypertension, because of increased lymphatic drainage. Absence of rales does not necessarily imply normal LV filling pressures.

Peripheral edema is found in >65% of patients admitted with acute heart failure and is less common in patients presenting with predominantly low-output heart failure or cardiogenic shock. The presence of edema has a reasonable positive predictive value for acute heart failure but a low sensitivity, so its absence does not exclude that diagnosis. Edema caused by acute heart failure is usually dependent, symmetric, and pitting. It is estimated that a minimum of 4 L of extracellular fluid is accumulated to produce clinically detectable edema.

34. **Ans. b. Minimum of 4 L**

Braunwald 11th Ed; Page - 469

Refer to explanation for Q. No 33.

35. **Ans. d. All are correct**

Braunwald 11th Ed; Page 469

The natriuretic peptides are counter regulatory hormones in heart failure with vasodilatory and other effects and they play an important role in differential diagnosis of patients presenting in the emergency department with dyspnea. For diagnostic natriuretic peptide testing in the setting of acute heart failure, it is found that negative predictive value (NPV; i.e., the ability to rule out heart failure a as a cause of dyspnea) is generally greater than positive predictive value (PPV) (i.e, the ability to definitively identify a diagnosis of heart failure as the cause of dyspnea). As with all biomarker testing, false positives (e.g., due to acute MI or pulmonary embolism) and false negatives (obesity) may occur. Although natriuretic peptide levels tend to be lower in patients with HfpEF than those with reduced systolic function, natriuretic peptide testing cannot reliably distinguish HfpEF from systolic heart failure in an individual patient.

36. **Ans. d. Blood urea nitrogen**

Braunwald 11th Ed; Page 469

Assessment of renal function is a critical component in the management of patients with acute heart failure. Estimated glomerular filtration rate (eGFR) should be calculated because serum creatinine may underestimate the degree of renal dysfunction, especially in elderly patients. Blood urea nitrogen (BUN) is more directly related to the severity of acute heart failure than creatinine and is typically elevated on admission in a large number of patients with acute heart failure. In addition to reflecting intrinsic renal function, serum BUN is approximately proportional to neurohormonal activation in acute heart failure.

37. **Ans. c. Elevated/High blood pressure**

Braunwald 11th Ed; Page 470

In a risk assessment model, among the variables, it has been identified that an elevated BUN, lower systolic BP and higher serum creatinine level at admission are the best predictor of in-hospital mortality. In a predictive model of post discharge event, it has been found that higher blood pressure is consistently associated with lower risk. In OPTIMIZE HF study, it was found that there was no evidence of increased risk even at a very high level of blood pressure (i.e., > 180 mm Hg).

Renal function (estimated by BUN, creatinine, GFR) is an important predictor of prognosis in patients with acute heart failure. BUN has consistently been shown to be a stronger predictor of outcome than creatinine. BUN appears to integrate a variety of important prognostic aspects, including intrinsic renal function and neurohormonal activation (due to impaired urea clearance). BNP and NT-proBNP have been demonstrated to be powerful predictors of risk in heart failure. In the setting of acute heart failure, natriuretic peptide levels at initial presentation are important predictors of both short and long-term outcomes.

38. **Ans. b. ACE inhibitor or ARBs should be used only in patients with MI who have reduced ejection fraction (< 35%)**

Braunwald 11th Ed; Page 517

Patients with left ventricular dysfunction who have not developed symptoms are placed in stage B heart failure. The goal of therapy in stage B heart failure is to reduce the risk of further damage to the heart and to minimize the rate of progression of LV dysfunction. In the absence of contraindication, beta blockers and angiotensin converting enzymes inhibitors or angiotensin receptor antagonist in the people who have intolerance of ACEIs are recommended for all patients with history of myocardial infarction regardless ejection fraction, and for all patients with diminished ejection fraction regardless history of MI. Calcium channel blockers with negative inotropic effect should not be used in these population. Guidelines directed therapy also recommend use of ICD in patients with asymptomatic ischemic cardiomyopathy who have had recent (> 40 days) MI with an EF of 30% or less, who are on an appropriate medical therapy and who have reasonable expectation of life longer than one year.

39. **Ans. d. Nebivolol**

Braunwald 11th Ed; Page 519

Use of one of the three beta blockers proven to reduce mortality (i.e. bisoprolol, carvedilol, and sustained release metoprolol succinate) is recommended for all patients with current or prior history of heart failure with reduced ejection fraction unless contraindicated to reduce morbidity and mortality.

ACC/AHA guidelines for treatment of patients with prior or current symptoms of chronic HFrEF (Stage C)

Class	Indication	Level of evidence
	Nonpharmacologic interventions	
I	• Patients with HF should receive specific education to facilitate HF self-care	B
	• Exercise training (or regular physical activity) is recommended as safe and effective for patients with HF who are able to participate to improve functional status	A
IIa	• Cardiac rehabilitation can be useful in clinically stable patients with HF to improve functional capacity, exercise duration, health-related quality of life, and mortality	B
	• Sodium restriction is reasonable for patients with symptomatic HF to reduce congestive symptoms	C
	• Continuous positive airway pressure (CPAP) can be beneficial to increase LVEF and improve functional status in patients with HF and sleep apnea	B
	Pharmacologic interventions	
I	• Measures listed as class I recommendations for patients in stages A and B are recommended where appropriate	A, B, C
	• GDMT as depicted in should be the mainstay of pharmacologic therapy for HFrEF	A
	Diuretics	
I	Diuretics are recommended in patients with HFrEF who have evidence of fluid retention, unless contra indicated, to improve symptoms	C
	ACEIs/ARBs/ARNIs	
I	• The use of ACE inhibitors is beneficial for patients with prior or current symptoms of chronic HFrEF, to reduce morbidity and mortality	A
	• The use of ARBs to reduce morbidity and mortality is recommended in patients with prior or current symptoms of chronic HFrEF who are intolerant of ACE inhibitors because of cough or angioedema	A
I	ARNIs are recommended in patients with HFrEF unless contraindicated, to reduce morbidity and mortality	B-R
I	ARNIs are recommended in patients with HFrEF NYHA Class II–III who are tolerant of an ACE inhibitor or ARB; replacement by a ARNI is recommended to further reduce morbidity and mortality	B-R
IIa	ARBs are reasonable to reduce morbidity and mortality as alternatives to ACE inhibitors as first-line therapy for patients with HFrEF, especially for patients already taking ARBs for other indications, unless contraindicated	A
IIb	Addition of an ARB may be considered in persistently symptomatic patients with HFrEF who are already being treated with an ACE inhibitor and a beta blocker in whom an aldosterone antagonist is not indicated or tolerated	A
IIa	Ivabradine can be beneficial to reduce HF hospitalizations in patients with NYHA Class II–IIIc HFrEF (LVEF <35%) who are receiving GDMT, including a beta blocker, and who are in sinus rhythm with a heart rate of ≥70 beats/min	B-R
III: Harm	Routinely combining an ACE inhibitor, an ARB, and an aldosterone antagonist is not recommended	C
III: Harm	ARNI should not be administered concomitantly with ACE inhibitors or within the last dose of an ACE inhibitor	B-R
III: Harm	ARNI should not be administered to patients with a history of angioedema	C-EO
	Beta-adrenergic blockers	
I	Use of one of the three beta blockers proven to reduce mortality (i.e., bisoprolol, carvedilol, and sustained-release metoprolol succinate) is recommended for all patients with current or prior symptoms of HFrEF, unless contraindicated, to reduce morbidity and mortality	A

Continued

Continued

Class	Indication	Level of evidence
	Aldosterone receptor antagonists	
I	Aldosterone receptor antagonists (or MRAs) are recommended in patients with NYHA Class II–IV and who have LVEF ≤35%. Unless contraindicated, to reduce morbidity and mortality	A
I	Aldosterone receptor antagonists are recommended to reduce morbidity and mortality following an acute MI in patients who have LVEF ≤40% who develop symptoms of HF or who have a history of diabetes mellitus, unless contraindicated	B
III: Harm	Inappropriate use of aldosterone receptor antagonists is potentially harmful because of life-threatening hyperkalemia or renal insufficiency when serum creatinine is >2.5 mg/dL in men or >2.0 mg/dL in women [or estimated glomerular filtration rate (eGFR) < 30 mL/min/173 m^2], and/or potassium >5.0 mEq/L	B
	Hydralazine and isosorbide dinitrate	
I	The combination of hydralazine and isosorbide dinitrate is recommended to reduce morbidity and mortality for patients self-described as African Americans with NYHA Class III–IV HFrEF receiving optimal therapy with ACE inhibitors and beta blockers, unless contraindicated	A
IIa	A combination of hydralazine and isosorbide dinitrate can be useful to reduce morbidity or mortality in patients with current or prior symptomatic HFrEF who cannot be given an ACE inhibitor or ARB because of drug intolerance, hypotension, or renal insufficiency, unless contraindicated	B
	Digoxin	
IIa	Digoxin can be beneficial in patients with HFrEF, unless contraindicated, to decrease hospitalizations for HF	B
	Anticoagulation	
I	Patients with chronic HF with permanent/persistent/paroxysmal AF and an additional risk factor for cardioembolic stroke (history of hypertension, diabetes mellitus, previous stroke or transient ischemic attack, or ≥75 years of age) should receive chronic anticoagulant therapy	A
I	The selection of an anticoagulant agent (warfarin, dabigatran, apixaban, or rivaroxaban) for permanent/persistent/paroxysmal AF should be individualized on the basis of risk factors, cost, tolerability, patient preference, potential for drug interactions, and other clinical characteristics, including time in the international normalized ratio (INR) therapeutic range if the patient has been taking warfarin	C
IIa	Chronic anticoagulation is reasonable for patients with chronic HF who have permanent/persistent/paroxysmal AF but are without an additional risk factor for cardioembolic stroke	B
III: No benefit	Anticoagulation is not recommended in patients with chronic HFrEF without AF, a prior thromboembolic event, or a cardioembolic source	B
	Statins	
III: No benefit	Statins are not beneficial as adjunctive therapy when prescribed solely for HF	A
	Omega-3 polyunsaturated fatty acids	
IIa	Omega-3 polyunsaturated fatty acid (PUFA) supplementation is reasonable to use as adjunctive therapy in patients with NYHA Class II–IV symptoms and HFrEF or HFpEF, unless contraindicated, to reduce mortality and cardiovascular hospitalizations	B
	Drugs of unproven value or that may cause harm	
III: No benefit	• Nutritional supplements as treatment for HF are not recommended in patients with current or prior symptoms of HFrEF	B
	• Hormonal therapies other than to correct deficiencies are not recommended for patients with current or prior symptoms of HFrEF	C
III: Harm	• Drugs known to adversely affect the clinical status of patients with current or prior symptoms of HFrEF are potentially harmful and should be avoided or withdrawn whenever possible (e.g., most antiarrhythmic drugs, most calcium channel blockers except amlodipine, NSAIDs, thiazolidinediones)	B
	• Long-term use of infused positive inotropic drugs is potentially harmful for patients with HFrEF, except as palliation for patients with end-stage disease who cannot be stabilized with standard medical treatment (see recommendations for stage D)	C
	Calcium channel blockers	
III: No benefit	Calcium channel blocking drugs are not recommended as routine therapy for patients with HFrEF	A

40. Ans. a. In all patients who are tolerant to ACEI/ARB to further reduce morbidity and mortality in patients with NYHA class II–III heart failure

Braunwald 11th Ed; Page 518

In ACC 2017 new guideline, there is a class I recommendation to replace an ACE inhibitor/ARB by a ARNI to further reduce morbidity and mortality in patients with NYHA class II–III heart failure. In 2016 ESC guideline, it was recommended that ACEI/ARB should not be replaced by an ARNI unless the patients remain symptomatic after an ACEI (equivalent to 10 mg twice daily of enalapril) or ARB, a beta blocker and mineralocorticoid receptor antagonist (MRA), and had elevated level of BNP or Pro-BNP or if there was a heart failure hospitalization within past 12 months with an elevated plasma level of BNP > 100 pg/mL or NT-ProBNP > 400 pg/mL.

41. Ans. d. Obese patients

Braunwald 11th Ed; Page 529

Circulating level of BNP and NT-ProBNP are elevated in patients with heart failure with preserved EF compared with the person without heart failure but are lower than in patients with heart failure with reduced ejection fraction. In patients with HfpEF, increased BNP is directly related to LV diastolic filling pressure and end diastolic wall stress. For any given LV diastolic filling pressure in patient with HfpEF, BNP levels are lower in obese patients and higher in women, older patient and in patient with concomitant pulmonary disease and renal dysfunction. There are several methods to allow adjustment of natriuretic peptide level for this concomitant state such as the adjustment for BMI. For everyone kg/m^2 increased in BMI above 25, NP level fall 4%. Because patient with HfpEF have a smaller LV cavity and thicker LV walls, their end diastolic wall stress is much lower than in HFeEF, even in setting of high systolic and diastolic pressure, thus producing a lower stimulus for BNP production. On average patients with HfpEF presenting with acute decompensation have a BNP value of 100–500 pg/mL Vs 500–1,500 pg/mL in patients with heart failure with reduced ejection fraction.

42. Ans. d. Digoxin

Braunwald 11th Ed; Page 519

Digoxin can be beneficial in patients with heart failure with reduced ejection fraction unless contraindicated, to decrease hospitalization for heart failure. However, it has not shown any mortality benefit. Contrary to that, ACEI/ARNI, Aldosterone receptor antagonist have shown to reduce morbidity and mortality. Hydralazine and isosorbide dinitrate combination is recommended to reduce morbidity and mortality for patients who are African, American with NYHA class III–IV heart failure.

43. Ans. d. Digoxin

Hurst's 14th Ed; Page 1694

The guideline directed medical therapy for heart failure with reduced ejection fraction now include four medications classes that includes SGLT-2i. The four groups are: (1) renin–angiotensin system inhibition with angiotensin receptor neprilysin inhibitor (ARNI), angiotensin converting enzyme inhibitors or angiotensin II receptor blocker alone; (2) beta blocker; (3) mineralocorticoid receptor antagonists (MRAs) and (4) the new group SGLT-2i.

44. Ans. b. Cardiac amyloidosis

Hurst's 14th Ed; Page 1503

Tafamidis affects a protein called transthyretin (TTR, mid primarily and liver). Transthyretin mediated amyloidosis is a condition in which abnormal deposit of TTR protein build up in many parts of body interfering normal function. Built up of TTR in the heart can lead to heart failure.

45. Ans. d. All of the above

Hurst's 14th Ed; Page 1430

Recovery of systolic function appears more common in those patients with LV systolic dysfunction occurring in the setting of adverse energetic circumstances (e.g., chronic tachycardia or thyroid disease), or dilated cardiomyopathy is associated with immune response (e.g., peripartum cardiomyopathy, acute myocarditis, systemic inflammatory response), are in those who have undergone revascularization or device therapy.

46. Ans. d. All of the above

Hurst's 14th Ed; Page 1430

Refer to explanation for Q. No 45.

47. Ans. d. Potassium sparing diuretic (spironolactone)

Hurst's 14th Ed; Page 1701–1704

Bumetanide, furosemide and torsemide inhibit reabsorption of sodium or chloride at the loop of Henle, whereas thiazide like diuretics act in the distal convoluting tubule and potassium sparing diuretics (spironolactone) in the collecting duct.

48. Ans. a. Thiazide

Hurst's 14th Ed; Page 1701 - 1704

Refer to explanation for Q. No 47.

49. Ans. c. Thiazide diuretic

Hurst's 14th Ed; Page 1701 - 1704

Refer to explanation for Q. No 47.

50. **Ans. a. Hepatic failure**

Braunwald 11th Ed; Page 500

In patient with heart failure, diuretic therapy is commonly initiated with low doses and the dose is increased until urine output increases and weight decreases, generally by 0.5 to 1 kg daily. Patient may become unresponsive to high doses of diuretic drugs, if they consume large amount of dietary sodium, are taking agents that can block the effects of diuretics (e.g., NSAIDs) or have significant impairment of renal function or perfusion.

51. **Ans. b. Intravenous administration of diuretic (bolus or continuous infusion)**

Braunwald 11th Ed; Page 503

Diuretic resistance is common in patient with congestive heart failure. It can be overcome in several ways, including escalation of loop diuretic dose, intravenous administration of diuretics (bolus or continuous infusion) or combination of different diuretics classes. The use of a thiazide or thiazide like diuretic (metolazone) in combination with a loop diuretic inhibits compensatory distal tubular sodium reabsorption, leading to enhanced natriuresis. However, addition of metolazone to loop diuretic is found to increase the risk of hypokalemia, hyponatremia, worsening renal function and mortality, whereas use of high dose of loop diuretics was not found to adversely affect survival. In DOSE (Diuretic Optimization Strategies Evaluation) trial it was found that use of intravenous loop diuretic offers benefits in terms of reducing the diuretic resistance.

52. **Ans. c. Spironolactone**

Braunwald 11th Ed; Page 506–507

MRA, also known as aldosterone antagonists or antimineralocorticoids, they have shown consistent improvements in all cause mortality, heart failure hospitalization and sudden cardiac death across a wide range of patients with heart failure with reduced EF. It should be used cautiously in patient with renal dysfunction or hyperkalemia (eGFR < 30 mL/min/1.73 m^2 or serum potassium > 5.0 mEq/L). Because of the higher selectivity of eplerenone for the aldosterone receptor, adverse effects such as gynecomastia and vaginal bleeding are seen less often in patients who take eplerenone than in those who take spironolactone.

53. **Ans. a. Benefit of ACE inhibition is seen only in the patient with moderate to severe symptoms of heart failure**

Braunwald 11th Ed; Page 504

ACEI reduce morbidity and mortality in heart failure with reduced ejection fraction. Randomized control trials (RCTs) clearly establish the benefits of ACE inhibition in patients with mild, moderate or severe symptoms of heart failure and in patients with or without CAD.

54. **Ans. d. Omega-3 PUFA**

Braunwald 11th Ed; Page 511

In pharmacological management of heart failure with reduced ejection fraction, several classes of medications have either unproven value or potential for harm. These drugs are calcium channel blocker, antiarrhythmic drugs, NSAIDs, medications for treatment of type 2 diabetes mellitus including thiazolidinediones, DPP-4 inhibitors and vitamins, hormones, and nutritional supplement. Supplementation with omega-3 PUFA has been evaluated as an adjunctive therapy for CVD and heart failure. The GISSI-HF (effect of n-3 polyunsaturated fatty acids in patients with chronic heart failure) trial showed a reduction in death among post MI patients taking 1 g of omega-3 PUFA. Trials in prevention of CVD including heart failure showed that omega-3 PUFA supplementation results in a 10–20% risk reduction in fatal and nonfatal cardiovascular events when used with other evidence-based therapies.

55. **Ans. c. Both of the above**

Braunwald 11th Ed; Page 501

Hyperkalemia is common in heart failure and can lead to arrhythmia. Two newer gastrointestinal potassium binding agents, patiromer and sodium zirconium cyclosilicate, have been shown to lower potassium level and enable treatment with a RAAS in patients with heart failure.

56. **Ans. d. NSAIDs**

Braunwald 11th Ed; Page 503

NSAIDs inhibits the synthesis of renal prostaglandins, which mediate vasodilation in the kidneys and directly inhibit sodium resorption in thick ascending loop of Henle and collecting tubule. Hence, NSAIDs can cause sodium and water retention and blunt the effect of diuretics. Several observational cohort studies have revealed increased morbidity and mortality in patients with heart failure using either nonselective or selective NSAIDs.

57. **Ans. b. If symptom improved at lower doses, the medication dose need not be titrated to the trial defined target dose**

2022 ACC/AHA Guidelines for Management of Heart Failure

Clinical trials of ACEI, ARB, ARNI, beta blockers and most other HFrEF medications had therapy initiated at low dose by trial protocol. If the initial dose is well tolerated, then the guidelines state that up-titration of medication dose should be done over time to a specified target dose unless not well tolerated. Even if symptoms improved or other indicators of response were shown at lower doses, medication dose should be increased to the trial defined target doses. Use of all four classes of drugs has been estimated to reduce all cause mortality by 73% compared with no treatment. If the target cannot be achieved or is not well tolerated, then the highest tolerated dose is recommended. In patients with HFrEF, beta blockers provide dose dependent improvement in LVEF, reduction in heart failure hospitalization and reduction in all cause mortality. Trials of lower versus higher doses of ACEI and ARB have shown, lower risk of cardiovascular death or heart failure hospitalization with higher doses, with similar safety and tolerability.

58. Ans. d. Simultaneous initiation and sequencing should be done based on patient's symptoms, vital signs, functional status, tolerance and renal function

2022 ACC/AHA Guidelines for Management of Heart Failure

Initiation and titration should be individualized and optimized according to patient's symptoms, vital signs, functional status, tolerance, renal function, electrolytes, comorbidities, specific cause of heart failure and regularity of follow-up. In patient with HFrEF, simultaneous initiation or sequencing, and order of guideline directed medications are usually individualized according to above mentioned factors.

59. Ans. d. SHIFT

2022 ACC/AHA Guidelines for Management of Heart Failure

Heart rate is a strong predictor of cardiovascular outcome in general population and in patients with cardiovascular disease including heart failure. The SHIFT (ivabradine and outcomes in chronic heart failure) trial tested the hypothesis that reducing heart rate in patients with heart failure improves cardiovascular outcomes. SHIFT demonstrated the efficacy of ivabradine, a sinoatrial node modulator that selectively inhibits the I_f current, in reducing the composite endpoint of cardiovascular death or heart failure hospitalization in patient with heart failure.

60. Ans. d. All are correct

2022 ACC/AHA Guidelines for Management of Heart Failure

In SHIFT trial, though the primary outcome was a composite of hospitalization and cardiovascular death, the greatest benefit with ivabradine was a reduction in heart failure hospitalization. SHIFT included patients with HFrEF and LVEF < 35% who were in sinus rhythm with a resting heart rate of > 70 bpm. The target of ivabradine therapy is heart rate and the benefits of ivabradine results from reduction in heart rate. Given the well proven mortality benefit of beta blocker therapy, these agents should be initiated and up titrated to target doses, as tolerated, before assessing the resting heart rate for consideration of ivabradine initiation.

61. Ans. d. Digoxin

2022 ACC/AHA Guidelines for Management of Heart Failure

Digoxin has been used for treatment of heart failure for > 5 decades. However, there is only one large, RCT of digoxin in patients with heart failure. This trial showed that treatment with digoxin for 2–5 years had no effect on mortality but modestly reduced the combined risk of death and hospitalization. It also showed no significant benefit on health-related quality of life. Digoxin helps in improving symptoms and exercise tolerance in mild-to-moderate heart failure, however, without any mortality benefit.

62. Ans. c. Vericiguat

2022 ACC/AHA Guidelines for Management of Heart Failure

Oral soluble guanylyl cyclase stimulator (vericiguat) directly binds and stimulates sGC and increases cGMP production. cGMP has several potential beneficial effects in patients with HF, including vasodilation, improvement in endothelial function, as well as decrease in fibrosis and remodeling of the heart. The VICTORIA (Vericiguat Global Study in Subjects with Heart Failure with Reduced Ejection Fraction) trial studied high-risk patients with heart failure with reduced ejection fraction comparing vericiguat to placebo.

63. Ans. d. Should be ischemic cardiomyopathy only

Braunwald 11th Ed; Page 548

The ICD is recommended for patients with non-ischemic DCMP or ischemic heart disease at least 40 days post MI with LVEF < 35% and NYHA Class II or III symptoms on chronic GDMT, who have reasonable expectation of meaningful survival of > 1 year. ICD therapy is recommended for this set up of patients for primary prevention of SCD to reduce total mortality. In the MADIT-I (Multicenter Automatic Defibrillator Implantation Trial) patient with previous MI, LVEF < 35% with non-sustained VT had a mortality benefit with ICD. Similar population in MUSTT (Multicenter Unsustained Tachycardia Trial) also showed benefit.

64. Ans. a. Patient with wider QRS duration (> 150 msec) and with LBBB

Braunwald 11th Ed; Page 546

The previous trials have shown that most benefit of ICD is gained with wider QRS duration and with LBBB. It has been proved in the trials like COMPANION, CARE-HF, MEDIT CRT, REVERSE, RAFT. QRS duration of > 150 msec was a predictor of response. The subgroup analysis of CRT trials have shown no benefit for those with LVEF < 35%, non-LBBB 120–149 msec and NYHA class I–II heart failure.

65. Ans. c. Benefit enhances with increasing with age

Braunwald 11th Ed; Page 554-555

CABG has been shown to improve outcome in patients with left main or left main equivalent disease and heart failure. Long term follow-up showed a reduction in all cause cardiovascular and heart failure hospitalization and all cause cardiovascular mortality in patients with LV dysfunction, who receives CABG and GDMT compared with GDMT alone. The long-term survival benefit is greater in those with more advanced ischemic cardiomyopathy (lower EF or 3 vessel disease) and diminishes with increasing age. CABG also improve quality of life compared with GDMT alone.

66. Ans. d. All

Braunwald 11th Ed; Chapter 26-27

GDMT including RAAS inhibition, beta blocker and biventricular pacing improved mitral regurgitation and LV dimension in patients with heart failure with reduced ejection fraction and secondary mitral regurgitation, particularly mitral regurgitation that is proportionate to LV dilatation. In a small, randomized control trial, Sacubitril–Valsartan resulted in significant reduction in effective regurgitant area, and in regurgitant volume when compared to valsartan alone.

67. Ans. d. Following remission in patients with HFrEF and HFmrEF, it is important to withdraw GDMT

Braunwald 11th Ed; Chapter 25-26

Continuation of GDMT for patients with improved HFrEF or HFmrEF is important to reduce the risk of recrudescent heart failure. In open label randomized, controlled trial, phased withdrawal of heart failure medications in patients with previous DCM, who were now asymptomatic and whose LVEF had improved from < 40 to > 50%, whose left ventricular end diastolic volume had normalized and who had an NT-proBNP concentration < 250 ng/L, resulted in relapse of cardiomyopathy and heart failure in 40% of patients within 6 months. Relapse is defined as at least one of these: (a) reduction in LVEF by > 10% and < 50%, (b) an increased in LVEDV by > 10% and to higher than the normal range, (c) a twofold raised in NT-pro BNP concentration and to > 400 ng/L or 4 clinical evidences of heart failure.

68. Ans. d. Amyloidosis

2022 ACC/AHA Guidelines for Management of Heart Failure

Cardiac amyloidosis is a restrictive cardiomyopathy with extra cellular myocardial protein deposition, most commonly monoclonal immunoglobulin light change (amyloid cardiomyopathy) or transthyretin amyloidosis. Transthyretin amyloidosis can be caused by pathogenetic variant in the transthyretin gene *TTR* (variant transthyretin amyloidosis). Diagnosis of this transthyretin amyloidosis is based on demonstration of LV thickening (wall thickness > 14 mm) along with symptom of fatigue, dyspnea or edema. There is often a discordance between wall thickness on echocardiogram and QRS voltage on ECG and also LV longitudinal strain impairment on echocardiography and diffused late gadolinium enhancement on cardiac MRI. Transthyretin amyloidosis is prevalent in severe aortic stenosis, HFpEF, Carpal–Tunnel syndrome, lumbar spinal stenosis and autonomic or sensory neuropathy.

69. Ans. d. All of the above

2022 ACC/AHA Guidelines for Management of Heart Failure

Refer to explanation for Q. No 68.

70. Ans. d. Cardiac amyloidosis

2022 ACC/AHA Guidelines for Management of Heart Failure

Refer to explanation for Q. No 68.

71. Ans. d. All of the above

2022 ACC/AHA Guidelines for Management of Heart Failure

In patient with cardiac amyloidosis due to transthyretin gene and EF < 40%, GDMT may be poorly tolerated. The vasodilating effect of ARNI, ACEI, and ARB may exacerbate hypotension especially with amyloid associated autonomic dysfunction. Beta blocker may worsen heart failure symptom as the patient with amyloid cardiomyopathy rely on heart rate response to maintain cardiac output. Intracardiac thrombosis occurs in approximately one-third of patients with cardiac amyloidosis, in some cases in absence of diagnosed AF and regardless of CHA_2DS_2-VASc score. The use of anticoagulation reduces the risk of intracardiac thrombosis. Patients with cardiac amyloidosis may have acquired hemostatic abnormalities including coagulation factor deficiencies, hyperfibrinolysis and platelet dysfunction. However, they are often not associated with hemostatic defects.

72. Ans. c. Disproportionate elevation of left sided filling pressure

2022 ACC/AHA Guidelines for Management of Heart Failure

Majority of patients with acute heart failure have clinical evidence of congestion without hypoperfusion. Elevation of right and left sided cardiac filling pressure are usually proportional in decompensation of chronic heart failure with low ejection fraction. However, in 25% of patients have a mismatched between right and left sided filling pressure. Disproportionate elevation of right sided pressure, particularly with tricuspid regurgitation, hinders effective decongestion. Disproportionate elevation of left sided filling pressure may be a cause of dyspnea in the absence of jugular venous distention and edema. Elevated natriuretic peptide can help identify.

73. Ans. b. Disproportionate elevation of right sided pressure especially in presence of TR

2022 ACC/AHA Guidelines for Management of Heart Failure

Refer to explanation for Q. No 72.

74. Ans. b. Weekly Intravenous Ferric carboxymaltose

2022 ACC / AHA Guidelines for Management of Heart Failure

Anemia is independently associated with heart failure disease severity and mortality and iron deficiency appears to be associated with reduced exercise capacity. Repletion of iron has been shown to improve exercise tolerance and quality of life. The FAIR-HF (Ferric carboxymaltose Assessment in patients with IRon deficiency and chronic Heart Failure) trial showed significant improvement in NYHA classification, 6 minutes' walk test and quality of life in patients with chronic heart failure, who received weekly intravenous ferric carboxymaltose or oral iron supplementation. However, the IRONOUT-HF (Iron Repletion Effect on Oxygen Uptake in Heart Failure) trial showed no such improvement with oral iron supplementation. This is attributed to the poor absorption of oral iron and inadequacy of oral iron to improve iron store in patients with heart failure. Therefore, oral iron is not adequate to treat iron deficiency anemia in patients with heart failure. Various trials have shown that Erythropoietin stimulating agents shows a trend toward improvement in functional capacity and reduction in hospitalization. However, the largest trial with Darbepoetin showed no benefit and an increased risk in thrombotic events including stroke.

75. Ans. a. Continuous positive air pressure ventilation

2022 ACC/AHA Guidelines for Management of Heart Failure

Patient with heart failure often have concomitant obstructive sleep disorder breathing. Patient with heart failure can have both obstructive sleep apnea and central sleep apnea. Sleep study can help in decision making in patients with heart failure. In patients with heart failure and central sleep apnea, continuous positive airway pressure is associated with better sleep quality and nocturnal oxygen saturation but has not been shown to affects survival. In adult with heart failure with reduced EF and sleep disorder breathing, meta-analysis of different RCTs have shown that positive air pressure therapy results in moderate reduction in BNP and improvement in blood pressure and LVEF. Adaptive servo ventilation was associated with increased mortality in several trials involving patient with heart failure with reduced ejection fraction and central sleep apnea. The weight of evidence does not support the use adaptive servo ventilation for central sleep apnea in heart failure with reduced EF.

76. Ans. c. SGLT-2i

2022 ACC/AHA Guidelines for Management of Heart Failure

The American Diabetes Association guidelines recommend the use of SGLT-2i as first line agent for treatment of hyperglycemia in patients with diabetes with heart failure or at high risk of heart failure. Use of this class of drugs is associated with reduction in major adverse cardiovascular event including hospitalization for heart failure and cardiovascular death.

77. Ans. c. AV nodal ablation with implantation of a CRT device

2022 ACC/AHA Guidelines for Management of Heart Failure

If a rhythm-controlled strategy fails or it's desired in patients with heart failure and atrial fibrillation, and ventricular rate remains high rapid despite medical therapy after all other options are exhausted, atrioventricular nodal ablation with implantation CRT device can be considered as treatment option. Ablate and pace is an old strategy for difficult to control AF. Early studies with RV pacing showed benefit. However, when RV pacing was compared with cardiac resynchronization in more recent trials especially in those with reduced LVEF, CRT generally proved produced more benefit than RV pacing.

78. Ans. b. Anticoagulation should be used in all patients with heart failure with or without AF

2022 ACC/AHA Guidelines for Management of Heart Failure

The interplay between atrial fibrillation (AF) and heart failure is complex. AF may worsen heart failure but also heart failure increases the risk of AF. Data from randomized trial support the use of anticoagulation among those with heart failure and AF, but not in patients with heart failure without AF. Anticoagulation may be accomplished by DOAC or with warfarin. Heart failure is a hypercoagulable state and serve as an independent risk factor for stroke, systemic embolization and mortality in setting of AF. Anticoagulation is indicated in most patients with heart failure and concomitant AF barring contraindication. In patient with heart failure and CHA_2DS_2-VASc score of 1, those with AF had a three folds higher risk compared with individual without concomitant AF. In a post hoc analysis of two contemporary heart failure trials, paroxysmal and new onset atrial fibrillation are associated with a greater risk for hospitalization caused by heart failure or stroke. Regardless of whether patient received rhythm or rate control for AF anticoagulation is recommended for patients with heart failure in AF for stroke prevention with CHA_2DS_2-VASc score > 2 for men and > 3 for women.

79. Ans. c. Dabigatran

2022 ACC/AHA Guidelines for Management of Heart Failure

Among the NOAC available the factor Xa inhibitors includes apixaban, rivaroxaban, edoxaban while the direct thrombin inhibitor is dabigatran.

80. Ans. b. ACEI and beta blockers

2022 ACC / AHA Guidelines for Management of Heart Failure

Heart failure secondary to cancer therapy related cardiomyopathy is associated with significant worse outcomes. Patients who developed heart failure while receiving potentially cardiotoxic therapy should have this therapy discontinued while a diagnostic workup is undertaken to understand the cause of heart failure and initiate GDMT. Trastuzumab is associated with asymptomatic decrease in LVEF in around 10% of the patients and shows high rate of recovery and low rate of discontinuation of therapy. Trastuzumab is often continued in patients deemed low risk while neurohormonal blockade is initiated. While patient diagnosed with anthracycline related cardiomyopathy typically the agent should be discontinued given the associated high mortality. Available data in patients with anthracycline and trastuzumab induced cardiomyopathy suggests beta blockers and ACEI are effective in improving LV dysfunction.

81. Ans. c. Serial biomarkers estimation (troponin) may be useful in risk stratification

2022 ACC/AHA Guidelines for Management of Heart Failure

Trastuzumab induced asymptomatic LV dysfunction is seen in > 10% of patients but is often associated with high recovery rate. Pre-emptive use of ACE, ARB, spironolactone or selected beta blockers use was investigated in number of clinical trials with conflicting results. As such there is no conclusive data that pre-emptive use of this drug prevents the development of cardiomyopathy. Cardiovascular biomarkers notably troponin have been studied for cardiovascular risk stratification in patients undergoing potentially cardio-toxic therapy. In one of the studies of 452 patients with breast cancer showed that elevated pre treatment level (>14 ng/L) was associated with fourfold increase in the risk of cancer therapy related cardiomyopathy. However, other smaller studies have found no advantage in measuring troponin or natriuretic peptide pretherapy. Overall, these biomarkers studies were observational and small in sample in size and number of events. Serial biomarkers may be useful in risk stratification. In a study of 703 patients receiving anthracycline and increase in the troponin within 24 hours of chemotherapy and 1 month after completion of treatment course were associated with greater risk of cancer therapy related cardiomyopathy.

82. Ans. c. Peripartum cardiomyopathy

2022 ACC/AHA Guidelines for Management of Heart Failure

Heart failure may complicate pregnancy either secondary to an existing pre-pregnancy cardiomyopathy or as a result of peripartum cardiomyopathy. The peripartum cardiomyopathy risk factors include maternal age > 30 years, African ancestry, multiparity, multi-gestation, pre-eclampsia/eclampsia, anemia, diabetes, obesity, and prolonged tocolysis. A genetic contribution is recognized, particularly titan gene mutations.

83. Ans. c. Furosemide, beta blockers, Hydralazine, and nitrates

2022 ACC/AHA Guidelines for Management of Heart Failure

As per the 2015 FDA Pregnancy and Lactation Labelling Rules, ACEI and ARB are found to be associated with second and third trimester renal and tubular dysplasia, oligohydramnios, fetal growth restriction, ossification disorders of the skull, lung hypoplasia, contractures of large joints, anemia, and intrauterine fetal death and are, therefore, strictly contraindicated. There are no specific data for ARNi or ivabradine. For spironolactone, there are evidence of dose-dependent feminization of male rabbit and rat offspring. Data are limited for eplerenone. HFrEF medications considered acceptable during pregnancy include furosemide, beta blocker (most commonly metoprolol), hydralazine and nitrate.

CHAPTER 12

Sleep Disorder Breathing and Cardiovascular Disease

1. **Normal apnea-hypopnea index (AHI) is:**
   a. Up to 5 events per hour
   b. Up to 5–10 events per hour
   c. 10–15 events per hour
   d. > 30 events per hour

2. **In a person who has apnea hypopnea index of 15–30 events per hour would be defined as:**
   a. Normal
   b. Mild OSA
   c. Moderate OSA
   d. Severe OSA

3. **Which of the following is *not* a risk factor for sleep disordered breathing?**
   a. Age
   b. Obesity
   c. Smoking
   d. Heart failure

4. **Physiological consequences of sleep disordered breathing (SDB) include all the following *except*:**
   a. Intermittent hypoxia
   b. Alteration in intrathoracic pressure
   c. Decrease in left ventricular muscle mass
   d. Increase in urinary norepinephrine excretion

5. **Which statement is *not* correct regarding sleep disordered breathing?**
   a. Sleep disordered breathing (SDB) is seen in both heart failure with reduced ejection fraction and heart failure with preserved ejection fraction.
   b. SDB has not been documented in heart failure with preserved ejection fraction
   c. Heart failure patients with SDB do not have daytime somnolence
   d. All are correct

6. **Which of the following drug used in heart failure is known to reduced daytime sleepiness and the prevalence of central sleep apnea?**
   a. Alpha blockers
   b. Beta blockers
   c. ACE inhibitors
   d. Calcium channel blockers

7. **CPAP treatment of OSA reduces all the following *except*:**
   a. Intrathoracic pressure
   b. Left ventricular preload
   c. Left ventricular afterload
   d. Transmural cardiac pressure gradient

8. **What is *correct* regarding the prevalence of sleep disordered breathing (SDB) by symptomatic severity of heart failure?**
   a. There is no relation between prevalence of SDB and severity of heart failure
   b. With increasing severity of heart failure, central sleep apnea increases
   c. With increasing severity of heart failure, prevalence of obstructive sleep apnea increases
   d. With increasing symptom of heart failure central sleep apnea increases and obstructive sleep apnea prevalence decreases

9. **Which of the following statement is *correct*?**
   a. In patient with heart failure with sleep disordered breathing, there is lack of daytime somnolence
   b. With increasing severity of heart failure, central sleep apnea increases
   c. With increasing heart failure severity, obstructive sleep apnea diminishes
   d. All of the above

10. **Which is *not* correct regarding central sleep apnea in patients with heart failure?**
    a. Daytime somnolence is absent in these patients
    b. Patients with heart failure have severe (AHI > 30)
    c. It is predictor of hospital readmission and mortality
    d. CSA improves with resolution of acute decompensated heart failure

11. All the following are correct regarding pulmonary hypertension in sleep disordered breathing *except*:
   a. PAH is associated with SDB is usually mild to moderate in severity
   b. More commonly seen in obese patients
   c. Right ventricular failure is common
   d. All are incorrect

12. Which of the following is *correct* regarding pulmonary hypertension in sleep disordered breathing?
   a. Pulmonary arterial hypertension is precapillary in nature
   b. SDB has no relationship with severity and presence of diastolic dysfunction
   c. Right ventricular failure is common
   d. All are incorrect

13. Which of the following is *not* a disease modifying therapy in patients with heart failure?
   a. ACEI/sacubitril-valsartan combination
   b. Beta blockers
   c. Aldosterone antagonists
   d. Diuretics

14. Which is the most effective treatment for Central sleep apnea?
   a. CPAP
   b. Oxygen therapy
   c. Bilevel positive airway pressure (BIPAP)
   d. Assisted servo-ventilation (ASV)

15. Which of the following drug has been found to reduce AHI and improve oxygen saturation in patient with heart failure and central sleep apnea?
   a. Furosemide
   b. Chlorthalidone
   c. Metolazone
   d. Acetazolamide

16. Which of the following is contraindicated in treatment of PAH due to interstitial lung disease?
   a. Oxygen therapy
   b. Pirfenidone
   c. Nintedanib
   d. Endothelin 1 antagonist ambrisentan

ANSWERS WITH EXPLANATIONS

1. Ans. a. Up to 5 events per hour

Hurst's 14th Ed; Page 1841

The severity of sleep disordered breathing is generally defined by average number of apneic and hypopneic events per hour of sleep, or the apnea-hypopnea index (AHI). Normal is defined as up to 5 events per hour, mild as 5–15 events per hour, moderate as 15–30 events per hour, and severe as > 30 events per hour.

2. Ans. c. Moderate OSA

Hurst's 14th Ed; Page 1841

Refer to explanation for Q. No 1.

3. Ans. c. Smoking

Hurst's 14th Ed; Page 1842

Risk factor for sleep disordered breathing (SDB) includes age, sex, ethnicity, obesity, smoking and alcohol use. Although exposure to tobacco smoke may increase upper airway inflammation and snoring, smoking is not a family established risk factors for SDB. Alcohol use may exacerbate SDB especially during the first 2 hours after ingestion, as a result of a decrease in upper airway muscle tone and perhaps a reduction in central respiratory drive.

4. Ans. c. Decrease in left ventricular muscle mass

Hurst's 14th Ed; Page 1845

Physiological consequences of sleep disordered breathing (SDB) includes intermittent hypoxia, sympathetic nervous system activation, alteration in intrathoracic pressure, cardiac remodeling, sleep reduction and fragmentation, metabolic dysregulation, endothelial dysfunction and thrombosis. Sleep disordered breathing brings left ventricular remodeling. Long-term SDB may lead to development of hypertension, left ventricular hypertrophy and reduced left ventricular ejection fraction. It has been found that there is a progressive increase in left ventricular mass index with AHI level, independent of BMI as reported in sleep heart health study which was an observational study. More severe SDB as defined by higher AHI and more hypoxemia was associated with greater left ventricular systolic dimension and lower ventricular ejection fraction. Left ventricular diastolic dysfunction also appears to be poorer in patients with more severe systolic disorder breathing, independent of obesity diabetes and hypertension. Sleep disordered breathing may more adversely affect myocardial function in patients with underlying coronary artery disease than in those without coronary artery disease.

5. Ans. b. SDB has not been documented in heart failure with preserved ejection fraction

Hurst's 14th Ed; Page 1850

Sleep disordered breathing (SDB) is common in patients with heart failure, with prevalence rates of 50-75%. SDB has been documented in patients with both heart failure with reduced ejection fraction or heart failure with preserved ejection fraction with no difference in prevalence between the two groups, and in patients with acute decompensated heart failure, where the prevalence may be even higher. The prevalence of central sleep apnea (CSA)/obstructive sleep apnea appears to increase as the symptomatic severity of the heart failure syndrome increases, and the severity of CSA/obstructive sleep apnea seems to mirror underlying cardiac dysfunction. In patients with SDB with heart failure compared to general SDB patients is a relative lack of symptoms, especially of daytime somnolence, which could contribute to the lack of recognition and detection of SDB in heart failure patients. Possible mechanism for a lack of daytime sleepiness in heart failure patients with SDB is the increased sympathetic nervous system activity in heart failure patients compared with healthy subjects, which is increased even further in the presence of OSA. Increased sympathetic stimulation could stimulate alertness to counteract the effects of sleep fragmentation and sleep deprivation.

A significant inverse correlation between the degree of subjective daytime sleepiness and daytime muscle sympathetic nervous system activity has been documented in patients with heart failure and obstructive sleep apnea. Patients with heart failure are often taking variety of medications that cross the blood-brain barrier, and these could also impact on sleep and SDB. β-blockers are known to reduce daytime sleepiness and the prevalence of central sleep apnea.

6. Ans. b. Beta blockers

Hurst's 14th Ed; Page 1850

Refer to explanation for Q. No 5.

7. Ans. a. Intrathoracic pressure

Hurst's 14th Ed; Page 1851-1852

Continuous positive airway pressure (CPAP) therapy delivered through a nasal or nasal-oral mask stabilizes the airway and thus prevents collapse and is the standard treatment for sleep disordered breathing. The CPAP treatment reduces the number of apneas/hypopneas during sleep, improves hypoxia and sleep architecture, and reduces arousals. Additional beneficial cardiovascular effects of CPAP include increased intrathoracic pressure, reduced left ventricular preload and afterload, and reduced transmural cardiac pressure gradients. All of which can ameliorate impaired cardiac function. CPAP improves daytime somnolence, measures of quality of life, and physical vitality scores.

8. Ans. d. With increasing symptom of heart failure central sleep apnea increases and obstructive sleep apnea prevalence decreases

Hurst's 14th Ed; Page 1850-1852

SDB or sleep disordered breathing is common in patients with heart failure, with prevalence rates of 50% to 75%. SDB is documented in both patients with heart failure with reduced ejection fraction and heart failure with preserved ejection fraction (HFpEF). Its prevalence is higher in patients who have acute decompensated heart failure. The prevalence of central sleep apnea (CSA)/CSR appears to increase as the symptomatic severity of the heart failure syndrome increases, and the severity of CSA/CSR seems to mirror underlying cardiac dysfunction. One of the important features of SDB in patients with heart failure compared to general SDB patients is a relative lack of symptoms, especially daytime somnolence. It is attributed to the increased sympathetic nervous system activity in patients with heart failure and SDB. Increased sympathetic stimulation could stimulate alertness to counteract the effects of sleep fragmentation and sleep deprivation.

9. Ans. d. All of the above

Hurst's 14th Ed; Page 1850-1852

Refer to explanation for Q. No 8.

10. Ans. d. CSA improves with resolution of acute decompensated heart failure

Hurst's 14th Ed; Page 1852

Effective treatment of heart failure may improve central sleep apnea (CSA)/Cheyne-Stokes respiration (CSR) breathing. But its negative prognostic impact persists even in patients who are receiving maximal and optimal heart failure therapy, including cardiac resynchronization. When present, CSA in acute decompensated heart failure patients is usually severe (AHI > 30) and has been shown to be a predictor of hospital readmission and mortality. Even with optimal medical management, resolution of acute decompensation, and return to baseline cardiopulmonary status, the severity of CSA may not change.

11. Ans. c. Right ventricular failure is common

Hurst's 14th Ed; Page 1850-1851

Pulmonary hypertension is seen in 20-40% of patients with SDB in absence of other known cardiopulmonary disorders. The pulmonary hypertension associated with SDB appears to be mild to moderate in severity and it is as a result of a combination of precapillary and postcapillary factors, including pulmonary arteriolar remodeling and hyperreactivity to hypoxia, left ventricular diastolic dysfunction, and left atrial enlargement. Individuals with SDB and pulmonary hypertension are usually obese and have hypoxemia and hypercapnia while awake, and some may have had underlying pulmonary disease. Severe SDB is independently associated with pulmonary hypertension in direct relationship with disease severity and presence of diastolic dysfunction. Although measurable changes in the structure and function of the right ventricle have been reported in association with SDB, clinical significance of these changes is uncertain. Right ventricular failure in SDB appears to be uncommon and it is seen more often when there is a coexisting left-sided heart disease or chronic hypoxic respiratory disease.

12. Ans. d. All are incorrect

Hurst's 14th Ed; Page 1850–1851

Refer to explanation for Q. No 11.

13. Ans. d. Diuretics

Hurst's 14th Ed; Page 1852–1853

ACEI/sacubitril-valsartan combination, beta blockers, aldosterone antagonists and SGLT-2 inhibitor are disease modifying therapy of heart failure. Diuretics do not modify basic pathological features of heart failure.

14. Ans. d. Assisted servo ventilation (ASV)

Hurst's 14th Ed; Page 1853

A number of treatments for central sleep apnea have been studied, including oxygen, carbon dioxide, CPAP, bilevel positive airway pressure (BiPAP), and ASV (assisted servo ventilation). Although CPAP improves CSA by increasing functional residual capacity and, as a result, oxygen stores, decreasing blood volume in the lungs and upper airway when lying down, and reduces hyperventilation via a direct effect on the paravasal J-receptors of the lung. In addition, CPAP reduces preload and afterload and the cardiac transmural pressure and may benefit cardiac function in some patients. It has additional benefits in heart failure, as positive end-expiratory pressure prevents alveoli collapsing secondary to pulmonary edema and maintains alveoli at a greater diameter, and therefore, reduces the work of breathing. It also increases alveolar recruitment, improves gas exchange, and reduces right-to-left intrapulmonary shunt of blood. However, a high proportion of patients with CSA have residual apnea events despite CPAP therapy. ASV has been shown to be the most effective intervention for controlling SDB in patients with heart failure. Studies have shown that ASV brings improvements in AHI, sleep quality, quality of life, left ventricular ejection fraction, NYHA Class, oxygen uptake, serum natriuretic peptide concentrations, inflammatory markers, and exercise capacity.

15. Ans. d. Acetazolamide

Hurst's 14th Ed; Page 1855

Two small trials of medical therapy with acetazolamide have been reported, showing reductions in AHI and improved oxygen saturation in patients with heart failure and CSA. It may be due to respiratory stimulating properties as well as diuretic action of acetazolamide.

16. Ans. d. Endothelin 1 antagonist ambrisentan

Ann Intern Med 2013; 7: 158: 641–649

There is no specific treatment of pulmonary hypertension in interstitial pulmonary fibrosis. Oxygen therapy is the main stay of therapy. Newer drugs like pirfenidone, a small-molecule anti-inflammatory drug, and nintedanib, a tyrosine kinase inhibitor, is approved for treatment of idiopathic pulmonary fibrosis. A trial (Randomized Placebo-Controlled Study to Evaluate Safety and Effectiveness of Ambrisentan in IPF [ARTEMIS]) using the endothelin-1 antagonist ambrisentan for IPF was halted prematurely because of an increase in the disease progression. An increase in ventilation/perfusion mismatch may be the underlying cause for the adverse effects of ambrisentan.

CHAPTER 13

Atherosclerosis and Coronary Artery Disease

ATHEROSCLEROSIS AND CORONARY ARTERY DISEASE

1. Which of the following anticoagulation is *not* recommended to support primary PCI?
   a. Unfractionated heparin
   b. Bivalirudin
   c. LMWH
   d. Fondaparinux

2. The scientific basis for inhibiting platelet aggregation in all patients with STEMI regardless of the reperfusion management strategy is because of:
   a. Platelet plays crucial role in thrombus formation
   b. Fibrinolysis can activate platelet
   c. Platelet rich thrombi resist fibrinolysis
   d. All of the above

3. Which of the following is a drug of choice for management of patients with heart failure despite treatment with diuretics and who are not hypotensive?
   a. Dopamine
   b. Dobutamine
   c. Norepinephrine
   d. Epinephrine

4. Kussmaul sign in the setting of inferior STEMI is predictive of:
   a. Cardiogenic shock
   b. Ventricular septal rupture
   c. Mitral regurgitation
   d. Concomitant RV infarct

5. In patient with inferior wall infarction the lead V_4R, demonstrating ST segment elevation of >1 mm and positive T wave then the probable site of occlusion is:
   a. Proximal occlusion of right coronary artery
   b. Distal occlusion of right coronary artery
   c. Anywhere in the right coronary artery
   d. Occlusion of the left circumflex artery

6. If lead V_4R in setting of inferior MI demonstrate ST segment depression >1 mm and negative T wave (in lead V_4R) then the probable site of occlusion is:
   a. Proximal occlusion of right coronary artery
   b. Distal occlusion of right coronary artery
   c. Occlusion of circumflex coronary artery
   d. Occlusion of obtuse marginal branch of circumflex artery

7. Which of the following drug should *not* be used in case of suspected RV infarct?
   a. Nitrate
   b. Morphine
   c. Diuretics
   d. All

8. Which of the following treatment modality has been found to improve RV mechanical function and lower in hospital mortality in patients with right ventricular infarct?
   a. Combination of diuretics and vasodilators
   b. Plasma volume expansion
   c. Reperfusion of right coronary artery
   d. All of the above

9. In STEMI, free wall rupture is associated with all the following *except*:
   a. Anterior or first MI
   b. Single vessel disease
   c. Reperfusion with fibrinolytic agent
   d. Reperfusion with PCI

10. Inferior myocardial wall infarction is associated with which of the following?
    a. Right ventricular infarction
    b. Rupture of interventricular septum in the basal portion
    c. Rupture of posteromedial papillary muscle
    d. All of the above

11. What is secondary prevention strategy in a patient in whom sustained VT/VF develops later in the course after STEMI (e.g., more than 48 hours) without evidence of reversible cause?
    a. Prophylactic beta-blocker only
    b. Prophylactic oral mexiletine only
    c. Oral amiodarone only
    d. ICD therapy

12. Which is treatment of choice in patients with post-MI Dressler syndrome?
    a. Glucocorticoids
    b. Nonsteroidal anti-inflammatory drugs
    c. Aspirin in higher doses
    d. Methotrexate

13. The negative and positive predictive value of any noninvasive tests are defined by:
    a. Its sensitivity
    b. Its specificity
    c. By the prevalence of disease in the population under study
    d. All of the above

14. If stress test is performed for risk stratification in a patient with known CAD, which of the following drugs should be discontinued before test?
    a. Beta-blockers
    b. Calcium channel blocker
    c. Long-acting nitrate
    d. Discontinuation of medication is not necessary

15. Which is *not* correct regarding exercise stress testing?
    a. Exercise ECG is useful in patients with chest pain syndrome who are considered to have strong probability of CAD.
    b. Antianginal therapy may reduce the sensitivity of exercise testing.
    c. Women have higher frequency of false positive stress test than men
    d. Exercise imaging modality have greater diagnostic accuracy in both men and women

16. Stress myocardial perfusion imaging is considered superior to be an exercise ECG alone because of:
    a. SPECT yield higher sensitivity and specificity
    b. It helps in localizing disease vessels
    c. It helps in determining the magnitude of ischemic and infarcted myocardium
    d. All of the above

17. Which is *not* correct regarding discrete coronary artery aneurysm?
    a. They are almost never found in arteries without severe stenosis
    b. LAD coronary artery is the most common site
    c. These are usually associated with extensive CAD
    d. These aneurysms can rupture and warrant resection

18. Which of the following is *not* correct regarding coronary collateral vessel?
    a. It protects against MI when total arterial occlusion occurs
    b. MI size is smaller in patients with collaterals
    c. Collateral dependent myocardial segments have normal baseline blood flow and O_2 consumption.
    d. Collateral protects against resting and exercise induced angina

19. What is the annual mortality rate of a patient with stable ischemic heart disease who is put on current guideline directed medical therapy?
    a. 1–3%
    b. 2–4%
    c. 4–6%
    d. 8–10%

20. All the following medical therapies have been shown to reduce mortality and morbidity in patients with stable ischemic heart disease *except*:
    a. Beta-blocker
    b. Aspirin
    c. Statin
    d. Angiotensin-converting enzyme inhibitor

21. Patients with atrial fibrillation undergoing PCI which combination of antiplatelet and anticoagulant provides the best balance of safety and efficacy?
    a. Oral anticoagulant + Aspirin + Clopidogrel
    b. Oral anticoagulant + Aspirin
    c. Oral anticoagulant + Clopidogrel
    d. Clopidogrel + Aspirin

22. In patients with stable angina, who are not considered to be at high risk, survival is better with:
    a. PCI
    b. Surgery
    c. Medical management
    d. Survival is similar with surgery, PCI and medical management

23. In STEMI, all the following are elevated *except*:
    a. Plasma and urinary catecholamine
    b. B-type natriuretic peptide
    c. Serum insulin
    d. Tissue RAAS

24. All the following are increased in the STEMI *except*:
    a. Natriuretic peptide
    b. Plasma and urinary catecholamine
    c. Tissue RAAS
    d. Affinity of hemoglobin for oxygen

25. The occurrence of nausea and vomiting during the onset of STEMI is due to activation of:
    a. Hering Breuer reflex
    b. Bezold–Jarisch reflex
    c. Bainbridge reflex
    d. Treppe phenomenon

26. Which of the following ECG changes in setting of acute STEMI often indicates left main coronary artery disease or multivessel disease with worse outcome?
    a. New onset LBBB
    b. New onset RBBB
    c. Abnormal R wave in V_1 in absence of preexcitation
    d. ST segment elevation in aVR

27. Which of the following statement regarding management of acute MI is *incorrect*?
   a. Chewable aspirin (nonenteric coated tablet) should be used in emergency room
   b. Long-acting oral nitrates preparation should be avoided in early course of STEMI
   c. Treating all patients hospitalized for STEMI with oxygen for 24–48 hours is beneficial
   d. All are correct

28. The most important factor to govern the short- and long-term survival after STEMI is:
   a. Resting LV function
   b. Residual potentially ischemic myocardium
   c. Susceptibility to serious ventricular arrhythmia
   d. All of the above

29. Which of the following is *incorrect* statement regarding the secondary prevention after acute myocardial infarction?
   a. Nitrate should be prescribed on routine basis to reduce long-term mortality
   b. The impact of beta-blocker in preventing mortality occurs in the first week and therefore it should be started as soon as possible
   c. Beta-blockers should be continued for at least 2–3 years
   d. ACE inhibitor should be used in all patients of acute MI even in presence of a normal global EF

30. Which of the following is *not* recommended for secondary prevention of coronary artery disease?
   a. Beta-blocker
   b. ACE inhibitors
   c. Statins
   d. Calcium channel antagonist

31. Which of the following chest pain descriptor has low likelihood of acute MI?
   a. Radiation to both shoulder or arms
   b. Associated with the exertion
   c. Associated with nausea or vomiting
   d. Chest pain described as pleuritic

32. In a patient with chest pain, diffuse ST segment elevation and PR segment depression suggest diagnosis of:
   a. Acute MI
   b. Pericarditis
   c. Dissection of aorta
   d. Pulmonary embolism

33. Which is *not* an independent predictor of risk for individuals within a population of the incidence of atherosclerosis?
   a. Plasma cholesterol concentration
   b. Cigarette smoking
   c. Elevated blood pressure
   d. Diabetes mellitus

34. The abdominal aorta in humans is particularly vulnerable to atherogenesis because:
   a. It is a wide caliber vessel
   b. The flow velocity is higher in abdominal aorta
   c. It has thick medial muscular layer
   d. It lacks vasa vasorum in its outer most aspect

35. The receptors for platelet derived growth factor (PDGF) is absent on endothelial cell lining of:
   a. Arteries
   b. Veins
   c. Capillaries
   d. Lymphatics

36. Which is *not* correct regarding atherosclerosis?
   a. The abdominal aorta is most extensively involved than thoracic aorta
   b. Renal artery appears to be spared from atherosclerosis except at their ostia
   c. Coronary arteries have most extensive atherosclerosis in their first 6 cm course
   d. All are correct

ANSWERS WITH EXPLANATIONS

1. Ans. d. Fondaparinux

Braunwald 11th Ed; Page 1136–1137

Either unfractionated heparin or bivalirudin is recommended as an anticoagulant to support primary PCI, with preference for bivalirudin or heparin without a concomitant Gp IIb/IIIa inhibitor for patient at high risk of bleeding. Fondaparinux is not recommended as the sole anticoagulant in this setting. Low molecular weight heparin (LMWH) has not had sufficient evaluation in primary PCI. There is no large data to support LMWH, however it has been used to support primary PCI for STEMI at a dose of 0.5 mg/kg intravenously at the time of procedure by many operators. Fondaparinux in OASIS-6 trial resulted in increased risk of catheter thrombosis and therefore it is not a choice of anticoagulant for during PCI.

2. Ans. d. All of the above

Braunwald 11th Ed; Page 1138

Platelet plays a major role in response to disruption of coronary artery plaque, especially in early phase of thrombus formation. Fibrinolysis can activate platelet, and platelet rich thrombi resist fibrinolysis more than fibrin and erythrocyte rich thrombi and therefore all patients with STEMI regardless of perfusion management strategy should receive antiplatelet drugs. The agent most extensively tested has been aspirin, and treatment with aspirin and a second antiplatelet agent, such as clopidogrel, prasugrel, ticagrelor, or cangrelor, is the standard of care for patients with STEMI.

3. Ans. b. Dobutamine

Braunwald 11th Ed; Page 1148

Dobutamine is a drug with positive inotropic action comparable to that of dopamine, but a slightly less positive chronotropic effect, and vasodilatory rather than vasoconstrictor activity. It is useful in patients in whom heart failure persists despite treatment with diuretics, who are not hypotensive, and who are likely to benefit from both an enhancement in contractility and afterload reduction. Dobutamine must be given with constant monitoring of the ECG and systemic arterial pressure.

4. Ans. d. Concomitant RV infarct

Braunwald 11th Ed; Page 1153

The hemodynamic feature of right ventricular infarction is normal LV filling pressure and depressed cardiac index with accompanying inferior LV infarct. The hemodynamic picture of RV infarct resembles that of pericardial disease which includes elevated RV filling pressure, a steep right atrial *y* descent, and an early diastolic dip and plateau (resembling the square root sign) in the RV pressure tracing. Patients with RV infarction may display the Kussmaul sign (increase in jugular venous pressure with inspiration) and pulsus paradoxus (decrease in systolic BP >10 mm Hg with inspiration). The Kussmaul sign in the setting of inferior STEMI is highly predictive of concomitant right ventricular infarct.

5. Ans. a. Proximal occlusion of right coronary artery

Braunwald 11th Ed; Page 1154

The recording of lead V$_4$R in setting of inferior wall infarction helps in localizing the site of occlusion as per the following diagram:

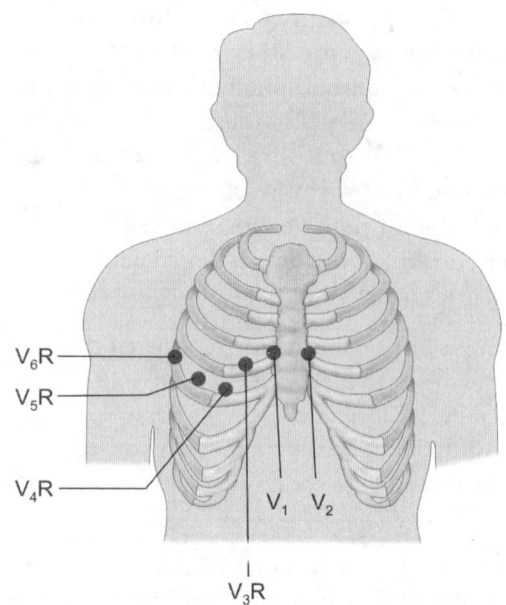

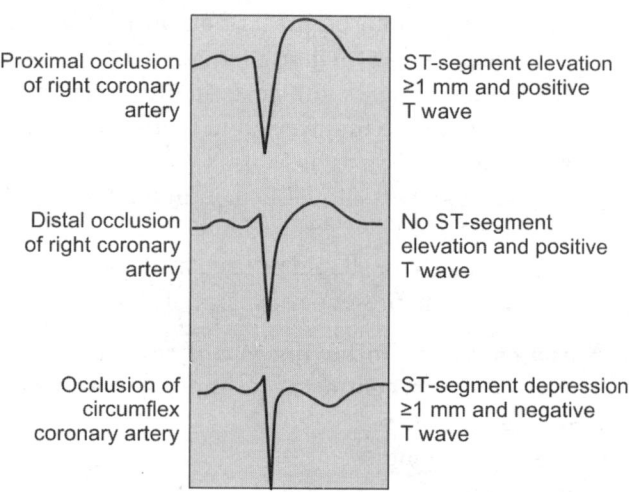

6. Ans. c. Occlusion of circumflex coronary artery

Braunwald 11th Ed; Page 1154

Refer to explanation for Q. No 5.

7. Ans. d. All

Braunwald 11th Ed; Page 1154-1155

Right ventricular infarction management requires judicious control of preload. Medications routinely prescribed for LV infarction may produce profound hypotension in patients with RV infarction and therefore, drugs such as nitrates, morphine, and diuretics should be avoided. In patients with hypotension caused by RV MI, hemodynamic can improve with a combination of expansion of plasma volume to augment RV preload and cardiac output and, when LV failure is present, arterial vasodilators is to be added.

8. Ans. c. Reperfusion of right coronary artery

Braunwald 11th Ed; Page 1155

Successful reperfusion of right coronary artery significantly improves RV mechanical function and lowers in-hospital mortality in patients with RV infarction. However, supportive treatment with expansion of plasma volume to augment RV preload and cardiac output and when LV failure is present arterial vasodilators indicated under hemodynamic monitoring.

9. Ans. d. Reperfusion with PCI

Braunwald 11th Ed; Page 1155

The free wall rupture following acute myocardial infarction can be catastrophic with an acute tear leading to tamponade and immediate death. Sometime the rupture is subacute in nature with nausea, hypotension, and pericardial discomfort. Rupture is more common in the left ventricle (specifically, the anterior or lateral wall) than in the right ventricle and seldom occurs in the atria. Other features associated with rupture include reperfusion with a fibrinolytic agent versus PCI, old age, female sex, hypertension, single vessel disease without collateral circulation, and an anterior or first MI. Mortality can be as high as 75-90% following free wall rupture.

10. Ans. d. All of the above

Braunwald 11th Ed; Page 1155-56

Inferior wall infarction is associated with RV infarction in 33% of cases. The rupture of interventricular septum is seen in inferior infarction and often it affects the basal septum and have a worse prognosis than those in an anterior location. Inferior wall infarction can also lead to the rupture of posteromedial papillary muscle which because of its singular blood supply occurs more frequently than the rupture of anterolateral muscle, often seen in setting of anterolateral MI.

11. Ans. d. ICD therapy

Braunwald 11th Ed; Page 1160

In patient in whom sustained VT/VF develops later in the course after STEMI (e.g., more than 48 hours) without evidence of a reversible cause, ICD therapy for secondary prevention should be considered before discharge. This situation differs from that in patients with VT/VF before reperfusion therapy, in whom antiarrhythmic therapy other than a beta blocker is not indicated.

12. Ans. c. Aspirin in higher doses

Braunwald 11th Ed; Page 1163

Postmyocardial infarction syndrome (Dressler syndrome) usually occurs 1-8 weeks after infarction, seen in 3-4% of all patients following MI. Usually presents as malaise, fever, pericardial discomfort, leukocytosis, an elevated erythrocyte sedimentation rate (ESR), and a pericardial effusion. Treatment is with Aspirin 650 mg 4 hourly and it may be effective. Glucocorticosteroid and NSAIDs are best avoided in patients with Dressler syndrome within 4 weeks of STEMI because of their potential to impair infarct healing, cause ventricular rupture, and increase coronary vascular resistance.

13. Ans. d. All of the above

Braunwald 11th Ed; Page 1214

Noninvasive stress testing can provide useful and important information to establish the diagnosis and estimate prognosis in patients with suspected angina pectoris. Appropriate application of noninvasive tests requires consideration of bayesian principles, which state that the negative and positive predictive values of any test are defined not only by its sensitivity and specificity but also by the prevalence of disease (or pretest probability) in the population under study.

14. Ans. d. Discontinuation of medication is not necessary

Braunwald 11th Ed; Page 1215

Antianginal therapy may reduce the sensitivity of exercise testing as a screening tool. If the purpose of the exercise test is to diagnose ischemia, it should be performed, if possible, in the absence of antianginal medications, especially long-acting beta-blocking agents, which should be stopped for 2-3 days before testing. For long-acting nitrates, calcium antagonists, and short-acting beta blockers, discontinuing use of the medications the day before testing usually suffices. If the test is being performed for risk stratification in a patient with known CAD, discontinuation of medications is not necessary.

15. Ans. a. Exercise ECG is useful in patients with chest pain syndrome who are considered to have strong probability of CAD

Braunwald 11th Ed; Page 1215

Exercise ECG is particularly helpful in patients with chest pain syndrome who are considered to have moderate probability of CAD and in whom the resting ECG is normal, provided that they are capable of achieving and adequate workload. Antianginal therapy may reduce the sensitivity of exercise as a screening tool. Earlier studies have indicated a much higher frequency of false-positive stress test results in women than in men. The Exercise imaging modalities have greater diagnostic accuracy than exercise electrocardiography in both men and women.

16. Ans. d. All of the above

Braunwald 11th Ed; Page 1215

Stress myocardial perfusion imaging (MPI) is particularly helpful in the diagnosis of CAD in patients with abnormal resting ECGs and in those in whom ST-segment responses cannot be interpreted accurately, such as patients with repolarization abnormalities caused by LV hypertrophy and those receiving digitalis. Exercise myocardial perfusion imaging (MPI) with simultaneous ECG recording is generally considered to be superior to an exercise ECG alone in detecting CAD, in identifying multivessel CAD, in localizing diseased vessels, and in determining the magnitude of ischemic and infarcted myocardium. Exercise SPECT yields higher sensitivity and specificity than exercise electrocardiography alone.

17. Ans. d. These aneurysms can rupture and warrant resection

Braunwald 11th Ed; Page 1219

Discrete coronary artery aneurysms are localized dilatation of the coronary artery, which are almost never found in arteries without severe stenosis. Discrete coronary artery aneurysms are most common in LAD territory and are usually associated with extensive CAD. These discrete atherosclerotic coronary artery aneurysms do not appear to rupture and do not warrant resection.

18. Ans. d. Collateral protects against resting and exercise induced angina

Braunwald 11th Ed; Page 1219

Coronary collaterals when they are of adequate size, it protects against MI when total occlusion occurs. In patients with abundant collateral vessels, MI size is smaller than in patients without collaterals, and total occlusion of a major epicardial coronary artery may not lead to LV dysfunction. In patients with chronic occlusion of a major coronary artery but without MI, collateral-dependent myocardial segments show almost normal baseline blood flow and O_2 consumption but severely limited flow reserve. This explains the ability of collateral vessels to protect against resting ischemia but not against exercise-induced angina.

19. Ans. a. 1–3%

Braunwald 11th Ed; Page 1219

The data from the Framingham study, obtained before the widespread use of aspirin, beta-blocking agents, and aggressive modification of risk factors, revealed an average annual mortality rate of 4% in patients with stable ischemic heart disease. The combination of these treatments has improved the prognosis, with a current annual mortality rate of 1–3% and a rate of major ischemic events of 1–2%.

20. Ans. a. Beta-blocker

Braunwald 11th Ed; Page 1219

Comprehensive management of stable ischemic heart disease requires reduction of coronary risk factors and application of pharmacological and nonpharmacological intervention for secondary prevention. Of the medical therapies, aspirin, statins and angiotensin-converting enzyme inhibitors shown have been shown to reduce mortality and morbidity in patients with stable ischemic heart disease. Other therapies, such as nitrates, beta blockers, calcium antagonists, and ranolazine, have been shown to improve symptoms and exercise performance, but their effect, on survival in patients with stable ischemic heart disease has not been demonstrated.

21. Ans. c. Oral anticoagulant + Clopidogrel

Braunwald 11th Ed; Page 1223

For patients with AF assessment of the risk and benefit of oral anticoagulant should be performed after considering the increased bleeding risk associated with combination therapy. Among patients at lower stroke risk, it may be preferable to defer OAC after MI and/or stenting and reinitiate OAC once the patient can safely be withdrawn from DAPT. When triple therapy is necessary, recommendations include: (1) limiting exposure to triple therapy to the shortest possible duration, (2) targeting the lower range of international normalized ratio (INR) for warfarin, (3) avoiding the more potent P2Y12 antagonism of prasugrel and ticagrelor (clopidogrel is preferred in combination with OAC), and (4) routinely administering proton pump inhibitors (PPIs) to prevent gastrointestinal (GI) bleed. A small trial has shown that withdrawing aspirin after coronary stenting is associated with favorable bleeding and efficacy compared with triple therapy. Two trials, PIONEER AF-PCI and RE-DUAL PCI trials both have shown that for patients with atrial fibrillation undergoing PCI dual therapy with an anticoagulant (preferably a reduced dose of a direct oral anticoagulant) and clopidogrel without aspirin provide the best balance of safety and efficacy.

22. Ans. d. Survival is similar with surgery, PCI and medical management

Braunwald 11th Ed; Page 1248

Indication for Coronary Revascularization in Stable Coronary Artery Disease

Certain anatomic subsets of patients are candidates for coronary artery bypass surgery, regardless of the severity of symptoms or LV dysfunction. Such patients include those with significant left main CAD and most patients with three vessel CAD that includes the proximal LAD, especially those with LV dysfunction (EF <50%). Patients with chronic stable angina and two-vessel CAD with significant proximal disease of the LAD and either LV dysfunction or high-risk findings on noninvasive testing may also be best considered for CABG. In patients with angina who are not considered to be at high risk, survival is similar with surgery, PCI, and medical management.

23. Ans. c. Serum insulin

Braunwald 11th Ed; Page 1111

Hyperglycemia is common in patient presenting with STEMI and it is associated with worse outcome. Abnormalities in insulin secretion and resultant impaired glucose tolerance appear to result from a reduction in pancreatic blood flow caused by the splanchnic vasoconstriction accompanying acute MI and cardiogenic shock. In addition, increased activity of the sympathetic nervous system with augmented catecholamines also inhibits insulin secretion and increases glycogenolysis. Plasma and urinary catecholamine levels peak in the first 24 hours after onset of chest pain, with the greatest rise in the plasma catecholamine secretion occurring during the first hour after onset of STEMI. The peptides atrial natriuretic peptide (ANP) and B-type natriuretic peptide (BNP) are released from cardiac atria in response to elevation in atrial pressure. Similarly, the non-infarcted regions of the myocardium appear to exhibit activation of the tissue RAAS with increased production of angiotensin II.

24. Ans. d. Affinity of hemoglobin for oxygen

Braunwald 11th Ed; Page 1111

In patients with MI, particularly when complicated by left ventricular failure or cardiogenic shock, the affinity of hemoglobin for oxygen falls. Due to increase in P50. The increase in P50 results from increased levels of erythrocyte 2,3-diphosphoglycerate, which is an important compensatory mechanism that mediates an estimated 18% increase in release of oxygen from oxyhemoglobin in patients with cardiogenic shock.

25. Ans. b. Bezold–Jarisch reflex

Braunwald 11th Ed; Page 1113

Nausea and vomiting may occur in the setting of acute MI, the underlying mechanism is activation of the vagal reflex or stimulation of LV receptor as a part of Bezold–Jarisch reflex. This symptom occurs more frequently in patients with inferior STEMI than with anterior STEMI.

26. Ans. d. ST segment elevation in aVR

Braunwald 11th Ed; Page 1118-1119

The ECG remains the most important diagnostic test in evaluation of patients with suspected ischemic symptoms. Established criteria aid the diagnosis of STEMI in LBBB, evidence of RBBB in setting of acute MI also portends a similar poor prognosis. Patients with an abnormal R wave in V_1 in the absence of pre-excitation or RV hypertrophy and inferior or lateral Q waves have an increased incidence of isolated occlusion of a dominant left circumflex coronary artery without collateral circulation. ST-segment elevations in aVR, reflecting the basal intraventricular septum, can be observed in up to 30% of STEMIs and identifies patients with a higher likelihood of left main coronary artery or multivessel disease and worse outcome.

27. Ans. c. Treating all patients hospitalized for STEMI with oxygen for 24–48 hours is beneficial

Braunwald 11th Ed; Page 1126

Aspirin is to be used in all patients with ACS and is a part of initial management strategy for patients with STEMI. Because low doses take several days to achieve a full antiplatelet effect, recommended dose is 162 to 325 mg administered on first medical contact. To achieve therapeutic blood levels rapidly, the patient should chew a nonenteric-coated tablet to promote buccal absorption bypassing the gastric mucosa.

Nitrates are indicated in most patients with acute coronary syndrome except the patients who were hypotensive or those who have right ventricular infarction. Long-acting oral nitrate preparation should be avoided in early course of STEMI because of frequent changing hemodynamic status of the patient. It has been in a practice to use oxygen for all patients with STEMI but however, using oxygen in patients who do not have hypoxemia may increase systemic vascular resistance and arterial pressure, promote coronary vasoconstriction and result in greater oxidative stress and therefore oxygen should be used only when the arterial oxygen saturation (SaO_2 is less than 90%).

28. Ans. a. Resting LV function

Braunwald 11th Ed; Page 1165

Both short-term and long-term survival after STEMI depend on three major factors i.e., resting LV function, residual potentially ischemic myocardium, and susceptibility to serious ventricular arrhythmias. The most important of these factors is the state of LV function. The second most important factor is how the severity and extent of the obstructive lesions in the coronary vascular bed perfusing residual viable myocardium affect the risk for recurrent infarction and serious ventricular arrhythmias. The survival is related to the quantity of myocardium that has become necrotic and the portion remaining in ischemic jeopardy.

29. Ans. a. Nitrate should be prescribed on routine basis to reduce long-term mortality

Braunwald 11th Ed; Page 1168

Although nitrates are suitable for management of specific conditions after STEMI like recurrent angina or as a part of treatment regimen for heart failure, there is no definite evidence that long-term nitrates therapy reduces mortality. Beta-adrenergic blocking agent have well-documented benefits. The impact of beta-blocker in preventing mortality occurs in the first week and therefore treatment should commence as soon as possible. The collective data from several trials on long-term follow-up of patients treated with beta-blockers after infarction suggest that therapy should be continued for at least 2 to 3 years. If the beta-blocker is well tolerated and there is no reason to discontinue therapy, then such therapy should be continued in the most of patients. To prevent late remodeling of left ventricle and to decrease the likelihood of recurrent ischemic events, indefinite therapy with ACE inhibitor in patients with heart failure, a moderate decrease in global EF, or a large regional wall motion abnormality, even in the presence of a normal global EF is recommended.

30. Ans. d. Calcium channel antagonist

Braunwald 11th Ed; Page 1168

Calcium channel antagonist are not recommended for secondary prevention of acute MI. It is used for the patients who cannot tolerate a beta-blocker because of adverse effect and contraindication and who have well preserved LV function.

31. Ans. d. Chest pain described as pleuritic

Braunwald 11th Ed; Page 1062

Value of elements of the chest pain history for the diagnosis of acute coronary syndrome

Pain descriptor	Positive likelihood ratio (93% CI)
Increased likelihood of AMI	
Radiation to the right arm or shoulder	4.7 (1.9–12.0)
Radiation to both arms or shoulders	4.1 (2.5–6.5)
Associated with exertion	2.4 (1.5–3.8)
Radiation to the left arm	2.3 (1.7–3.1)
Associated with diaphoresis	2.0 (1.9–2.2)
Associated with nausea or vomiting	1.9 (1.7–2.3)
Worse than previous angina or similar to previous MI	1.8 (1.6–2.0)
Described as pressure	1.3 (1.2–1.5)
Decreased likelihood of AMI	
Described as pleuritic	0.2 (0.1–0.3)
Described as positional	0.3 (0.2–0.5)
Described as sharp	0.3 (0.2–0.5)
Reproducible with palpation	0.3 (0.2–0.4)
Inframammary location	0.8 (0.7–0.9)
Not associated with exertion	0.8 (0.6–0.9)

32. Ans. b. Pericarditis

Braunwald 11th Ed; Page 1062

Diffuse ST segment elevation and PR segment depression is suggestive of diagnosis of pericarditis.

33. Ans. d. Diabetes mellitus

Braunwald 7th Ed; Page 1105

Risk factor is defined as a causative agent or a condition that can be used to predict an individual probability of developing a disease. Used in this fashion, there are at least three independent predictors of risk for individuals within a population of the incidence of atherosclerosis, i.e., plasma cholesterol concentration, cigarette smoking and elevated blood pressure.

34. Ans. d. It lacks vasa vasorum in its outer most aspect

Braunwald 7th Ed; Page 1106

The normal artery consists of an intima lined by endothelium on the inner (luminal) aspect of the vessel and bounded by the internal elastic lamina on its outer aspect. The media is bounded by the internal elastic lamina and in well developed muscular and elastic artery by an external elastic lamina. The adventitia is bounded by external elastic lamina and exterior of vessel itself. The adventitia, i.e., the outer wall consists of dense collagenous structure containing numerous bundles of collagen fibrils, elastic fibers and many fibroblasts, together with some smooth muscle cells. It is a highly vascular tissue and contains many nerve fibers as well. The adventitia provides the outer most portions of the media of large elastic arteries with much of their nutrition via vasa vasorum as well as with lymphatic channel innervations. It has been observed that the abdominal aorta in human lacks vasa vasorum in its outermost aspect and have been suggested as one of the reasons the abdominal aorta is particularly vulnerable to atherosclerosis.

35. Ans. a. Arteries

Braunwald 7th Ed; Page 1107

The endothelial cells has been seen enface by light and scanning electron microscopy and in cross section appears to be highly similar morphologically in different part of arterial tree. There may be functional differences in these lining cells in different anatomical sites. Capillary endothelial cells contain receptors on their surface for a potent growth regulatory peptide, platelet derived growth factor (PDGF), whereas these receptors are absent on arterial endothelium.

36. Ans. c. Coronary arteries have most extensive atherosclerosis in their first 6 cm course

Braunwald 7th Ed; Page 1114

There appears to be a general pattern in the distribution of advanced lesion of atherosclerosis in human. Generally, the abdominal aorta is more extensively involved than the thoracic aorta. Lesions in the aorta are usually most prominent near the ostia of major branches that leave the aorta. Some arteries such renal arteries appear to be spared from atherosclerosis, except at their ostia. The coronary arteries demonstrate the most intense involvement with lesion of atherosclerosis located within the first 6 cm of the artery. In hypertensive patients, lesion of the carotids, cerebral and basilar arteries are more common. It has been suggested that the severity of lesion formation in a given artery may be related in part to the particular nature of characteristic of blood flow in the artery and that rheological forces play major role in determining the localization, extend and severity of lesion in susceptible individual.

CAD/CABG

1. Which of the following pathological changes are found in the venous graft which gets occluded 1 to 2 months following bypass surgery?
   a. Thrombosis
   b. Endothelial disruption
   c. Intimal fibroplasia
   d. Vein graft atherosclerosis

2. Which of the following characteristics differentiates vein graft atherosclerosis from native coronary atherosclerosis?
   a. It's circumferential distribution
   b. It's eccentric location
   c. Lack of fibrous capsule and friable nature
   d. All of the above

3. Which of the following lipid lowering drug has been shown to decrease the progression of angiographic lesion in vein grafts and decrease in graft attrition?
   a. Lovastatin
   b. Atorvastatin
   c. Simvastatin
   d. Pravastatin

4. Which of the following is a commonly used arterial conduit for coronary artery bypass surgery?
   a. Left internal mammary artery
   b. Right internal mammary artery
   c. Radial artery
   d. Gastroepiploic artery (GEA)

5. Which of the following factor does *not* influence the early vein graft patency following coronary artery bypass surgery?
   a. Surgical technique
   b. Size of vessel grafted
   c. Coronary risk factors
   d. Gender

6. The most common cause of low cardiac output syndrome following coronary artery bypass surgery is:
   a. Hypovolemia
   b. Use of cardiopulmonary bypass
   c. Pre-existing low LVEF
   d. Intra- or postoperative myocardial ischemia

7. The most common rhythm disturbance immediately following cardiac surgery is:
   a. Ventricular ectopy
   b. Ventricular tachycardia
   c. Atrial fibrillation
   d. Sinus tachycardia

8. The prophylactic use of which of the following drug has been shown to have a protective effect against development of atrial flutter/fibrillation following cardiac surgery:
   a. Digoxin
   b. Verapamil
   c. Diltiazem
   d. Beta blockers

9. The most common conduction disturbance following cardiac surgery is:
   a. Left bundle branch block
   b. Right bundle branch block
   c. Bifascicular block
   d. Complete AV block

10. Which is *not* a major determinant of myocardial oxygen demand?
    a. Heart rate
    b. Inotropic state
    c. Preload
    d. Afterload

11. Which of the following pathogens have been identified within a human atherosclerotic lesion?
    a. *Chlamydia pneumoniae*
    b. Cytomegalovirus
    c. *Helicobacter pylori*
    d. All of the above

12. Which of the following statement is *correct* regarding cardiac troponin?
    a. Troponin levels may be normal early after the onset of acute coronary syndrome
    b. Cardiac troponin are less useful for the diagnosis of unstable angina
    c. Troponin are most useful for risk stratification in cases with acute coronary syndrome
    d. All are correct

13. The presence of right bundle branch block along with ST segment elevation in lead V_1 indicates the occlusion of LAD:
   a. Proximal to the first septal and first diagonal branch
   b. Distal to these two branches
   c. Proximal to the first diagonal but distal to the septal branch
   d. Proximal to the septal but distal to the first diagonal branch

14. The occurrence of left anterior fascicular block in the setting of acute inferior wall infarction indicates:
   a. Additional left circumflex artery disease
   b. Additional left anterior descending artery disease
   c. Disease in RCA proximal to RV branch
   d. Disease in RCA distal to RV branch

15. Which of the following statement is *not* correct regarding acute myocardial infarction:
   a. The majority of early deaths are as a result of ventricular arrhythmia
   b. The biological state of atherosclerotic lesion is the major determinant of myocardial infarction
   c. The majority of myocardial infarctions occur with the arterial lesion that are not significant (less than 60%)
   d. In spite of use of thrombolysis, aspirin, coronary intervention and ACE inhibitors the mortality of patients with acute MI is 15–30%

16. Which of the following is *not* correct?
   a. Acute myocardial infarction occurs without chest pain in 20–25% of cases
   b. Acute mortality rate for Q wave myocardial infarction is 10–12%
   c. Acute myocardial infarction cannot be diagnosed by ECG in presence of a left bundle branch block
   d. The resting ECG is a sensitive tool for detecting the presence of atherosclerotic coronary heart disease

17. What is the approximate incidence of early reinfarction following a non Q wave MI?
   a. 80%   b. 75%
   c. 15–25%   d. 5–8%

18. Which of the following drug has been recommended for treatment of patients with non Q wave myocardial infarction?
   a. Verapamil   b. Diltiazem
   c. Beta blockers   d. Thrombolysis

19. Which of the following is the preferred marker to establish the diagnosis if a patient is admitted beyond 72 hours, from the onset of infarction?
   a. Myoglobin   b. CPK MB
   c. LDH   d. Troponin

20. Which of the following is the most specific marker for diagnosing myocardial infarction in presence of skeletal muscle injury?
   a. Myoglobin   b. CPK MB
   c. LDH   d. Troponin I

21. All the following biochemical parameters are altered following acute myocardial infarction *except*:
   a. Blood glucose level
   b. White blood cell count
   c. Serum cholesterol and lipoprotein fractions
   d. Growth hormone and catecholamine level

22. Which of the following is the most specific or reliable marker for diagnosing myocardial infarction after noncardiac surgery?
   a. Troponin T   b. Troponin I
   c. CPK MB   d. LDH

23. Which is *not* correct regarding pseudoaneurysm following myocardial infarction?
   a. It has a narrow base
   b. Its wall is composed only of a thrombus and pericardium
   c. The risk of rupture is very high
   d. It does not require surgical intervention often

24. Which of the following is *not* seen due to occlusion of right coronary artery?
   a. Activation of vagal nervous system
   b. Ischemia of the sinus and atrioventricular node leading to sinus bradycardia and AV block
   c. Ischemia of the papillary muscles
   d. Right bundle branch block

25. An electrocardiographic pattern of ST elevation in lead aVR and lead V_1 along with ST segment depression in inferior lead and in V_5–V_6 indicates the LAD occlusion:
   a. Proximal to the septal and first diagonal branch
   b. Distal to these two branches
   c. Proximal to the first diagonal but distal to the septal branch
   d. Proximal to the septal branch but distal to the first diagonal

26. The advance lesion of atherosclerosis is due to which fundamental biological process:
   a. Accumulation of intimal smooth muscle cell, macrophages and lymphocytes
   b. Formation of connective tissue matrix by proliferation of smooth muscle cells
   c. Accumulation of lipids inform of cholesteryl esters and free cholesterol
   d. All of the above

27. Which of the following is *not* an independent predictor of risk for individuals within a population of the incidence of atherosclerosis?
   a. Plasma cholesterol concentration
   b. Cigarette smoking
   c. Elevated blood pressure
   d. Obesity

28. Which of the following vessel in humans lacks vasa vasorum in its outer aspect?
   a. Coronary artery   b. Cerebral artery
   c. Abdominal aorta   d. Renal artery

29. All of the following factors released from endothelium are important in vasoconstriction *except*:
   a. Endothelin
   b. Angiotensin converting enzyme
   c. Platelet derived growth factor
   d. EDRF

30. Which of the following is *incorrect* regarding endothelial cells lining the arterial tree?
   a. They produce vasoactive substances
   b. Has a nonthrombogenic surface
   c. Can form procoagulant materials
   d. Can crawl over one another at sites of injury to facilitate the repair of de-endothelialized surface

31. Platelet derived growth factor (PDGF) is a growth factor for all *except*:
   a. Fibroblasts
   b. Smooth muscle cells
   c. Mesenchymal derived cells
   d. Arterial endothelium

32. Vascular cells adhesions molecule-1 (VCAM-1) and intercellular adhesion molecule-1 (ICAM-1) formation is induced by:
   a. EDRF   b. PDGF
   c. Prostacyclin   d. Oxidized LDL

33. Which of the following arteries is relatively spared from atherosclerosis?
   a. Vertebral artery   b. Cerebral artery
   c. Renal artery   d. Basilar artery

34. The lesion of atherosclerosis in coronary artery is located mostly in:
   a. Ostial portion   b. Middle portion
   c. First 6 cm of artery d. Uniformly throughout

35. The normal myocardial oxygen consumption in a healthy human heart is:
   a. 3–5 cc/min/100 g
   b. 6–8 cc/min/100 g
   c. 10–12 cc/min/100 g
   d. 14–16 cc/min/100 g

36. Which of the following group of drugs have dilatory effect on coronary collaterals?
   a. Beta adrenergic agonists
   b. Calcium artery antagonists
   c. Alpha adrenergic agonists
   d. Beta blockers

37. Which is *not* correct regarding myocardial stunning?
   a. It may occurs following exercise induced ischemia
   b. It effect both systolic and diastolic functions
   c. It is seen following cardiopulmonary bypass
   d. It occurs in regionally ischemic heart

38. Which of the following is a adverse reaction noted following reperfusion?
   a. Acceleration of myocyte necrosis
   b. No reflow phenomenon
   c. Reperfusion induced hemorrhage
   d. All of the above

ANSWERS WITH EXPLANATIONS

1. Ans. a. Thrombosis

Hurst's 10th Ed; Page 1511

Much of the late attrition of SVGs appears to be related to intrinsic pathologic changes in those grafts: intimal fibroplasia and vein graft atherosclerosis. Almost all SVGs examined within a few months after operation exhibit intimal fibroplasias, a hypercellular proliferative hyperplasia that involves the intima, is usually concentric, and is distributed throughout the length of the graft. With time, it becomes less cellular and more fibrotic. Intimal hyperplasia may cause stenoses and occlusions, but it usually does not.

2. Ans. d. All of the above

Hurst's 10th Ed; Page 1511

Vein graft atherosclerosis is characterized by lipid infiltration and areas of intimal fibroplasia. It is different in distribution and character than native coronary atherosclerosis. Native coronary artery atherosclerosis is a proximal, eccentric and intermittent lesion, i.e., usually covered by a fibrous cap. Vein graft atherosclerosis is distributed throughout the length of vein graft. It is circumferential, not encapsulated and extremely friable. With time, the early circumferential lesion will often progress to eccentric lesion causing severe stenosis. Vein graft atherosclerosis is a dangerous lesion. Because of the friability and nonencapsulated nature of the lesion, embolization of atherosclerotic debris is a major risk during percutaneous intervention on vein graft and during reoperations and it is probable that spontaneous embolization may occur. Vein graft atherosclerosis is usually not recognize before 2–3 years after operation and does not appear to cause much graft attrition before 5 postoperative years. However, the increase rate of graft attrition seen more than 5 years after operation appears to be a large part due to vein graft atherosclerosis and the presence of late stenosis in vein graft predicts adverse clinical event.

3. Ans. d. Pravastatin

Hurst's 10th Ed; Page 1511

Since the early saphenous vein graft atherosclerosis study, substantial progress has been made in extending the effectiveness of vein grafts. Perioperative treatment with platelet inhibitors have decreased the occlusion rate of vein graft at 1 year after operation. Such that approximately 90% of saphenous vein graft are found to be functioning at the end of first postoperative year. Lipid lowering regimen including use of statins have been shown to decrease the rate of vein graft atherosclerosis 5–15 years after operation and have decreased the risk of death and nonfatal myocardial infarction during a 5-year follow-up after bypass surgery.

4. Ans. a. Left internal mammary artery

Hurst's 10th Ed; Page 1513

The various graft which are used during bypass surgery as conduits are internal thoracic artery grafts (right and left internal thoracic artery), radial artery, gastroepiploic artery and inferior epigastric artery. The internal thoracic artery is a commonly used conduit during bypass surgery. Early patency rate of internal thoracic artery grafts are better than those for vein graft. But more importantly, the late attrition of internal thoracic artery graft is extremely low. Early occlusion of internal thoracic artery graft is usually technically related and today is uncommon. BARI (Bypass Angioplasty Revascularization Investigation) trial noted a 98% 1 year patency rate for internal thoracic artery graft. A 20 years patency rate of left internal thoracic artery (LITA) to LAD graft is still approximately 90%. The most common cause of late internal thoracic artery graft failure appears to be the competition in blood flow through a native coronary artery, i.e., only moderately stenotic. That may produce a diffuse internal thoracic artery narrowing or string sign. The success of left internal thoracic artery to LAD graft has led to the use of right internal thoracic artery (RITA) as a bypass graft usually simultaneously with LITA (bilateral internal thoracic artery grafting). The RITA has been used as an in situ graft and as a free graft with proximal anastomosis constructed either to LITA or to the aorta.

5. Ans. c. Coronary risk factors

Hurst's 10th Ed; Page 1510

Patency rate of saphenous vein graft within the first postoperative year are 80–90% and are influenced by surgical technique, gender (men more than women), coronary artery size (bigger more than smaller), and the coronary artery grafted (left anterior descending artery greater than circumflex or right coronary artery), but they were not influenced by coronary risk factors.

6. Ans. a. Hypovolumia

Hurst's 10th Ed; Page 1528

Satisfactory cardiac performance following cardiac surgery is usually indicated by a cardiac index greater than 2.2 L/min/m^2 with a heart rate below 100 bpm. Marginal cardiac function is present with a cardiac index between 2.0 and 2.2 L/min/m^2. A cardiac index below 2.0 L/min/m^2 is unacceptably low and therapeutic intervention is indicated. The most common cause of low cardiac output postoperatively are related to a decreased left ventricular preload. The decreased preload inturn can be attributed to hypovolemia (due to bleeding or to vasodilatation) or as a consequence of weaning of the drugs), cardiac tamponade or right ventricular dysfunction. Alternative explanation for low cardiac output includes decrease cardiac contractility due to a pre-existing low ejection fraction or to intra or postoperative ischemia or infarction. Tachy or bradyarrhythmia decrease cardiac output by reducing ventricular preload or by reducing the number of effective ventricular contraction per minute. Substantial increase in systemic vascular resistance (i.e., vasoconstriction) impedes ventricular ejection and lowers the cardiac ouput. Vasodilatation from sepsis or anaphylaxis resulting in systemic hypotension can lead to reduced coronary blood flow and myocardial ischemia. Sepsis is also associated with production of myocardial depressant factors. Anemia may result in reduced blood viscosity leading to hypotension and decreased oxygen delivery to the heart.

7. Ans. d. Sinus tachycardia

Hurst's 10th Ed; Page 1529 & 1530

The most common rhythm disturbance immediately after cardiac surgery is sinus tachycardia. This condition is appropriately treated by searching for and correcting the underlying cause (pain, anxiety, low cardiac output, anemia, fever or β-blocker withdrawl). The second most common arrhythmia is ventricular ectopy. Again an underlying cause such as myocardial ischemia, hypokalemia, hypomagnesemia, hypoxia or administration of sympathomimetic drugs must be sought and corrected if possible. After cardiac surgery a few patient develops sustained ventricular tachycardia or ventricular fibrillation. These profound rhythm disturbances may develop in the absence of evidence of acute myocardial ischemia or infarction or electrolyte imbalance. In most cases the patients have had previous myocardial infarction and have undergone complete revascularization including for regions likely to be nonviable. Reperfusion of these areas that probably includes viable as well as nonviable myofibrils embedded in the healed infarct may lead to altered dispersion of repolarization and these changes results into the reentrant arrhythmias. The ventricular tachycardia in these patients uncommonly respond to lidocaine and usually require Amiodarone. In some cases, a combination of amiodarone and β-blockers is required. The most common supraventricular dysrhythmia with exception of sinus tachycardia are atrial fibrillation and atrial flutter and these rhythm disturbances occurs in 10-30% of patients following cardiac surgery. The predominate predisposing factor in the development of atrial fibrillation is the patient age. The prevalence of atrial fibrillation in postoperative cardiac patient less than 40 years of age is as lower 3.7% while the prevalence is at least 28% in patients over 70 years. Atrial fibrillation is most likely to appear on the second postoperative day. Within 1-3 days 80% of these patients will return to sinus rhythm with only digoxin or β-blocker therapy. The prophylactic use of β-blockers has a protective effect against the development of atrial fibrillation or flutter. These beneficial effect has been demonstrated with anyone of the several β-blocker, administered in low or high dose and started preoperatively or postoperatively. Neither digoxin nor verapamil has demonstrated effective prophylaxis against atrial fibrillation or flutter. Preoperative oral administration of amiodarone also reduces the prevalence of postoperative atrial fibrillation.

The prevalence of intraventricular conduction abnormality after coronary artery bypass surgery is reported to be 1-45% with approximately 10% being the most commonly reported frequency. The most common conduction defect is right bundle branch block which may be due to selective sensitivity of right bundle to the effect of hypothermia and the extracorporeal circulation process. Only about 5% of the patients are left with a permanent conduction abnormality and the prognosis for these patients is no worse than it is for comparable patient with no conduction defect.

8. Ans. d. Beta blockers

Hurst's 10th Ed; Page 1529 & 1530

Refer to explanation for Q. No 7.

9. Ans. b. Right bundle branch block

Hurst's 10th Ed; Page 1529 & 1530

Please refer to explanation for Q. No 7 (last paragraph)

10. Ans. c. Preload

Hurst's 10th Ed; Page 1237

There is direct correlation between coronary blood flow and myocardial oxygen consumption. The physiological rationale is based on the requirement for coronary blood flow to meet the energy requirement of the heart. The main parameters dictating cardiac oxygen consumption are heart rate (chronotropy), cardiac contractility (inotropy) and left ventricular wall stress. The coronary perfusion at rest in human is about 200 mL/min, it can increase up to 1000 mL/min on maximal exercise. The difference between value at rest and maximal level of coronary flow represent the coronary flow reserve. The mechanism by which the coronary bed adopts the blood flow to cardiac workload represents one component of coronary autoregulation, i.e., the recruitment of coronary flow reserve to match coronary blood flow to energy needs.

11. Ans. d. All of the above

Hurst's 10th Ed; Page 1240

Atherothrombosis as defined by response to injury hypothesis, a chronic low grade inflammatory condition. Controversy persists as to whether infectious agents play a primary role either in atherothrombosis or in the transformation of stable to unstable coronary artery disease. *Chlamydia, pneumoniae* and cytomegalovirus, and *Helicobacter pylori* have been identified within human atherosclerotic lesions. Antibodies against *Chlamydia* heat shock protein can cross-react against heat shock proteins produced by endothelium resulting in endothelial damage and accelerated atherosclerosis. Although antibodies to *Chlamydia*, cytomegalovirus and *Helicobacter* pylori are found more often in patient with atherothrombosis than in controls, these associations do not indicate causality. Antibodies to these agents due to prior infection are found in a high proportion of population particularly the elderly.

12. Ans. d. All are correct

Hurst's 10th Ed; Page 1244

The widespread availability of more sensitive biochemical cardiac marker particularly troponin has improved the ability to diagnose lesser degree of myocardial necrosis. As many as 25 to 33% of patients with unstable angina will have elevated level of troponin T or troponin I on admission or soon thereafter. Many of these patients have normal level of CPK—MB. Troponin T or troponin I measurement may be normal early after the onset of acute coronary syndrome and becomes positive later. Patient with elevated level of troponin should be treated as high-risk case compared with unstable angina patients with normal troponin level. These high-risk patients should be classified having non ST elevation MI even in presence of normal CPK-MB level.

13. Ans. a. Proximal to the first septal and first diagonal branch

Hurst's 10th Ed; Page 1363

Right bundle branch block is a very specific marker of an occlusion before the first septal branch as well as ST segment elevation in lead V_1 more than equal to 2.5 mm, any ST segment elevation in lead aVR, and ST segment depression in lead V_5.

14. Ans. b. Additional left anterior descending artery disease

Hurst's 10th Ed; Page 1370

Right bundle branch block with or without hemiblock during acute anterior MI indicate proximal LAD occlusion. Bundle branch block or complete AV block indicate a poor prognosis. Left anterior fascicular block in acute inferior wall MI suggest additional LAD disease.

15. Ans. d. In spite of use of thrombolysis, aspirin, coronary intervention and ACE inhibitors the mortality of patients with acute MI is 15-30%

Hurst's 10th Ed; Page 1277

The important general facts about myocardial infarction are:

- Majority of patients of acute MI who die, approximately half of them do so within 1 hour of onset of symptom before reaching to the hospital;
- The majority of early deaths are the result of ventricular arrhythmias that can be readily aborted by defibrillation either during prehospital care or in the hospital coronary care unit;
- The major cause of myocardial infarction is atherosclerotic disease of the epicardial coronary arteries. Although luminal narrowing resulting in hemodynamically significant obstruction of blood flow is the major cause of symptoms of coronary ischemia, the majority of myocardial infarction occurs as a result of disruption of arterial lesions that are not hemodynamically significant (<60%). This breakdown of the structural integrity of arterial intima occur because of weakening induced by proteolytic degradation of matrix protein byproducts released from inflammatory leukocytes and result in exposure of blood to thrombogenic intimal material causing obstructive clot formation. The biological state of atherosclerotic lesion and not the extent of stenosis is the major determinant whether or not plaque rupture and myocardial infarction occurs;
- Episode of ischemia preceding coronary occlusion enhance the survivability of myocardial cells (ischemic preconditioning);
- Irreversible cardiac injury occurs if occlusion is complete for at least 15-20 minutes. Irreversible injury occurs maximally in the area at risk when occlusion is sustained for 4-6 hours but most of the damage occurs in first 2-3 hours. Thus, restoration of flow within first 4-6 hours is associated with the salvage of myocardium but salvage is exponentially greater if restoration of blood flow occurs in 1-2 hours;
- Restoration of the blood flow by thrombolysis results in myocardial salvage and improve mortality. The extent of benefit depends on restoration of near normal blood flow (open artery hypothesis) and is inversely related to the time between the onset of occlusion (symptom) and restoration of blood flow;
- Because of their salutary effects on thrombus formation and ventricular arrhythmia, aspirin and β-adrenergic blocker drugs have proved to be effective for secondary prevention in patients who have had a myocardial infarction. Aspirin has also been shown to be modestly effective for primary prevention in middle aged male;
- Lipid lowering and smoking cessation have both been shown to be effective in primary and secondary prevention of myocardial infarction. The mortality following acute MI has been estimated to come down to about 30% in the pre CCU era. The mortality rate has dropped dramatically to about 15% in the CCU era with the use of hemodynamic monitoring and defibrillation and β-blockers. The increase use of thrombolytics, coronary intervention, aspirin and angiotensin converting enzyme inhibitors have decrease the mortality of patients treated for the conventional ST segment elevation MI to 6-7%.

16. Ans. d. The resting ECG is a sensitive tool for detecting the presence of atherosclerotic coronary heart disease

Hurst's 10th Ed; Page 1281

Myocardial infarction has typically been diagnosed on the basis of the triad of chest pain, electrocardiographic changes and elevated plasma enzyme activity. Although acute myocardial infarction can occur without chest pain in 20-25% of cases, chest pain remains the most common symptoms and is usually responsible for patients seeking medical help. Acute myocardial infarction is difficult to diagnose electrocardiographically in the presence of left bundle block because of the unpredictability of depolarization and repolarization patterns. It has been suggested that marked ST segment deviation beyond what could be anticipated from conduction abnormality could be useful in the diagnosis of acute myocardial infarction in the setting of left bundle branch block. The resting electrocardiogram is insensitive for detecting the presence of atherosclerotic coronary heart disease. It is normal in 50% of patients with angiographically significant coronary obstruction. The mortality rate for Q wave infarction is about 10–12%.

17. **Ans. c. 15–25%**

Hurst's 10th Ed; Page 1283

Approximately 15–25% of patients with non-Q wave MI have evidence of early reinfarction and therefore aggressive management is needed to prevent and control the symptom and to prevent the further episode of myocardial ischemia and necrosis. Calcium channel antagonists are used to control ongoing or recurring ischemia related symptoms in patients who are already receiving adequate doses of nitrates and β-blockers, in patients who are unable to tolerate adequate doses of one or both of these agents or in those with variant angina. Several randomized trials assessing the use of calcium antagonist in acute coronary syndrome generally confirm that these agents relieve or prevent symptoms and related ischemia to a degrees similar to that of β-blockers.

18. **Ans. b. Diltiazem**

Hurst's 10th Ed; Page 1283

Refer to explanation for Q. No 17.

19. **Ans. d. Troponin**

Hurst's 10th Ed; Page 1287, 1288 & 1290

Elevated plasma CPK-MB as a diagnostic marker for myocardial infarction is associated with a very low incidence of false negative results when samples are collected frequently and appropriately within 48–72 hours of the onset of symptoms. However, false positive result do occur since trace amount of CPK-MB can also be released from tissue other then the heart. Skeletal muscle injury as noted may induce the synthesis CPK-MB and has been documented after crash injury, electrical injury, dermatomyositis and polymyositis as well as in professional athletes and marathon runners. Troponin I has not been found to be elevated in patient with normal skeletal muscle despite severe exercise or injury or in blood of the marathon runners. Troponin I is not elevated in chronic renal failure. An increase in troponin T has been reported in patient with polymyositis without cardiac involvement.

In patients admitted 48–72 hours after onset of symptoms particularly when associated with minimal myocardial damage, plasma CPK-MB may have return to normal level. In this situation, it has been traditional to utilize LDH isoenzymes, since LDH-1 activity peaks between 48 and 72 hours and remains elevated for 10–14 days. But the preferred diagnostic marker is now troponin I and T. Patient who had myocardial infarction after non cardiac surgery is also reliably determined from serial analysis of plasma, CPK-MB, troponin T or troponin I every 4–6 hours. There is marked elevated of other enzymes due to tissue trauma including total CPK, but not CPK-MB troponin T and troponin I are highly specific to the myocardium.

The stress of myocardial infarction elicits numerous hormonal and metabolic responses. Both catecholamine and growth hormones are elevated, however serum cholesterol and lipoproteins faction are relatively unchanged in the initial 1–2 days but decrease significantly over subsequent days and weeks. In establishing the baseline level of these values for guiding future therapeutic interventions measurement should be performed on admission or should be delayed for 6–8 weeks. The other abnormalities seen on occasion is that of increase in the blood glucose following myocardial infarction which in some cases particularly in patient with mild or moderate diabetes may be associated with development of significant ketoacidosis. It has been observed that in early days following myocardial infarction, the glucose tolerance curve is abnormal and it returns to normal after a few weeks. The white blood cell count is usually mildly to moderately elevated for 3–5 days.

20. **Ans. d. Troponin I**

Hurst's 10th Ed; Page 1287, 1288 & 1290

Refer to explanation for Q. No 19.

21. **Ans. c. Serum cholesterol and lipoprotein fractions**

Hurst's 10th Ed; Page 1287, 1288 & 1290

Refer to explanation for Q. No 19.

22. **Ans. b. Troponin I**

Hurst's 10th Ed; Page 1287, 1288 & 1290

Refer to explanation for Q. No 19.

23. **Ans. d. It does not require surgical intervention often**

Hurst's 10th Ed; Page 1328

A pseudoaneurysm is a rare complication of myocardial infarction. Its prevalence is not known. The probable sequence of events in the development of pseudoaneurysm is: (1) occurrence of a transmural MI with localized pericarditis arising at the site of infarction; (2) development of adhesion between the visceral and parietal pericardium; (3) rupture of infarcted myocardium with the extra vasted blood confined by the visceral pericardium; (4) progressive enlargement of the aneurysmal sac and (5) the development of thrombus within the sac.

Unlike a true ventricular aneurysm, a pseudoaneurysm has a narrow base. The wall is composed only of a thrombus and pericardium and the risk of rupture is high. While the neck is small (its diameter is <50% of the diameter of the fundus), the pseudoaneurysm may progressively enlarge to become larger than the left ventricle. The pseudoaneurysm may be clinically silent or may present as progressively worsening heart failure, an abnormal bulge on the cardiac border, persistent ST segment elevation in the area overlying the infarction or systolic murmur. The diagnosis of pseudoaneurysm can be established by 2D echocardiographic studies, radionuclide studies, MRI or left ventriculographic contrast studies. Surgical resection is always indicated.

24. Ans. d. Right bundle branch block

Hurst's 10th Ed; Page 1361

The presentation of acute myocardial infarction varies depending on the coronary artery involved. The left anterior descending (LAD) branch supplies the anterior, lateral, septal and frequently the inferoapical segment of the left ventricle, including the proximal part of the bundle branches leading to large myocardial infarction. Right coronary artery (RCA) perfuses the sinus node (55% of patients), the right ventricle, the AV node, the posteromedial papillary muscle, the inferior part of the left ventricle and variably also the posterior and lateral segments. The clinical picture may be impressive due to: (1) activation of vagal nervous system; (2) ischemia of the sinus and AV node leading to sinus bradycardia and delay or block in AV node; (3) right ventricular involvement and cardiogenic shock; (4) ischemia of the papillary muscle leading to the mitral regurgitation.

The circumflex branch perfuses the posterior wall and variably the inferior and lateral segments. In case of posterior wall involvement following occlusion, abnormalities in ventricular activation occurs in the 2nd half of the QRS complex and are therefore difficult to pick up on 12 lead ECG frequently causing under estimation of the area at-risk and under treatment of the patient.

25. Ans. a. Proximal to the septal and first diagonal branch

Hurst's 10th Ed; Page 1362

The ECG signs of an anterior myocardial infarction are ST segment elevation in precordial leads V_2, V_3 and V_4. The behavior of the ST segment in the other precordial and frontal leads depends on the presence of ischemia in three vectorially opposite areas: (1) the basoseptal area perfused by proximal septal branch; (2) basolateral area perfuse by the 1st diagonal branch; (3) inferoapical area when the distal LAD wraps around the apex. This leads schematically to occlusion either (1) proximal to the septal and 1st diagonal branch (40% of cases); (2) distal to this two branches (40%) or (3) proximal to the first diagonal but distal to the septal branch (10%) or (4) proximally to the septal but distal to the 1st diagonal branch (10%). Whenever there is a dominance of basal area, i.e., the occlusion of proximal LAD, the typical feature in ECG includes ST elevation in lead aVR and ST elevation of more than 2.5 mm in lead V_1, ST segment depression in inferior leads and in lead V_5 and abnormal Q wave in lead aVL.

26. Ans. d. All of the above

Braunwald 7th Ed; Page 1105

Atherosclerosis is a progressive disease process that generally begins in childhood and has clinical manifestation in middle to late adulthood. It is a multifactorial process which if it leads to clinical sequelae requires extensive accumulation of a smooth muscle cell within the intima of the affected artery. The form and content of the advanced lesion of atherosclerosis demonstrate the result of three fundamental processes. These are: (1) accumulation of intimal smooth muscle cell together with variable numbers of accumulated macrophages and T-lymphocytes; (2) formation by the proliferated smooth muscle cell of large amount of connective tissue matrix including collagen, elastic fibers and proteoglycans and (3) accumulation of lipids, principally in the form of cholesteryl esters and free cholesterol within the cells as well as in surrounding connective tissues.

27. Ans. d. Obesity

Braunwald 7th Ed; Page 1105

The risk factor for coronary artery disease is a causative agent or condition that can be used to predict an individual probability of developing disease. There are three independent predictors of risk for individuals within a population of the incidence of atherosclerosis, i.e., plasma cholesterol concentration, cigarette smoking and elevated blood pressure.

28. Ans. c. Abdominal aorta

Braunwald 7th Ed; Page 1106

Refer to explanation for Q. No 27.

29. Ans. d. EDRF

Braunwald 7th Ed; Page 1108 & 1114

The endothelial lining of the arterial wall normally provides a nonthrombogenenic surface because of its capacity to form prostaglandin derivatives, particularly prostacyclin (PGI II), a potent vasodilator, i.e., an effective inhibitor of platelet aggregation and because of its surface coat of heparin sulfate, endothelial cell also make the most potent vasodilator, i.e., endothelial derived relaxing factor (EDRF). EDRF formation by endothelium may be critical in maintaining a balance between vasoconstriction and vasodilatation. Endothelial cell can also secrete agents that are effective in lysing fibrin clot including plasminogen as well as procoagulant materials such as von willebrand factor. They also secrete a number of vasoactive agents such as endothelin, angiotensin converting enzyme and platelet derived growth factor which may be important in vasoconstriction.

A particular characteristic of endothelium lining the arterial wall is that endothelial cell grows in an obligate monolayer. Such growth representative of cells that line most body surfaces including epithelial surfaces and is characterized by the fact that endothelial cell can not crawl over one and other sites of injury to facilitate repair of a surface that has been de-endothelialized. In other words, only the cell at the margin of an injury can participate in the regenerative response. Thus, if a particular anatomical site is repeatedly injured over a prolonged period and if the endothelial cell that regenerate lose their replication capacity, cells distal to the site capable of replicating may not be able to participate simply because they cannot reach the site to do so.

Arterial endothelial cells are capable of synthesizing and secreting several mitogens, one of which is a form of PDGF. PDGF is a growth factor for mesenchymal derived connective tissue forming cells such as fibroblast and smooth muscle cells but not for arterial endothelial cells. Endothelial cells have receptor for many different molecular on their surface including receptor for low density lipoprotein (LDL), for growth factors and probably for a number of pharmacological agents. A special capacity of endothelium that may be particularly important in atherogenesis is its ability to modify lipoproteins. LDL appears to be modified by a process of low level oxidation when they are bound to LDL receptor, internalized and transported through the endothelium. Such modified LDL can bind to a specific type of receptor termed a scavenger receptor, on the surface of macrophages where they are ingested and contribute to the formation of foam cells. This activity is important in atherosclerosis. Oxidized LDL may play an important initiative role in inducing atherosclerosis and migration of monocytes and T lymphocytes from the lumen into the artery wall. Oxidized LDL can induce the formation of at least 2 macro molecules on the surface of endothelium, vascular cell adhesion molecule 1 (VCAM-1) and intercellular adhesion molecule 1 (ICAM-1). This two molecules can participate in the increased migration of monocytes and T cells to the endothelium through receptor ligant type interactions with appropriate molecules on the surface of the leukocytes.

30. Ans. d. Can crawl over one another at sites of injury to facilitate the repair of de-endothelialized surface

Braunwald 7th Ed; Page 1108 & 1114

Refer to explanation for Q. No 29.

31. Ans. d. Arterial endothelium

Braunwald 7th Ed; Page 1108 & 1114

Refer to explanation for Q. No 29.

32. Ans. d. Oxidized LDL

Braunwald 7th Ed; Page 1108 & 1114

Refer to explanation for Q. No 29.

33. Ans. c. Renal artery

Braunwald 7th Ed; Page 1108 & 1114

Refer to explanation for Q. No 29.

34. Ans. c. First 6 cm of artery

Braunwald 7th Ed; Page 1108 & 1114

Refer to explanation for Q. No 29.

35. Ans. b. 6–8 cc/min/100 g

Braunwald 7th Ed; Page 1162

The heart is an aerobic organ, i.e., it relies almost exclusively on the oxidation of substrate for the generation of energy and it can develop only small oxygen debt. Therefore, in steady state determination of rate of myocardial oxygen consumption (MVO_2) provides an accurate measure of its total metabolism. The myocardial oxygen consumption in a healthy human heart 6–8 cc/min/100 g of the heart muscle.

36. Ans. a. Beta adrenergic agonists

Braunwald 7th Ed; Page 1174

Coronary collaterals dilate in response to nitrates and β-adrenergic agonists. On the other hand, calcium antagonists, β-blockers and β-adrenergic agonists have no detectable direct effect on collateral function. Vasopressin and serotonin are potent constrictor of the collateral circulation.

37. Ans. d. It occurs in regionally ischemic heart

Braunwald 7th Ed; Page 1176

Myocardial stunning is a process whereby after a brief episode of severe ischemia prolonged myocardial dysfunction with gradual return of contractile activity occurs. Stunning may occur following exercise induced ischemia, and coronary spasm. It affects both systolic and diastolic function and can occur in the globally as well as the regionally ischemic heart. Clinically myocardial stunning probably occur more frequently in patients who have undergone ischemic cardiac arrest during cardiopulmonary bypass. Such heart may not recover normal function for days. In patient with myocardial infarction (both with and without the administration of reperfusion thrombolytic therapy) reversibly injured, functionally stunned myocardial lies adjacent to infarcted myocardium. Myocardial stunning is an important feature of unstable angina. The severity of ischemic stress is an important influence in the genesis of myocardial stunning. The severity of stunning is always greater in the subendocardial layers of the left ventricular wall which are more ischemic than the subepicardial layer. The duration of ischemia is a second important factor.

38. Ans. d. All of the above

Braunwald 7th Ed; Page 1176-1177

Despite the unequivocal utility of reperfusion in limiting cell death in the presence of severe ischemia, reperfusion can elicit and a number of adverse reaction that may limit its beneficial action.
1. Acceleration of myocytes necrosis—after reperfusion ischemic cells often suddenly develop ultra structural changes indicative of cell death including "explosive swelling" and widespread architectural disruption;
2. The no reflow phenomena—this refers to the failure to achieve sustained reperfusion after a prolonged period of ischemia. The areas of reduced or absent reflow often appear to result from ischemia induced microvascular damage and myocardial contracture. However, the no reflow phenomena does not appear to augment myocytes death because the zone of reflow is content within the areas in which myocytes were already necrotic at the time of onset of reperfusion. Reperfusion induced hemorrhage-reperfused infarct frequently contain hemorrhagic areas. Reperfusion induced hemorrhage like the no reflow phenomena is caused largely by microvascular damage. It is generally contain within the areas of myocardium already necrotic at the time of reperfusion.

Reperfusion can be detrimental by causing arrhythmias and can contribute to myocardial stunning.

HYPERLIPIDEMIA

1. Which of the following is *correct* regarding Fredrickson classification of the hyperlipidemias?
   a. It is not an etiological classification
   b. It does not differentiate primary and secondary hyperlipidemia
   c. It does not consider the levels of high density lipoprotein (HDL) cholesterol
   d. All are correct

2. Which is the commonest variety of hyperlipidemia according to Fredrickson classification?
   a. Type I
   b. Type II
   c. Type III
   d. Type IV

3. Atherogenicity is *not* seen in which variety of hyperlipidemia:
   a. Type I   b. Type II
   c. Type III   d. Type IV

4. Which of the lipoprotein is *not* atherogenic?
   a. Chylomicrons   b. Chylomicron remnant
   c. VLDL   d. LDL

5. Which of the following observational studies demonstrated positive relation between total cholesterol level and CAD?
   a. MRFIT (Multiple Risk Factor Interventional Trial)
   b. The lLRC-CPPT (Lipid Research Clinics Coronary Primary Prevention Trial)
   c. Helsinki heart study
   d. West of Scotland Coronary Prevention Study (WOSCOPS)

ANSWERS WITH EXPLANATIONS

1. Ans. d. All are correct

Braunwald 5th Ed; Page 1127

Dyslipidemia can be classified according to which lipoprotein levels are abnormal as in the Fredrickson classification system. The Fredrickson classification system is not diagnostic and does not consider HDL or Lp(a). Fredrickson classification is not an etiological classification and does not differentiate primary and secondary hyperlipidemia.

Fredrickson Classification of the Hyperlipidemias

Pheno-type	Lipo-protein(s) elevated	Plasma cholesterol level	Plasma tri-glyceride level	Athero-genicity	Relative frequency
I	Chylo-microns	Normal to ↑	↑↑↑↑	Not seen	<1%
IIa	LDL	↑↑	Normal	+++	10%
IIb	LDL and VLDL	↑↑	↑↑	+++	40%
III	IDL	↑↑	↑↑↑	+++	<1%
IV	VLDL	Normal to ↑	↑↑	+	45%
V	VLDL and chylo-microns	↑ to ↑↑	↑↑↑↑	+	5%

2. Ans. d. Type IV

Braunwald 5th Ed; Page 1127

Refer to explanation for Q. No 1.

3. Ans. a. Type I

Braunwald 5th Ed; Page 1127

Refer to explanation for Fredrickson classification of the hyperlipidemias in Q. No 1.

4. Ans. a. Chylomicrons

Braunwald 5th Ed; Page 1127

Refer to explanation for Q. No 1.

5. Ans. b. The LRC-CPPT (Lipid Research Clinics Coronary Primary Prevention Trial)

Braunwald 5th Ed; Page 1128

The LRC-CPPT (Lipid Research Clinics Coronary Primary Prevention Trials) provided the first major clinical substantiation of the lipid hypothesis. It results were the first to give rise to the rule of thumb that a 1% decrease in the total cholesterol reduces the incidence of coronary artery disease events 2–3%.

CARDIOVASCULAR SURGERY

1. Direct anastomosis of the end of subclavian artery to the side of the pulmonary artery is known as:
   a. Glenn shunt
   b. Waterston shunt
   c. Blalock–Taussig Shunt
   d. Modified Blalock–Taussig shunt

2. Modified Blalock–Taussig shunt is:
   a. A direct anastomosis of the end of subclavian artery to the side of pulmonary artery
   b. PTFE graft between subclavian artery and pulmonary artery
   c. Direct anastomosis of SVC to pulmonary artery
   d. None of the above

3. First open heart surgery using heart lung machine was performed by:
   a. John Gibbon   b. Walton Lillehei
   c. John Kirklin   d. Albert Starr

4. First successful heart transplant was performed by:
   a. John Gibbon   b. John Kirklin
   c. Norman Shumway   d. Christian Barnard

5. Selective coronary angiography was introduced by:
   a. Mason Sones   b. Judkins
   c. Amplatz   d. Gruentzig

6. Operative procedures on the heart or major intrathoracic vessels done when the heart is beating and supporting the effective circulation comes under category of:
   a. Open heart surgery
   b. Surgery under hypothermia
   c. Surgery on cardioplegia
   d. Closed heart surgery

7. All the following surgeries are done through left thoracotomy *except*:
   a. Repair of coarctation of aorta
   b. Blalock–Taussig Shunt
   c. Closed mitral valvotomy
   d. Waterston shunt between pulmonary artery and posterior aspect of ascending aorta

8. Which of the following is *not* a closed heart surgery?
   a. Closed mitral valvotomy
   b. Repair of coarctation of aorta
   c. OPCAB
   d. All of the above

9. Which of the following serves the function of lungs during extracorporeal circulation (ECC)?
   a. Blood pump
   b. Oxygenator
   c. Heat exchangers
   d. Left ventricular assist device (LVAD)

10. **Which of the following is an essential component of equipments to maintain effective circulation and carry out function of lungs during an open heart surgery?**
    a. Blood pump
    b. Oxygenator
    c. Heat exchangers
    d. All are essential

11. **Which of the following oxygenator is more physiological and similar to natural lungs?**
    a. Film oxygenators
    b. Disc oxygenators
    c. Bubble oxygenators
    d. Membrane oxygenators

12. **To neutralize each mg of heparin, what is the usual dose of protamine sulfate:**
    a. 0.5–1 mg/kg/wt
    b. 1–1.5 mg of protamine for each mg of heparin administered
    c. 2–3 mg of protamine for each mg of heparin administered
    d. None of the above

13. **The very safe period of arrest during deep hypothermia and circulatory arrest (DHCA) is to avoid brain damage is:**
    a. 30 minutes or less
    b. 45 minutes or less
    c. 60 minutes or less
    d. 90 minutes or less

14. **Retrograde cardioplegia is administered through:**
    a. Ascending aorta, proximal to the site of clamp
    b. Direct coronary ostial cannulation
    c. Through coronary sinus
    d. Through IVC

15. **Which is the commonly used circulatory assist device?**
    a. Left ventricular assist device (LVAD)
    b. Right ventricular assist device (RVAD)
    c. Total artificial heart
    d. Intra-aortic balloon pump (IABP)

16. **Octopus and Starfish are:**
    a. Types of artificial heart
    b. Type of ventricular assist device
    c. Types of aortic stents
    d. Mechanical stabilizers to be used for OPCAB

17. **Which is the most commonly used conduits during coronary artery bypass surgery?**
    a. Left internal mammary artery
    b. Saphenous vein
    c. Radial artery
    d. Gastroepiploic artery

18. **All the following factors makes Internal mammary artery an ideal conduit for CABG except:**
    a. Its size matches the coronary artery
    b. It is resistant to atherosclerosis
    c. Has excellent long-term patency
    d. Its' location in chest helps in easy harvesting

19. **Which is current regarding radial artery conduit's unpopularity?**
    a. It is a small caliber vessel
    b. It's length is often inadequate
    c. Radial artery spasm is frequent problem
    d. Its' harvesting often leads to ischemic in hand

20. **Gastroepiploic artery graft is used for bypass all of the following except:**
    a. Right coronary artery
    b. Posterior descending artery
    c. Obtuse marginal artery
    d. Left anterior descending artery

21. **Which of the following is *not* a biological conduit for CABG?**
    a. Borine IMA
    b. Human umbilical vein
    c. Dacron
    d. Cryopreserved umbilical vein

22. **Which of the following conduit have lower long-term patency?**
    a. IMA graft
    b. Radial artery
    c. Inferior epigastric artery
    d. Vein grafts

23. **What is definition of left main equivalent disease?**
    a. When there is critical block in all three major epicardial arteries
    b. When there is total block of all the three arteries
    c. When there is significant block in proximal LAD (proximal to first septal and first diagonal) and proximal left circumflex artery
    d. When there is significant block in proximal left circumflex artery and total occlusion of left anterior descending artery

24. **CABG is indicated for all the following subset of patients *except*:**
    a. Left main coronary artery disease
    b. Triple vessel disease
    c. Double vessel disease (LCx + RCA) with good LV function
    d. Double vessel disease (LAD + RCA) with impaired LV function

25. **Which of the following factor influences selection for CABG and its long-term results?**
    a. LV function
    b. Diabetes mellitus
    c. Extent and severity of CAD
    d. All of the above

26. In a patient with effort angina who is found to have significant proximal LAD lesion and ejection fraction is <50% and noninvasive test showing extensive reversible ischemia. The best treatment option is:
a. Medical treatment
b. CABG with LIMA graft
c. PTCA with stent of LAD
d. Medical treatment with PTCA and stent of LAD

27. In the current days, the incidence of perioperative myocardial infarction is:
a. Less than 2.5%
b. Less than 4%
c. Less than 5%
d. Less than 10%

28. Which is *incorrect* regarding perioperative myocardial infarction following CABG?
a. The incidence is <2.5%
b. Incidence is higher after endarterectomy
c. There is no difference in the incidence of perioperative MI between CABG on pump and off pump
d. The incidence of perioperative MI is higher with CABG on pump compare to off pump CABG

29. Which is the commonest arrhythmia seen in the perioperative case after CABG?
a. AV block
b. Ventricular tachycardia
c. Atrial fibrillation
d. Paroxysmal atrial tachycardia

30. The early recurrence of angina around 3 months after bypass surgery is unlikely to be due to?
a. Acute graft closure
b. Inadequate revascularization
c. Progression of disease in the native arteries distal to the graft
d. Spasm of arterial conduit

31. Which of the following is a biological valve?
a. Starr–Edwards ball valve
b. Medtronic–Hall valve
c. Carbomedics valve
d. Medtronic–Hancock valve

32. Which of the following prosthetic heart valve has lowest effective orifice areas?
a. Medtronic–Hall valve
b. Bjork–Shiley valve
c. Starr–Edwards valve
d. Chitra valve

33. Which is *not* a complication of mechanical prosthetic valve?
a. Valve thrombosis
b. Hemolysis
c. Degeneration and calcification
d. Paravalvular leak

34. The normal mitral valve area is:
a. 1–2 cm^2
b. 2–3 cm^2
c. 3–4 cm^2
d. 4–5 cm^2

35. A person who is found to have mitral valve area of 1–2 cm^2 with a mean pressure gradient 6–9 mm Hg would be classified as:
a. Mild mitral stenosis
b. Moderate mitral stenosis
c. Severe mitral stenosis
d. Critical mitral stenosis

36. The commonest cause of pulmonary stenosis is:
a. Carcinoid syndrome
b. Extrinsic pulmonary obstruction by cardiac tumors
c. Rheumatic involvement along with disease of cardiac valve
d. Congenital

37. A child with pulmonary valve area on echocardiogram of 1.5 cm^2 and gradient of 80 mm Hg will be classified as:
a. Trivial pulmonary stenosis
b. Mild pulmonary stenosis
c. Moderate pulmonary stenosis
d. Severe pulmonary stenosis

38. The treatment of choice for congenital pulmonary stenosis is:
a. Closed pulmonary valvotomy
b. Open pulmonary valvotomy
c. Pulmonary valvotomy with infundibular resection
d. Balloon pulmonary valvotomy

39. The pericardiectomy for constrictive pericarditis is a:
a. Open heart surgery
b. Closed heart surgery
c. Off pump surgery
d. None of them

40. In the current era, the mortality is:
a. 20%
b. 10–15%
c. 3–5%
d. 0%

41. The most commonest cause of left ventricular aneurysm is:
a. Transmural myocardial infarction
b. Trauma
c. Chagas disease
d. Sarcoidosis

42. Which is the commonest location of ventricular aneurysm?
a. Anterolateral wall of LV
b. Posterolateral wall of LV
c. Lateral wall of LV
d. Inferior wall of LV

43. Which is *not* correct regarding false left ventricular aneurysm?
   a. It often develop after acute rupture of an infarct
   b. It is formed due to the adhesions between parietal pericardium and epicardium
   c. The mouth is usually wide
   d. They occur more often on the diaphragmatic surface

44. Which is *not* true regarding postmyocardial infarction ventricular septal defect?
   a. The incidence has come down due to thrombolysis
   b. The location is 40% anterior and 60% posterior
   c. A posterior septal rupture is often association with mitral regurgitation
   d. It may occur within 2 days of MI or as late as 2 weeks

45. Which of the following is *not* an absolute indication for surgery in native valve endocarditis?
   a. Heart failure unresponsive to medical treatment due to MR or AR
   b. Evidence of aortic root abscess and true or false aneurysm of sinus of Valsalva
   c. Evidence of valve dysfunction and persistent infection after a week of appropriate antibiotic treatment
   d. Mobile vegetations more than 10 mm

46. Prosthetic heart valve endocarditis is called early if symptoms begin:
   a. Within 30 days of surgery
   b. Within 60 days of surgery
   c. Within 90 days of surgery
   d. Within 4 months of surgery

47. The commonest positive organism for early prosthetic valve endocarditis is:
   a. Coagulase positive *Staphylococcus*
   b. Coagulase negative *Staphylococcus–Staphylococcus epidermidis*
   c. Gram-negative bacilli
   d. Fungi (*Candida* species)

48. Which is *not* correct regarding prosthetic valve endocarditis?
   a. In early prosthetic valve endocarditis the organism responsible is usually a nosocomial one and while for late endocarditis, a community acquired organism is often the culprit
   b. During the initial months after implantation, a mechanical valve is at higher risk for SABE then bioprosthetic valve. However, after 12 months the incidence of SABE is more on bioprosthetic valve
   c. At 5 years, the incidence of SABE is comparable among mechanical and bioprosthetic valve
   d. All are correct

49. The report mortality for surgery following prosthetic valve endocarditis is:
   a. 2–4%   b. 6–8%
   c. 8–10%   d. 22%

50. A moderate size ventricular septal defect is one which has a diameter:
   a. Equal to the aorta
   b. Above 50% of aorta
   c. Less than one-third of aorta
   d. None of the above

51. Which is *true* regarding ventricular septal defect?
   a. There is an inverse relationship between the probability of VSD closure and age at which the patient is seen
   b. Infant with large VSD intractable heart failure during the first 3 months requires prompt closure
   c. In children having pulmonary resistance <4 U/m^2, surgery could be postponed up to 1 year
   d. All of the above

52. Pulmonary artery banding is the procedure of choice for all of the following *except*:
   a. Isolated VSD
   b. Multiple muscular VSD (Swiss cheese defects)
   c. Tricuspid atresia with VSD
   d. All of the above

53. An atrial septal defect which is <5 mm in diameter is a risk for:
   a. Pulmonary hypertension
   b. Cardiac failure
   c. Infective endocarditis
   d. Paradoxical embolism

54. The most common type of ASD is:
   a. Ostium secundum type
   b. Sinus venosus type
   c. Ostium primum type
   d. Coronary sinus type

55. Atrial Switch operation (Senning or Mustard operation) is performed for correction of:
   a. Tricuspid atresia with VSD in pulmonary stenosis
   b. Total anomalous pulmonary venous return
   c. Tetralogy of Fallots
   d. Transposition of great arteries

ANSWERS WITH EXPLANATIONS

1. Ans. c. Blalock–Taussig Shunt

IGNOU, MCC 005; Page 6

Alfred Blalock, Cardiac surgeon at John Hawkins University did the first palliative shunt between subclavian artery and pulmonary artery for cyanotic heart disease. This is known as Blalock-Taussig shunt. This was a direct anastomosis of the end of subclavian artery to the side of pulmonary artery. Marc de Leval in 1981 used a Polytetrafluoroethylene (PTFE) graft between subclavian artery and pulmonary artery (modified BT shunt).

2. Ans. b. PTFE graft between subclavian artery and pulmonary artery

IGNOU, MCC 005; Page 6

Refer to explanation for Q. No 1.

3. Ans. a. John Gibbon

IGNOU, MCC 005; Page 7

The first open heart surgery using heart lung machine was performed by John Gibbon. He successfully closed atrial septal defect in a young girl.

4. Ans. d. Christian Barnard

IGNOU, MCC 005; Page 7

Christian Barnard did successful heart transplantation in 1967 at Cape Town.

5. Ans. a. Mason Sones

IGNOU, MCC 005; Page 8

Mason Sones in 1959 introduced selective coronary angiography.

6. Ans. d. Closed heart surgery

IGNOU, MCC 005; Page 8

Operative procedures on the heart or major intrathoracic vessels done when the heart is beating and supporting effective circulation comes under the category of closed heart surgery. Depending on the type of surgery planned the heart may be approached through median sternotomy, left or right thoracotomy. Through this closed heart surgery, the first operation conducted was ligation of a patent ductus arteriosus through a left thoracotomy. Same approach is used for repair of coarctation of aorta, a few of interrupted aortic arches, pulmonary artery bending and palliative aortopulmonary shunts. BT shunt either classical or modified, Potts shunt between the left pulmonary artery and descending thoracic aorta are also done through left thoracotomy. This is also approach for closed mitral valve valvotomy (CMV). Right thoracotomy is used for classic or modified BT shunt, Waterston shunt between pulmonary artery and posterior aspect of ascending aorta and Blalock-Hanlon atrial septectomy are done through this approach. Partial pericardiectomy can be done through a left thoracotomy or a median sternotomy. Central aortopulmonary shunt with Goretex grafts, pulmonary artery bending, closed mitral valvotomy and infundibular resection can be done through a median sternotomy approach. The latest addition to the list of closed heart surgery is coronary artery bypass surgery on a beating heart, i.e. off pump coronary artery bypass (OPCAB).

7. Ans. d. Waterston shunt between pulmonary artery and posterior aspect of ascending aorta

IGNOU, MCC 005; Page 8

Refer to explanation for Q. No 6.

8. Ans. d. All of the above

IGNOU, MCC 005; Page 8

Refer to explanation for Q. No 6.

9. Ans. b. Oxygenator

IGNOU, MCC 005; Page 9–10 & 13

Open heart surgery is considered as one of the most significant advances in medicine of 20th century. Establishment of safe cardiopulmonary bypass (CPB) by extracorporeal circulation (ECC) has helped the surgeons to stop the heart, open it, carry out intricate corrections or do cardiac transplantation.

Equipment

To main effective circulation and carry out functions of the lungs during an open heart operation the equipment should have:
- Blood pump
- Oxygenators
- Heat exchangers

Blood Pump

Ideal Characteristics

- It should be able to pump up to seven liters of blood per minute.
- It should not damage cellular and acellular components of blood.
- All parts coming in contact with blood should have a smooth surface.
- Assuring no turbulence and no stagnation.

- Parts like tubing, oxygenators and heat exchangers, which come in contact with blood, should be disposable without contaminating permanent parts of the pump.
- It should be able to monitor blood flow accurately.
- Availability of manual operation facility at times of power failure.

Types of Pumps

- *Roller pump*: This is the type most commonly used in clinical perfusion. It has a circular metal housing inside which there is a rotating arm with two rollers fixed at 180° apart. Polyvinyl chloride (PVC) tubing which is resilient, passing through the inner perimeter of the housing is compressed by the rollers effecting nonpulsatile forward flow. The occlusion of the rollers are checked routinely and adjusted to optimum level. Too much occlusion will cause hemolysis; too less will reduce forward flow.
- *Centrifugal pump*: This is available for clinical perfusion from 1976 (Bio Medicus Pump). It is disposable, causes less blood trauma and reduces the risk of massive air embolism. It is useful for prolonged mechanical circulatory support like ventricular assist devices (VADs), percutaneous cardiopulmonary support and extra corporeal membrane oxygenation (ECMO).
- *Pulsatile perfusion*: Conventional pumps give continuous flow with very little pulsatile property. Pulsatile perfusion is likely to result in better postoperative renal and cardiac function. A simple method of achieving pulsatile perfusion is by adding intra aortic balloon pump (IABP) to the bypass circuit.

Oxygenators

They serve the function of lungs during extracorporeal circulation (ECC)—oxygenation removal of carbon dioxide and transport of gaseous anesthetic agents. The oxygenator will have a reservoir for venous blood and the blood sucked from cardiac chambers as well as pericardium (cardiotomy suckers). It will have facility to cool and rewarm blood (heat exchanger).

Ideal Characteristics

- Maximize gas transfer (oxygen, carbon dioxide and anesthetic gases).
- Minimize blood trauma
- Good heat transfer efficiency.
- Minimize priming volume (amount of fluid required to fill the oxygenator and the tubing).

Types of Oxygenators

- Film oxygenators
- Disk oxygenators
- Bubble oxygenators
- Membrane oxygenators
- Film and disk oxygenators are not used for clinical perfusion now.
    a. *Bubble oxygenators*—these have a mixing chamber where venous blood is collected and from the bottom end microbubbles of oxygen are passed and as they rise to the top, gas exchange takes place. The oxygenated blood is then defoamed using silicon antifoam A (dimethylpolysiloxane) before pumping into the circulation. Bubble oxygenators are used rarely and that too for only short bypass procedures.
    b. *Membrane oxygenator*—they are more physiological and are similar to natural lungs. There is separation of blood and gas by membrane across which gas exchange takes place. There are two types: (i) True membrane; (ii) Microporous membrane oxygenators.
        i. True membrane oxygenator—there is no contact between blood and gas at any time. It is more expensive and needs larger priming volume.
        ii. Microporous membrane oxygenator—at the beginning of perfusion, there is contact between blood and gas across the micropores. In a short time, protein coating of micropores occurs, severing direct contact. However after several house of use, the functional capacity of the membrane decreases. So they are not useful for prolonged use as in extracorporeal membrane oxygenator (ECMO).

Heat Exchangers

This is an integral part of cardiopulmonary bypass and is designed to cool and warm the perfusate. Non sterile water from ice bath or warm water passed through the tubing made of stainless steel or aluminium is immersed in blood flowing in opposite directions (counter current heat exchange). Rapid cooling is desirable at the beginning of perfusion with the circulating water kept at 0°C. Rewarming has to be done slowly to avoid damage to blood elements and to avoid bubble formation in the perfusate. The temperature gradient between water and blood should always be less than 10°C, while rewarming. The maximum temperature of the bath should be less than 42°C.

Open Heart Surgery

When patient is connected to cardiopulmonary bypass for an operative procedure, it is considered to be open-heart operation. In a routine coronary artery bypass, no cardiac chamber is opened. Yet, as the patient is connected to heart lung machine and heart is stopped, it is considered as open heart surgery.

Hypothermia

Hypothermia reduces the metabolic requirements of the body thereby reducing oxygen consumption. It also preserves high-energy phosphate stores of the body. At normal temperature, if there is circulatory arrest for three minutes, brain suffers hypoxic damage. At 30°C, this period extends up to 10 minutes. If the temperature is brought down to 18°C, this period extends up to 45 minutes. In 1953, John Lewis used surface hypothermia up to 28°C and by inflow occlusion method closed atrial septal defect while the heart was arrested for 5.5 minutes. Japanese surgeons started surface cooling followed by short-period of core cooling to achieve deep hypothermia (18°C) to have circulatory arrest to correct complicated intra cardiac lesions in babies. Surface cooling being a cumbersome procedure, these days both cooling and rewarming are done on the pump. In this technique of deep hypothermia and circulatory arrest (DHCA), it is safe if the period of arrest is 30 minutes or less. Between 30 and 45 minutes, it is relatively safe. Above one hour, brain damage is likely to occur. IN adults, the same technique is used for aortic arch anerurysms and pulmonary thromboendarterectomy. At the time of circulatory arrest, retrograde cerebral perfusion with cold perfusate through superior vena cava (cerebroplegia) is practised.

Myocardial Protection

To a great extent, the result of cardiac surgery depends on how well the myocardium is protected during cardiopulmonary bypass. Temporary depression of myocardium (stunning) or myocardial necrosis resulting in low cardiac output may occur after bypass. Subendocardial layer is particularly vulnerable to injury. A still heart, free of blood is essential for accurate intracardiac repair. In the earlier era, fibrillatory arrest or ischemic arrest by cross clamping the aorta was used to facilitate open heart surgery. These days, diastolic arrest of the heart is achieved by administration of cold cardioplegic solution, proximal to aortic clamp. When there is aortic regurgitation, aorta is opened and direct coronary ostial cannulation is required for giving cardioplegia. When there are multiple blocks in coronary arteries, antegrade cardioplegia will not ensure uniform distribution of the solution. Such cases will need retrograde cardioplegia administered through a coronary sinus cannula. Special retrograde cardioplegia cannulae are available with balloons, which will-fill up at the time of cardioplegia. The coronary sinus can be cannulated blindly through a purse string on the right atrium. The coronary sinus pressure should be kept below 30 mm Hg at the time of cardioplegia.

The cardioplegic solution could be cold asanguinous (clear) or with blood. The commonly used one is St Thomas solution that essentially contains 20 mEq of potassium cooled down to 4°C. Cardioplegia is usually supplemented with topical cold saline or ice slush.

Cardioplegia may be cold or warm. At times patients are operated at normothermia with warm blood cardioplegia. If the patient has recent myocardial infarction or when the ejection fraction is low, it is good to give warm blood (hotshot) just before releasing aortic clamp, to reduce reperfusion injury. The cardioplegic solution is slightly hyperosmola and buffered with sodium bicarbonate or THAM. Amino acids like Glutamate and Aspartate added to the solution reduces reperfusion injury. Adenosine adds to further protection. To reduce the injury due to oxygen free radicals, super oxide dismutase (SOD) and dimethyl sulfoxide (DMSO) can be added to the cardioplegic solution.

Venting of the Heart

It is important that heart does not distend during cardiopulmonary bypass. This is prevented by venting of the left side of the heart by inserting a cannula into the left atrium, left ventricle, pulmonary artery or aortic root below the cross clamp. The cannula is connected to low suction and the same cannula is used for deairing of the chambers of the left heart at the end of the intracardiac procedure.

Blood Salvage and Bloodless Open Heart Surgery

At the time of cardiopulmonary bypass, cardiotomy suckers blood from the chambers of the heart and pericardium back into the reservoir. In operations like repair of aneurysm of aorta, an equipment called cell saver can be used. This sucks all the spilled blood, washes, centrifuges and packs into red cell concentrate ready to be administered to the patient.

Blood transfusion is not without harm: (1) it may lead to transfer of infections like HIV. Hepartitis B or C, cytomegalovirus, malaria, etc. (2) Febrile reaction; (3) Incompatibility and (4) Limited supply. Conservation of blood could be achieved by autologus blood donation. In a fit patient, blood could be collected preoperatively, up to 10 days before surgery. Intraoperatively one or two units can be collected, just before bypass.

With these methods, it is now possible to do bloodless open heart surgery.

Hemofiltration

Ultrafiltration during open heart surgery helps in removing excess fluid, especially in renal failure patients. Patients are hemodiluted (hematocrit 18-20) during bypass. Hemofiltration helps in blood preservation, especially platelets and coagulation factors. It reduces postoperative complement activation and cardiopulmonary bypass induced inflammatory response. There is also improvement in pulmonary and neurological function. Ultrafiltration equipment is connected to the circuit. In children and babies, it is carried out just before coming off bypass. This is called modified ultrafiltration (MUF).

CHAPTER 13 | Atherosclerosis and Coronary Artery Disease

10. Ans. d. All are essential

IGNOU, MCC 005; Page 9, 10 & 13

Refer to explanation for Q. No 9.

11. Ans. d. Membrane oxygenators

IGNOU, MCC 005; Page 9, 10 & 13

Refer to explanation for Q. No 9.

12. Ans. b. 1–1.5 mg of protamine for each mg of heparin administered

IGNOU, MCC 005; Page 9, 10 & 13

Refer to explanation for Q. No 9.

13. Ans. a. 30 minutes or less

IGNOU, MCC 005; Page 9, 10 & 13

Refer to explanation for Q. No 9.

14. Ans. c. Through coronary sinus

IGNOU, MCC 005; Page 9-10 & 13

Refer to explanation for Q. No 9.

15. Ans. d. Intra-aortic balloon pump (IABP)

IGNOU, MCC 005; Page 13-14

Intra-aortic balloon pump (IABP) was introduced by Kantrowitz (1968). It is also known as counter pulsation or diastolic augmentation.

Indication
Intra-aortic balloon pump is commonly used to support failing left ventricle after open heart surgery or in cardiogenic shock after myocardial infarction. It is at times used in unstable angina and as a supportive measure for urgent PTCA or revascularization. In patients with postinfarction ventricular septal defect and hemodynamic instability, IABP is indicated before surgery.

Contraindication
It is absolutely contraindicated if there is more than trivial aortic regurgitation. Aortic aneurysm and severe aorta iliac disease are also contraindications for use of IABP.

Equipment
Basically, it has an intra-aortic balloon pump. A balloon with a capacity of 40 mL is passed percutaneously through the femoral artery up to the upper end of descending thoracic aorta. The tip of the balloon has radio-opaque marker and should be placed below the left subclavian artery. An inert gas like helium is pumped into the balloon, to synchronize with diastole. The balloon is deflated during systole. Synchronization is achieved by ECG trigger or aortic pressure wave. This will cause diastolic augmentation of blood pressure (counter pulsation) causing augmentation of coronary and cerebral blood flow. When the pump deflates during systole, there is reduction in the afterload and of myocardial oxygen consumption. This improves cardiac output by 10% and helps recovery of myocardium.

Complications
Intra-aortic balloon pump can compromise blood flow to the leg at the time of insertion, pumping or after removal of balloon. It may also cause perforation, bleeding, thrombosis, embolism or dissection of the artery. It is important to check the vascularity of the leg frequently, both clinically and by Doppler.

Ventricular Assist Devices
These come handy when IABP has failed or when prolonged circulatory support is needed. Now left ventricular (LVAD), right ventricular (RVAD) and biventricular assist devices are available. Implantable assist devices can be fitted in when patient is awaiting heart transplantation (bridge to transplantation).

Total Artificial Heart
Jarvik seven was the first successful total artificial heart supporting the patient for 112 days. The disadvantage is that the patient has to be connected to a power source outside and the patient's heart has to be removed. Totally implantable heart is still a distant dream.

16. Ans. d. Mechanical stabilizers to be used for OPCAB

IGNOU, MCC 005; Page 14-15

CABG is done on epicardial vessels. Cardiopulmonary bypass is used only to get a still heart for accurate anastomosis. If there is a method of stabilizing a small area of the heart over the coronary artery with the rest of heart beating and maintaining reasonable hemodynamics, it is possible to do the operation off pump (OPCAB) or beating heart surgery. A few ingenious mechanical stabilizers achieve the local stabilization. The most commonly used one currently is "Octopus", which has two blades with suckers. The two blades are placed on equipment "Starfish" which resembles its namesake in the ocean, when applied to the apex of the heart helps in exposing any surface of the heart as required without much hemodynamic compromise.

When partially occluded coronary or a 100% blocked artery with good collaterals is opened, there will be considerable bleeding. To control that, suitably sized intraluminal shunt devices are available. They help to control bleeding, permit distal perfusion and do not interfere with the anastomosis. While the last few sutures are being applied, the shunt is removed and anastomosis is completed. When a shunt is not used, a carbon dioxide blower will help in keeping the field free of blood.

To perform successful OPCAB good cooperation between the surgeon and the anesthesiologist is needed. Controlled hand ventilation is needed at crucial stages. Arterial pressure and ECG changes like ST-T changes are monitored when heart is rotated or translocated into the right pleura. Transesophageal ECHO helps in monitoring region wall motion of left ventricle.

Usually the operation is done through median sternotomy. Minimally invasive techniques or a left thoracotomy may be used in selected cases. Before grafting, heparin is administered in doses of 1–3 mg/kg. Hypothermia is to be avoided.

A pump is kept standby which could be assembled, primed and got ready in a matter of few minutes. It is important to make the anastomosis accurate. The advantage of OPCAB is that recovery is faster. Patient can be extubated same day, transferred from ICU next day and discharged in 6–7 days time. This brings down the cost of hospitalization significantly.

17. Ans. b. Saphenous vein

IGNOU, MCC 005; Page 15-19

Various conduits used for coronary artery bypass surgery:
- *Venous conduits*: Reverse saphenous vein was first conduit used for CABG. It is usually harvested from the leg starting above the ankle going up to a desired length. It could also be harvested from thigh. Either a single, long skin incision or multiple skin incisions are made. The branches are ligated. The vein is removed and distended with heparinized blood or a solution containing glyceryl trinitrate (GTN).
- *Arterial conduits*:
  - Internal mammary artery—the internal mammary arteries arise from the first part of subclavian and courses 1 cm. lateral to the sternal edge on either side. In the 6th intercostal space, it divides into two branches. It is accompanied by two venae comitantes. LIMA is an ideal conduit for CABG because: (i) size matches the coronary artery; (ii) it is resistance to atherosclerosis; (iii) it has excellent long-term patency.
  - Left internal mammary artery (LIMA graft)—it is most often used for bypassing left anterior descending (LAD) coronary artery and its diagonal branch. The right internal mammary artery is used for bypassing right coronary artery or posterior descending branch. Internal mammary artery can be used as in C2 graft without disconnecting it from the subclavian artery. It can also be used as a pregraft between aorta and coronary artery. For total arterial revascularization (TAR) using mammary arteries, preRIMA end is anastomosed to the side of LIMA as Y or T grafts. The LIMA is then used for bypassing diagonal and LAD branches, RIMA is then taken around the heart for side to side anastomosis with obtuse marginal branches and its anastomose to PDA, thereby achieving total arterial revascularization. In the place of RIMA a radial artery graft can be used the same way for total arterial revascularization.
- *Radial artery*: It has been used as a conduit for CABG. The main problem with the radial artery is spasm. Radial artery is taken from the nondominant hand after performing Allen's test to ensure ulnar artery adequacy to support palmar arch circulation. It is harvested by a long incision overlying the course of artery. To avoid spasm papaverine (30 mg/20 mL of saline) is liberally applied at the time of dissection and later on conduit is tipped in the same solution until it is used. Patient is kept on Diltiazem to prevent spasm of radial artery.
- *Other arterial conduits*:
  - Gastroepiploic artery (GE)—gastroepiploic artery is a less popular arterial conduit now. The midline chest incision is extended to the umbilicus and the right gastroepiploic artery along with its venae comitantes is raised. The pedicle is passed behind duodenum and through the diaphragm. It is then used to bypass RCA, PDA or OM branches.
  - Inferior epigastric artery (IEA)—this is a branch of external iliac artery supplying the abdominal wall. It is raised as a free graft for CABG. The usual length available is 6–8 cm.
  - Biological conduits—freeze dried arterial, bovine IMA, human umbilical vein, cryopreserved umbilical vein or artery and omniflow sheep collagen tube grafts also have poor short- and long-term patency.

Longevity of Conduits (Long-term Patency)

Vein grafts—at the end of 10 years only 50% of saphenous vein grafts are patent 50% of the rest may have significant atherosclerotic changes. In a large series 93% of the grafts were patent at 5 years, 54% at 10 years and 16% at 15 years. To a certain extent patency depends on the atraumatic handling at the time of harvesting. Strict control of risk factors for development of atherosclerosis will also improve long-term patency of venous grafts.

Internal mammary artery (IMA)—this is an excellent graft. When the left internal mammary artery (LIMA) is anastomosed to LAD, which has >70% block, patency at the end of 2 years is 99%. It falls to 92% at the end of 10 years. The right internal mammary artery (RIMA) can be used in situ to bypass RCA, PDA or LAD. It can also be used as a free graft with proximal end anastomosed to aorta or left internal mammary artery (LIMA) as a T or Y graft. Long-term patency of free IMA is slightly lower than in situ IMA. In another large series IMA patency was

90% at 10 years. After 10 years there was no further fall when followed up to 20 years. Internal mammary artery is particularly resistant to atherosclerosis.

Radial artery (RA)—patency of RA is less than that of IMA but much superior to a venous graft. One of the studies showed 90% patency at 13 months and 83% at the end of 7 years. LIMA patency was 91% for the same period.

Gastroepiploic artery (GEA) is seldom used now. Patency has been reported as 94% at one year, 88% at 5 years and 83% at 10 years.

Inferior epigastric artery—IEA is also not used frequently these days. Reported patency is 93% at 5 years.

18. Ans. d. Its' location in chest helps in easy harvesting

IGNOU, MCC 005; Page 15-19

Refer to explanation for Q. No 17.

19. Ans. c. Radial artery spasm is frequent problem

IGNOU, MCC 005; Page 15-19

Refer to explanation for Q. No 17.

20. Ans. d. Left anterior descending artery

IGNOU, MCC 005; Page 15-19

Refer to explanation for Q. No 17.

21. Ans. c. Dacron

IGNOU, MCC 005; Page 15-19

Refer to explanation for Q. No 17.

22. Ans. d. Vein grafts

IGNOU, MCC 005; Page 15-19

Refer to explanation for Q. No 17.

23. Ans. c. When there is significant block in proximal LAD (proximal to first septal and first diagonal) and proximal left circumflex artery

IGNOU, MCC 005; Page 19-21

Indications for coronary artery bypass surgery: The modalities of treatment for coronary artery disease are: 1. medical, 2. angioplasty and stenting, and 3. coronary artery bypass surgery.

The patient's symptoms, nature and number of blocks, suitability of distal vessels for grafting and left ventricular function have to be taken into account before deciding on surgical treatment. Assessment of viability of myocardium will help in identifying patients who will benefit from surgery.

Left main coronary artery disease (LMCAD)—stenosis of 50% or more of the left main coronary artery is an indication for surgery. Results of medical management are very poor and angioplasty is hazardous in these patients. Even if patient is asymptomatic or when angina is well-controlled with medication, early surgery is indicated. The operation has to be done urgently if there is critical left main lesion.

Triple vessel disease (TVD)—patients with TVD and impaired left ventricular function do badly on medical treatment. They are candidates for CABG. Operation is a better choice compared to triple vessel angioplasty and stenting. If a triple vessel disease patient has significant block in proximal LAD (Proximal to first septal and first diagonal) and proximal circumflex it will amount to left main equivalent disease. They will have to undergo CABG. In spite of triple vessel disease if the symptoms are mild, blocks are <70% and left ventricular function good; they can be put on medical treatment with close follow-up.

Double vessel disease (DVD)—percutaneous intervention with stenting is usually advised for these patients. However, if it is left main equivalent disease or when block is close to a major branch or if left ventricle is impaired, surgery is a better choice.

Single vessel disease (SVD)—they do well on medical treatment or with angioplasty. However if proximal LAD is significantly blocked and LIMA can be used as a conduit, surgery gives excellent results. In a patient with proximal LAD lesion if the ejection fraction (EF) is less than 50% and noninvasive tests show extensive reversible ischemia, surgery is the best choice.

Unstable angina—it is indicative of important reversible myocardial ischemia that needs urgent evaluation and treatment. Medical management usually relieves symptoms and if the patient settles down, further investigations can be done electively. Urgent intervention is required in patients with left main coronary artery disease (LMCAD) and severe TVD. Angina at rest suggests ongoing ischemia, which might lead to myocardial infarction (MI).

Acute myocardial infarction—patients with acute Non-Q myocardial infarction may need urgent intervention as indicated for cases of unstable angina.

Uncomplicated Q wave MI—CABG has very little place in cases of uncomplicated Q wave myocardial infarction. However, the place of urgent surgery has to be compared to thrombolytic therapy and primary PTCA. The risk of surgery reduces with passage of time. If it is safe, it is better to postpone the surgery for 48 hours.

Acute MI with hemodynamic deterioration—these patients may require urgent insertion of intra-aortic balloon pump (IABP) followed by PTCA or surgery. Fifty percent of them can be salvaged by surgery or angioplasty. Single most important factor for successful surgery is myocardial protection at the time of surgery. Reperfusion injury has to be avoided at the end of revascularization. Cold or warm cardioplegic arrest, controlled aortic reperfusion with warm blood (hot shot) and allowing an empty beating heart time for full recovery of myocardium have improved surgical results.

Acute complications of PTCA—The incidence of complications after PTCA that require emergency surgery has reduced considerably in the present era. Introduction of stents, perfusion catheters and excellent medical management have all contributed to this. In the initial periods of angioplasty surgical team and operating room used to be stand-by when angioplasty is done. If there is hemodynamic collapse after angioplasty, insertion of IABP, percutaneous cardiopulmonary bypass and emergency CABG may be required.

Influence of LV function—LV function, whether normal or impaired is important while selecting a patient for CABG and for long-term results of surgical revascularization. If left ventricular function is normal even in the presence of less than critical blocks in all three coronary arteries, medical treatment gives good results. Depressed LV function is an indication for surgery. IF the ejection fraction (EF) is more than 0.3, surgical results are good. However, when ejection fraction is less than that risk of surgery becomes greater with poor long-term benefits. Exercise or resting thallium 201 scintigraphy, dobutamine stress echocardiography or positron emission tomography (PET) scanning will help in distinguishing ischemic viable myocardium from a scar.

Influence of diabetes mellitus—diabetes causes microvascular obstructive disease in heart, kidney, retina and peripheral nerves. Scrupulous rather than casual control of diabetes helps in protecting these organs. Coronary artery and cardiovascular disease are more prevalent in diabetic patients. In diabetic patients coronary artery disease is more diffuse and the target vessels for grafting usually smaller in these patients. Patient's perception of angina is modified in diabetes and they usually come for treatment in more advanced condition. Statistics shows that 25–30% of patients coming up for CABG are diabetic. Hyperglycemia has to be well controlled before and after coronary artery bypass surgery.

24. Ans. d. Double vessel disease (LAD + RCA) with impaired LV function

IGNOU, MCC 005; Page 19-21

Refer to explanation for Q. No 23.

25. Ans. d. All of the above

IGNOU, MCC 005; Page 19-21

Refer to explanation for Q. No 23.

26. Ans. b. CABG with LIMA graft

IGNOU, MCC 005; Page 19-21

Refer to explanation for Q. No 23.

27. Ans. a. Less than 2.5%

IGNOU, MCC 005; Page 23

Perioperative myocardial infarction: It is diagnosed by the appearance of fresh Q waves. Non-Q, myocardial infarction is suspected when there is serial rise in cardiac enzymes. Initial reading of cardiac enzymes after CABG on bypass may show elevation, which settles down if there is no perioperative MI. With better myocardial protection these days, the incidence of perioperative MI which was 5.8% in CASS report has come down to 2.5% or even less. The incidence is higher after endarterectomy. In recent reports, there is no difference in the incidence of perioperative MI between CABG on pump and off pump (OPCAB).

Last follow-up shows that 95% of the patients are free of fatal or non-fatal MI 5 years after CABG. This falls to 85% at 10 years and 65% at 15 years.

28. Ans. d. The incidence of perioperative MI is higher with CABG on pump compare to off pump CABG

IGNOU, MCC 005; Page 23

Refer to explanation for Q. No 27.

29. Ans. c. Atrial fibrillation

IGNOU, MCC 005; Page 24

Perioperative arrhythmias—cardiac arrhythmias are not uncommon after CABG. These may be ventricular or atrial.

Ventricular arrhythmias—these include premature ventricular contractions (PVC), ventricular tachycardia (VT) and ventricular fibrillation (VF). At times they may be responsible for sudden cardiac death in the postoperative period. These patients are closed monitored in the first 48 hours. Electrolyte imbalance or ischemia of the myocardium may trigger ventricular irritability. Correction of electrolyte and acid base imbalance and judicious use of antiarrhythmic agents help in the management of ventricular arrhythmias.

Atrial arrhythmias—atrial fibrillation is the most common rhythm abnormality after CABG. Paroxysmal atrial tachycardia and atrial flutter are less common. Increased sympathetic stimulation and withdrawal of β-blockers may be causative factors. The treatment is based on two principles:
1. Rate control, and 2. Rhythm control. Rapid intravenous digitalization is seldom used these days. If hemodynamics

is stable, β-blockers are used intravenously with caution. Propranolol 0.5 mg IV every 2 minutes up to a maximum dose of 4 mg will help in most cases. Verapamil 40 mg through nasogastric tube or up to 5 mg IV are considered dangerous to treat AF. The currently favored drug is amiodarone in doses of 5 mg/kg given over 20 minutes as an infusion followed by continuous infusion for 4–8 hours. Oral amiodarone therapy is then continued.

30. Ans. c. Progression of disease in the native arteries distal to the graft

IGNOU, MCC 005; Page 28

Recurrence of Angina following CABG

- *Early*: Recurrence of angina soon after the patient resumes activities is either due to inadequate revascularization or acute graft closure. In the immediate postoperative period if ECG shows significant fresh changes or if there is unexplained hypotension acute graft occlusion has to be suspected. The best treatment is immediate reoperation and regrafting for the occluded conduit. Very often, regrafting can be done off pump or on cardiopulmonary bypass. Early recurrence of angina peaks around 3rd month when patient has resumed normal activities. Coronary angiogram has to be done again and patient should have either angioplasty or repeat surgery depending on the findings.
- *Late recurrence of angina*: This is a reflection of progress of disease in the native coronary arteries distal to the grafts or narrowing or blockage of one or more of the grafts. This occurs more frequently when only saphenous vein grafts are used as conduits. Such patients should have angiogram followed by either angioplasty or surgery.

31. Ans. d. Medtronic–Hancock valve

IGNOU, MCC 005; Page 31–34

Types of Valves
Prosthetic Valves
- Starr–Edwards (S-E) Silastic Ball valve prosthesis
- St. Jude Medical valve (SJM)
- Medtronic–Hall valve
- Carbomedics valve
- Bjork-Shiley valve (B-S)
- Omni Science valve
- Chitra valve

Biological Valves
Biological valves are available for all positions. Mitral position they are usually mounted on a stent (stent mounted), whereas for aortic position they may be stentless or stented. The different varieties that have been tried are allograft (homograft) aortic valves, xenograft (porcine or bovine) aortic valves, pericardial, fascia lata or durameter valves. The latter two types have been discontinued because of structural failure.

Carpentier-Edwards Valve (C-E)
This is porcine aortic valve preserved in glutaraldehyde and mounted on flexible stent made of cobalt-chromium-nickel alloy (ELGILOY). Glutaraldehyde, a chemical used for tanning of leather causes stability to valve leaflets due to cross linkage of collagen fibres and it reduces antigenicity. It has sewing silicon rubber. Valves are available for aortic and mitral position in various sizes. Biological deterioration will occur after 7–10 years but mechanical failure is uncommon. The rate of biological deterioration is faster in children.

Medtronic–Hancock (Standard Model)
These are glutaraldehyde preserved xenograft aortic valve, which are mounted. The modified orifice version (M-O) is one where the right coronary cusp (which in a porcine valve has a muscular ridge) is excised and replaced with another leaflet of a valve of the same size. A new variety of second generation Hancock valve in which the fixation pressure is zero and toluidine blue is added to inhibit calcium deposition is now available.

Pericardial Valves Carpentier Edwards (Perimount Valve)
Pericardium preserved in glutaraldehyde and mounted on flexible stent is available for mitral and aortic positions. (Perimount) C—E aortic valves have been tested for longer period and are considered to the best among stent mounted bioprosthetic valves.

Stentless Devices
A bioprosthesis mounted on a stent reduces the effective orifice area (EOA). The newer version (third generation) stentless glutaraldehyde preserved porcine valves are now available for clinical use. The commonly used one is Toronto stentless prosthetic valve (SPV) made by St. Jude Medical. The other type is Medtronic free style porcine bioprosthesis.

Aortic Allograft (Homograft)
In the earlier years fresh antibiotic preserved aortic allografts were tried. As the shelf life is limited, availability of all sizes at all times could not be guaranteed. At present cryopreservation is preferred.

Pulmonary Autograft and Ross Procedure
Sir Donald Ross in 1967 introduced the concept of using patient's own pulmonary valve (autograft) for aortic valve replacement and pulmonary allograft to replace the excised pulmonary valve. This cryopreserved pulmonary

allograft does not deteriorate in the low-pressure pulmonary circulation. The pulmonary autograft in aortic position has functioned well over a long period of follow up.

Mitral Valve Replacement with Allograft (Mitral Homograft)

C. Acar and colleagues used mitral allograft for mitral valve replacement using a new technique of fixation of papillary muscles. They also inserted an annuloplasty ring along with the cryopreserved mitral valve. This complex procedure is yet to be universally accepted.

Prosthetic valve hemodynamics

Valve	Effective orifice area (EOA–aortic)	Effective orifice area (EOA–mitral)
Native	3–4 cm^2	4–5 cm^2
Free homograft (Edwards)	3–4 cm^2	4–5 cm^2
Starr–Edwards	1.2–1.6 cm^2	1.4–3.1 cm^2
Single leaflet (disk)	1.5–2.1 cm^2	1.9–3.2 cm^2
Bi leaflet	2.4–3.2 cm^2	2.8–3.4 cm^2
Heterograft (mounted)	1.0–1.7 cm^2	1.3–2.7 cm^2

Postoperative Anticoagulation

Thromboembolism remains a serious complication after valve replacement. Lifelong anticoagulation is required for all patients with a prosthetic valve and in a few cases with bioprosthesis.

Bioprosthetic Valves

The risk of thromboembolism is limited to the first 3 months, until the sewing ring gets endothelialized. The recommendation is to have less intense regimen of anticoagulation (INR 2–2.5) for all mitral bioprosthetic valves. As the incidence of thromboembolism is less for aortic bioprosthesis anticoagulation is considered to be optional in many center. They are put on aspirin and persantin. However, patients with mitral bioprosthesis who are in AF, who has very large LA and has LA thrombus with history of thromboembolism should have long-term low level anticoagulation.

Mechanical Prosthetic Valves

These patients should have life long anticoagulation. In the absence of anticoagulation systemic embolism and strokes have been reported to be 5–50%. Anticoagulation have reduced this incidence to 1–3 % per year. However, the treatment itself can cause complications. This is related to the level of anticoagulation. Low level of anticoagulation (INR 2–2.5) has shown to have fewer complications and at the same time as effective in preventing thromboembolism. Standard anticoagulation (INR 3–4.5) which gives rise to more complications should be limited to high-risk group. It is generally believed that patients with prosthetic aortic valves in sinus rhythm need only lower levels of anticoagulation. In our country, where control of anticoagulation is more difficult, a low level of anticoagulation is advisable.

Anticoagulation in prosthetic valves

Valve	INR mitral	INR aortic
Bi leaflet	2.5–3.5	2.0–2.5
Tilting disk	2.5–3.5	2.0–2.5
Ball valves	3.0–3.5	2.5–3.0
History of embolism	INR 2.5–3.5 with anticoagulants plus aspirin persantin	INR 2–2.5 with anticoagulants plus aspirin plus persantin

The usual anticoagulants used are: 1. Warfarin sodium, and 2. Acitrom (coumarin derivative).

In patients who had thromboembolism previously, addition of low dose aspirin (75 mg/day) is found to be useful along with anticoagulation.

32. Ans. c. Starr–Edwards valve

IGNOU, MCC 005; Page 31–34

Refer to explanation for Q. No 31.

33. Ans. c. Degeneration and calcification

IGNOU, MCC 005; Page 31–34

Refer to explanation for Q. No 31.

34. Ans. d. 4–5 cm^2

IGNOU, MCC 005; Page 37

The normal mitral valve area is 4–5 cm^2. Usually symptoms appear when the valve area has become <2.5 cm^2. Symptoms are present at rest when the valve area is <1.5 cm^2. Mitral stenosis is classified as mild, moderate or severe based on: 1. pressure gradient across the valve on echo or cardiac catheterization; 2. calculated valve area.

Degree of MS	Mean pressure gradient	Valve area
Mild MS	< 5 mm Hg	> 2 cm^2
Moderate MS	6–9 mm Hg	1–2 cm^2
Severe MS	> 10 mm Hg	< 1 cm^2

35. Ans. b. Moderate mitral stenosis

IGNOU, MCC 005; Page 37

Refer to explanation for Q. No 34.

36. Ans. d. Congenital

IGNOU, MCC 005; Page 54–55

Pulmonary Valve Disease

Pulmonary stenosis—The obstruction may be valvular, infundibular or supravalvular.

Indications for surgery: Congenital pulmonic stenosis is the most common lesion requiring relief. Very rarely it could be due to rheumatic involvement along with disease of other cardiac valves. Carcinoid syndrome can cause thickening and fusion of the valve cusps and also produce outflow obstruction. Extrinsic pulmonary obstruction could be caused by cardiac tumors or aneurysm of sinus of Valsalva.

Quantification of Pulmonary Stenosis by Echo

By Valve Area

- Mild: > 1.5 cm^2
- Moderate: 0.5–1.5 cm^2
- Severe: < 0.5 cm^2

By Peak Pressure Gradient

- Trivial: < 25 mm Hg
- Mild: 25–50 mm Hg
- Moderate: 50–80 mm Hg
- Severe: > 80 mm Hg

Neonates presenting with critical pulmonary stenosis and intact ventricular septum usually present within 2 weeks and need urgent treatment.

Pulmonary stenosis may be present in infants, children or adults. Mild stenosis can be left alone and followed up. Moderate stenosis is treated at the time of surgery of associated lesions. If the stenosis is severe and isolated, it has to be treated by balloon valvotomy.

37. Ans. c. Moderate pulmonary stenosis

IGNOU, MCC 005; Page 54-55

Refer to explanation for Q. No 36.

38. Ans. d. Balloon pulmonary valvotomy

IGNOU, MCC 005; Page 54-55

Refer to explanation for Q. No 36.

39. Ans. b. Closed heart surgery

IGNOU, MCC 005; Page 57

Pericardiectomy is a closed heart surgery. Pericardiectomy used to have a mortality of 10–15% in the earlier era. At present it is around 3–5% and does not approach 0% even though it is a closed heart operation.

40. Ans. c. 3–5%

IGNOU, MCC 005; Page 57

Refer to explanation for Q. No 39.

41. Ans. d. Sarcoidosis

IGNOU, MCC 005; Page 59

Ventricular aneurysm: 95% of ventricular aneurysms occur after transmural myocardial infarction. Trauma, Chaga's disease, sarcoidosis and congenital causes are the other etiological factors. 85% of them are on the anterolateral wall of the LV, 5–10% posterolaterally and less than 5% are on the lateral wall. The clinical presentation may be with congestive cardiac failure, angina pectoris, ventricular arrhythmias, and dyspnea or thromboembolism. Rarely, it could be asymptomatic. Diagnosis is confirmed by chest X-ray, ECG, ECHO and cardiac catheterization and LV and coronary angio. Special investigations like MRI, MUGA scan, thallium/PET scan and electrophysiological study will be required in some cases before surgery.

42. Ans. a. Anterolateral wall of LV

IGNOU, MCC 005; Page 59

Refer to explanation for Q. No 41.

43. Ans. c. The mouth is usually wide

IGNOU, MCC 005; Page 61

False left ventricular aneurysm: False aneurysm develops after acute rupture of an infarct. It is usually fatal, but a few survive because of previous adhesions between parietal pericardium and epicardium. The mouth is usually narrow and the aneurysm may expand and rupture. They occur more often on the diaphragmatic surface. Doppler color flow imaging and transesophageal echocardiography help in diagnosing a false aneurysm. Resection is always recommended and carries higher risk than surgery for true aneurysm.

44. Ans. b. The location is 40% anterior and 60% posterior

IGNOU, MCC 005; Page 66

Postmyocardial infarction VSD (septal rupture): The correct terminology is septal rupture as the defect formed is not a direct through and through defect, but irregular as a result of necrosed muscle. It is most common after anteroseptal myocardial infarction. The location is 60% anterior and 40% posterior. A posterior septal rupture is often associated with mitral regurgitation. The incidence in patients who are thrombolyzed has come down to 0.2% from a previously quoted 2%. It may occur within 2 days of MI or as late as 2 weeks.

45. Ans. d. Mobile vegetations more than 10 mm

IGNOU, MCC 005; Page 71

Indications for surgery in native valve endocarditis: About two-thirds of patients with native valve endocarditis can be cured with proper medical treatment. In the rest of the patients, early surgical treatment improves the prognosis.

Indications	Class of evidence
Heart failure unresponsive medical treatment due to MR or AR	I
Acute AR with tachycardia and early closure of mitral valve	I
Fungal endocarditis	I
Evidence of aortic root abscess and true or false aneurysm of sinus of Valsalva	I
Evidence of valve dysfunction and persistent infection after 7–10 days of appropriate antibiotic treatment	I
Recurrent emboli after appropriate antibiotic therapy	IIa
Infection with gram-negative organism with poor response to antibiotics and evidence of valve dysfunction	IIa
Mobile vegetations > 10 mm	IIb
Early infection of mitral valve that can be repaired	III
Persistent pyrexia and leukocytosis with negative blood cultures	III

For patients with native valve endocarditis who get cured on medical treatment, indications for surgery are the same as patients without endocarditis.

46. Ans. b. Within 60 days of surgery

IGNOU, MCC 005; Page 71

Prosthetic valve endocarditis (PVE) is called Early when symptoms begin within 60 days of surgery and Late when the onset is after 2 months. The most common organism for early PVE is coagulase negative *Staphylococcus—Staphylococcus epidermidis*. Less commonly the causative organism could be *Staphylococcus aureus*, gram-negative bacilli, diphtheroids or fungi (*Candida* species).

In early PVE the organism responsible could be a nosocomial one and for late endocarditis a community acquired organism is often the culprit. Data suggests that during the initial after implantation, a mechanical valve is at higher risk than bioprosthetic valve. However, after twelve months the incidence is more on bioprosthetic valves. At 5 years the incidence is comparable.

47. Ans. b. Coagulase negative *Staphylococcus-Staphylococcus epidermidis*

IGNOU, MCC 005; Page 71

Refer to explanation for Q. No 46.

48. Ans. d. All are correct

IGNOU, MCC 005; Page 71

Refer to explanation for Q. No 46.

49. Ans. d. 22%

IGNOU, MCC 005; Page 73

Results: The hospital mortality for valve replacement for endocarditis varies between 4–30%. Operative mortality is higher for urgent operations. It also depends on the patient's preoperative status. For PVE the mortality is higher. The experience of Brigham and Women's Hospital in Boston showed a mortality of 6% for native valve endocarditis and 22% for PVE.

50. Ans. b. Above 50% of aorta

IGNOU, MCC 005; Page 74

Indications for surgery in VSD: Some VSDs close spontaneously or become smaller in size. This has to be taken into consideration before surgery is advised. Spontaneous closure can be complete by 1 year of age or the defect narrowed considerably. There is an inverse relationship between the probability of closure and age at which the patient is seen. 80% of patients with large VSD seen at 1 month of age may close spontaneously. 60% of those seen at 3 months and 50% seen at 6 months and 25% of those presenting at 12 months. A large VSD will have a diameter equal to aorta and a moderate one about 50% and a small one less than one-third of its diameter. When infants with large VSDs have severe and intractable heart failure or respiratory symptoms during the first 3 months, prompt closure is advised. Most often these babies have other associated cardiac anomalies that are also corrected. Operation is not advised in the first 3 months, if the symptoms are not serious, as spontaneous closure may occur. In infants older than 3 months significant growth failure and increase in pulmonary vascular resistance are indications for surgery. An infant presenting at 6 months with severe symptoms and a pulmonary vascular resistance index of 4–8 wood U/m^2 needs early repair. In children having pulmonary resistance (Rp) less than 4 U/m^2 surgery could be postponed up to 1 year. There is no advantage in waiting further as the results of surgery at 1 year is as good as at a later stage in experienced centers. In older children with large VSD with severe pulmonary vascular disease, cardiac catheterization and calculations of shunt and pulmonary vascular resistance with isoproterenol infusion and 100% oxygen inhalation are done to decide operability. Moderate VSD with no elevation of pulmonary artery pressure may be advised surgery at 2–3 years of age. When smaller VSDs are seen at a later age, the consensus is to close surgically as there is possibility of endocarditis and prolapse of aortic cusp. There is also the social and psychological stigma of a harsh murmur creating problems at school check up, preemployment and preinsurance medical examination. Surgery carries negligible risk and there is complete cure.

51. Ans. d. All of the above

IGNOU, MCC 005; Page 74

Refer to explanation for Q. No 50.

52. Ans. a. Isolated VSD

IGNOU, MCC 005; Page 75

Pulmonary artery banding: Banding of pulmonary trunk is done to reduce pulmonary flow in a baby. It is seldom done for isolated ventricular septal defect. Multiple muscular ventricular septal defects (Swiss cheese defects) are difficult to close in infancy and so pulmonary artery banding may treat them. It is also the procedure of choice for tricuspid atresia with VSD and other types of univentricular hearts without pulmonary stenosis. Pulmonary artery banding is done with a view to Fontan type of correction at a later stage.

53. Ans. d. Paradoxical embolism

IGNOU, MCC 005; Page 76

The presence of an ASD or partial anomalous pulmonary venous connection (PAPVC) with right ventricular volume overload and a significant left right shunt (Qp/Qs of < 1.5:1) is an indication for closure. The optimal age for operation is usually 1-2 years. Surgery can be done at very young and very old age. Pulmonary vascular disease which raises pulmonary vascular resistance to > 8 U/m^2 at rest makes an ASD inoperable. Associated mitral and tricuspid regurgitations are not contraindications for surgery and they might need valve repair. Generally a very small defect that is less than 5 mm in diameter does not require surgery. However, there is a possibility of paradoxical embolism even in such small defects. If the patient has a history of stroke, closure is advised. Surgical closure is indicated in such cases if device closure is contraindicated or it has failed.

54. Ans. a. Ostium secundum type

IGNOU, MCC 005, Page 76

The most common type of atrial septal defect is ostium secundum defect.

55. Ans. d. Transposition of great arteries

IGNOU, MCC 005; Page 85

Atrial switch operation (Senning and mustard operation): In transposition of the great arteries there is ventriculoarterial discordance whereby aorta arises from right ventricle and pulmonary artery from left ventricle. In atrial switch operation a baffle is placed in the atrium in such a way that blood from SVC and IVC flows under the baffle to mitral valve and left ventricle and to the pulmonary artery. Pulmonary venous return flows over the patch to tricuspid valve and RV and then to aorta.

CHAPTER 14

Acute Rheumatic Fever and Infective Endocarditis

1. **In which part of the World there is lowest prevalence of rheumatic heart disease in school age children?**
   a. South America
   b. Asia
   c. Africa
   d. United States

2. **Which is *not* correct regarding rheumatic fever?**
   a. Initial attack of RF occur most commonly between ages of 6 and 15 years
   b. RF is rarely seen before the age of 5 years
   c. The incidence of ARF is higher in female
   d. It is more common in warm tropical climates

3. **What is the approximate incidence of rheumatic fever, following streptococcal pharyngitis in a patient who had previous episode of rheumatic fever?**
   a. 3%
   b. 13%
   c. 33%
   d. 50%

4. **Which of the following pathological feature differentiate rheumatic fever from other connective tissue disorders?**
   a. Exudative and inflammatory reaction involving connective tissue
   b. Fibrinoid necrosis of collagen tissue
   c. There is generalized vasculitis
   d. Thrombotic lesions are not seen in RF

5. **Which is *correct* regarding Aschoff nodule?**
   a. Its presence is pathognomonic of rheumatic carditis
   b. It is found almost invariably in all cases of patients with rheumatic fever in biopsy
   c. Aschoff nodules are seen in all organs
   d. They are most often noted in the wall of right ventricle and RA appendages

6. **The formation of 'verrucae' at the edges of valvular leaflet in RF is due to:**
   a. Edema and cellular infiltration
   b. Hyaline degeneration
   c. Fibrosis
   d. Calcification

7. **The most specific manifestation of rheumatic fever is:**
   a. Arthritis
   b. Chorea
   c. Carditis
   d. Subcutaneous nodules

8. **Which is the most characteristic component of rheumatic carditis?**
   a. Pericarditis
   b. Valvulitis
   c. Myocarditis
   d. Pancarditis

9. **Which is the most common major manifestation of ARF?**
   a. Carditis
   b. Arthritis
   c. Erythema marginatum
   d. Chorea

10. **Which of the following is least specific clinic manifestation of ARF?**
    a. Erythema marginatum
    b. Subcutaneous nodules
    c. Fever
    d. Arthritis

11. **The most striking feature of rheumatic arthritis is:**
    a. It is always asymmetric and migratory
    b. Only the larger joints are involved
    c. It does not result in permanent joint deformity
    d. Its dramatic response to salicylates

12. **ESR is usually normal with which of the following manifestation of ARF?**
    a. Polyarthritis
    b. Chorea
    c. Carditis
    d. Fever

13. **All of the following conditions are associated with normal ESR in rheumatic heart disease *except*:**
    a. Without rheumatic activity
    b. Chorea
    c. CHF
    d. Anemia

14. **In what percent of patients with acute RF, throat culture is positive for Group A streptococci?**
    a. 5–6%
    b. 10–11%
    c. 30–33%
    d. >90%

15. Which is *not* correct regarding Group A streptococcal antigen detection tests in diagnosis of ARF?
  a. Most of tests have high degree of specificity
  b. A negative test excludes the presence of group A *Streptococcus* in pharynx
  c. These tests do not distinguish between a recent infection and chronic pharyngeal carrier of the organism
  d. All are correct

16. Which is the most reliable evidence of a recent streptococcal infection in a case of ARF?
  a. Elevated ASO titre
  b. Positive throat culture
  c. Positive rapid antigen test
  d. Elevated acute phase reactants

17. The optimal dose of aspirin for treating ARF in:
  a. 75 mg/kg/day
  b. 50 mg/kg/day
  c. 100 mg/kg/day
  d. 800–1,000 mg/kg/day

18. Which is *incorrect* in treatment of ARF?
  a. Salicylates are effective only in cases with mild or no carditis
  b. Salicylates are particularly effective in relieving joint pain
  c. Patients with cardiac involvement respond more with steroids than salicylates
  d. Salicylates or corticosteroid therapy have a very positive effect on the course of carditis and diminishes the incidence of residual heart disease

19. For preventing primary attacks of rheumatic fever following onset of acute streptococcal pharyngitis, appropriate antimicrobial therapy should be started:
  a. Within 48 hours   b. Within 6 days
  c. Within 9 days   d. Up to 21 days

20. Which antimicrobial agent is *not* recommended for treatment of streptococcal upper respiratory tract infection?
  a. Cephalosporins
  b. Sulfonamides
  c. Azithromycin
  d. Erythromycin

21. Patient with rheumatic carditis in initial attack of ARF should have secondary antimicrobial prophylaxis for:
  a. At least 10 years after last episode
  b. 5 years after last attack
  c. Until age of 21 years
  d. Lifelong

22. In countries with high incidence of rheumatic fever, recommended regimen for secondary prevention is:
  a. Injection benzathine penicillin G every 3 weeks
  b. Injection benzathine penicillin G every 4 weeks
  c. Oral penicillin V
  d. Oral sulfisoxazole

23. In a pregnant women, who is allergic to penicillin, the drug of choice for secondary prevention of rheumatic fever is:
  a. Cephalosporins
  b. Erythromycin
  c. Sulfonamides
  d. Tetracyclines

24. Which of the following is mandatory to prove the diagnosis of acute rheumatic fever?
  a. Presence of one major and two minor criteria
  b. Presence of two major criteria
  c. Evidence of a preceding group A streptococcal infection
  d. a or b + c

ANSWERS WITH EXPLANATIONS

1. Ans. d. United States

Braunwald 6th Ed; Chapter 66; Page 2192

The incidence of RF and prevalence of RHD are markedly variable in different countries. The currently estimated prevalence of rheumatic heart disease in United States of America is 2 per 100,000. There has been a steady decline in the incidence of RF in the industrialized countries. However, in the nonindustrialized countries there has been a persistent high incidence of the disease.

RHD in school age children

Location	Prevalence per 1,000
United States	0.6
Japan	0.7
Asia (other)	0.4–21.0
Africa	0.3–15.0
South America	1.0–17.0

2. Ans. c. The incidence of ARF is higher in female

Braunwald 6th Ed; Chapter 66; Page 2192

There is a causal relationship between RF and group A streptococcal pharyngitis. The epidemiologies of the two illnesses are very similar. Initial attack of RF occurs most commonly between the age of 6 and 15 years and RF is rarely seen before the age of 5 years. The risk of RF is increased in the population at high-risk of streptococcal pharyngitis such as military recruits, person living in crowded condition and those in close contact with school age children. An untreated group A streptococcal tonsillopharyngitis is the antecedent event that precipitates RF. RF does not follow streptococcal skin infection. Proper antimicrobial treatment of the streptococcal pharyngitis with eradication of organism virtually eliminates the risk of RF. In situation producing epidemic streptococcal pharyngitis (such as the military population, crowding) as many as 3% of untreated acute streptococcal sore-throat may be followed by RF. Endemic infections results in much lower attack rate. It has been documented that about 1/3rd of all cases of acute RF follow mild or almost asymptomatic pharyngitis.

3. Ans. d. 50%

Braunwald 6th Ed; Chapter 66; Page 2192

Refer to explanation for Q. No 2.

4. Ans. d. Thrombotic lesions are not seen in RF

Braunwald 6th Ed; Chapter 66, Page 2193

The acute phase of RF is characterized by exudative and proliferative inflammatory reactions involving connective tissue or collagen tissue. Although the disease process is diffused, it affects monthly the heart, joints, brain and cutaneous and subcutaneous tissues. A generalized vasculitis affecting a small blood vessel is commonly noted but unlike the vasculitis of some other connective tissue disorder, thrombotic lesions are not seen in RF. The basic structural change in collagen is fibrinoid degeneration. The interstitial connective tissue become edematous and eosinophilic, with frail fragmentation and disintegration of collagen fiber. This is associated with infiltration of mononuclear cells including large modified fibrohistiocytic cells (Aschoff cells). Some of the histiocytes are multinucleated and form Aschoff giant cell. The Aschoff nodule in the proliferative stage is considered pathognomonic of rheumatic carditis. These nodules have been described almost invariably in autopsies of patients who died of rheumatic carditis. Recent observation indicates that aschoff nodules are observed in only 30-40% of biopsies from patients with primary or recurrent episode of RF. Aschoff bodies may be seen in any area of myocardium but not in other affected organs such as joints or brain. They are most often noted in interventricular septum, the wall of the left ventricle or left atrial appendages. Aschoff nodules persist for many years after a rheumatic attack even in patients with no evidence of recent or active inflammation.

5. Ans. a. Its presence is pathognomonic of rheumatic carditis

Braunwald 6th Ed; Chapter 66, Page 2193

Refer to explanation for Q. No 4.

6. Ans. b. Hyaline degeneration

Braunwald 6th Ed; Chapter 66, Page 2193

The inflammation of valvular tissues accounts for the more commonly recognized clinical manifestations of rheumatic carditis. Initial inflammation leads to valvular insufficiency. The histological findings in endocarditis consist of edema and cellular infiltration of the valvular tissue and the chordae tendineae. Hyaline degeneration of the affected valve leads to the formation of verrucae at its edge, preventing total approximation of the leaflets. Fibrosis and calcification of the valve occur if inflammation persists. Eventually this causes may lead to valvular stenosis.

7. Ans. c. Carditis

Braunwald 6th Ed; Chapter 66, Page 2193

Rheumatic carditis is a pancarditis affecting the endocardium, myocardium and pericardium to varying degree. Clinically rheumatic carditis is almost always associated with a murmur of valvulitis. The severity of carditis is variable. In its most severe form death from cardiac failure may occur. More commonly carditis, is less intense and predominant effect is subsequent scarring of the heart valve. Evidence of carditis may be very subtle; signs of valvular involvement may be mild and transient and may be easily missed on auscultation. Patients who show no clear evidence of carditis on initial examination should be monitored closely over a few weeks to ascertain cardiac involvement. Carditis is often the regarded as the most specific manifestation of rheumatic fever and it is noted in at least 50% of patients with acute rheumatic fever.

Valvulitis (endocarditis) involving mitral and aortic valves and the chordae of mitral valve is the most characteristic component of rheumatic carditis. Mitral insufficiency is the hallmark of rheumatic carditis. Aortic insufficiency is less common and usually associated with mitral insufficiency. The pulmonary and tricuspid valves are rarely involved. Residual valvular damage is a major concern in patients with rheumatic fever and may lead to intractable cardiac failure requiring surgical intervention. Myocarditis or pericarditis in the absence of valvulitis is not likely to be due to rheumatic fever.

8. Ans. b. Valvulitis

Braunwald 6th Ed; Chapter 66, Page 2193

Refer to explanation for Q. No 8.

9. Ans. b. Arthritis

Braunwald 6th Ed; Chapter 66, Page 2194

Polyarthritis is the most common major manifestation of rheumatic fever but is the least specific. It is always asymmetric, migratory and involves larger joints (knees, ankles, elbows and wrist). Characteristically, there is swelling, redness, heats, severe pain and limitation of motion and tenderness to touch. The arthritis of rheumatic fever is benign and does not result in permanent joint deformity. Joint fluid shows a finding characteristic of inflammation (not infection). In untreated cases, arthritis usually last for 2-3 weeks. A striking feature of rheumatic arthritis is its dramatic response to salicylates. Indeed if a patient does not improve substantially after 48 hours of adequate salicylate therapy, the diagnosis of rheumatic fever should be in doubt.

10. Ans. d. Arthritis

Braunwald 6th Ed; Chapter 66, Page 2194

Refer to explanation for Q. No 9.

11. Ans. d. Its dramatic response to salicylates

Braunwald 6th Ed; Chapter 66, Page 2194

Refer to explanation for Q. No 9.

12. Ans. b. Chorea

Braunwald 6th Ed; Chapter 66, Page 2194

Elevated acute phase reactants offer objective but nonspecific indications of tissue inflammation.

The erythrocyte sedimentation rate (ESR) and C-reactive protein (CRP) level are almost always elevated during the acute stages of the disease in patients with carditis or polyarthritis but are usually normal in patient with chorea. The ESR is very useful in following the course of disease. It usually returns to normal as the rheumatic activity subsides. The ESR may be elevated in patient with anemia and may be suppressed to normal levels in patient with congestive heart failure. Unlike the ESR, the CRPs are unaffected by anemia or cardiac failure.

13. Ans. d. Anemia

Braunwald 6th Ed; Chapter 66, Page 2194

Refer to explanation for Q. No 12.

14. Ans. b. 10-11%

Braunwald 6th Ed; Chapter 66, Page 2195

A number of illnesses mimic acute rheumatic fever and there is no laboratory test or tests that allow the specific diagnosis of RF. It is important to establish an antecedent streptococcal infection in the form of demonstrating a group 'A' streptococcal pharyngitis in the tonsillopharynx or an elevated or rising streptococcal antibody titer. Evidence of an antecedent streptococcal infection is required for the confirmation of the initial diagnosis of acute RF. At the time of diagnosis of acute RF only about 11% of patients have throat culture positive for group "A" streptococci. The paucity of positive culture is due to elimination of the organism by host defense mechanism during the latent period between the onset of infection and subsequent development of RF. Several rapid group A streptococcal antigen detection methods are commercially available. Most of these tests have a high degree of specificity but low sensitivity in the clinical setting. A negative test does not exclude a presence of group "A" streptococci in pharynx. A positive throat culture or rapid antigen test does not distinguish between a recent infection that can be associated with acute RF and chronic pharyngeal carriage of the organism. Because the presence of group 'A' *Streptococcus* in the pharynx may not represent active infection, elevated or rising anti streptococcal antibody titres provide more reliable evidence of a recent streptococcal infection than a positive culture or a positive rapid antigen tests. The most commonly used antibody tests are antistreptolysin O (ASO) and the antideoxyribonuclease B (anti DNaseB). The ASO test is usually obtained first and if not elevated the anti DNaseB test is done. Elevated titers for both tests may persist for several weeks or months. ASO titre rise and fall more rapidly than Anti-DNase B. A slide agglutination test is commercially available and measures antibodies to several streptococcal antigens. It is simple to perform, rapid and widely available; however, the test is not well-standardized and not very reproducible and is not recommended as a definitive test for evidence of preceding group "A" streptococcal infection.

15. Ans. b. A negative test excludes the presence of group A *Streptococcus* in pharynx

Braunwald 6th Ed; Chapter 66, Page 2195

Refer to explanation for Q. No 14.

16. Ans. a. Elevated ASO titre

Braunwald 6th Ed; Chapter 66, Page 2195

Refer to explanation for Q. No 14.

17. Ans. c. 100 mg/kg/day

Braunwald 6th Ed; Chapter 66, Page 2195

There is no specific treatment for the inflammatory reaction initiated by RF. Supportive therapy is aimed at reducing constitutional symptoms, controlling toxic manifestation and improving cardiac function. Patient with mild or no carditis usually respond well to salicylates. Salicylates are particularly effective in relieving joint pain. Such pain usually abates within 24 hours of starting salicylates. For optimal anti-inflammatory effect serum salicylates levels around 20 mg% are required and therefore aspirin at doses of 100 mg/kg/day given 4-5 times daily, usually results in adequate serum level to achieve a clinical response. Patient with significant cardiac involvement particularly those with pericarditis or congestive heart failure respond more promptly to corticosteroid than to salicylates alone; indeed steroid may be life saving in very ill patients. Occasionally, patients who do not respond to adequate dose of salicylates may benefit from a trial course of corticosteroids, i.e., prednisolone 1-2 mg/kg/day is the usual dose. There is no evidence that salicylates or corticosteroids therapy affect the course of carditis or diminishes the incidence of residual heart disease. Therefore, the duration of therapy with anti-inflammatory agents is arbitrarily based on an estimate of the severity of episode and the promptness of the clinical response. Mild attack with little or no cardiac involvement may be treated with salicylates for about 1 month or until there is sufficient clinical and laboratory evidence of inflammatory inactivity. In more severe cases therapy with corticosteroids may be continued for 2-3 months. The medication is then gradually reduced over the next 2 weeks. Even with prolonged therapy some patients (~ 5%) will continue to demonstrate evidence of rheumatic activity for 6 or more months. A rebound is manifested by the reappearance of mild symptom or of acute phase reactant, may occur in some patients after anti-inflammatory medications have been discontinued usually within 2 weeks. Moderate symptoms usually subside without treatment. More severe symptom may require treatment with salicylates. Some physicians recommend the use of salicylates (aspirin 75 mg/kg/day) during the period when corticosteroids are being tapered and believe that such an approach may reduce the likelihood of a rebound.

18. Ans. d. Salicylates or corticosteroid therapy have a very positive effect on the course of carditis and diminishes the incidence of residual heart disease

Braunwald 6th Ed; Chapter 66, Page 2195

Refer to explanation for Q. No 17.

19. Ans. c. Within 9 days

Braunwald 6th Ed; Chapter 66, Page 2196

Prevention of primary attacks of RF depends on the prompt recognition and proper treatment of Group 'A' streptococcal pharyngitis. Eradication of group A *Streptococcus* from the throat is essential. Although appropriate antimicrobial therapy started up to 9 days after the onset of acute streptococcal pharyngitis is effective in preventing primary attacks of RF, early therapy is advisable because it reduces both morbidity and period of infectivity. Penicillin is the antimicrobial agent of choice for the treatment of group 'A' streptococcal pharyngitis except in patient with history of allergy to penicillin. Penicillin has a narrow spectrum of activity, a long standing proven efficacy and is least expensive regimen. Penicillin may be administered intramuscularly or orally depending on patients likely adherence to an oral regimen. Intramuscular benzathine penicillin G is preferred particularly for patients who are unlikely to complete a 10 days course of oral therapy and patient with a personal or family history of RF or rheumatic heart disease. Benzathine penicillin G injection should be given as a single dose in a large muscle mass. The oral antibiotic of choice is penicillin V. Patient should take oral penicillin regimen for entire 10 days period although they are likely to be asymptomatic after first few days. Although the broader spectrum amoxicillin is often used in the treatment of group 'A' phrayngitis, it offers no microbiological advantage over penicillin. Oral erythromycin is acceptable for patient allergic to penicillin. Treatment should also be prescribed for 10 days. Erythromycin estolate (20-40 mg/kg/day in two or four divided doses) or erythromycin ethyl succinate (40 mg/kg/day in two to four divided doses) is effective in treating in streptococcal pharyngitis. The new macrolide Azithromycin has similar susceptibility pattern to the data of erythromycin against group "A" streptococcal pharyngitis but may cause fewer gastrointestinal side effect. Azithromycin can be administered once daily and produces high tonsillar tissue concentration and a 5 days course of azithromycin is approved by Food and Drug Administration as a second line therapy for the treatment of patients 16 years of age or older with group 'A' streptococcal pharyngitis. The recommended dosage is 500 mg as a single dose on first day followed by 250 mg daily for 4 days. A ten days course of an oral cephalosporin is acceptable alternative particularly in patient for penicillin allergy. Certain antimicrobials are not recommended for treatment of streptococcal upper respiratory tract infection. Tetracyclines should not be used because of high prevalence of resistant strains. Sulfonamides and trimethoprim—sulfamethoxazole will not eradicate group A *Streptococcus* in patient with pharyngitis and should not be used to treat active infection. Chloramphenicol is not recommended because of unpredictable efficacy and potential serious toxicity.

20. Ans. b. Sulfonamides

Braunwald 6th Ed; Chapter 66, Page 2196

Refer to explanation for Q. No 19.

21. Ans. d. Lifelong

Braunwald 6th Ed; Chapter 66, Page, 2193, 2196–2197

Guidelines for the diagnosis of the initial attack of rheumatic fever (Jones Criteria*)

Major manifestations	Minor manifestations	Supporting evidence for antecedent group A streptococcal infection
• Carditis • Polyarthritis • Chorea • Erythema marginatum • Subcutaneous nodules	• Clinical findings • Arthralgia fever • Laboratory findings • Elevated acute phase reactants • Erythrocyte sedimentation rate • C-reactive protein • Prolonged P-R interval	• Positive throat culture or rapid Streptococcal antigen test • Elevated or rising Streptococcal antibody titer

*If supported by evidence of preceding group A streptococcal infection, the presence of two major manifestations or one major and two minor manifestations indicates a high probability of acute rheumatic fever.

Secondary prevention of rheumatic fever (Prevention of recurrent attacks)

Agent	Dose	Mode
Benzathine penicillin G	1,200,000 U every 4 weeks* or	Intramuscular
Penicillin V	250 mg twice daily or	Oral
		Continued

Continued

Agent	Dose	Mode
Sulfadiazine	• 0.5 g once daily for < 27 kg (60 lb) • 1.0 g once daily for patients > 27 kg (60 lb)	Oral
For individuals allergic to penicillin and sulfadiazine		
Erythromycin	250 mg twice daily	Oral

* In high-risk situations, administration every 3 weeks is justified and recommended.

Duration of secondary rheumatic fever prophylaxis

Category	Duration
Rheumatic fever with carditis and residual heart disease (persistent valvular disease*)	At least 10 years since last episode and at least until age 40 years, sometimes lifelong prophylaxis
Rheumatic fever with carditis but no residual heart disease (no valvular disease*)	10 years or well into adulthood, whichever is longer
Rheumatic fever without carditis	5 years or until age 21 years, whichever is longer

*Clinical or echocardiographic evidence.

22. Ans. a. Injection benzathine penicillin G every 3 weeks

Braunwald 6th Ed; Chapter 66, Page, 2193, 2196–2197

Refer to explanation for Q. No 21.

23. Ans. b. Erythromycin

Braunwald 6th Ed; Chapter 66, Page, 2193, 2196–2197

Refer to explanation for Q. No 21.

24. Ans. d. a or b + c

Braunwald 6th Ed; Chapter 66, Page, 2193, 2196–2197

Refer to explanation for Q. No 21.

ACUTE RHEUMATIC FEVER AND SUBACUTE INFECTIVE ENDOCARDITIS

1. Patients presenting with which of the following symptom in acute rheumatic fever may have normal streptococcal serology testing?
   a. Arthritis
   b. Carditis
   c. Subcutaneous nodules
   d. Chorea

2. Which is *not* correct regarding Carey Coombs murmur?
   a. It is a mid-diastolic rumble heard at apex
   b. It may be associated with murmur of mitral regurgitation
   c. It is preceded by opening snap
   d. It disappears as the valvulitis improves

3. The milking sign is seen in:
   a. Infective endocarditis
   b. Aorta arthritis
   c. Restrictive cardiomyopathy
   d. Rheumatic fever

4. Which of the following country has been labeled as Rheumatic fever/RHD "Hot spot" of the world?
   a. Australia
   b. India
   c. Bangladesh
   d. Kyrgyzstan

CHAPTER 14 | Acute Rheumatic Fever and Infective Endocarditis

5. The inflammatory process and acute rheumatic fever damages which of the following structure?
   a. Collagen fibrils
   b. Connective tissue
   c. Both of them
   d. None of them

6. Which of the following is *not* correct regarding the pathogenesis of acute rheumatic fever?
   a. Streptococcal skin infection does not cause rheumatic fever
   b. Lifetime cumulative incidence of rheumatic fever in population remains 3–6% regardless of geography or ethnicity
   c. Hereditary place a major susceptibility factor of the disease
   d. It is associated with low socioeconomic strata

7. Which of the following feature support the diagnosis of post streptococcal reactive arthritis rather than acute rheumatic fever in a patient with streptococcal pharyngeal infection?
   a. Shorter latent period
   b. Less response to NSAIDs
   c. Associated renal manifestation
   d. All of the above

8. All the following are correct regarding carditis in acute rheumatic fever *except*:
   a. Carditis may be asymptomatic in some patients
   b. Incidence of carditis varies with the age of the patient
   c. Myocarditis in the absence of valvulitis is unlikely
   d. The most common valvular lesion n ARF is mitral stenosis

9. In a patient with a history of previous RHD, a change in the character of the murmurs or appearance of new murmur indicates:
   a. Presence of acute rheumatic carditis
   b. Infective endocarditis
   c. Both of the above
   d. None of the above

10. Which is *not* correct regarding acute rheumatic fever?
   a. Chorea Sydenham does not occur simultaneously with arthritis
   b. Chorea does not occur with carditis
   c. Multiple crops of subcutaneously nodules are related to the severity of rheumatic carditis
   d. Erythema marginatum usually occurs in patients with carditis

11. Which is *not* correct regarding erythema marginatum in acute rheumatic fever?
   a. It is pathognomonic of the disease
   b. It occurs on upper arms or trunk but spare the face
   c. It occurs in patients with carditis
   d. It may occur early or late in the course of disease

12. Which of the following is a must for the diagnosis of recurrent rheumatic fever?
   a. Two major criteria
   b. One major and two minor criteria
   c. Three minor criteria
   d. Presence of preceding GAS infection

13. Evidence of preceding GAS infection in suspected case of acute rheumatic fever can be obtained from which of the following method?
   a. Throat swab culture
   b. Rising titre of ASO or anti-DNase B
   c. Positive rapid group A streptococcal carbohydrate antigens
   d. All of the above

14. All the statements are correct regarding treatment and prevention of acute rheumatic fever *except*:
   a. The use of corticosteroids reduces the risk of heart valve lesion in patients with acute rheumatic fever
   b. IM penicillin reduces the attack rate by as much as 80% when given as a primary preventive measure
   c. IM penicillin is superior to oral penicillin in the prevention of rheumatic fever recurrence
   d. More frequent injections are more effective in preventing rheumatic fever recurrence than injections every 4 weeks

ANSWERS WITH EXPLANATIONS

1. Ans. d. Chorea

Hurst's 14th Ed; Page 1189

Acute rheumatic fever usually has an acute febrile onset and presents with variable combinations of major and minor manifestations. Major manifestations include arthritis, carditis, chorea and erythema marginatum. The diagnosis of acute rheumatic fever is made when patients develop two major manifestations or one major manifestation and at least two minor manifestations. In addition, evidence of preceding infection with Group A Streptococcus must be demonstrated using streptococcal serology. The exceptions are patients who present with chorea or indolent carditis because these manifestations may only become apparent months after the inciting streptococcal infection so that additional manifestations may not be present and streptococcal serology testing may be normal.

2. Ans. c. It is preceded by opening snap

Hurst's 14th Ed; Page 1191

The auscultatory hallmark of acute rheumatic carditis is appearance of new murmurs or changing murmurs. In acute rheumatic carditis, stenotic lesions are uncommon in the early stages of the disease, but a transient apical mid-diastolic murmur (Carey Coombs) may occur in association with murmur of mitral regurgitation. This murmur occurs in patients with mitral valvulitis due to acute rheumatic fever. It is a short, mid-diastolic rumble best heard at the apex, and disappears as the valvulitis improves. It can be distinguished from the diastolic murmur of mitral stenosis by the absence of an opening snap before the murmur. The murmur is caused by increased blood flow across a thickened mitral valve.

3. Ans. d. Rheumatic fever

Hurst's 14th Ed; Page 1192

Sydenham Chorea is one of the features of acute rheumatic fever. It is a neurological disorder characterized by involuntary, purposeless, rapid, and abrupt movements associated with muscular weakness and emotional lability. Chorea occurs in up to 30% of cases of acute rheumatic fever. The abnormal movements disappear during the sleep. Mild chorea may best be demonstrated by asking the patient to squeeze the examiner's hand. This results in repetitive irregular squeezes labeled as the "milking sign".

4. Ans. d. Kyrgyzstan

Braunwald 11th Ed; Page 1511

The rheumatic fever and RHD incidence are decreasing in the developed countries however, it is still higher in some of the developing countries especially of the Asian region. Among developing countries, Kyrgyzstan probably has the highest incidence of rheumatic fever and RHD approximately 543 per 100,000 population per year and thus is labeled as rheumatic fever "hot spot" of the world.

5. Ans. c. Both of them

Braunwald 11th Ed; Page 1510

Rheumatic fever is initiated by a pharyngeal infection with group A beta-hemolytic streptococci (GAS) and following a latent period of approximately 2-3 weeks, the illness is characterized by acute inflammation of the heart, joints, skin, subcutaneous tissue, and central nervous system. Pathologically, the inflammatory process causes damage to collagen fibrils and connective tissue ground substance (fibrinoid degeneration), and thus rheumatic fever is classified as a connective tissue or collagen vascular disease.

6. Ans. a. Streptococcal skin infection does not cause rheumatic fever

Braunwald 11th Ed; Page 1511

The untreated group A hemolytic streptococcal pharyngitis leads to rheumatic fever. Streptococcal skin infection is believed not to cause rheumatic fever. However, a report of rheumatic fever following streptococcal wound infection, as well as the high prevalence of pyoderma with relative paucity of streptococcal pharyngitis in aboriginal communities of Australasia with a high incidence of rheumatic fever has raised about the link between streptococcal skin infection and rheumatic fever. Several lines of epidemiologic evidence support the role of hereditary factors in susceptibility to rheumatic fever. The lifetime cumulative incidence of rheumatic fever in populations exposed to rheumatogenic GAS infection is constant at 3 – 6% regardless of geography or ethnicity. This suggests that the proportion of susceptible individuals is the same in all continental populations of the world. The familial aggregation of rheumatic fever has been reported. The heritability of rheumatic fever is 60%, which highlights the importance of heredity as a major susceptibility factor of the disease. The rheumatic fever is associated with low socioeconomic status. The incidence of rheumatic fever has been falling consistently in industrialized countries since mid-19th century, independently of the advent of penicillin, possibly because of less crowding, improved housing and nutritional conditions, higher levels of parental employment, and better access to healthcare.

7. Ans. d. All of the above

Braunwald 11th Ed; Page 1513

Post streptococcal reactive arthritis is diagnosed in patients who have an arthritis that is not typical of rheumatic fever but who have evidence of recent streptococcal infection. This condition is said to occur after a shorter latent period than rheumatic fever, is less responsive to NSAIDs, may be associated with renal manifestations, and evidence of carditis is usually not seen.

8. Ans. d. The most common valvular lesion n ARF is mitral stenosis

Braunwald 11th Ed; Page 1513

Carditis is the most serious manifestation of rheumatic fever, because it may lead to chronic RHD with its attendant complications of atrial fibrillation, stroke, heart failure, infective endocarditis, and death. In some patients the carditis may be asymptomatic and is detected during the clinical examination of a patient with arthritis or chorea. The incidence of carditis in rheumatic fever varies with the age of the patient. It is reported in 90–92% of children under age 3 years, in 50% of children age 3–6 years, in 32% of teenagers age 14–17 years, and only in 15% of adults with a first attack of rheumatic fever. Myocarditis in the absence of valvulitis is unlikely to be rheumatic in origin. The most common valvular lesion is mitral regurgitation causing an apical pansystolic murmur. Aortic regurgitation is less common. Stenotic lesions are uncommon in the early stages of the disease, but a transient apical mid-diastolic murmur (Carey Coombs) may occur in association with the murmur of mitral regurgitation.

9. Ans. c. Both of the above

Braunwald 11th Ed; Page 1513

In patients with a history of previous RHD, a change in the character of the murmurs or the appearance of a new murmur indicates either the presence of acute rheumatic carditis or development of infective endocarditis.

10. Ans. b. Chorea does not occur with carditis

Braunwald 11th Ed; Page 1513

Chorea may be the only presenting manifestation of rheumatic fever in some patients, it is more common in females. Chorea may last for 1 week to 2 years but usually lasts for 8–15 weeks.

Because of the long latent period and resolution of the original infection, chorea does not occur simultaneously with arthritis but may coexist with carditis. The subcutaneous nodules of rheumatic fever resemble the nodules of rheumatoid arthritis and may be detected over the occiput, elbows, knees, ankles, and Achilles tendons. The Nodules are usually seen in children with prolonged active carditis rather than in the early stages of rheumatic fever. Multiple crops of nodules may be related to the severity of the rheumatic carditis. Erythema marginatum is a less common manifestation of rheumatic fever and occurs on the upper arms or trunk but not the face. Erythema marginatum usually occurs in patients with carditis and may occur early or later in the course of the disease.

11. Ans. a. It is pathognomonic of the disease

Braunwald 11th Ed; Page 1514

Erythema marginatum is a less common manifestation of rheumatic fever and occurs on the upper arms or trunk but not on the face. It is not pathognomonic of the disease. The rash is evanescent, pink, and nonpruritic. It extends centrifugally while the skin at the center returns to normal and has an irregular, serpiginous border. The rash may also become more prominent after a hot shower. Erythema marginatum usually occurs in patients with carditis and may occur early or later in the course of the disease.

12. Ans. d. Presence of preceding GAS infection

Braunwald 11th Ed; Page 1514

No specific clinical, laboratory, or other method exists to confirm a diagnosis of rheumatic fever. Diagnosis is usually made by using the clinical criteria formulated by T. Duckett Jones.

The initial diagnosis of acute rheumatic fever is made if, in the presence of preceding GAS infection, two major criteria or one major and two minor criteria are present. The diagnosis of recurrent acute rheumatic fever requires two major, one major and two minor, or three minor criteria in the presence of preceding GAS infection. Evidence of preceding GAS infection, essential for the diagnosis, may be obtained from throat swab culture (only positive in ~ 11% of patients) or by demonstrating a rising titer of antistreptococcal antibodies, either antistreptolysin O (ASO) or anti-deoxyribonuclease B (anti-DNase B), or by a positive rapid group A streptococcal carbohydrate antigen test in a child whose clinical presentation suggests a high pretest probability of streptococcal pharyngitis.

13. Ans. d. All of the above

Braunwald 11th Ed; Page 1514

Refer to explanation for Q. No 12.

14. Ans. a. The use of corticosteroids reduces the risk of heart valve lesion in patients with acute rheumatic fever

Braunwald 11th Ed; Page 1516

The choice of treatment in acute rheumatic fever is anti-inflammatory agent including salicylates, NSAIDs, and corticosteroids. All these anti-inflammatory agents have been compared with placebo or controls, or compared with one another, in systemic randomized controlled trials and there is little evidence of benefit from using corticosteroids or IV immunoglobulin to reduce the risk of heart valve lesion in patient with acute rheumatic fever.

Antibiotic treatment of proven or presumed GAS pharyngitis is effective in reducing the attack rate of rheumatic fever by 70%. IM penicillin appears to reduce the attack rate by as much as 80%. Evidence from clinical trials is strongly in support of superiority of IM compared to oral penicillin in the prevention of rheumatic fever recurrence. More frequent injections are more effective in preventing rheumatic fever recurrence than injections every 4 weeks. The evidence is strong for injection every two weeks, with an almost 50% reduction in the risk of rheumatic fever recurrence compared to the injection every 4 weeks. The evidence for injection every 3 weeks is less strong. Despite this evidence, the WHO recommends intervals of 3–4 weeks for the secondary prevention of rheumatic fever.

INFECTIVE ENDOCARDITIS

1. Which of the following is usual causative organism of infective endocarditis in patients with colonic cancer?
   a. Beta hemolytic Streptococci
   b. *Staphylococcus aureus*
   c. *Streptococcus gallolyticus*
   d. Enterococci

2. Infective endocarditis manifest with definite vegetation in which of the following location?
   a. Aortic valve position
   b. Mitral valve position
   c. Tricuspid valve
   d. Pulmonary valve

3. Which of the following is the most common predisposing condition for infective endocarditis?
   a. Rheumatic mitral valve disease
   b. Degenerative mitral valve prolapse
   c. Aortic regurgitation
   d. Bicuspid aortic valve

4. Which of the following is *not* correct regarding infective endocarditis?
   a. Valvular regurgitant lesions are more prone to infection than stenotic lesion
   b. Functional mitral regurgitation associated with left ventricular remodeling leading to MR is uncommonly affected by infective endocarditis
   c. *Staphylococcus aureus* can cause infective endocarditis in normal valve
   d. Bicuspid aortic valve is commonest congenital heart disease predisposed to infective endocarditis

5. Which is the commonest portal of pathogen entry in causation of infective endocarditis?
   a. Cutaneous such as vascular access or surgical site
   b. Oral/dental
   c. Gastrointestinal source
   d. Respiratory or otorhinolarynglottic portal

6. Infective endocarditis affecting which of the following location is associated with high incidence of periannular complication?
   a. Mitral valve
   b. Aortic valve
   c. Tricuspid valve
   d. Pulmonary valve

7. Fever as a presenting symptom of infective endocarditis may be absent in which of the following conditions?
   a. Elderly people
   b. Immunocompromised patient
   c. Patient with CIED infection
   d. All of the above

8. Janeway lesion in infective endocarditis are associated with infection of which of the following organism?
   a. *Streptococcus hemolyticus*
   b. Staphylococcal endocarditis
   c. Enterococci
   d. Fungal infection

9. Which of the following peripheral manifestations of infective endocarditis is not due to the immune complex deposition?
   a. Osler nodes
   b. Roth spots
   c. Janeway lesion
   d. Diffuse glomerulonephritis

10. In modified Duke criteria for diagnosis of infective endocarditis, which of the following is taken as a major criteria?
   a. Predisposing heart condition
   b. Immunological phenomenon such as glomerulonephritis
   c. Mycotic aneurysm
   d. Positive blood culture for infective endocarditis

11. According to modified Duke criteria for diagnosis of infective endocarditis which of the following is considered as a major criteria?
   a. Echocardiographic findings of vegetation
   b. Vascular phenomenon such as mycotic aneurysm
   c. Immunological phenomenon such as glomerulonephritis
   d. Predisposing heart condition

12. In the community acquired infective endocarditis which is the commonest organism?
   a. *Staphylococcus aureus*
   b. *Streptococcus viridans*
   c. *Staphylococcal pneumoniae*
   d. *Streptococcus gallolyticus*

13. Which of the following is a commonest offending organism implicated in healthcare associated infective endocarditis?
   a. *Streptococcus viridans*
   b. *Staphylococcus aureus*
   c. *Streptococcus gallolyticus*
   d. *Candida albicans*

14. Which of the following hematological parameter is found to be a predictor of early adverse outcomes in infective endocarditis?
   a. Anemia
   b. Leukopenia
   c. Thrombocytopenia
   d. Elevated ESR

15. Heart failure is most frequently associated with infective endocarditis involving:
   a. Mitral valve
   b. Aortic valve
   c. Tricuspid valve
   d. Pulmonary valve

16. Which is an imaging of choice for diagnosis of prosthetic valve endocarditis?
   a. CT Scan
   b. X-ray chest
   c. Transthoracic echocardiography
   d. Transesophageal echocardiography

17. Which is the commonest site of embolic event in infective endocarditis?
   a. Spleen
   b. Renal
   c. Peripheral artery
   d. CNS

18. Which is the rarest site of embolization in infective endocarditis?
   a. CNS
   b. Spleen
   c. Mesenteric
   d. Coronary

19. Which is *not* correct regarding embolization in infective endocarditis?
   a. Aortic valve vegetation are more likely to embolize than mitral valve
   b. Embolic risk is equivalent in native & in prosthetic valve
   c. Vegetations >10 mm in dimension are more likely to embolize
   d. All of the above

20. Which of the following is a high-risk predictor for embolization in infective endocarditis (IE)?
   a. *Staphylococcus aureus* IE
   b. Vegetations in mitral valve
   c. Vegetations >10 mm in diameter
   d. All of the above

21. Which of the following statement is *not* correct regarding infective endocarditis?
   a. Mitral valve vegetation are more likely to embolize than those in aortic position
   b. Embolic risk is higher in prosthetic valve IE than native IE.
   c. The risk of embolism decreases within one week after initiation of appropriate antibiotic therapy.
   d. All are incorrect

22. Which is antibiotic of choice for patients who have history of immunoglobulin E (IgE) mediated allergic reaction?
   a. Aqueous crystalline penicillin G sodium
   b. Cephalosporin
   c. Gentamycin
   d. Vancomycin

23. For Enterococcal strains resistant to vancomycin and penicillin which is optimal treatment regimen for infective endocarditis?
   a. Daptomycin
   b. Linezolid
   c. Both of them
   d. None of them

24. In a patient with infective endocarditis when the isolate organism is resistant to all aminoglycoside which is the preferred antibiotic?
   a. Penicillin
   b. Combination of high dose ceftriaxone with ampicillin
   c. Linezolid
   d. Daptomycin

25. Which of the following is antibiotic of choice for infective endocarditis due to HACEK organism?
   a. Penicillin
   b. Ceftriaxone
   c. Cefotaxime
   d. Fluoroquinolone

26. Intervalvular fibrosa invasion is reported in which of the following location endocarditis?
   a. Aortic valve
   b. Posterior mitral valve
   c. Pseudoaneurysm
   d. Fistula

27. Which is the commonest indication for surgery in infective endocarditis?
   a. Heart failure
   b. Uncontrolled infection
   c. Periannular extension of infection
   d. Embolization

28. Which is *not* correct regarding embolization in infective endocarditis?
   a. Occult embolism may occur in approximate 20% of patients
   b. Risk of embolization is highest in the first week after initiation of antibiotic therapy
   c. Surgery is recommended in presence of large mobile vegetation (>10 mm).
   d. All of the above

29. Which is the common site of vegetation in patients with aortic regurgitation and infective endocarditis?
   a. Ventricular side of aortic leaflet
   b. Aorta side of aortic leaflet
   c. Mitral chordae
   d. Over anterior mitral leaflet

30. Which is the common site of vegetation formation in patient with ventricular septal defect with infective endocarditis?
   a. LV side of VSD
   b. RV side of VSD
   c. Pulmonary valve
   d. Septal leaflet of tricuspid valve

31. Which is the commonest site of involvement in infective endocarditis caused by Rickettsial organism/*Coxiella Burnetii*?
   a. Tricuspid valve
   b. Pulmonary valve
   c. Mitral valve
   d. Aortic valve

32. A large bulky vegetation that can obstruct valve orifice and can embolize large vessel (e.g., femoral artery) is seen with:
   a. Staphylococcal endocarditis
   b. Streptococcal endocarditis
   c. Rickettsial organism endocarditis
   d. Fungal infective endocarditis

33. The complex infective endocarditis is defined as situation including all *except*:
   a. There is an infection with virulent organism (*Staphylococcus aureus*)
   b. Severe hemodynamic compromise
   c. Aortic valve involvement
   d. Mitral valve involvement

ANSWERS WITH EXPLANATIONS

1. Ans. c. *Streptococcus gallolyticus*

Braunwald 11th Ed; Page 1484

Streptococcus gallolyticus is usually found in gastrointestinal tract. It is a cause of infective endocarditis in patients with underlying GI lesion especially colonic cancer. It is seen more in aging population.

2. Ans. b. Mitral valve position

Braunwald 11th Ed; Page 1486

According to the International Collaboration on Endocarditis – Prospective Cohort Study (ICE – PCS) the native valve endocarditis is most common (72%) followed by prosthetic valve endocarditis (21%) and pacemaker or implantable cardioverter defibrillator (ICD) infective endocarditis (7%). This study also found that infective endocarditis manifests with definite vegetations most frequently in the mitral valve position (41%), followed by aortic valve position (38%), whereas the tricuspid valve (12%) and pulmonary (1%) valves were much less frequently involved. Preexisting valvular regurgitant lesions are much more prone to infection than stenotic lesions. Incidence of infective endocarditis is directly related to the impact of pressure on the closed valve, with shear stress disruption of the valvular endothelium in the vicinity of the egressing regurgitant jet. In the presence of the Venturi effect, circulating organisms are deposited within the high-velocity, lowered pressure eddy zones of the regurgitant orifice of the receiving chamber, leading to the typical localization of vegetations on the upstream aspect of the infected valve.

Mitral regurgitation associated with degenerative mitral valve prolapse (MVP), particularly with advanced myxomatous leaflet thickening, is the most common predisposing condition for infective endocarditis and is much more common than rheumatic mitral valve disease. Second most common native valve lesion predisposing to infective endocarditis is aortic regurgitation.

The risk of infective endocarditis in patients with bicuspid aortic valve (BAV) is very low.

3. Ans. b. Degenerative mitral valve prolapse

Braunwald 11th Ed; Page 1486

Refer to explanation for Q. No 2.

4. Ans. d. Bicuspid aortic valve is commonest congenital heart disease predisposed to infective endocarditis

Braunwald 11th Ed; Page 1486

The Functional mitral regurgitation, associated with left ventricular (LV) remodeling causing malcoaptation of intrinsically normal mitral leaflets in a low pressure, low-cardiac-output state, is quite uncommonly complicated by infective endocarditis. Congenital heart disease, other than bicuspid aortic valve disease, is a predisposing condition to infective endocarditis. Unrepaired ventricular septal defects are the most frequent congenital heart disease lesions associated with infective endocarditis, followed by ventricular outflow tract obstructive lesions, such as with tetralogy of Fallot. Structurally normal valves may also be affected in infective endocarditis, with risk associations of advanced age, renal failure requiring hemodialysis, and infection caused by *Staphylococcus aureus* or enterococci.

5. Ans. a. Cutaneous such as vascular access or surgical site

Braunwald 11th Ed; Page 1486

A study have demonstrated that a portal of pathogen entry responsible for infective endocarditis could be identified in almost 75% of patients. The most common entry site was cutaneous (40%), associated with healthcare delivery, such as vascular access or a surgical site, or sites used for intravenous drug abuse. The second most common (29%) portal of entry is oral/dental, with an active infection implicated much more frequently than a prior dental procedure. Thirdly, a GI source was detected in 23% of patients, in the majority with colonic neoplasm, or less commonly, ulcerative or inflammatory disease. Far less (<5%) frequently, a genitourinary, otorhinolaryngottic, or respiratory portal of entry was detected.

6. Ans. b. Aortic valve

Braunwald 11th Ed; Page 1486

Infective endocarditis affecting bicuspid aortic valve is not uncommon. Aortic valve endocarditis is associated with high incidence of periannular complication of infective endocarditis.

7. Ans. d. All of the above

Braunwald 11th Ed; Page 1486

Fever is the most common presenting symptoms in up to 95% of cases with infective endocarditis but may be absent in up to 20% of patients, especially elderly persons, the immunocompromised, patients treated with previous empiric antibiotic therapy, or patients with CIED infections. Fever start subsiding usually after 5–7 days of appropriate antibiotic therapy. Persistence of fever may indicate progressive infection with perivalvular extension such as abscess, septic embolization, an extracardiac site of infection (native or prosthetic), infected indwelling catheters or devices, inadequate antibiotic treatment of a resistant organism.

8. Ans. b. Staphylococcal endocarditis

Braunwald 11th Ed; Page 1487

Janeway lesions are painless hemorrhagic macules with a predilection for the soles or palms and are sequelae of peripheral septic embolization, most often associated with staphylococcal infective endocarditis.

9. Ans. c. Janeway lesion

Braunwald 11th Ed; Page 1487

The classical peripheral manifestation of infective endocarditis includes Petechiae, Janeway lesion, Splinter subungual hemorrhages, Osler notes, Roth spots and glomerulonephritis. Petechiae are most common, occurring on the conjunctivae, oral mucosa, or extremities. Janeway lesions are painless hemorrhagic macules with a predilection for the soles and palms and are sequelae of peripheral septic embolization, most often associated with staphylococcal infective endocarditis. Splinter subungual hemorrhages also are painless, dark-red linear lesions in the proximal nailbed. Osler nodes are painful, erythematous, nodular lesions usually located in the pads of the fingers and toes and are the result of immune complex deposition and focal vasculitis. Roth spots are retinal hemorrhages with a pale center of coagulated fibrin and also are related to immune complex–mediated vasculitis secondary to infective endocarditis. An immune complex–mediated diffuse glomerulonephritis may be associated with these findings.

10. Ans. d. Positive blood culture for infective endocarditis

Braunwald 11th Ed; Page 1488

Duke criteria for diagnosis of infective endocarditis

Definite infective endocarditis
Pathologic criteria
• Microorganisms demonstrated by results of cultures or histologic examination of a vegetation, a vegetation that has embolized, or an intracardiac abscess specimen; or
• Pathologic lesions; vegetation, or intracardiac abscess confirmed by results of histologic examination showing active endocarditis
Clinical criteria
• 2 major criteria or
• 1 major criterion and 3 minor criteria, or
• 5 minor criteria
Possible infective endocarditis
• 1 major criterion and 1 minor criterion, or
• 3 minor criteria
Rejected diagnosis of infective endocarditis
• Firm alternate diagnosis explaining evidence of suspected IE, or
• Resolution of IE syndrome with antibiotic therapy for ≤4 days, or
• No evidence of IE at surgery or autopsy, on antibiotic therapy for ≤4 days, or
• Does not meet criteria for possible IE

11. Ans. a. Echocardiographic findings of vegetation

Braunwald 11th Ed; Page 1488

Definition of term used in the modified duke criteria for diagnosis of infective endocarditis

Major criteria
- Blood culture findings positive for IE
  - Typical microorganisms consistent with IE from two separate blood cultures:
    - Viridans streptococci. *Streptococcus gallolyticus* (formerly known as *S. bovis*). *Staphylococcus aureus*, HACEK group, or
    - Community-acquired enterococci, in the absence of a primary focus, or
  - Microorganisms consistent with IE from persistently positive blood culture findings, defined as:
    - ≥2 positive culture findings of blood samples drawn >12 hours apart, or
    - 3 or most of ≥4 separate culture findings of blood (with first and last sample drawn ≥1 hour apart)
    - Single positive blood culture for *Coxiella burnetii* or anti-phase I IgG titer ≥1:800
- Evidence of endocardial involvement
  - Echocardiography findings positive for IE [TEE recommended in patients with prosthetic valves, rated at least possible IE by clinical criteria or complicated IE (paravalvular abscess); TTE as first test in other patients], defined as follows:
    - Oscillating intracardiac mass on valve or supporting structures, in the path of regurgitant jets, or on implanted material in the absence of an alternative anatomic explanation, or
    - Abscess, or
    - New partial dehiscence of prosthetic valve
    - New valvular regurgitation: Worsening or changing of preexisting murmur not sufficient

Minor criteria
- Predisposition, predisposing heart condition, or intravenous drug use
- Fever—temperature >38°C
- Vascular phenomena, major arterial emboli, septic pulmonary infarcts, mycotic aneurysm, intracranial hemorrhage, conjunctival hemorrhages, and Janeway lesions
- Immunologic phenomena: Glomerulonephritis, Osler nodes, Roth spots, and rheumatoid factor
- Microbiologic evidence: Positive blood culture finding but does not meet a major criterion as noted above (excludes single positive culture findings for coagulase-negative staphylococci and organisms that do not cause endocarditis) or serologic evidence of active infection with organism consistent with IE

12. Ans. b. *Streptococcus viridans*

Braunwald 11th Ed; Page 1489

The complete blood count often is abnormal in infective endocarditis. In patients with subacute infective endocarditis, a normochromic normocytic anemia of variable severity is detected in a majority of patients. A leukocytosis may be detected in 50-60% of patients and it is more common with acute than with subacute infective endocarditis. Leukopenia also may infrequently occur with subacute infective endocarditis and usually is associated with splenomegaly. Thrombocytopenia may occur in approximately 10% of patients and has been found to be a predictor of early adverse outcome. The ESR usually is elevated in patients with infective endocarditis in almost >61% of patients. An elevated ESR is found to be independently associated with a decreased risk of in-hospital death, presumably because of an association with subacute infective endocarditis with a more indolent course.

13. Ans. b. *Staphylococcus aureus*

Braunwald 11th Ed; Page 1489

Refer to explanation for Q. No 12.

14. Ans. c. Thrombocytopenia

Braunwald 11th Ed; Page 1489

Refer to explanation for Q. No 12.

15. Ans. b. Aortic valve

Braunwald 11th Ed; Page 1492

Local valvular destruction is very frequently seen in left-sided valvular regurgitant lesions, and heart failure may complicate the course of approximately 30-40% of patients with infective endocarditis and is three times more common in native than in prosthetic valve infective endocarditis. According to a registry heart failure most frequently is associated with aortic valve infective endocarditis (30%), followed by mitral valve (20%) and tricuspid valve (<10%).

Echocardiography is a very helpful imaging for a suspected case of infective endocarditis. However, there are multiple limitations in form of poor acoustic window, body habitus, pulmonary disease may not help in diagnosing infective endocarditis. TEE circumvent all these potential impediments to transthoracic imaging. The TEE is a procedure of choice for diagnosing prosthetic valve endocarditis.

16. Ans. d. Transesophageal echocardiography

Braunwald 11th Ed; Page 1492

Refer to explanation for Q. No 15.

17. Ans. d. CNS

Braunwald 11th Ed; Page 1494

The various site of embolization with infective endocarditis are CNS (38%), spleen (30%), renal (13%), lung (10%), peripheral artery (6%), mesenteric (2%) and coronary (1%).

18. Ans. d. Coronary

Braunwald 11th Ed; Page 1494

Refer to explanation for Q. No 17.

19. Ans. a. Aortic valve vegetation are more likely to embolize than mitral valve

Braunwald 11th Ed; Page 1494-1495

Echocardiographic analysis have shown that vegetations >10 mm in greatest dimension are independent predictors of embolism, with considerably higher risk with dimensions above 15 mm. Pedunculated and highly mobile vegetations also are independently associated with embolic risk. Both vegetation length of >10 mm and severe vegetation mobility are predictors of embolism. Mitral valve vegetations, particularly on the anterior leaflet in native valve infective endocarditis, are more likely to embolize than those in the aortic position. The embolic risk generally is equivalent in native and in prosthetic valve infective endocarditis.

The infecting organism also has an impact on embolic risk. *Staphylococcus aureus* IE has been consistently implicated as an independent risk predictor for embolism. IE from *Streptococcus gallolyticus* and VGS is less implicated. The presence of intracardiac perivalvular abscess is another independent risk for stroke associated with infective endocarditis.

20. Ans. d. All of the above

Braunwald 11th Ed; Page 1494-1495

Refer to explanation for Q. No 19.

21. Ans. b. Embolic risk is higher in prosthetic valve IE than native IE

Braunwald 11th Ed; Page 1494-1495

Refer to explanation for Q. No 19.

22. Ans. d. Vancomycin

Braunwald 11th Ed; Page 1496

Vancomycin is recommended in patients who cannot tolerate penicillin or cephalosporin therapy because of a history of immunoglobulin E (IgE) mediated allergic reactions.

23. Ans. c. Both of them

Braunwald 11th Ed; Page 1496-1498

Usual treatment of infective endocarditis caused by strains that are susceptible to both penicillin and gentamicin, 4 weeks of antibiotic treatment is recommended in patients with symptoms for 3 months or less; 6 weeks is recommended for symptoms of infective endocarditis longer than 3 months or for prosthetic valve endocarditis. Enterococci are common causative organisms in infective endocarditis, particularly in the elderly population, and treatment requires both penicillin or ampicillin and an aminoglycoside. If an isolate is gentamicin resistant and streptomycin susceptible, streptomycin should be given with either ampicillin or penicillin. When the isolate is resistant to all aminoglycosides or the patient is unable to tolerate an aminoglycoside-containing regimen, a combination of "high-dose" ceftriaxone (4 g daily in two divided doses) with ampicillin has been successfully used.

24. Ans. b. Combination of high dose ceftriaxone with ampicillin

Braunwald 11th Ed; Page 1496-1498

Refer to explanation for Q. No 23.

25. Ans. b. Ceftriaxone

Braunwald 11th Ed; Page 1499

The primary choice of therapy for IE caused by the HACEK group of organisms is ceftriaxone, given for 4 weeks for native valve infection and 6 weeks for prosthetic valve endocarditis. Cefotaxime and ampicillin sulbactam are acceptable alternative therapeutic agents. Fluoroquinolones should be efficacious as second-line agents.

26. Ans. a. Aortic valve

Braunwald 11th Ed; Page 1501

The current guidelines states that surgery should be considered in patients with infective endocarditis in presence of (1) heart failure, (2) features suggestive of high risk embolism, and (3) uncontrolled infection. Heart failure is the most frequently encountered reason for consideration of urgent surgical treatment. Heart failure may because by severe regurgitation (aortic or mitral), intracardiac fistula or less often vegetation related valve obstruction.

Uncontrolled infection is the second most common reason for surgical intervention, can be characterized broadly by increasing vegetation size, abscess formation, false aneurysm or creation of fistula.

Persistent fever frequently is associated with these anatomic findings. Early surgery indicated in setting of uncontrolled infection, associated with persistent fever and positive blood culture despite an appropriate antibiotic regimen. Perivalvular extension of infection is more common in aortic valve endocarditis. Perivalvular abscess is more frequently occur in posterior or lateral portion of mitral annulus where is an aortic infective endocarditis extension can occur through the intervalvular fibrosa. Predictors of intervalvular fibrosa invasion includes presence of a prosthetic valve, aortic location and infection with coagulase negative staphylococci.

Infective endocarditis related embolism is common (20–50% of cases) and can be fatal. Occult embolism may occur in approximately 20% of the patients.

27. Ans. a. Heart failure

Braunwald 11th Ed; Page 1501

Refer to explanation for Q. No 26.

28. Ans. d. All of the above

Braunwald 11th Ed; Page 1501

Refer to explanation for Q. No 26.

29. Ans. c. Mitral chordae

Hurst's 14th Ed; Page 1624

The endothelial damage is the inciting event for infective endocarditis to occur. The vegetations are most likely to form in areas where blood-flow injury is likely to occur—on the ventricular side of semilunar valves and the atrial side of AV valves. Jet lesions from regurgitant valves or intracardiac shunts may also damage endothelium, and vegetations may form on such sites of injury, including the mitral chordae with aortic regurgitation, the mural left atrial endocardium with mitral regurgitation, or the septal leaflet of the tricuspid valve with ventricular septal defect.

30. Ans. d. Septal leaflet of tricuspid valve

Hurst's 14th Ed; Page 1624

Refer to explanation for Q. No 29.

31. Ans. d. Aortic valve

Hurst's 14th Ed; Page 1626

The rickettsial organism *Coxiella burnetii* is the causative agent of Q fever and is a cause of infective endocarditis in areas where cattle, sheep, and goat farming are common. The aortic valve is affected in >80% of cases, and the infection is difficult to eradicate with antibiotics.

32. Ans. d. Fungal infective endocarditis

Hurst's 14th Ed; Page 1626

Fungal endocarditis is associated with high mortality. Fungal endocarditis develops in patients who have multiple predisposing conditions such as an immunocompromised state, the use of endovascular devices, and previous reconstructive cardiac surgery. *Candida* and *Aspergillus* species are the most common causes of fungal infective endocarditis and are associated with large, bulky vegetations that can obstruct valve orifices and can also embolize to large vessels (e.g., the femoral artery).

33. Ans. d. Mitral valve involvement

Hurst's 14th Ed; Page 1632–1633

Complex infective endocarditis is defined as infection with a virulent organism (e.g., *Staphylococcus aureus*), severe hemodynamic compromise, aortic valve involvement, persistent fever or bacteremia, clinical change during therapy, or symptomatic deterioration.

Chapter 15: Valvular Heart Disease and Prosthetic Heart Valves

VALVULAR DISEASE

1. In fetus oxygenated blood from placenta is returned to left heart by:
   a. SVC
   b. IVC
   c. Pulmonary vein
   d. Bronchial vein

2. Valvular AS is feature of which type of hypercholesterolemia?
   a. Type I
   b. Type II
   c. Type III
   d. Type IV

3. Survival is shortest with which of the following symptoms in AS?
   a. Dyspnea
   b. Syncope
   c. Angina
   d. Equal with all

4. Gastrointestinal bleeding, idiopathic or due to angiodysplasia of right colon or other vascular malformation occurs commonly in which lesion:
   a. Valvular AS
   b. Aortic regurgitation
   c. Tricuspid regurgitation
   d. Mitral stenosis

5. Which of the following is a sensitive indicator of myocardial function in aortic regurgitation?
   a. End systolic volume
   b. End diastolic volume
   c. Wall thickness
   d. Ejection fraction

6. Which of the following troublesome symptom is most frequently observed in patient of aortic regurgitation?
   a. Syncope
   b. Angina
   c. Nocturnal angina accompanied by diaphoresis
   d. Palpitation

7. Pulsus Bisferien's is best recognized in:
   a. Carotid pulse
   b. Brachial pulse
   c. Femoral pulse
   d. Radial pulse

8. Which of the following is most sensitive echocardiographic finding in cases of aortic regurgitation?
   a. Dilatation of aortic root
   b. Increased end systolic and end diastolic diameter of left ventricle
   c. Reduced fractional shortening
   d. Diastolic fluttering of anterior leaflet of mitral valve

9. The most precise method to assess left ventricular performance is:
   a. Serial roentgenogram
   b. Echocardiogram
   c. Radionuclide ventriculogram
   d. Biplane left ventriculography

10. Organic tricuspid stenosis is most common in:
    a. India
    b. Japan
    c. North America
    d. Western Europe

11. Severe tricuspid regurgitation has been reported to be the presenting manifestation of:
    a. Cushing syndrome
    b. Thyrotoxicosis
    c. Acromegaly
    d. Myxedema

12. Which of the following hemodynamic features are seen in tricuspid regurgitation?
    a. Absence of 'X' descent
    b. Prominent 'V' or CV wave (ventricularization of atrial pressure)
    c. Elevation of mean atrial pressure
    d. All of the above

13. Which of the following is most prominent event in JVP in cases of tricuspid regurgitation?
    a. Prominent 'A' wave
    b. Absent X wave
    c. Prominent CV wave
    d. Prominent Y descent

14. Which of the following is a sensitive and precise tool for assessing the tricuspid regurgitation?
   a. ECG
   b. Contrast echo with saline and demonstration of microbubble traversing to and fro across the tricuspid valve
   c. Indicator dilution technique
   d. RV angiography

15. Which of the following is treatment of choice for tricuspid valve endocarditis in heroin addicts?
   a. Antibiotic alone
   b. Antibiotic with resection of valve without replacement
   c. Ab + resection and immediate valve replacement
   d. Ab + resection of valve with valve replacement few weeks to months letter

16. The most common cause of pulmonary regurgitation is:
   a. Congenital
   b. SABE
   c. Post surgical
   d. Secondary to pulmonary hypertension

17. Most common symptom of aortic stenosis is:
   a. Angina
   b. Syncope
   c. Dyspnea
   d. Palpitation

18. Which of the following is most common cause of valvular aortic stenosis?
   a. Bicuspid valve
   b. Congenital AS
   c. Rheumatic AS
   d. SABE

19. Reduced pulse pressure in aortic stenosis is due to:
   a. Reduced systolic BP
   b. Elevated diastolic BP
   c. Both a and b
   d. None of them

20. Prominent A wave in JVP is seen most commonly with:
   a. Supravalvular aortic stenosis
   b. Valvular aortic stenosis
   c. Subaortic stenosis
   d. Not seen in AS

21. The most constant physical finding of AS is:
   a. Presence of aortic ejection click
   b. Presence of aortic systolic murmur
   c. Presence of delayed aortic closure
   d. Presence of aortic diastolic murmur

22. Which of the following is *true* regarding aortic ejection click?
   a. Intensity of ejection click is correlated with intensity of A2
   b. Aortic ejection click is heard in <1/3 of adults
   c. Presence of ejection click helps in localization of valvular level of stenosis
   d. All are true

23. Which of the following feature of murmur of aortic stenosis helps in deciding the severity of AS?
   a. Intensity of murmur
   b. Duration of murmur
   c. Configuration of murmur
   d. All of the above

24. Which of the following is most common alteration seen in second heart sound in significant AS?
   a. Delay in aortic closure, leading to single second sound without inspiratory splitting
   b. Delay in A2 leading to paradoxical splitting of 2nd HS
   c. Presence of normal inspiratory splitting
   d. Decreased or absent A2

25. Which of the following is *true* regarding the early diastolic murmur of aortic stenosis?
   a. 50–75% of 'pure' aortic stenosis is accompanied by early diastolic murmur at base
   b. It is uncommon with supravalvular AS or subaortic stenosis
   c. It is accompanied by normal pulse pressure and absence of peripheral signs of aortic stenosis
   d. All are true

26. What is the incidence of sudden death in patient with aortic stenosis?
   a. 3–5%
   b. 5–10%
   c. 15–20%
   d. 25%

27. The most common cause of aortic regurgitation is:
   a. Rheumatic fever
   b. Syphilis
   c. Bacterial endocarditis
   d. Myxomatous degeneration

28. Due to which disorder pathological changes similar to the syphilis is seen in aortic wall in aortic regurgitation?
   a. Ankylosing spondylitis
   b. Rheumatoid arthritis
   c. Reiter's syndrome
   d. Pseudoxanthoma elasticum

29. Which of the following valve is most commonly involved in rheumatoid arthritis?
   a. Mitral
   b. Aortic
   c. Tricuspid
   d. Pulmonary

30. Which of the following is determinant of volume overload in case of aortic incompetence?
   a. Volume of regurgitant blood flow
   b. Area of regurgitant orifice
   c. Diastolic pressure gradient between aorta and LV
   d. All of the above

31. Which of the following is most important determinant of severity of reflux in aortic regurgitation?
   a. Size of orifice
   b. Duration of diastole
   c. Diastolic pressure gradient between aorta and LV
   d. Volume of regurgitation

32. Which of the following is most common presenting manifestation of aortic regurgitation?
   a. Palpitation   b. Angina
   c. Dyspnea   d. Syncope

33. Angina pectoris in aortic regurgitation differs from that occurring in aortic stenosis in which of the following manner:
   a. More often occurs at rest and last longer
   b. It is preceded by symptom of left ventricular failure
   c. It more often occurs in night and accompanied by vasomotor phenomenon such as flushing, perspiration and dyspnea
   d. All are true

34. Bilateral neck pain associated with tenderness over the carotids is seen most often in:
   a. Aortic stenosis
   b. Aortic incompetence
   c. Idiopathic hypertrophic subaortic stenosis
   d. Supravalvular AS

35. Which of the following sign observed in AR is more specific for aortic regurgitation?
   a. Corrigan's pulse   b. Duroziez's murmur
   c. Hill sign   d. De Musset sign

36. Severity of aortic regurgitation is best judged by:
   a. Location of murmur
   b. Intensity of murmur
   c. Duration of murmur
   d. Shape of murmur

37. Which of the following hemodynamic feature is specific for acute AR?
   a. Premature closure of mitral valve
   b. Presence of S3
   c. Presence of S4
   d. Short early diastolic murmur

38. Which of the following ECG finding differentiate aortic regurgitation from aortic stenosis?
   a. Presence of sinus rhythm
   b. Increased QRS amplitude with depressed ST segment and T wave inversion
   c. Presence of conduction disturbance
   d. Horizontal axis in ECG

39. Which of the following radiological feature is specific for aortic regurgitation?
   a. Posterior and inferior elongation of cardiac apex
   b. LA enlargement
   c. Aortic dilatation
   d. Calcification of aortic valve

40. Which of the following features of mitral valve seen in echo is specific for AR?
   a. Fast, fine vibration or fluttering during diastole of AML
   b. Extremely rapid diastolic closure rate of mitral leaflet
   c. Mitral valve closure occurring prior to the QRS
   d. Thickening of mitral leaflet

41. Long-term survival after valve replacement is better in:
   a. Isolated aortic stenosis
   b. Isolated aortic regurgitation
   c. Combined aortic stenosis/aortic regurgitation
   d. Equal in all 3 subsets

42. The total removal of which of the following cardiac valve without replacement is well-tolerated hemodynamically:
   a. Mitral valve   b. Aortic valve
   c. Tricuspid valve   d. Pulmonary valve

43. Which of the following cardiac valve has tendency to get incompetent often?
   a. Mitral valve   b. Aortic valve
   c. Pulmonary valve   d. Tricuspid valve

44. What percentage of patients with rheumatic fever has organic tricuspid involvement?
   a. <5%
   b. 10–15%
   c. >25%
   d. Tricuspid valve is not involved

45. Right upper quadrant abdominal pain which is often worst in the morning and improves as the day goes on is often seen in which condition?
   a. Mitral stenosis
   b. Tricuspid valve disease
   c. Pulmonary hypertension
   d. Inferior vena cava thrombosis

46. The pulmonary circulation is a low resistance circuit because of:
   a. Absence of high resistance muscular arterioles
   b. Voluminous, diffusely anastomotic capillary bed
   c. A large reserve capacity with little resistance to passive distention by increased pulmonary blood flow
   d. All of the above

47. Which valvular lesion the intestinal lymphangiectasia leading to malabsorption is feature of?
   a. Severe mitral regurgitation
   b. Severe tricuspid regurgitation
   c. Severe aortic regurgitation
   d. Severe pulmonary stenosis

48. Which of the following feature point it to be of organic nature in a patients with tricuspid insufficiency?
   a. Associated tricuspid stenosis
   b. Absence of pulmonary hypertension
   c. Rheumatic involvement of other cardiac valve
   d. Both a and b

49. Which is *not* correct regarding tricuspid endocarditis?
   a. Most often seen in heroin addicts
   b. Streptococcus viridans is most common organism
   c. Multiple septic pulmonary embolism often seen
   d. Chest X-ray reveals multiple infiltrates

50. In what percentage of patients with rheumatic mitral valvular disease there is accompanying tricuspid stenosis?
   a. 3–5%   b. 8–10%
   c. 10–15%   d. >25%

51. Which of the following clinical feature is unusual with tricuspid stenosis?
   a. Orthopnea   b. Edema
   c. Ascites   d. Hepatomegaly

ANSWERS WITH EXPLANATIONS

1. Ans. b. IVC

Hurst's 8th Ed; Page 1762

The fetus obtains all metabolic necessities, including oxygen, from the placenta. The fetal circulation is an adaptation to allow most of the right ventricular output to bypass the lungs and instead to perfuse the placenta. The fetal circulation is arranged in parallel fashion rather than in series, with mixing at the atrial (foramen ovale) and great vessel (ductus arteriosus) levels. Normally, systemic venous blood enters the right atrium via the superior or inferior vena cava. From the inferior vena cava, blood is diverted by the crista dividens though the foramen ovale into the left atrium, so that approximately 27% of combined ventricular output reaches the left ventricle, with the remainder passing through the tricuspid valve to the right ventricle. This left atrial flow mixes with a small volume of pulmonary venous return to enter the left ventricle and the ascending aorta. Most of this output perfuses the coronary arteries, head, and upper body vessels, with a small proportion crossing the aortic arch to the descending aorta. Right ventricular output enters the main pulmonary artery, where approximately 90% (59% of combined ventricular output) is diverted through the ductus arteriosus to the descending aorta. Thus, approximately two-thirds of the combined cardiac output passes through the right side of the heart and one-third passes through the left side of the heart.

The oxygen saturation of fetal blood is considerably lower than that in a newborn or infant because of the placenta's less efficient oxygen exchange compared with that the lungs. The blood with the highest saturation (approximately 70%) is that returning from the placenta. As described above, some of this higher saturation blood is diverted across the foramen ovale, so that saturation on the left side of the heart (65%) is somewhat higher than it is on the right side (55%). As a result, lower-saturation blood (some 55%) passes preferentially through the ductus arteriosus to the placenta, thus increasing the efficiency of oxygen pickup.

2. Ans. b. Type II

Braunwald 5th Ed; Page 1036

In severe atherosclerosis there is involvement of aortic valve, aorta and other major arteries. This form of aortic stenosis occur more frequently in patients with severe hypercholesterolemia and is observed in children with homozygous type II hyperlipoproteinemia and is an extremely rare condition.

3. Ans. a. Dyspnea

Braunwald 5th Ed; Page 1039

In the natural history of adult with aortic stenosis, a long latent period exist during which there is gradually increasing obstruction and an increase in the pressure load on the myocardium while the patient remain asymptomatic. The cardinal manifestation of aortic stenosis, which commences most commonly in the sixth decade of life are angina pectoris, syncope and heart failure. In patient in whom the obstruction remains unrelieved, once this symptoms become manifest, the prognosis is poor. Survival curve shows that interval from

4. Ans. a. Valvular AS

Braunwald 5th Ed; Page 1040

Gastrointestinal bleeding, idiopathic or due to angiodysplasia (most commonly of the right colon) or other vascular malformation occurs more often in patient with calcific aortic stenosis than in person without this condition. It may cease after aortic valve replacement.

5. Ans. a. End systolic volume

Braunwald 11th Ed; Page 1420

In patient with aortic regurgitation, as left ventricular function deteriorates the left ventricle dilates. Ventricular end diastolic volume increases without further elevation of aortic regurgitant volume. The ratio of left ventricular end diastolic thickness to radius declines, systolic wall tension rises, reducing ejection fraction, forward stroke volume and ventricular emptying while end systolic volume rises. As the left ventricle decompensates interstitial fibrosis increases and compliance may decline and left ventricular end diastolic pressure rises. In advance stages, there may be considerable elevation of left atrial, pulmonary artery wedge, pulmonary arterial, right ventricular and right atrial pressures and lowering of the effective cardiac output, first during exercise and then even at rest. There is failure of the normal decline in end systolic volume or rise in the ejection fraction during exercise. The end systolic volume provides a useful overall index of myocardial function in patients with AR and correlates with operative mortality and postoperative left ventricular dysfunction. Both the immediate and long-term results are excellent in patient with normal left ventricular end systolic volumes (<40 mL/m$_2$) and is poor in patient in whom index is elevated (>80 mL/m$_2$), and variable in patients with intermediate values.

6. Ans. c. Nocturnal angina accompanied by diaphoresis

Braunwald 5th Ed; Page 1048

In patients with chronic severe aortic regurgitation, the left ventricle gradually undergoes enlargement while the patients remains asymptomatic or almost so. Symptoms of reduced cardiac reserve or myocardial ischemia develop most often in the fourth or fifth decade and usually only after considerable cardiomegaly and myocardial dysfunction have occurred. Exertional dyspnea, orthopnea or paroxysmal nocturnal dyspnea are the principal complaint. Syncope is rare and although angina pectoris is less frequent than it is in patient with aortic stenosis, nocturnal angina often accompanied by diaphoresis that occur when the heart rate slows and arterial diastolic pressure falls to extremely low levels may be the troublesome symptom. These episodes are occasionally accompanied by abdominal discomfort presumably caused by splanchnic ischemia. Patient with severe aortic regurgitation often complains of an uncomfortable awareness of the heart beat especially on lying down and disagreeable thoracic pain due to pounding of the heart against the chest wall.

onset of symptoms to the time of death is approximately 2 years in the patient with heart failure, 3 years in those with syncope and 5 years in those with angina.

7. Ans. a. Carotid pulse

Braunwald 5th Ed; Page 22

A bisferiens pulse is characterized by two systolic peaks, the percussion and tidal waves separated by a distinct mid systolic dip. This type of pulse is detected most readily by palpation of carotid and less commonly of the brachial arteries. It occurs in condition in which a large stroke volume is ejected rapidly from left ventricle and is observed most commonly in patient with pure aortic regurgitation or with a combination of aortic regurgitation and stenosis. It may disappear as heart failure supervenes. A bisferiens pulse also occurs in patient with hypertrophic obstructive cardiomyopathy but the bifid nature may only be recorded not palpated.

8. Ans. d. Diastolic fluttering of anterior leaflet of mitral valve

Braunwald 5th Ed; Page 1050

Echocardiography is helpful in identifying the cause of aortic regurgitation. It may show thickening of the valve cusp, prolapse of the valve, a thickened leaflet, vegetation or dilatation of aortic root. Two dimensional studies are useful for the measurement of left ventricular end diastolic and end systolic dimension, volume and ejection fraction. These measurements when made serially and are of immense value in selecting the optimal timing for surgical intervention and is a method of choice for a precise assessment of left ventricular performance in patients with aortic regurgitation. In acute aortic regurgitation, the echocardiogram reveal a reduction in amplitude of the opening movement of the mitral valve, premature closure and delayed opening of the mitral valve and on the M-mode study a reduction in the EF slope, indicating that the left ventricle is operating on the steep portion of the pressure volume curve. Left ventricular end diastolic dimensions are not markedly increased and fractional shortening is normal. This contrast with the findings in chronic aortic regurgitation in which end-diastolic dimension and wall motions are increased. Occasionally with equilibration of aortic and left ventricular pressure in diastole, premature opening of aortic valve may be detected. High frequency diastolic fluttering of the anterior leaflet of the mitral valve during diastole is an important echocardiographic finding in both acute and chronic regurgitation. However, it does not occur when the mitral valve is rigid. This sign occurs even in mitral regurgitation resulting from movement imparted to the anterior leaflet of mitral valve by the jet of blood regurgitating from the aorta.

CHAPTER 15 | Valvular Heart Disease and Prosthetic Heart Valves

9. Ans. b. Echocardiogram

Braunwald 5th Ed; Page 1050

Refer to the answer of Q. No 8.

10. Ans. a. India

Braunwald 5th Ed; Page 1054

Tricuspid stenosis is almost always rheumatic in origin. Other causes of obstruction to right atrial emptying are unusual and includes congenital tricuspid stenosis, right atrial tumor and carcinoid syndrome (which more frequently produces tricuspid regurgitation). Rarely obstruction to right ventricular inflow can be due to endomyocardial fibrosis, tricuspid valve vegetation and extracardiac tumor. The majority of cases of rheumatic tricuspid valve disease present with tricuspid regurgitation or a combination of stenosis and regurgitation. Rheumatic tricuspid stenosis is uncommon and almost never occurs as an isolated lesion but generally accompanies mitral valve disease. In many patients with tricuspid stenosis the aortic valve is also involved. Tricuspid stenosis is found at autopsy in about 15% of patients with rheumatic heart disease but is of clinical significant in only about 5% of cases. Organic tricuspid valve disease is more common in India than in North American or Western Europe. It has been reported to occur in the heart of more than 1/3rd of patient with rheumatic heart disease studied at autopsy in the subcontinent.

11. Ans. b. Thyrotoxicosis

Braunwald 5th Ed; Page 1056

The most common cause of tricuspid regurgitation is the dilatation of the right ventricle and of the tricuspid annulus due to right ventricular failure of any cause which causes secondary functional tricuspid regurgitation. This is observed in patient with right ventricular hypertension secondary to any form of cardiac and pulmonary vascular diseases, most commonly mitral valve disease, right ventricular infarction, congenital heart disease which pulmonary stenosis and pulmonary hypertension, primary pulmonary hypertension and rarely cor pulmonale. Severe TR has been reported to be the presenting manifestation of thyrotoxicosis. In infants, tricuspid regurgitation may complicate right ventricular failure secondary to neonatal pulmonary disease and pulmonary hypertension with persistence of the fetal pulmonary circulation. Functional regurgitation may diminish or disappear as right ventricle decrease in size with the treatment of heart failure. Tricuspid regurgitation can also occur as a consequence of dilatation of the annulus in Marfans syndrome in which it is associated with right ventricular dilatation secondary to pulmonary hypertension.

12. Ans. d. All of the above

Braunwald 5th Ed; Page 1057

On physical examination in patient with tricuspid regurgitation there is evidence of jugular venous distention, the normal X and X disappear and prominence systolic (S) wave, i.e., C-V wave is apparent. The S wave and Y descent become more prominent during inspiration. A venous systolic thrill and murmur in neck may be present in patient with severe TR. The right ventricular impulse is hyperdynamic and thrusting in quality. Rarely a right atrial systolic impulse may be observed or palpated along the right lower sternal edge.

13. Ans. c. Prominent CV wave

Braunwald 5th Ed; Page 1057

Refer to the answer of Q. No 12.

14. Ans. b. Contrast echo with saline and demonstration of microbubble traversing to and fro across the tricuspid valve

Braunwald 5th Ed; Page 1058

Contrast echocardiography involves rapid injection of saline or indocyanine green dye into an antecubital vein made while a two dimensional echocrdiography is being recorded. It is both sensitive and specific for tricuspid regurgitation. The injection produces micro cavities that are usually readily visible on echocardiography and normally travels as a bolus through the circulation. In tricuspid regurgitation, these microcavities can be seen to travel back and fourth across the tricuspid orifice and to pass into the inferior vena cava and hepatic veins during systole.

15. Ans. d. Ab + resection of valve with valve replacement few weeks to months letter

Braunwald 5th Ed; Page 1058

In treatment of patient with tricuspid endocarditis in heroine addicts, it has been noted that total excision of the tricuspid valve without immediate replacement can be tolerated by those patients who usually do not have associated pulmonary hypertension. When antibiotic therapy is unsuccessful, valvular replacement frequently results in reinfection or continued infection. Therefore, diseased valvular tissue should be excised to eradicate the endocarditis and antibiotic treatment can be continued. Initially most patients tolerate loss of tricuspid valve without great difficulty although reduction in left ventricular ejection fraction may occur. Later-right ventricular dysfunction usually occurs. Therefore, a bioprosthetic valve may be inserted six to nine months after valve excision and control of the infection.

16. Ans. d. Secondary to pulmonary hypertension

Braunwald 5th Ed; Page 1059

By far the most common cause of pulmonary regurgitation is the dilatation of the valve ring secondary to pulmonary hypertension (of any etiology) or to dilatation of the pulmonary artery, either idiopathic or consequent to a connective tissue disorder such as Marfan's syndrome. The second most common cause of pulmonary regurgitation is infective endocarditis. Less frequently, it is iatrogenic and is induced at the time of surgical treatment of congenital pulmonary stenosis or tetralogy of Fallots. Pulmonary regurgitation may also result from the variety of lesions directly affecting the pulmonary valve including congenital malformation such as absent, malformed, fenestrated or supernumerary leaflets, less common causes includes trauma, carcinoid syndrome, rheumatic involvement, injury produced by pulmonary artery flow directed catheter, syphilis and chest trauma.

17. Ans. a. Angina

Braunwald 5th Ed; Page 1039

The cardinal manifestations of aortic stenosis, which commences most commonly in the 6th decade of life are angina pectoris, syncope and heart failure. The interval from the onset of symptoms to the time of death is approximately 2 years in patient with heart failure, 3 years in those with syncope and 5 years in those with angina. Angina occurs in approximately 2/3rd of patients with critical aortic stenosis and usually resembles that observed in patient with CAD in that it is commonly precipitated by exertion and relieved by rest. In patients without CAD, it results from combination of increased oxygen needs by the hypertrophied myocardium and reduction of oxygen delivery secondary to excessive compression of coronary vessels. Syncope is most commonly due to the reduction of cerebral perfusion that occurs during exertion when arterial pressure declines consequent to the systemic vasodilatation in presence of fixed cardiac output. Syncope has also been attributed to the malfunction of baroreceptor mechanism and to vasodepressor response to a greatly elevated left ventricular systolic pressure during exercise.

Exertional dyspnea with orthopnea, paroxysmal nocturnal dyspnea and pulmonary edema reflects varying degree of pulmonary venous hypertension. These are relatively late symptoms in aortic stenosis and their presence for more than 5 years suggest the possibility of associated mitral valvular disease.

18. Ans. a. Bicuspid valve

Braunwald 5th Ed; Page 1039

Obstruction to left ventricular outflow tract is localized most commonly at aortic valve. However, obstruction may also occur above the valve (supravalvular aortic stenosis) or below the valve (discrete subvalvular aortic stenosis) and may be caused by hypertrophic obstructive cardiomyopathy. Valvular aortic stenosis without accompanying mitral valve disease is more common in men and very rarely occur on a rheumatic basis but instead is usually either a congenital bicuspid valve or is degenerative in origin.

19. Ans. c. Both a and b

Braunwald 5th Ed; Page 1040

The arterial pulse characteristically rises slowly and is small and sustained (pulsus parvus et tardus). In the advanced stage, systolic and pulse pressure are both reduced however in patients with mild AS with associated AR and older patient with an inelastic arterial bed both systolic and pulse pressure may be normal or even increased. A systolic pressure exceeding 200 mm Hg is rare in patient with critical aortic stenosis.

20. Ans. b. Valvular aortic stenosis

Braunwald 5th Ed; Page 1040

On physical examination, the jugular venous pulse in patient with aortic stenosis usually shows prominent A wave reflecting reduce right ventricular compliance consequent to hypertrophy of the ventricular septum. With pulmonary hypertension and secondary right ventricular failure and tricuspid regurgitation, V or CV waves may be prominent. Prominent A wave is more commonly seen with valvular aortic stenosis.

21. Ans. b. Presence of aortic systolic murmur

Braunwald 5th Ed; Page 1041

In patient with valvular aortic stenosis auscultatory features are very specific. S1 is normal or soft and S4 is prominent, presumably because atrial contraction is vigorous and mitral valve is partially closed during presystole. Second heart sound may be single because calcification and immobility of aortic valve making A2 inaudible or because P2 is buried in the prolonged aortic ejection murmur or may be due to prolongation of left ventricular systole which makes A2 coincide with P2. Paradoxical splitting of S2 which suggest associated left ventricular dysfunction may also occur. With left ventricular failure and secondary pulmonary hypertension P2 may become accentuated. When the valve is rigid A2 may be inaudible. An aortic ejection sound occurs simultaneously with the halting of upward movement of aortic valve. It is depended on mobility of the valve cusp and disappear when they becomes severely calcified. Thus, it is common in children with congenital aortic stenosis but is rare in elderly adults with acquired calcific aortic stenosis and rigid valves. This sound occurs approximately 0.06 second after the onset of S1 and has a frequency similar to that of S1. The ejection sound is heard most readily with the diaphragm of stethoscope along the left sternal border. In contrast to pulmonary ejection sound aortic ejection sound usually do not vary with respiration. The systolic murmur of aortic stenosis is usually late peaking and best heard at the base of the heart but is often well-transmitted along the carotid vessel and to the apex. Cessation of the murmur before A2 is helpful in differentiating it from the pan systolic mitral murmur. In patient with calcified aortic valve the murmur is harsh and rasping at the base but high frequency component selectively radiate to apex (Gallavardin phenomenon), where it may actually be more prominent and where it may be mistaken for murmur of mitral regurgitation. In general, the more severe the stenosis the longer the duration of the murmur and more likely that it peaks in mid systole. High pitch decrescendo diastolic murmur secondary to aortic regurgitation are common in many patients with dominant aortic stenosis, though it is not found in supravalvular and subvalvular aortic stenosis. There is no accompanying peripheral sign of aortic regurgitation and pulse pressure is normal.

22. Ans. d. All are true

Braunwald 5th Ed; Page 1041

Refer to the answer of Q. No 21.

23. Ans. b. Duration of murmur

Braunwald 5th Ed; Page 1041

Refer to the answer of Q. No 21.

24. Ans. a. Delay in aortic closure, leading to single second sound without inspiratory splitting

Braunwald 5th Ed; Page 1041

Refer to the answer of Q. No 21.

25. Ans. d. All are true

Braunwald 5th Ed; Page 1041

Refer to the answer of Q. No 21.

26. Ans. a. 3-5%

Hurst's 8th Ed; Page 1700

Most patients with valvular aortic stenosis including some with severe aortic stenosis are often asymptomatic. The symptoms of aortic stenosis are angina pectoris, syncope, exertional presyncope, dyspnea and the symptom of heart failure. Once symptom occurs in patient with severe aortic stenosis, the life span of the patient is very short without surgical treatment. Sudden cardiac death is stated to occur in 5% of patients with aortic stenosis. It occurs only in those with severe valvular aortic stenosis, most of whom have had some cardiac symptom before the fatal episode. Typical angina pectoris occurs with or without associated with CAD in patient with aortic stenosis.

27. Ans. a. Rheumatic fever

Braunwald 5th Ed; Page 1045

Aortic regurgitation may be caused by primary disease of either the aortic valve leaflets or the wall of the aortic root or both. Among patients with pure aortic regurgitation coming to valve replacement, the percentage with aortic root disease has been increasing. Rheumatic fever is a common cause of primary disease of the valve leading to the aortic regurgitation. Other primary valvular causes of aortic regurgitation include infective endocarditis, trauma, congenital bicuspid aortic valve with aortic regurgitation. Less common causes of aortic regurgitation include a variety of forms of congenital aortic regurgitation, rupture of congenitally fenestrated valve, aortic regurgitation in association with systemic lupus erythematosus, rheumatoid arthritis, ankylosing spondylitis, Takayasu's disease, Whipple's disease and Crohn's disease.

28. Ans. a. Ankylosing spondylitis

Braunwald 5th Ed; Page 1703

The aorta in ankylosing spondylitis is histologically similar to that in syphilitic aortitis. There is adventitial scarring, intimal proliferation with the scarring of the media, and the vasa vasorum are narrowed and surrounded by lymphocytes and plasma cells. The adventitial scarring extends below the base of aortic valve. This thickening is particularly prominent behind the commissures of aortic valve cusp and form a bump. Aortic regurgitation therefore result from shortening and thickening of the aortic valve cusp, displacement of the cusp by the fibrous tissue bump and dilatation of the aortic root. Similarly, one can rarely observe mitral valve regurgitation secondary to the dilatation of left ventricle from aortic regurgitation and from thickening of the basal portion of anterior mitral leaflet. Aortic valvular disease has been reported in up to 10% patient with ankylosing spondylitis. Rarely aortic insufficiency may be the presenting manifestation. Aortic regurgitation may be progressive and require aortic valve replacement. Mitral regurgitation is relatively uncommon in ankylosing spondylitis.

29. Ans. a. Mitral

Braunwald 5th Ed; Page 1074

In autopsies studies, the prevalence of rheumatoid granuloma involving the heart valves ranges from 3 to 5% in patients with rheumatoid arthritis. Heart valve lesion in rheumatoid arthritis involves the valve leaflet and valve ring and may be pathologically identical to rheumatoid nodules. There may also be nongranulomatous valve inflammation with subsequent fibrosis and thickening of valve leaflets. The order of frequency of valvular involvement is similar to rheumatic fever, i.e., mitral, aortic, tricuspid and pulmonary. The process appears to begin within the core of the valve leaflets preserving the peripheral portions. This defer from rheumatic valvular disease in which the entire leaflet is involved. In an echocardiographic study, it was found that 13% of patients with rheumatoid arthritis had abnormality of mitral valve including mitral valve prolapse and mitral annular calcification. Despite the relative rarity of hemodynamic valve incompetence numerous cases of progressive aortic insufficiency has been reported and rarely patient may require mitral and/or aortic valve replacement.

30. Ans. d. All of the above

Braunwald 5th Ed; Page 1049

In patient with aortic regurgitation, it is the volume of regurgitant blood flow, areas of regurgitant orifice and the diastolic pressure gradient between aorta and left ventricle are the determinants of the volume overload. However, the determinant of severity of reflux in patient with aortic regurgitation, it is the diastolic pressure gradient between the aorta and left ventricle which is more important than the size the orifice, duration of diastole and volume of regurgitation.

31. Ans. c. Diastolic pressure gradient between aorta and LV

Braunwald 5th Ed; Page 1049

Refer to the answer of Q. No 30.

32. Ans. c. Dyspnea

Braunwald 5th Ed; Page 1035-36/1037

Patient with aortic regurgitation are asymptomatic for decade. Symptoms in patient with aortic regurgitation usually consists of angina pectoris or heart failure or both, angina pectoris may be the result of associated coronary atherosclerosis or it may occur with a widely patent coronary arteries. In the later situation, angina pectoris is the result of low aortic diastolic pressure that leads to decrease myocardial perfusion in the phase of increased oxygen demands, secondary to increase left ventricular volume and systolic pressure. Angina is not common in patient with aortic regurgitation. An unusual form of angina pectoris in patient with aortic insufficiency and normal coronary arteries occurs paroxysmally usually at night. These attacks are severe, frequently associated with nightmares, dyspnea, forceful and rapid heart action, skin flushing profuse sweating and a wide pulse pressure. Diffuse abdominal or epigastric pain has also been noted during such paroxysm. Sometime there is bilateral neck pain associated with tenderness over carotid seen in patient with aortic incompetence. Ostial coronary atherosclerosis narrowing may develop in patient with luetic aortic regurgitation. Such patients are prone to particularly, severe attacks of angina pectoris that are often associated with marked dyspnea. Congestive heart failure is the most common symptoms that develop in the patient with aortic regurgitation. It usually appears after decade during which the patient reported no symptoms whatsoever. Symptoms of heart failure may be of insidious onset with patient initially noting only slight decrease in exercise tolerance. Stable dyspnea on exertion may occur for a short period of time or it may be present for a number of years before more severe symptom of left ventricular failure (othopnea, paroxysmal nocturnal dyspnea) develops. Paroxysmal dyspnea may be severe and is more common in patient with luetic aortic regurgitation possibly because of the presence of ostial coronary arterial obstruction in later group of patients.

33. Ans. c. It more often occurs in night and accompanied by vasomotor phenomenon such as flushing, perspiration and dyspnea

Braunwald 5th Ed; Page 1035-36/1037

Refer to the answer of Q. No 32.

34. Ans. b. Aortic incompetence

Braunwald 5th Ed; Page 1035-36/1037

Refer to the answer of Q. No 32.

35. Ans. b. Duroziez's murmur

Braunwald 5th Ed; Page 22

Signs characteristic of severe aortic regurgitation includes: (a) the Corrigan or Water Hammer pulse; (b) Pistol-shot sound heard over the femoral artery when the stethoscope is placed on it (Traube's sign); (c) Duroziez's sign, i.e., a systolic murmur heard over the femoral artery when the arteries gradually compress proximally, a diastolic murmur when the artery is compressed distally; (d) Quincke's sign, i.e., phasic flushing of the nail bed. Of these Duroziez sign is the most predictive of severe aortic regurgitation. In Hill's sign of severe aortic regurgitation the indirectly recorded systolic pressure in the lower extremity exceeds that in arm by >20 mm. Other signs are of increased pulse pressure include Becker's sign (visible pulsation of the retinal arterioles) and Muller's sign (pulsatile uvula).

36. Ans. c. Duration of murmur

Braunwald 5th Ed; Page 1050

The diagnostic auscultatory feature of aortic regurgitation is the presence of aortic regurgitant murmur, i.e., one of the high frequency early diastolic murmur beginning soon after A2. It is heard best with the diaphragm of the stethoscope while the patient is sitting up and leaning forward with breath held in deep expiration. In severe aortic regurgitation, the murmur reaches an early peak and then has a dominant decrescendo pattern throughout diastole. The severity of regurgitations correlates better with the duration than with the intensity of murmur. In mild AR, murmur may be limited to the early diastole and is typically high pitch and blowing. In severe regurgitation, the murmur is holodiastolic and may have a rough quality. In severe aortic regurgitation and left ventricular decompensation, equilibration of aortic and left ventricular pressure in late diastole abolishes the late component of regurgitant murmur. When the regurgitation is due to primary valvular disease, the diastolic murmur is best heard along the left sternal border in 3rd and 4th intercostal spaces however when it

37. Ans. a. Premature closure of mitral valve

Braunwald 5th Ed; Page 1050

In patient with acute aortic regurgitation, the left ventricle has no opportunity to adopt to the increased load. In acute aortic regurgitation, the regurgitant volumes fills a ventricle of normal size that cannot accommodate the combined large regurgitant volume and inflow from the left atrium and because the ability of total stroke volume to rise acutely is limited, forward stroke volumes declines. The sudden increase in the left ventricular filling, causes the left ventricular diastolic pressure to rise rapidly to high level. As left ventricular pressure rises rapidly above left atrial pressure during early diastole, the mitral valve closes prematurely in diastole. Preclosure of mitral valve is accompanied by diastolic mitral regurgitation. This protect the pulmonary venous bed from backward transmission of the greatly elevated end diastolic pressure. Premature closure of the mitral valve together with the tachycardia that shorten diastole reduces the time interval during which the mitral valve is opened. Left ventricular and aortic systolic pressure exhibit little change. Because aortic diastolic pressure cannot decline below the elevated left ventricular end diastolic pressure the systemic arterial pulse pressure widens relatively little.

38. Ans. b. Increased QRS amplitude with depressed ST segment and T wave inversion

Braunwald 5th Ed; Page 1050

Chronic aortic regurgitation results in left axis deviation and a pattern of left ventricular diastolic volume overload characterized by an increase in initial forces (prominent Q wave in lead I, AVL and V3 to V6) and a relatively small R wave in lead V1. With the passage of time, this initial forces diminish but the total QRS amplitude increases. The T wave may be tall and upright in left precordial leads early in the course but more commonly they are inverted with ST segment depression. Left ventricular conduction defect occurs late in the course and are usually associated with left ventricular dysfunction.

39. Ans. c. Aortic dilatation

Braunwald 5th Ed; Page 1050

On X-ray examination in patient with aortic regurgitation, chronic aortic regurgitation cardiac size is a function of the duration and severity of regurgitation and the state of the left ventricular function. Marked enlargement of the cardiac shadow is a common finding in chronic aortic regurgitation. Typically, the left ventricle enlarges in an inferior and leftward direction causing a significant increase in the long axis. But sometimes, little or no increase in the transverse diameter of the heart.

Calcification of the aortic valve is uncommon in patient with pure aortic regurgitation but is often present in patient with combined aortic stenosis and regurgitation. Presence of distinct left atrial enlargement in the absence of heart failure suggests the possibility of associated mitral valve disease. Dilatation of ascending aorta is usually more marked than in patient with aortic stenosis and may involve the entire aortic arch including aortic knob. Severe aneurysmal dilatation of aorta should suggest the aortic root disease, i.e., Marfans syndrome or annuloaortic ectasia. Linear calcification in the wall of ascending aorta are seen in syphilitic aortitis but are nonspecific and are observed in degenerative disease as well.

40. Ans. a. Fast, fine vibration or fluttering during diastole of AML

Braunwald 5th Ed; Page 1050

Echocardiography is helpful in identifying the cause of aortic regurgitation. It may show the thickening of the valve cusp, prolapse of the valve, thickened leaflet, vegetation or dilatation of the aortic root. In acute aortic regurgitation, the echocardiogram reveals a reduction in the amplitude of the opening movement of the mitral valve, premature closure and delayed opening of the mitral valve and on the M-mode study a reduction in the EF slope, indicating that left ventricle is operating on steep portion of its pressure volume curve. Left ventricular end diastolic dimensions are not markedly increased and fractional shortening is normal. This contrast with the findings in chronic aortic regurgitation in which end diastolic dimension and wall motion are increased. Occasionally with equilibration of the aortic and left ventricular pressure diastolic premature opening of the aortic valve may be detected.

High frequency diastolic fluttering anterior leaflet of the mitral valve during diastole is an important echocardiographic findings in both acute and chronic aortic regurgitation. However, it does not occur when the mitral valve is rigid. This sign which unlike the Austin Flint murmur occurs even in mild aortic regurgitation, results from the movement imparted to the anterior leaflet of mitral valve by the jet of blood regurgitating from the aorta.

41. Ans. a. Isolated aortic stenosis

Braunwald 5th Ed; Page 1046-1053

In general, the result of aortic valve replacement in patient with aortic regurgitation are similar to those in patient with aortic stenosis, with a large percentage of exhibiting striking improvement in symptoms. Reduction in heart size and in left ventricular diastolic volume and mass occurs in majority of patients. However, the extent of improvement in left ventricular function may not be salutary in the patient with AR as it is in patient with aortic stenosis. Perhaps the ventricular dysfunction is more advanced and less reversible in patient with volume overload by the time they become symptomatic and are referred for surgical treatment than it is in patient with pressure overload. As in case of aortic stenosis, the operative risk of aortic valve replacement in patient with aortic regurgitation depends on the general condition of patients, the state of left ventricular function and skill and experience of surgical team. The mortality rate ranges from 3 to 8% in the most medical center. A late mortality of approximately 5 to 10% per year is observed in survivor in whom the cardiac enlargement was marked and impaired LV function was present preoperatively.

42. Ans. c. Tricuspid valve

Braunwald 5th Ed; Page 1054-1057

Tricuspid valve disease may be an incidental findings or its presence may provide a clue to otherwise unexplain cardiovascular signs or symptoms. Tricuspid regurgitation is the most commonly seen lesion and when present is most often functional. However, acquired and congenital defect must be excluded. Tricuspid stenosis is seen much less frequent but must be considered in patient with rheumatic heart disease who have involvement of both mitral and aortic valve especially if there is a failure to improve after corrective surgery. The clinical diagnosis of severe tricuspid valve disease particularly tricuspid regurgitation is usually not difficult. However, clinical signs of mild to moderate disease may be quite subtle and noninvasive techniques such as echo Doppler are often require to establish the diagnosis. Often the right upper quadrant abdominal pain which is often worst in the morning and improves as the day goes on is seen with patient with tricuspid valve disease. Similarly the intestinal lymphangiectasia leading to malabsorption is a feature of severe tricuspid regurgitation. In patient with tricuspid insufficiency, if there is associated tricuspid stenosis along with absence of pulmonary hypertension and involvement of other cardiac valves with rheumatic fever suggest that the tricuspid insufficiency is of organic in origin. In patient with tricuspid stenosis usual clinical feature is edema, ascites, hepatomegaly and feature suggestive of right heart failure. However, orthopnea is uncommon in patient with isolated tricuspid stenosis.

Tricuspid regurgitation in absence of pulmonary hypertension usually does not require surgical treatment. Indeed in both patients and experimental animals, normal pulmonary artery pressure may tolerate total excision of the tricuspid valve as long as right ventricular systolic pressure is normal for a period of time. Dilatation of right side of the heart usually occurs months or years after tricuspid valvotomy, and annuloplasty with insertion of prosthetic valve than can be carried out after adequate sterilization of the valve ring.

Tricuspid regurgitation resulting from infective endocarditis especially in narcotic addicts are particularly due to staphylococcal endocarditis and it is characterized by repeated episode of septic pulmonary embolism with multiple infiltrate on X-ray chest.

43. Ans. d. Tricuspid valve

Braunwald 5th Ed; Page 1054-1057

Refer to the answer of Q. No 42.

44. Ans. b. 10-15%

Braunwald 5th Ed; Page 1054-1057

Refer to the answer of Q. No 42.

45. Ans. b. Tricuspid valve disease

Braunwald 5th Ed; Page 1054-1057

Refer to the answer of Q. No 42.

46. Ans. d. All of the above

Braunwald 5th Ed; Page 1054-1057

Refer to the answer of Q. No 42.

47. Ans. b. Severe tricuspid regurgitation

Braunwald 5th Ed; Page 1054-1057

Refer to the answer of Q. No 42.

48. Ans. d. Both a and b

Braunwald 5th Ed; Page 1054-1057

Refer to the answer of Q. No 42.

49. Ans. b. Streptococcus viridans is most common organism

Braunwald 5th Ed; Page 1054-1057

Refer to the answer of Q. No 42.

50. Ans. a. 3-5%

Braunwald 5th Ed; Page 1054-1057

Refer to the answer of Q. No 42.

51. Ans. a. Orthopnea

Braunwald 5th Ed; Page 1054-1057

Refer to the answer of Q. No 42.

VALVULAR HEART DISEASE

1. Which of the following is *not* correct regarding opening snap?
   a. It is accompanied by an attenuated S1
   b. It can be heard even if there is calcification confined to the tip of mitral leaflets
   c. A2 OS interval varies inversely with LA pressure
   d. A2 OS is indicator of liability of valve

2. What would be an approximate trans mitral diastolic gradient in a patient with severe MS (mitral valve area 1.0 cm^2)?
   a. 10 mm
   b. 15 mm
   c. 20 mm
   d. >20 mm

3. Kerley B lines are seen in X-ray chest of patients with mitral stenosis, when resting pulmonary capillary wedge pressure is:
   a. >10 mm Hg
   b. >20 mm Hg
   c. >25 mm Hg
   d. >40 mm Hg

4. What is approximate rate of progression of untreated mitral stenosis (reduction in valve area)?
   a. 0.05 cm^2/year
   b. 0.09 cm^2/year
   c. 0.1 cm^2/year
   d. 1.2 cm^2/year

5. The prevalence of atrial fibrillation in patients with mitral stenosis is related to:
   a. Severity of valve obstruction
   b. Patient age
   c. Even when MS is severe, prevalence of AF is related to age
   d. None of the above

6. Medical management of patients with mitral stenosis and atrial fibrillation includes all the following, *except*:
   a. Penicillin prophylaxis for beta hemolytic streptococcal infection
   b. Prophylaxis for infective endocarditis
   c. Correction of anemia and infection
   d. Anticoagulation with vitamin K antagonist

7. Anticoagulation is indicated for patients with severe mitral stenosis and sinus rhythm when?
   a. LA enlargement (diameter >55 mm)
   b. Spontaneous contrast on echocardiogram
   c. History of prior embolization
   d. All of the above

8. A high likelihood of impaired LV systolic function is seen after mitral valve surgery, if the preoperative LV end systolic diameter is more than:
   a. 20 mm
   b. 30 mm
   c. 40 mm
   d. 50 mm

9. Which component of mitral annulus is prone to dilatation leading to mitral regurgitation?
   a. Anterior component
   b. Posterior component
   c. Septal component
   d. Lateral component

10. Primary atrial fibrillation leading to significant mitral regurgitation is classified as Carpentier dysfunction.
    a. Type I
    b. Type II
    c. Type IIIA
    d. Type IIIB

11. Pregnant patient with severe MS who are symptomatic the ideal time of performing BMV is:
    a. After 16th week
    b. After 20th week
    c. After 24th week
    d. After 28th week

12. The term juvenile mitral stenosis is used when the mitral stenosis develops before age of:
    a. 6 years
    b. 10 years
    c. 14 years
    d. 20 years

13. Which of the following is *not* a cause of primary tricuspid disease?
    a. Endocarditis
    b. Carcinoid heart disease
    c. Rheumatic heart disease
    d. Ischemic heart disease

14. Which is the most apically placed and largest orifice cardiac valve?
    a. Mitral
    b. Aortic
    c. Pulmonary
    d. Tricuspid

15. Which of the following is the commonest cause of tricuspid stenosis?
    a. Rheumatic heart disease
    b. Device leads
    c. Carcinoid syndrome
    d. Endomyocardial fibrosis

16. Clinically significant tricuspid stenosis is found in what percentage of patients with rheumatic heart disease?
    a. <2%
    b. <3%
    c. <5%
    d. <10%

17. The absence of symptoms of pulmonary congestion in a patient with obvious mitral stenosis suggest the coexistence of:
    a. Aortic stenosis
    b. Pulmonary stenosis
    c. Tricuspid stenosis
    d. Mitral regurgitation

18. What is approximate systolic pulmonary artery pressure to produce Graham steel murmur?
  a. Approximately >35 mm Hg
  b. Approximately >45 mm Hg
  c. Approximately >55 mm Hg
  d. Approximately >100 mm Hg

19. In combined valvular disease, hemodynamically poorly tolerated combination is:
  a. Mitral stenosis with aortic regurgitation
  b. Aortic stenosis with mitral regurgitation
  c. Aortic stenosis with aortic regurgitation
  d. Severe aortic and mitral regurgitation

20. Which of the following statement is *not* correct regarding severe aortic regurgitation?
  a. It is the intensity of murmur than the duration which correlates better with severity
  b. AR due to primary valvular disease has diastolic murmur heard best along left sternal border
  c. AR due to dilatation of ascending aorta murmur is heard readily along right sternal border
  d. When the diastolic murmur is musical, its' signifies perforation of aortic cusp

21. Which of the following patient with severe AR has best long-term outcome without surgery?
  a. Severe AR with end systolic diameter <40 mm
  b. Severe AR with end systolic volume <45 mm
  c. Severe AR with end systolic diameter >50 mm
  d. Severe AR with end systolic diameter >55 mm

22. Approximately what percentage of patients with rheumatic heart disease have isolated mitral stenosis?
  a. 10%
  b. 25%
  c. 30%
  d. 50%

23. The pathologic hallmark of rheumatic disease "Aschoff Bodies" are seen most frequently in:
  a. Pericardium
  b. Valve tissue
  c. Myocardium
  d. Conduction tissue

24. Which of the following can cause mitral stenosis?
  a. Carcinoid disease
  b. Methysergide therapy
  c. Radiotherapy for chest or breast cancer
  d. All of the above

25. Single aortic sound in aortic stenosis is because of:
  a. Calcification and immobility of aortic valve
  b. Closure of pulmonary valve being buried in prolonged aortic ejection murmur
  c. Prolongation of LV systole so A2 coincide with P2
  d. All of the above

26. Murmur of aortic stenosis is augmented by which of the following maneuver?
  a. Squatting
  b. Strain of Valsalva
  c. Standing
  d. All

27. What is the rate of progression from aortic sclerosis to stenosis?
  a. 0.81 to 0.9%/year
  b. 1.8 to 1.9%/year
  c. 2.8 to 3.9%/year
  d. 3.8 to 4.9%/year

28. Which of the following statement is *incorrect* regarding calcific aortic valve disease?
  a. There is epidemiological association between cardiovascular risk factor and calcific aortic valve disease
  b. Even in the absence of valve obstruction, known CV disease it is associated with increased risk of MI
  c. Statin is useful in preventing the progression of aortic valvular disease
  d. All of the above

29. Which of the following level is closely associated with occurrence of aortic stenosis?
  a. Serum HDL level
  b. Total cholesterol level
  c. Serum LDL level
  d. Lp(a)

30. Which of the following drug is known to reduce the progression of aortic stenosis without causing calcification?
  a. Statin
  b. Bempedoic acid
  c. PCSK9 inhibitors
  d. All

31. Which of the following is operating pathophysiological mechanism of severe low flow, low gradient aortic stenosis with preserved ejection fraction?
  a. Hypertrophic small LV
  b. Concurrent hypertension
  c. Atrial fibrillation
  d. All of the above

32. Dobutamine stress echocardiography is helpful in decision making in which of the following type of aortic valve disease?
  a. Aortic valve sclerosis
  b. Symptomatic severe high gradient aortic stenosis
  c. Low flow, low gradient AS with reduced LVEF
  d. Low flow, low gradient aortic stenosis with preserved LVEF

CHAPTER 15 | Valvular Heart Disease and Prosthetic Heart Valves

33. Which class of drug should be chosen to treat hypertension in patients with aortic stenosis?
  a. Beta blocker
  b. Calcium channel blocker
  c. Diuretic
  d. ACE inhibitor/ARBs

34. If aortic valve replacement is needed for stenosis or regurgitation in bicuspid aortic valve, concurrent aortic root replacement is recommended if aortic dimension exceeds:
  a. 40 mm   b. 45 mm
  c. 50 mm   d. 55 mm

ANSWERS WITH EXPLANATIONS

1. Ans. a. It is accompanied by an attenuated S1

Braunwald 11th Ed; Page 1418

Mitral opening snap is caused by a sudden tensing of the valve leaflet after the valve cusps have completed their opening excursion. The opening snap occurs when the movement of the mitral dome into left ventricle suddenly stops. It is audible best at the apex. The mitral valve cannot be totally rigid if it produces an opening snap, so an opening snap usually is accompanied by an accentuated S1. Calcification confined to the tip of the mitral valve leaflets does not preclude an opening snap, although calcification of the body and tip does. The mitral OS follows A2 by 0.04 to 0.12 second and this interval varies inversely with the LA pressure.

2. Ans. c. 20 mm

Braunwald 11th Ed; Page 1415

The normal cross-sectional area of mitral valve orifice is 4 to 6 cm^2. When the orifice is reduced to approximately 2 cm^2, which is considered to represent mild MS, blood can flow from the left atrium to the left ventricle only propelled by a small pressure gradient. When the mitral valve opening is reduced to 1 cm^2, which represent severe MS, a left atrioventricular pressure gradient (transmitral diastolic gradient) of approximately 20 mm Hg in presence of normal LVEF is required to maintain normal cardiac output at rest.

3. Ans. b. >20 mm Hg

Braunwald 11th Ed; Page 1419

Radiologic changes in the lung fields in patients with severity of mitral stenosis consists of Interstitial edema. It is manifested as Kerley B lines (dense, short, horizontal lines most frequently seen in costophrenic angles). This finding is present in 30% of patients with resting PCWP <20 mm Hg and in 70% with pressure >20 mm Hg. Severe longstanding mitral obstruction often results in Kerley A lines (straight, dense lines up to 4 cm in length, running toward the hilum), as well as the findings of pulmonary hemosiderosis and rarely, parenchymal ossification.

4. Ans. b. 0.09 cm^2/year

Braunwald 11th Ed; Page 1420

Serial echocardiographic data from the two largest series have shown that the approximate rate of progression of mitral stenosis is decreased in valve area by 0.09 cm^2/year. Approximately one third of patients showed rapid progression, which is defined as a decrease in MVA of >0.1 cm^2/year.

5. Ans. c. Even when MS is severe, prevalence of AF is related to age

Braunwald 11th Ed; Page 1420

The most common complication of mitral stenosis is atrial fibrillation. The prevalence of atrial fibrillation in patients with mitral stenosis is related to the severity of valve obstruction and patient age. In historical series, AF was present in 17% of patients age 21 to 30 years, 45% age 31 to 40 years, 60% age 41 to 50, and 80% older than 51. Even when mitral stenosis is severe, the prevalence of AF is related to age.

6. Ans. b. Prophylaxis for infective endocarditis

Braunwald 11th Ed; Page 1420

The medical management of mitral stenosis directed primarily towards (a) prevention of recurrent rheumatic fever, (b) prevention and treatment of complication of mitral stenosis (c) monitoring disease progression to allow intervention at the optimal time. Patients with MS caused by rheumatic heart disease should receive penicillin prophylaxis for beta-hemolytic streptococcal infections to prevent recurrent rheumatic fever, as per the guidelines. Prophylaxis for infective endocarditis is no longer recommended. Anemia and infections should be treated promptly and aggressively in patients with valvular heart disease. Anticoagulation with vitamin K antagonists (VKAs) for prevention of systemic embolism is warranted in any patient with mitral stenosis and AF, prior embolism, or known thrombus in the LA cavity or appendage.

7. Ans. d. All of the above

Braunwald 11th Ed; Page 1420

Anticoagulation with vitamin K antagonists (VKAs) for prevention of systemic embolism is warranted in any patient with mitral stenosis and atrial fibrillation, prior embolism, or known thrombus in the LA cavity or appendage. Anticoagulation also may be considered for patients with severe mitral stenosis and sinus rhythm when there is severe LA enlargement (diameter >55 mm) or spontaneous contrast on echocardiography. Treatment with warfarin is used to maintain with international normalized ratio (INR) between 2 and 3. Patients who have paroxysmal AF are repeated conversion, spontaneous or induced carry the risk of embolization and therefore they need to be on oral anticoagulants.

8. Ans. c. 40 mm

Braunwald 11th Ed; Page 1429

Preoperative myocardial contractility is an important determinant of the risk of operative death, cardiac failure perioperatively, and postoperative level of LV function. End systolic pressure-volume relationship is an important index for evaluating LV function in patients with mitral regurgitation. The simple measurement of end-systolic volume or diameter is found to be useful predictor of function and survival after mitral valve surgery. A preoperative LV end-systolic diameter that exceeds 40 mm identifies a patient with a high likelihood of impaired LV systolic function after surgery.

9. Ans. b. Posterior component

Hurst's 14th Ed; Page 1215

The mitral annulus is a fibromuscular ring located in the left atrioventricular groove. The mitral annulus is subjectively divided into anterior and posterior segments based on the attachments of the anterior and posterior mitral leaflets but can also be segmented by location into septal and lateral components. The anterior portion of the mitral annulus is in continuity with the fibrous skeleton of the heart, defined by the right and left fibrous trigones and the aortic mitral curtain. This portion of the mitral annulus is fibrous in nature, and much less prone to dilation in compared to the posterior portion of the annulus. Because the fibrous skeleton is discontinuous along the posterior portion of the mitral annulus, this portion dilates or increases its circumference in the setting of chronic mitral valve regurgitation with associated atrial and ventricular dilatation.

10. Ans. a. Type I

Pathophysiologic triad of mitral valve regurgitation composed of (top to bottom of each column): ventricular view, atrial view, leaflet dysfunction, valve lesions, and etiology—Carpentier classification

Hurst's 14th Ed; Page 1218

Type I	Type II	Type IIIA	Type IIIB
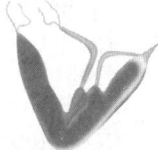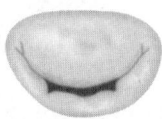	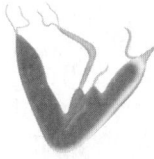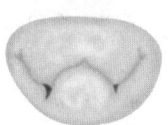	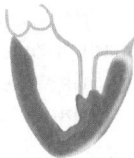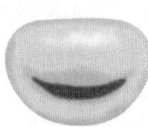	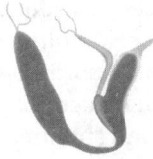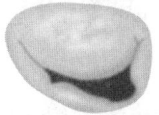
Normal leaflet motion (annular dilatation)	Increased leaflet motion (leaflet prolapse)	Restricted leaflet motion (restricted opening)	Restricted leaflet motion (restricted closure)
Annular dilatation Annular deformation Leaflet perforation Leaflet cleft	Myxomatous degeneration Chordal elongation Chordal rupture Papillary muscle elongation Papillary muscle rupture	Leaflet thickening, retraction Chordal thickening, retraction Chordal fusion Calcification Commissural fusion Ventricular fibrosis	Leaflet tethering Displacement of PM Ventricular dilatation Ventricular fibrosis
Ischemic cardiomyopathy Dilated cardiomyopathy Endocarditis Congenital	Degenerative disease Marfan's syndrome Endocarditis Rheumatic disease Trauma Ischemic cardiomyopathy Ehler–Danlos syndrome	Rheumatic disease Carcinoid disease Radiation Lupus erythematosus Ergotamine use Hypereosinophilic syndrome Mucopolysaccharidosis	Ischemic cardiomyopathy Dilated cardiomyopathy

Based on the combination of main dysfunction, lesion and etiology that can results in mitral regurgitation Carpentier classified it into four classes which helps in assessment of patient with mitral regurgitation. This dysfunction is classified on the basis of position of the leaflet margins in relationship to the plane of the mitral annulus. Type I dysfunction implies normal leaflet motion, is the most common cause of significant mitral valve regurgitation, and often results from isolated annular dilatation or leaflet perforation. The isolated annular dilatation is common in the setting of primary atrial fibrillation while leaflet perforation is common in setting of infective endocarditis leading to valve perforation and acute MI. Type II dysfunction implies excess leaflet motion and is most commonly associated with chordal elongation or rupture in the setting of degenerative mitral valve disease. Type IIIA dysfunction designates restricted opening and closing leaflet motion, and results typically from rheumatic valve disease or other inflammatory diseases that lead to chordal and leaflet scarring and calcification. Type IIIB dysfunction is associated with restricted leaflet motion in systole, and is most commonly associated with papillary muscle displacement and associated leaflet tethering in the setting of ischemic or nonischemic dilated cardiomyopathy.

11. Ans. b. After 20th week

Hurst's 14th Ed; Page 1256

Pregnant patients with severe MS (MVA < 1.5 cm^2) who continue to remain symptomatic (NYHA class III-IV) despite medical therapy should undergo BMV if the valve is suitable. The success rate of BMV reaches almost around 98–99% with maternal mortality rate was 1%. The procedure should be performed after 20 weeks in the second trimester if the patient's symptoms permit. Technical aspects include use of minimal fluoroscopy with avoidance of right heart study and LV angiogram, utilization of echo guidance and use of pelvic and abdominal shield.

12. Ans. d. 20 years

Hurst's 14th Ed; Page 1256

Rheumatic mitral stenosis presenting below 20 years is termed juvenile mitral stenosis. This is very common in developing countries. Heart failure/pulmonary edema is a frequent finding, while atrial fibrillation is uncommon. Severe PAH with gross pulmonary vascular obstruction is common.

13. Ans. d. Ischemic heart disease

Hurst's 14th Ed; Page 1260

Tricuspid regurgitation can be due to disease involving tricuspid valve or secondary to the left sided valvular lesion, ischemic heart disease and atrial fibrillation. Primary tricuspid disease is most commonly a result of endocarditis, carcinoid heart disease and rheumatic heart disease, with lead and catheter related pathology from cardiac devices as an increasingly recognized cause.

14. Ans. d. Tricuspid

Hurst's 14th Ed; Page 1260

The tricuspid valve is most epically placed valve with largest orifice among the four valves.

15. Ans. a. Rheumatic heart disease

Braunwald 11th Ed; Page 1445

Among the causes of tricuspid stenosis, rheumatic heart disease is the commonest reason although the rheumatic heart valve disease is more frequently affect left sided valve. Other causes are obstruction to the right atrial emptying due to tricuspid atresia, RA tumor, carcinoid syndrome or rarely endomyocardial fibrosis.

16. Ans. c. <5%

Braunwald 11th Ed; Page 1445

Tricuspid stenosis is found at autopsy in approximately 15% of patients with rheumatic heart disease but its clinical significance only approximately 5%.

17. Ans. c. Tricuspid stenosis

Braunwald 11th Ed; Page 1445

Tricuspid stenosis produces symptoms suggestive of low cardiac output in form of fatigue or discomfort caused by hepatomegaly ascites and anasarca. Some patient complaint of flattering discomfort in the neck caused by joint 'a' wave in jugular venous pulse. Occasionally, this symptom of mitral stenosis likely dyspnea, orthopnea and paroxysmal nocturnal dyspnea may be masked in the presence of severe TS because existence of TS prevents surges of blood into the pulmonary circulation behind the stenotic mitral valve. The absence of symptoms of pulmonary congestion in a patient with obvious mitral stenosis should suggest the possibility of tricuspid stenosis.

18. Ans. c. Approximately >55 mm Hg

Braunwald 11th Ed; Page 1451

When systolic pulmonary artery pressure exceeds approximately 55 mm Hg, dilation of the pulmonic annulus results in a high-velocity regurgitant jet, causing the audible murmur of pulmonary regurgitation, or Graham Steell murmur. This murmur is high-pitched, blowing, and decrescendo, beginning immediately after loud P2, and is most prominent in the left parasternal region in the second to fourth intercostal spaces.

19. Ans. d. Severe aortic and mitral regurgitation

Braunwald 11th Ed; Page 1453

The combination of severe aortic regurgitation with mitral regurgitation is a hemodynamically poorly tolerated lesion. The normal mitral valve ordinarily serves as a backup to the aortic valve, and premature (diastolic) closure of the mitral valve limits the volume of reflux that occurs in patients with acute AR. With severe combined regurgitant lesions, regardless of the cause of the mitral lesion, blood may reflux from aorta through both chambers of the left side of the heart into the pulmonary veins. Patients who operated on combined AR and MR have also poor outcomes than patients undergoing double-valve replacement for any other combinations of lesions, presumably because both AR and MR may produce irreversible LV damage.

20. Ans. a. It is the intensity of murmur than the duration which correlates better with severity

Braunwald 11th Ed; Page 1403

The diastolic murmur, main finding in AR, is of high frequency and begins immediately after A2. The severity of AR correlates better with the duration than with the intensity of the murmur. In mild AR, the murmur may be limited to early diastole and typically is high-pitched and blowing. In severe AR the murmur is holodiastolic and may have a rough quality. When the murmur is musical, it usually signifies eversion or perforation of an aortic cusp. In patients with severe AR and LV decompensation, equilibration of aortic and LV pressures in late diastole abolishes the late diastolic component of the regurgitant murmur. When aortic regurgitation is caused by primary valvular disease, the diastolic murmur is heard best along the left sternal border in the third and fourth intercostal spaces. However, when it is caused by dilation of the ascending aorta, the murmur often is heard best along the right sternal border.

21. Ans. a. Severe AR with end systolic diameter <40 mm

Braunwald 11th Ed; Page 1408

Asymptomatic patients with severe AR but normal LV function have an excellent prognosis and do not require prophylactic operation. On average, <6% of patients each year require surgery because of the development of symptoms or of LV dysfunction. The LV end-systolic dimension determined by echocardiography is valuable in predicting outcome in asymptomatic patients. Patients with severe AR and an end-systolic diameter <40 mm almost invariably remain stable and can be followed without need for surgery in the near term. However, patients with an end-systolic diameter of >50 mm have a 19% likelihood per year of developing symptoms of LV dysfunction, and those with an end-systolic diameter >55 mm are at increased risk for development of irreversible LV dysfunction if they do not undergo aortic valve replacement.

22. Ans. b. 25%

Braunwald 11th Ed; Page 1415

The predominant cause of mitral stenosis is rheumatic fever. Approximately 25% of all patients with rheumatic heart disease have isolated mitral stenosis and approximately 40% have combined mitral stenosis and mitral regurgitation. Multivalve involvement is seen in 38% of patients with mitral stenosis, with aortic valve affected in approximately 35% and tricuspid valve in approximately 6%. The pulmonary valve is rarely affected.

23. Ans. b. Valve tissue

Braunwald 11th Ed; Page 1415

Aschoff bodies, the pathologic hallmark of rheumatic disease, are seen most frequently in the myocardium, not the valve tissue, with Aschoff bodies identified in only 2% of autopsied patients with chronic valve disease.

24. Ans. d. All of the above

Braunwald 11th Ed; Page 1415

Mitral stenosis is a rare complication of malignant carcinoid disease, generally seen only with the pulmonary metastases or right to left shunting. Methysergide therapy is also an unusual but documented cause of mitral stenosis, as was the association with the diet drug fenfluramine. A troublesome form of mitral stenosis is seen following radiotherapy for chest or breast cancer, characterized by heavy calcification and thickening of the aortomitral curtain. It often requires multimodality imaging for full characterization.

25. Ans. d. All of the above

Braunwald 11th Ed; Page 1395

Splitting of S2 is helpful in excluding the diagnosis of severe aortic stenosis, because normal splitting implies the aortic valve leaflets are flexible enough to create an audible closing sound (A2). With severe AS, S2 may be single because (1) calcification and immobility of the aortic valve make A2 inaudible, (2) closure of the pulmonic valve (P2) is buried in the prolonged aortic ejection murmur, or (3) prolongation of LV systole makes A2 coincide with P2.

26. Ans. a. Squatting

Braunwald 11th Ed; Page 1395

The intensity of the aortic systolic murmur varies from beat to beat when the duration of diastolic filling varies, as in atrial fibrillation or after a premature contraction. This characteristic is helpful in differentiating AS from MR, in which the murmur usually is unaffected. The murmur of valvular AS is augmented by squatting, which increases stroke volume. It is reduced in intensity during the strain of the Valsalva maneuver and on standing, both of which reduce transvalvular flow.

27. Ans. b. 1.8 to 1.9%/year

Braunwald 12th Ed; Page 1100

The aortic sclerosis without stenosis, which is defined as irregular thickening or calcification of the aortic valve leaflets, increases with age and ranges from 9% in populations with a mean age of 54 years to 42% in populations with a mean age of 81 years. The rate of progression from aortic sclerosis to stenosis is 1.8 to 1.9%/year.

28. Ans. c. Statin is useful in preventing the progression of aortic valvular disease

Braunwald 12th Ed; Page 1101

Calcific aortic valve disease is the most common cause of aortic stenosis in adults. Aortic sclerosis, identified by echocardiography or computed tomography (CT), is the initial stage of calcific aortic valve disease and, even in the absence of valve obstruction or known cardiovascular disease, is associated with an increased risk of myocardial infarction (MI) and cardiovascular and all-cause mortality. Epidemiologic associations have been documented between cardiovascular risk factors and calcific aortic valve disease, suggesting that treating or preventing these risk factors may lessen the risk may lessen the risk of aortic stenosis.

The pathogenesis of aortic stenosis is processed similar to atherosclerosis where the initial lesion is plaque like with a central core of lipid and macrophages. Over time the plaque becomes calcified and it also contains some lamellar bone. The process holds in common many of the risk factors for atherosclerotic coronary artery disease including hyperlipidemia, hypertension, and the metabolic syndrome. Because of the resemblance of the aortic stenosis lesion to that of coronary atherosclerosis, it was postulated that statins, so effective in treating coronary artery disease, might retard the progression of aortic stenosis. Three randomized trials failed to show any benefit of statin use in aortic stenosis when applied to patients with a range of disease severity. It was argued that even earlier application of statins would be required to show benefit, or statin failure could be because of the tendency for statins to promote plaque calcification. Statin helps stabilizing the coronary plaque, avoiding rupture and subsequent coronary events; conversely this tendency in the aortic plaque might cause decreased leaflet mobility, worsening rather than retarding the progression. Statins therefore have failed to alter the progression of aortic stenosis, though in aortic stenosis active inflammation is involved.

29. Ans. d. Lp(a)

Braunwald 12th Ed; Page 1103

Lipoprotein (a) is more tightly associated with aortic stenosis than LDL. PCSK9 inhibitor can reduce both lipid moieties and also, it's not procalcific. Therefore, it may be future therapeutic choice for preventing aortic stenosis in preventing degenerative aortic stenosis.

30. Ans. c. PCSK9 inhibitors

Braunwald 12th Ed; Page 1103

Refer to the answer of Q. No 29.

31. Ans. d. All of the above

Braunwald 12th Ed; Page 1104

Multiple explanations have been put forward for low forward flow in the setting of normal ejection fraction. This group of patients generally have small LV volumes (concentric remodeling), so that a normal EF of a small end-diastolic volume generates a small stroke volume and hence a low gradient. Other etiologies of low flow have also been identified in this patient population. Hypertension has been shown to reduce the transaortic gradients in experimental models and in patients, primarily because of changes in transvalvular flow rates and not directly as a result of to changes in arterial compliance. Right ventricular dysfunction, atrial fibrillation, and mitral regurgitation are independently associated with low-flow low-gradient aortic stenosis.

32. Ans. c. Low flow, low gradient AS with reduced LVEF

Staging of the Aortic Valve Disease

Braunwald 12th Ed; Page 1411

Stage	Definition	Valve anatomy	Valve hemodynamics	Hemodynamic consequences	Symptoms
A	At risk of AS	• Bicuspid aortic valve (or other congenital valve anomaly) • Aortic valve sclerosis	Aortic V_{max} <2 m/sec	None	None
B	Progressive AS	Mild-to-moderate leaflet calcification of a bicuspid or trileaflet valve with some reduction in systolic motion or rheumatic valve changes with commissural fusion	*Mild AS:* Aortic V_{max} 2.0–2.9 m/sec or mean ΔP <20 mm Hg *Moderate AS:* Aortic V_{max} 3.0–3.9 m/sec or mean ΔP 20–39 mm Hg	• Early LV diastolic dysfunction may be present • Normal LVEF	None

Continued

Continued

Stage	Definition	Valve anatomy	Valve hemodynamics	Hemodynamic consequences	Symptoms
C	Asymptomatic severe AS				
C1	Asymptomatic severe AS	Severe leaflet calcification or congenital stenosis with severely reduced leaflet opening	Severe AS: Aortic V_{max} ≥4 m/sec, or mean ΔP ≥40 mm Hg AVA typically is ≤1 cm² (or AVAi ≤0.6 cm²/m²) Very severe AS is an aortic V_{max} ≥5 m/sec, or mean ΔP ≥ 60 mm Hg	• LV diastolic dysfunction • Mild LV hypertrophy • Normal LVEF	None Exercise testing is reasonable to confirm symptom status
C2	Asymptomatic severe AS with LV dysfunction	Severe leaflet calcification or congenital stenosis with severely reduced leaflet opening	Aortic V_{max} ≥4 m/sec, or mean ΔP ≥40 mm Hg AVA typically is ≤1 cm² (or AVAi ≤0.6 cm²/m²)	LVEF <50%	None
D	Symptomatic severe AS				
D1	Symptomatic severe high-gradient AS	Severe leaflet calcification or congenital stenosis with severely reduced leaflet opening	Severe AS: Aortic V_{max} ≥4 m/sec, or mean ΔP ≥40 mm Hg AVA typically is ≤1 cm² (or AVAi ≤0.6 cm²/m²), but may be larger with mixed AS/AR	• None–exercise • LV diastolic dysfunction • LV hypertrophy • Pulmonary hypertension may be present	• Exertional dyspnea or decreased exercise tolerance • Exertional angina • Exertional syncope or presyncope
D2	Symptomatic severe low-flow/low-gradient AS with reduced LVEF	Severe leaflet calcification with severely reduced leaflet motion	AVA ≤1 cm² with resting aortic V_{max} <4 m/sec, or mean ΔP <40 mm Hg Dobutamine stress echo shows AVA ≤1 cm² with V_{max} ≥4 m/sec at any flow rate	• LV diastolic dysfunction • LV hypertrophy • LVEF <50%	HF, angina, syncope or presyncope
D3	Symptomatic severe low-gradient AS with normal LVEF or paradoxical low-flow severe AS	Severe leaflet calcification with severely reduced leaflet motion	AVA ≤1 cm² with aortic V_{max} ≤4 m/sec, or mean ΔP <40 mm Hg AVAi ≤0.6 cm²/m² Stroke volume index <35 mL/m² Measured when patient is normotensive (systolic BP <140 mm Hg)	• Increased LV relative wall thickness • Small LV chamber with low-stroke volume • Restrictive diastolic filling • LVEF ≥50%	HF, angina, syncope or presyncope

33. Ans. d. ACE inhibitor/ARBs

Braunwald 11th Ed; Page 1397

Hypertension accompanies aortic stenosis in a majority of patients. Hypertension imposes an additional load on the left ventricle and is associated with more adverse hypertrophic LV remodeling. Therefore, hypertension should be treated according to established guidelines. There is no one class of medicines established as the preferred treatment of hypertension in patients with aortic stenosis, but because the renin-angiotensin system is upregulated in the valve and ventricle of patients with aortic stenosis, angiotensin-converting-enzyme (ACE) inhibitors or angiotensin receptor blockers (ARBs) are preferentially considered. Small studies have demonstrated their safety, and some suggest a clinical benefit, but larger-scale randomized studies are lacking.

34. Ans. b. 45 mm

Braunwald 11th Ed; Page 1397

Bicuspid aortic valve disease is associated with an aortopathy with the dilatation of ascending aorta related to accelerated degeneration of aortic media. The present location and severity of aortic dilatation are related to valve morphology but do not appear to be related to the severity of valve dysfunction. If AVR is needed for stenosis or regurgitation, concurrent aortic root replacement is recommended if the maximum aortic dimension (measured at end-diastole) exceeds 45 mm. Even in the absence of aortic valve disease, aortic root replacement is recommended when the aortic dimension is 55 mm or greater in adults with BAV and may be considered with an aortic diameter of 50 mm if there is a family history of dissection or evidence of rapid progression.

PROSTHETIC VALVE

1. Which of the following do *not* require lifelong anticoagulation?
   a. Mechanical valve prostheses
   b. Mechanical valve prosthesis with atrial fibrillation
   c. Bioprotheses with atrial fibrillation
   d. Transcatheter aortic valve implantation

2. Which of the following is most commonly implanted mechanical valve now a days?
   a. Ball and cage valve
   b. Monoleaflet valve
   c. Bileaflet valve
   d. All are equally used

3. Which of the following mechanical valve has low risk of pannus formation?
   a. Ball and Cage valve
   b. Monoleaflet valve
   c. Bileaflet valve
   d. Tissue valve

4. Use of which of the following has resulted into production of a durable bioprosthesis:
   a. Fascia lata
   b. Dura mater
   c. Pericardium
   d. Glutaraldehyde fixation

5. Which of the following tissue used in constructing bioprosthetic valve has greater durability?
   a. Fascia lata
   b. Dura mater
   c. Bovine pericardium
   d. Porcine aortic valves

6. Teratogenicity of Warfarin is a highest during:
   a. First trimester
   b. Second trimester
   c. Third trimester
   d. Uniform throughout pregnancy

7. Which of the statement regarding Warfarin is *not* correct?
   a. Teratogenicity of warfarin is the highest in first trimester
   b. Use of warfarin throughout pregnancy is less risky to mother and fetus than use of unfractionated heparin
   c. Risk of warfarin induced embryopathy is not dose related
   d. All are incorrect

8. In a patient with prosthetic heart valve on anticoagulation which level of INR increases risk of major bleed exponentially and requires rapid reversal?
   a. INR > 2.5
   b. INR > 3.5
   c. INR > 5
   d. INR > 6

ANSWERS WITH EXPLANATIONS

1. Ans. d. Transcatheter aortic valve implantation

Braunwald 11th Ed; Page 1455

Currently available mechanical valves have excellent long-term durability. However, all patients with mechanical valves require lifetime anticoagulation with a vitamin K antagonist. Moreso, if the patient has atrial fibrillation. Bioprosthetic valve does not require lifetime anticoagulation, but in presence of atrial fibrillation they also require anticoagulation. It is the transcatheter aortic valve implantation which does not require lifetime anticoagulation.

2. Ans. c. Bileaflet valve

Hurst's 14th Ed; Page 1277

Three types of mechanical prosthesis are seen in clinical practice: (a) Ball and cage valve—It is no longer in clinical use; (b) Monoleaflet valve—Again it is not much in clinical use; (c) Bileaflet mechanical valve—It is the most commonly implanted mechanical prosthesis.

3. Ans. a. Ball and cage valve

Hurst's 14th Ed; Page 1277

Ball-and-cage valves are no longer commercially available. The advantages of the ball-and-cage design stem from the fact that the silastic occluder travels completely out of the valve orifice in systole, reducing the risk of pannus or thrombus spreading from the sewing ring and interfering with the valve mechanism. Moreover, the continuously changing points of contact resulted into reduce wear and tear of this valve. With these first-generation mechanical prostheses was: (a) the high thrombogenic risk, attributed in part to the lack of central blood flow; (b) bulky profile of the prosthesis, which can result in left ventricular outflow tract obstruction when implanted in the mitral position.

4. Ans. d. Glutaraldehyde fixation

Hurst's 14th Ed; Page 1279

Bioprosthetic valves were developed to find a nonthrombogenic alternative to mechanical prostheses with the inherent avoidance of life-long anticoagulation. Porcine valves were implanted initially, which led to the structural failure. Subsequent to this alternative tissue, such as fascia lata, dura mater, and pericardium were used, though with the minimal improvement in prosthesis longevity. Alain Carpentier discovered that glutaraldehyde fixation could produce a durable bioprosthesis. Glutaraldehyde fixation extends tissue longevity by cross-linking collagen fibers and reducing cell viability, enzymatic degradation, and tissue antigenicity.

5. Ans. c. Bovine pericardium

Hurst's 14th Ed; Page 1279

Modern bioprosthetic valves are constructed from animal tissue, predominantly bovine pericardium or porcine aortic valves, both fixed in glutaraldehyde. Pericardial valves are known to have the potential for greater durability, primarily due to the greater amount of collagen in pericardium compared to porcine valve tissue; and secondly because of improved hemodynamics associated with more symmetrical function of the leaflets.

6. Ans. a. First trimester

Hurst's 14th Ed; Page 1287

The risk of miscarriage, fetal abnormalities, and fetal mortality is increased with any anticoagulant regimen. Warfarin crosses the placenta, but heparin does not. Warfarin can be teratogenic during the first trimester and its teratogenicity lesser in second and third trimester. The use of warfarin throughout pregnancy is associated with less risk to mother and fetus than the use of unfractionated heparin. This is because unfractionated heparin has the highest risk of thromboembolic events and maternal death in patients with mechanical valves, and is also associated with maternal thrombocytopenia, osteoporosis, and increased risk of infection from long-term intravenous administration. The risk of warfarin embryopathy is dose related, and in patients with mechanical valves who require > 5 mg warfarin daily to achieve a therapeutic INR, dose-adjusted low molecular weight heparin twice daily during the first trimester is the better choice.

7. Ans. c. Risk of warfarin induced embryopathy is not dose related

Hurst's 14th Ed; Page 1287

Refer to the answer of Q. No 6.

8. Ans. d. INR > 6

Hurst's 14th Ed; Page 1284

The complication of oral anticoagulation for mechanical prosthetic heart valve is bleeding complications. Therefore, these patients require constant monitoring of their INR. The risk of major bleeding increases exponentially with INR more than 6.0 and which therefore usually requires rapid reversal.

CHAPTER 16
Congenital Heart Disease

1. Which is the most common seen cardiac malformation at birth?
   a. Patent ductus arteriosus
   b. Atrial septal defects
   c. Ventricular septal defects
   d. Tetralogy of Fallot

2. Which of the following congenital anomalies is more common in males?
   a. Patent ductus arteriosus
   b. Ebstein anomaly of tricuspid valve
   c. Hypoplastic left heart syndrome
   d. Atrial septal defects

3. The most common cardiac anomalies seen in fetal alcohol syndrome is:
   a. Patent ductus arteriosus
   b. Ventricular septal defect
   c. Peripheral pulmonary artery stenosis
   d. Cardiomyopathy

4. Which of the following statement is *true* regarding genetics and cardiac malformation?
   a. Chromosomal aberrations or genetic mutations accounts for <10% cases of cardiac malformation
   b. Only one of a pair of monozygotic twins is affected by congenital heart disease.
   c. There is two or threefold increase in the incidence of congenital heart disease in siblings of affected patients
   d. All are true

5. Peripheral pulmonic stenosis is seen in:
   a. Rubella syndrome
   b. Cutis laxa
   c. Arteriohepatic dysplasia
   d. All of the above

6. Pulmonary valve is *not* affected in:
   a. Noonan's syndrome
   b. Rubella syndrome
   c. Apert syndrome
   d. Arteriohepatic dysplasia

7. Accelerated atherosclerosis is seen in:
   a. Progeria syndrome   b. Cockayne syndrome
   c. Both of the above   d. None of them

8. Coronary arterial involvement is seen in:
   a. Osteogenesis imperfecta
   b. Marfan syndrome
   c. Pseudoxanthoma elasticum
   d. Ehlers-Danlos syndrome

9. Multivalvular coronary and great artery disease is a feature of:
   a. Margnio syndrome
   b. Pompe disease
   c. Homocystinuria
   d. Mucopolysaccharidoses

10. Which of the following is *not* a feature of Turner syndrome?
    a. Coarctation of aorta
    b. Ventricular septal defect
    c. Aortic dilatation
    d. Bicuspid aortic valve

11. Which of the following teratogens produces obstructive valvular and great arterial lesion in fetus?
    a. Alcohol   b. Lithium
    c. Dilantin   d. Thalidomide

12. What percent of total cardiac output flows through lungs in fetus?
    a. 7-10%   b. 20-25%
    c. 30-40%   d. 50-60%

13. Which of the following statement is *not* correct regarding fetal circulation?
    a. Fetal circulation consists of parallel pulmonary and systemic pathways
    b. The RV contributes about 45% and the left ventricle 55% to the total fetal cardiac output.
    c. The pulmonary blood flow is low (7-10% of total cardiac output in fetus)
    d. The adaptation to cardiocirculatory stress is less effective in fetus than in adulthood

14. Following hemodynamic changes occur at birth *except*:
   a. Reduction in pulmonary vascular resistance
   b. Reduction in systemic vascular resistance
   c. Increase in arterial blood oxygen tension
   d. Constriction of the ductus arteriosus

15. In a healthy mature infants the ductus arteriosus is closed functionally by:
   a. 10–15 hours
   b. Within 72 hours
   c. Within a week
   d. Requires three weeks

16. In surviving preterm infants the ductus arteriosus closes spontaneously:
   a. Within 72 hours
   b. Within 2 weeks
   c. Two to four weeks
   d. Within four to twelve months of birth

17. The potential channel of blood flow after birth is:
   a. Ductus arteriosus
   b. Ductus venosus
   c. Foramen ovale
   d. All of the above

18. The cardinal findings of fetal heart failure on echocardiography includes all *except*:
   a. Scalp edema
   b. Pericardial effusion
   c. Ascites
   d. Increased fetal movements

19. The commonest cause of cardiac decompensation in preterm infant is:
   a. Patent ductus arteriosus
   b. Transposition of great arteries
   c. Tetralogy of Fallot
   d. Coarctation of aorta

20. The causes of cardiac decompensation in full-term new born includes all *except*:
   a. Hypoplastic left heart syndrome
   b. Myocarditis
   c. Hepatic arteriovenous fistula
   d. Ventricular septal defect

21. Which is the rare manifestation of heart failure in infants?
   a. Feeding difficulties and failure to gain weight
   b. Tachycardia, tachypnea
   c. Pleural and pericardial effusion
   d. Peripheral edema and ascites

22. Which statement is *incorrect* regarding heart failure in infants?
   a. A resting heart rate with little variability is characteristic
   b. Hepatomegaly is regularly seen although liver tenderness is uncommon
   c. Peripheral edema is unusual in spite of hepatomegaly
   d. All are correct

23. Cyanosis is produced, when the level of reduced hemoglobin exceeds:
   a. 3.9 mg/dL
   b. 5.9 mg/dL
   c. 8.9 mg/dL
   d. 2.9 mg/dL

24. Which of the following 'drugs' has no role in treatment of hypoxic spells?
   a. Morphine sulfate
   b. Alpha adrenoreceptor stimulants
   c. Beta adrenoreceptor blocking agents
   d. All are useful

25. Which is *not* correct regarding impaired growth in patients with congenital heart disease?
   a. Weight gain is slower than linear growth in acyanotic heart disease, while in cyanotic CHD, height and weight usually parallels each other
   b. Mental development is seldom affected
   c. Boys appears to be more retarded in growth than girls
   d. All are correct

26. The most accurate method for assessing the pulmonary vascular bed especially its reactivity is:
   a. Echocardiography and Doppler
   b. Cardiac catheterization
   c. Pulmonary wedge angiography
   d. Lung biopsy

27. Prophylactic regimens against SABE for Genito urinary procedure in low risk patient is:
   a. IV Ampicillin + IV Gentamicin ½ hours before procedure and repeated after 6 hours.
   b. IV Vancomycin over 1 hour + IV Gentamicin, before procedure and repeated after 6 hours.
   c. IV Ampicillin before procedure and to be repeated with oral preparation after 6 hours.
   d. Amoxycillin orally (3 g) before the procedure and repeated (1.5 g) after 6 hours.

28. Which is *correct* regarding neonatal heart?
   a. It contains fewer myofilaments to generate force and to shorten during contraction
   b. the chamber stiffness of ventricle is greater than that seen in adult life

c. It exhibits suboptimal response to drugs viz. Digitalis
d. All are correct

29. Which of the following is *correct* regarding Digoxin and neonatal heart?
a. Premature infants are more sensitive to digitalis than full term new borns.
b. Infants tolerates higher serum digoxin concentration than adults without developing sign and symptom of digitalis toxicity
c. Both (a+b)
d. None of the above

30. The therapeutic level of digoxin in infant is:
a. <1 ng/mL
b. <2 ng/mL
c. 1–5 ng/mL
d. >5 ng/mL

31. Which of the following congenital lesion produces reverse differential cyanosis?
a. Coarctation of aorta with PDA with normally related great arteries
b. Coarctation of aorta with PDA in transposition of great arteries
c. Ventricular septal defect with pulmonary hypertension
d. All of the above

32. The pattern of arterial blood gas showing decreased pH and pO_2 with normal pCO_2 and unchanged response to O_2 inhalation suggest diagnosis of:
a. Hyaline membrane disease
b. Hypoventilation
c. Decreased or ineffective pulmonary blood flow
d. Systemic hypoperfusion

33. A counter clockwise, superiorly oriented frontal QRS loop with absent or reduced right ventricular force suggests diagnosis of:
a. Pulmonary atresia
b. Ventricular inversion
c. Tricuspid atresia
d. Endocardial cushion defect

34. A boot-shaped heart with concavity of the pulmonary outflow tract suggests diagnosis of:
a. Tetralogy of Fallot
b. Pulmonary atresia
c. Tricuspid atresia
d. All of the above

35. Diagnostic quality images of the fetal heart in utero can be obtained by:
a. 12 weeks of gestation
b. 14 weeks of gestation
c. 16 weeks of gestation
d. 32 weeks of gestation

36. Left axis deviation of P wave in the frontal plane in EKG suggests the diagnosis of:
a. Ostium secundum ASD
b. Ostium primum variety of ASD
c. Sinus venosus ASD
d. Common AV canal defect

37. In ostium primum defect the echocardiographic goose neck deformity is seen in which view:
a. Apical four chamber
b. Subcostal view
c. Parasternal long axis
d. Parasternal short axis

38. Goose neck deformity is pathognomonic of:
a. Secundum variety of ASD
b. Sinus venosus ASD
c. Subaortic stenosis
d. Common AV canal defect

39. Which of the following is *not* correct regarding goose neck deformity seen on angiography?
a. It is pathognomonic of common AV canal defect
b. It is visualized best in right anterior oblique left ventriculogram
c. It is best seen in diastole
d. All are correct

40. The commonest site of defect in ventricular septum is:
a. Membranous septum
b. The inlet septum
c. The trabecular septum
d. The infundibular septum

41. The doubly committed subarterial VSD is due to deficiency in:
a. Membranous septum
b. Inlet septum
c. The trabecular septum
d. Infundibular septum

42. If a child with ventricular septal defect and poor growth, has sudden growth spurt, fewer respiratory infection and a diminution in intensity of murmur, it suggests:
a. Spontaneous closure of VSD
b. Appearance of pulmonary vascular obstructive disease
c. Appearance of right ventricular outflow tract obstruction
d. Closure of ductus

43. Which of the following phenomenon is rarely seen below the age of 5 years in patients with VSD?
a. Spontaneous closure
b. Appearance of pulmonary vascular disease

c. Appearance of RVOT obstruction
  d. Aortic regurgitation

44. Which of the following statement is *incorrect*?
  a. In most patients with VSD and aortic regurgitation, the ventricular septal defect is large
  b. In those infants, who develop RVOT obstruction, the incidence of spontaneous closure is low
  c. In patients with VSD and AR, mild RVOT obstruction, often exists
  d. Aortic regurgitation is more often seen in Japanese patients with VSD

45. Which of the following factor plays crucial role in final anatomic closure of ductus?
  a. Increase in partial pressure of oxygen accompanying ventilation
  b. Changes in synthesis and metabolism of vasoactive eicosanoids
  c. Intimal proliferation and fibrosis
  d. All of the above

46. Which is *not* correct regarding patency of ductus arteriosus in full term infants and children?
  a. Occurs particularly in females
  b. Mostly in pregnancy complicated by first trimester rubella
  c. Occurs most frequently in isolated form
  d. Occurs mostly with other congenital anomalies

47. Which is the commonest cardiac defect associated with aorticopulmonary septal defect?
  a. VSD
  b. PDA
  c. Interrupted aortic arch
  d. Aortic origin of right pulmonary artery

48. Which is the ideal time for corrective repair of Truncus arteriosus?
  a. Before 3 months of age
  b. Before 1 year of age
  c. Before school going age
  d. Anytime after diagnosis

49. Which of the following is most often involved in coronary AV fistula?
  a. Right coronary artery
  b. Left anterior descending artery
  c. Left circumflex artery
  d. Both are involved equally

50. Which is the commonest drain site for coronary AV fistula?
  a. Right atrium
  b. right ventricle
  c. Pulmonary artery
  d. Left ventricle

51. In an infant the EKG demonstration of deep Q waves is associated with ST segment elevation and T wave inversion in lead I, avL, V5 and V6 supports the diagnosis of:
  a. Anomalous origin of left coronary artery from pulmonary trunk
  b. Acute myocarditis
  c. Diphtheric myocarditis
  d. Acute myocardial infarction

52. The most important extracardiac anomaly associated with localized juxtaductal coarctation of aorta is:
  a. Gonadal dysgenesis (Turner syndrome)
  b. Bicuspid aortic valve
  c. Aneurysm of circle of Wills
  d. Patent ductus arteriosus

53. Which of the following anomaly is rarely associated with juxtaductal coarctation of aorta?
  a. Mitral stenosis
  b. Patent ductus arteriosus
  c. Tetralogy of Fallot
  d. Ventricular septal defect

54. The characteristic electrocardiographic changes observed in neonates and infants with coarctation of aorta is:
  a. Right ventricular hypertrophy and right axis deviation
  b. Left ventricular hypertrophy and left axis deviation
  c. Biventricular hypertrophy and normal axis
  d. No definite pattern is seen

55. Precise anatomic localization and hemodynamic severity of coarctation of aorta can be obtained by which of the following noninvasive diagnostic modality?
  a. Computed tomography
  b. Magnetic resonance imaging
  c. Two D-echocardiography and Doppler assessment
  d. Intravascular ultrasonography

56. Which of the following statement is *incorrect* regarding surgical management of coarctation of aorta?
  a. The surgical repair should be delayed until age of 4–6 years
  b. There is 5–10% risk of recurrence of coarctation after surgery
  c. Paradoxical hypertension is noted more often following balloon angioplasty than the surgery
  d. Necrotizing aortitis of small vessel of gut is rarely seen following surgery

57. The aortic isthmus is:
   a. Portion of aorta between the left subclavian artery and the ductus arteriosus
   b. Normally is narrowed in fetus and new born
   c. The lumen of isthmus is about 2/3 that of ascending and descending aorta
   d. All are correct

58. In aortic arch interruption, which is *correct*?
   a. Interruption distal to the left subclavian artery (Type A) occurs with equal frequency to interruptions distal to left common carotid (Type B)
   b. Subaortic ventricular septal defect is found in 80–90% cases.
   c. There is frequent association with DiGeorge Syndrome
   d. All are correct

59. Majority of the congenital anomalies of heart are present at what interval after conception
   a. 3 weeks
   b. 4 weeks
   c. 6 weeks
   d. 12 weeks

60. Which of the following congenital heart disease is *not* anatomic in the gross morphologic sense?
   a. Marfan syndrome
   b. Congenital complete AV block
   c. PDA
   d. VSD

61. Which of the following is a dynamic congenital heart disease?
   a. Perimembranous VSD
   b. Bicuspid aortic valve
   c. Patient ductus arteriosus in a premature infant
   d. All of the above

62. Which of the following is an essential intrinsic component of the fetal circulation
   a. Ductus arteriosus
   b. Ductus venosus
   c. Foramen ovale
   d. All of the above

63. When the functional closure of ductus arteriosus takes place after birth?
   a. Within first 24 hours
   b. Within 48 hours
   c. Within 72 hours
   d. Within 7 days

64. All normal systolic murmurs are mid systolic *except*:
   a. Vibratory systolic murmur
   b. Pulmonary systolic murmur
   c. Systolic mammary soufflé
   d. Cardiorespiratory systolic murmur

65. Which is *not* true regarding still's murmur?
   a. It is seldom heard in infancy
   b. The murmur is maximal between apex and the lower left sternal edge
   c. It is prevalent after age of 3 years
   d. Its incidence increases towards adolescence

66. Which is *true* regarding venous Hum?
   a. It is universal in children
   b. Maximal intensity of hum is at supraclavicular fossa lateral to sternocleidomastoid muscle.
   c. The venous hum may disappear with movement of head
   d. All of the above

67. Which is *true* regarding mammary soufflé?
   a. It is heard during late pregnancy and early postpartum period
   b. It is best heard in supine position and may disappear in upright position
   c. Valsalva maneuver does not alter intensity
   d. All of the above

68. Which of the following feature helps in differentiating the murmur of ductus from mammary soufflé?
   a. Peaking at second heart sound
   b. Location of murmur
   c. Obliteration by local compression
   d. None of the above

69. In congenital complete AV block an increase in cardiac output with exercise is:
   a. Rate dependent
   b. Stroke volume dependent
   c. Atrial contribution dependent
   d. None of the above

70. There is high incidence of congenital complete AV block in offspring of mothers with:
   a. Diabetes mellitus
   b. Rheumatic heart disease
   c. Complete AV block
   d. Systemic lupus erythematosus

71. The complete AV block in utero can be diagnosed by:
   a. Fetal echocardiography
   b. Holter monitoring
   c. Fetal electrocardiography
   d. Fetal auscultation

72. Which is *true* regarding association between maternal lupus erythematosus and congenital AV block?
   a. Mother with SLE who had one child with neonatal heart block are at greater risk of subsequent offspring with AV block

b. Children of mothers with lupus may subsequently develop overt connective tissue disease
c. Maternal lupus may not became manifest for years after the birth of an infant with congenital complete heart block
d. All are correct

73. Which is *not* correct regarding the fetus with isolated congenital complete heart block?
a. Generally they do not develop hydrops
b. They are born alive
c. Survive the neonatal period with good outcome
d. All are correct

74. Which is *not* correct regarding EKG in congenital complete AV block?
a. Accrochage (Period of Synchronization) is uncommon
b. Atrial rate tends to decrease with age
c. Congenital atrial flutter may coexist
d. All are correct

75. Which of the following feature in EKG helps in differentiating isolated congenital AV block from congenital AV block associated with corrected transposition of great arteries?
a. Voltage criteria for LVH together with prominent left precardial Q waves
b. Absent left precardial Q waves
c. Pattern of RVH
d. Biventricular hypertrophy

76. Major variable that relates to long-term survival in corrected TGA is presence of:
a. Complete AV block
b. Ventricular septal defect
c. Atrioventricular valve regurgitation
d. Pulmonic stenosis

77. The most common co-existent malformation in corrected transposition of great arteries is:
a. VSD b. Pulmonic stenosis
c. Ebstein's anomaly d. Complete AV block

78. Which of the following lesion is obligatory in Truncus arteriosus?
a. ASD
b. VSD
c. Right sided aortic arch
d. Absent pulmonary arteries

79. Which is the commonest variety of Truncus arteriosus?
a. Truncus with short main pulmonary artery and giving right and left pulmonary arteries

b. Truncus with right and left pulmonary arteries taking origin from separate ostia
c. Truncus with a single pulmonary arterial branch
d. All are equally common

80. Which of the following feature differentiate the normal tri-leaflet aortic valve from that of Truncus arteriosus?
a. Presence of raphe
b. Cuspal inequality
c. Focal or diffuse thickening
d. All of the above

81. When a Bounding arterial pulse occurs in a mildly cyanotic infant with congestive heart failure, which of the following is possible diagnosis?
a. Tetralogy of Fallot with aortic regurgitation
b. Truncus arteriosus
c. Absent pulmonary valve
d. All of the above

82. What is the mechanism of bounding arterial pulse in truncus arteriosus?
a. Low pulmonary vascular resistance
b. Truncal valve regurgitation
c. Both a and b
d. None of the above

83. The left hilar coma is a useful radiologic sign of:
a. Corrected transposition of great arteries
b. Interrupted aortic arch
c. Truncus arteriosus
d. Tricuspid atresia

84. All the following are characteristic auscultatory feature of congenital MS *except*:
a. Loud 1st heart sound
b. Apical rumbling diastolic murmur
c. Mitral opening sharp
d. None of the above

85. In which category of patients of MS restoration of sinus rhythm by oral Quinidine/DC shock indicationed:
a. In younger patients
b. In patients without severe LA enlargement
c. In patients with recent onset atrial fibrillation
d. All of the above

86. MVP is associated most commonly with which of the following condition:
a. Ehlers–Danlos syndrome
b. Osteogenesis imperfecta
c. Marfan Syndrome
d. Noonan syndrome

87. **Most common cause of isolated mitral regurgitation requiring valve replacement is:**
    a. MVP
    b. Rheumatic endocarditis
    c. Trauma
    d. AMI

88. **Which is *true* regarding the auscultatory finding of MVP?**
    a. Most important finding is mid systolic click occurring after 14 second after S1
    b. As opposed to systolic ejection click it occur after the beginning of upstroke of carotid pulse
    c. MVP also produces an early diastolic sound heard at apex or at left sternal edge 0.7–0.11 second following A2 due one to return of prolapsed posterior leaflet from LA to its normal position.
    d. All are true

89. **Which of the following maneuvers best differentiates the murmur of IHSS and MVP?**
    a. Valsalva Strain phase
    b. Amyl nitrite Inhalation
    c. Premature beat
    d. Handgrip

90. **The most common location of infective endocarditis in cases with coarctation of aorta is:**
    a. Site of coarctation
    b. VSD
    c. Circle of Willis
    d. Bicuspid aortic valve

91. **Which of the following is *not* true regarding rupture of aneurysm in circle of Willis in coarctation of aorta?**
    a. Majority of cerebral hemorrhage occurs in second or third decade
    b. Hypertension is necessary precondition
    c. It can occur long after repair of coarctation
    d. None of the above

92. **Which of the following is *not* correct regarding pregnancy in coarctation of aorta?**
    a. The incidence of toxemia is high in women with coarctation
    b. Cardiac failure is rare
    c. There is increased risk of aortic rupture and intracranial hemorrhage
    d. There is increased risk of developing infective endocarditis

93. **Which is *correct* regarding rib notching in coarctation of aorta?**
    a. Anterior ribs are not affected
    b. It seldom appears before the age of 6 years
    c. It is rare above the third and below ninth rib
    d. All are correct

94. **Rib notching confined to the lower ribs is seen in:**
    a. Coarctation of aorta located distal to the left subclavian artery
    b. Coarctation causing narrowing of orifice of the left subclavian artery
    c. Anomalous origin of the right subclavian artery distal to the coarctation
    d. Abdominal coarctation

95. **Retrosternal notching or scalloping in lateral X-ray chest in coarctation is caused by:**
    a. Coarctated segment of aorta
    b. Dilated subclavian artery
    c. Postcoarctation segment of aorta
    d. Tortuous internal mammary artery

96. **Which of the following radiological feature is *not* seen in Pseudocoarctation?**
    a. "Figure 3" sign in X-ray chest PAV
    b. Mirror image "E sign" in barium filled esophagus
    c. Rib notching
    d. None of the above

97. **The eponym Steidele's complex is applied for:**
    a. Coarctation of aorta
    b. Tubular hypoplasia of aortic arch
    c. Subaortic stenosis with parachute mitral valve
    d. Complete interruption of aortic arch

98. **Which is the commonest site of interruption of aortic arch?**
    a. Interruption between the left common carotid and left subclavian artery
    b. Isthmic interruption distal to the left subclavian artery
    c. Interruption between the innominate and left carotid arteries
    d. All are equally common

99. **DiGeorge syndrome (Thymic aplasia) is associated with:**
    a. Type A interrupted aortic arch
    b. Type B interrupted aortic arch
    c. Type C interrupted aortic arch
    d. Coarctation of aorta

100. **Which of the following variety of the pulmonic stenosis has strong tendency to coexist with VSD?**
    a. Valvular pulmonic stenosis
    b. Infundibular pulmonic stenosis
    c. Subinfundibular pulmonic stenosis
    d. Double chambered right ventricle

101. Bilateral stenosis of the pulmonary arterial branches with supravalvular aortic stenosis is a component of:
   a. Turner syndrome
   b. Williams syndrome
   c. Noonans syndrome
   d. Leopard syndrome

102. Which of the following is *not* correct regarding maternal Rubella infection and fetal damage?
   a. Most cases occur following primary disease rather than rubella reinfections
   b. Maternal Viremia is not a prerequisite for placental and fetal rubella infections
   c. The risk of fetal damage is small if maternal rubella occurs after 16th week
   d. Cardiac defects consistently occurs in infants infected during the first 10 weeks of gestation

103. Which of the following is most common cardiac lesion due to maternal rubella?
   a. Patent ductus arteriosus
   b. Ventricular septal defect
   c. Peripheral pulmonary artery stenosis
   d. Pulmonary valve stenosis

104. Which of the following is ductus dependent lesion?
   a. Interrupted aortic arch
   b. Pulmonary atresia with VSD
   c. Hypoplastic left heart syndrome
   d. All of the above

105. Which of the following lesion is less common in male?
   a. Transposition of great arteries
   b. Congenital aneurysm of sinus of Valsalva
   c. Coarctation of aorta
   d. Atrial septal defect

106. Which of the following is *not* true regarding congenital heart disease?
   a. The approximate incidence of CHD is 8/1,000 live births
   b. It includes congenital bicuspid valve and MVP
   c. Extracardiac anomalies occurs in approximately 50% of infants
   d. None of the above

107. Which of the following is *not* a cardiac teratogen?
   a. Thalidomide
   b. Diphenylhydantoin
   c. Amiodarone
   d. Lithium Carbonate

108. Primitive cardiac tube is formed at which age of gestation?
   a. 4th week   b. 6th week
   c. 7th week   d. 8th week

109. Which of the following aortic arches regresses completely in human embryo?
   a. 1, 2 and 6   b. 1, 2 and 5
   c. 1, 3 and 6   d. 2, 4 and 6

110. Ductus arteriosus develops from:
   a. Distal half of left 4th aortic arch
   b. Distal half of right 4th aortic arch
   c. Distal half of right 6th aortic arch
   d. Distal half of left 6th aortic arch

111. What is the approximate contribution of right ventricle in total fetal cardiac output?
   a. 25%   b. 40%
   c. 55%   d. 72%

112. What is the total pulmonary blood flow in fetus?
   a. 8% of total cardiac output
   b. 10% of total cardiac output
   c. 12% of total cardiac output
   d. 15% of total cardiac output

113. The functional closure of ductus arteriosus occurs at:
   a. 6–8 hours after birth
   b. 10–15 hours after birth
   c. 24–48 hours after birth
   d. 48–72 hours after birth

114. The spontaneous closure of ductus in preterm infants occurs within:
   a. 2–4 months of birth
   b. 4–6 months of birth
   c. 4–8 months of birth
   d. 4–12 months of birth

115. Which of the following is commonest cause of cardiac decompensation in preterm infant?
   a. Transposition of great arteries
   b. Ventricular septal defect
   c. Hypoplastic left heart syndrome
   d. Patent ductus arteriosus

116. Which of the following is least commonly observed physical sign in infants with CHF?
   a. Tachypnea
   b. Tachycardia
   c. Gallop rhythm
   d. Hepatomegaly

117. Which is the most common complication in patients with cyanotic congenital heart disease?
   a. Cerebral thrombosis
   b. Brain abscess
   c. Paradoxical embolism
   d. Retinopathy

118. Which of the following is *not* used in treatment of hypoxic spells?
   a. Sodium bicarbonate
   b. Alpha-adrenoceptor stimulants
   c. Beta-adrenoceptor blockers
   d. Alpha-adrenoceptor blockers

119. All of the following are true regarding brain abscess in cyanotic congenital heart disease *except*:
   a. It is rare under 2 years of age
   b. It occurs in approximately 2% of population with cyanotic congenital heart disease
   c. Seizures and paralysis frequently heralds the onset of a brain abscess
   d. A mortality rate of 30–40% is often related to delay in diagnosis and treatment

120. Retinopathy in cyanotic congenital heart disease is *not* related to:
   a. Decreased arterial oxygen saturation
   b. Erythrocytosis
   c. Hypercapnia
   d. None of the above

121. Which of the following reserve mechanism is limited in neonatal heart?
   a. Preload reserve
   b. Contractile reserve
   c. Systolic reserve
   d. Heart rate reserve

122. The therapeutic level of digoxin in infants range from:
   a. 1–2 ng/mL
   b. 1–3 ng/mL
   c. 1–5 ng/mL
   d. 2–5 ng/mL

123. Which of the following drug is *not* used in treatment of infants with congestive heart failure?
   a. Digoxin
   b. Indomethacin
   c. Prostaglandins E1
   d. All of the above are used

124. Which of the following congenital heart disease produces differential cyanosis with upper part of body pink and the lower part of the body blue?
   a. Patent ductus arteriosus with reversed shunt
   b. Coarctation of aorta with PDA
   c. Interrupted aortic arch with PDA
   d. All of the above

125. Reversed differential cyanosis is a feature of:
   a. TGA with coarctation of aorta with PDA
   b. TGA with interrupted aortic arch
   c. Both of the above
   d. None of the above

126. In a newborn with cyanotic CHD, a counter clockwise superiorly oriented frontal QRS loop with absent or reduced right ventricular forces suggest diagnosis of:
   a. Tricuspid atresia
   b. Pulmonary atresia
   c. Double outlet right ventricle
   d. All of the above

127. Which of the following laboratory investigation is most useful in differentiating between cardiac and respiratory cause of cyanosis?
   a. Clinical examination
   b. Blood gas and pH patterns
   c. Electrocardiogram
   d. Radiographic examination

128. In a plain skiagram of chest, a boot shaped heart with concavity of the pulmonary outflow tract suggest the diagnosis of:
   a. Tetralogy of Fallot
   b. Pulmonary atresia
   c. Tricuspid atresia
   d. All of the above

129. An ovoid heart with a narrow base with increased pulmonary vascular marking is suggestive of:
   a. Transposition of great arteries
   b. Total anomalous pulmonary venous return
   c. Tricuspid atresia
   d. Single ventricle with inverted rudimentary chamber

130. Diagnostic quality image of fetal heart in utero can be obtained as early as by:
   a. 12th week of gestation
   b. 14th week of gestation
   c. 16th week of gestation
   d. After 18th week of gestation

131. What percentage of patient with atrial septal defect have associated mitral valve abnormality?
   a. 4–10%
   b. 5–12%
   c. 10–20%
   d. 15–20%

132. Which of the following factor determines the magnitude of left to right shunt through an ASD?
   a. Size of the defect
   b. Relative compliance of the ventricle

c. Relative resistance of pulmonary and systemic circulation
d. All of the above

133. Left-to-right shunt in ASD occurs predominantly during:
a. Late diastolic and early ventricular systole
b. Late ventricular systole and early diastole
c. Throughout ventricular systole
d. Throughout ventricular diastole

134. Left axis deviation of the P wave in the frontal plane (manifested by negative P wave in lead III) suggests the diagnosis of:
a. Ostium primum ASD
b. Ostium secundum ASD
c. Sinus venosus type of ASD
d. Complete endocardial cushion defect

135. Left axis deviation and superior orientation and counter clockwise rotation of the QRS loop in the frontal plane suggests the presence of:
a. Tricuspid atresia
b. Ostium primum ASD
c. Secundum ASD with mitral valve prolapse
d. All of the above

136. Goose neck deformity as evident angiographically suggests the diagnosis of:
a. Ostium primum ASD
b. Sinus venosus ASD
c. Ostium secundum ASD
d. Complete AV canal defect

137. What percentage of patients with VSD closes by age of 3 years?
a. 60%
b. 50%
c. 40%
d. 30%

138. What percentage of patients with large VSD and history of congestive heart failure in infancy experiences spontaneous closure?
a. 15–20%
b. 10–15%
c. 10–12%
d. 7–8%

139. Atrial septal defect is found in patients with tetralogy of Fallot in about:
a. 4% of cases
b. 5–6% of cases
c. 10% of cases
d. 12% of cases

140. Appearance of systolic click preceding pansystolic murmur in a case of VSD is suggestive of:
a. Pulmonary hypertension
b. Right ventricular outflow tract obstruction
c. Formation of septal aneurysm
d. None of the above

141. Which is *not* true regarding the aortic regurgitation in patients with VSD?
a. It occurs in approximately 5% of patients
b. It is rare below 5 years of age
c. In most patients VSD is small to moderate size
d. It is rare complication in Japanese

142. Which is the commonest associated anomalies in patients with aorticopulmonary septal defect?
a. PDA
b. VSD
c. Coarctation of aorta
d. Right aortic arch

143. Which is the commonest associated anomaly with persistent truncus arteriosus?
a. VSD
b. Right sided aortic arch
c. Truncal valve stenosis
d. None of the above

144. Which is *not* true regarding congenital aneurysm of sinus of Valsalva?
a. It is an uncommon anomaly
b. Right coronary sinus is often involved
c. Unruptured aneurysm is always asymptomatic
d. The receiving chamber of aorticocardiac fistula is usually the right ventricle

145. Which of the following anomalies is never seen in association with juxtaductal coarctation of aorta?
a. Pulmonary atresia
b. Tricuspid atresia
c. Tetralogy of Fallot
d. All of the above

146. The most important extracardiac anomaly in association with coarctation of aorta is:
a. Gonadal dysgenesis
b. Aneurysm of sinus of Valsalva
c. Aneurysm of circle of Willis
d. Down syndrome

147. Which of the following is most common variety of aortic arch interruption?
a. Type A
b. Type B
c. Type C
d. All are equally common

148. What is the recurrence rate following the repair of coarctation in infancy?
a. 2–4%
b. 5–10%
c. 10–14%
d. >20%

149. Which of the following is most commonly found congenital anomaly in patients with DiGeorge syndrome?
 a. Hypoplasia of aortic arch
 b. Coarctation of the aorta
 c. Interrupted aortic arch
 d. Patent ductus arteriosus

150. Which of the following is the cause of aortic regurgitation in patients with subaortic stenosis?
 a. Thickening of aortic valve and impaired mobility of cusps secondary to trauma of jet
 b. Destruction of aortic leaflet by vegetation
 c. Poststenotic dilatation of aortic root causing aortic regurgitation
 d. Dilatation of left ventricle

151. In type A aortic arch interruption the defect is:
 a. Distal to left subclavian artery
 b. Between left common carotid and subclavian artery
 c. Between innominate and left common carotid artery
 d. Proximal to innominate artery

152. At cardiac catheterization, if the pulmonary artery wedge pressure is higher than a simultaneous left atrial pressure, the possible diagnosis is:
 a. Pulmonary AV fistula
 b. Cor triatriatum
 c. Supravalvular mitral diaphragm
 d. Parachute mitral valve

153. In majority of patients with tetralogy of Fallot the site of outflow tract obstruction is?
 a. Infundibular
 b. Valvular
 c. Supravalvular
 d. Peripheral pulmonary arterial narrowing

154. Which of the following factor is of fundamental significance in the hemodynamics of tetralogy of Fallot?
 a. Severity of RVOT obstruction
 b. Degree of over ride of aorta
 c. Size of VSD
 d. Right ventricular function

155. During cardiac catheterization the catheter enters into aorta from right ventricle in all *except*:
 a. Transposition of great arteries
 b. Tetralogy of Fallot
 c. Large VSD
 d. All of the above

156. Which of the following is most specific electrocardiographic feature of hypothermia?
 a. Sinus bradycardia
 b. Presence of "J" wave
 c. Somatic tremor effect
 d. QT prolongation

157. The most commonly associated defect in patients with Ebstein anomaly is:
 a. Ostium secundum ASD
 b. Pulmonary stenosis or atresia
 c. Ventricular septal defect
 d. None of the above

158. Cyanosis in infancy, which disappears early in life and recurs at a later age is diagnostic of:
 a. Pulmonary atresia with VSD
 b. Tetralogy of Fallot
 c. Ebstein anomaly
 d. Corrected transposition of great arteries

159. Which of the following is characteristic electrocardiographic finding of Ebstein anomaly?
 a. "Himalayan" P waves
 b. Type B WPW syndrome
 c. 'Second QRS' complex
 d. Prolonged PR interval

160. Which of the following EKG pattern is uncommon in Ebstein's anomaly:
 a. Right bundle branch block pattern
 b. Left bundle branch block pattern
 c. Complete heart block
 d. LV dominance

161. Most accurate method to diagnose Ebstein's anomaly is?
 a. Echocardiography
 b. Angiocardiography
 c. Electrocardiography
 d. Hemodynamic study with intracardiac electrogram

162. The relative infrequency of left ventricular hypertrophy in the electrocardiogram despite a thick walled left ventricle is a feature of:
 a. Aortic atresia without VSD
 b. Aortic atresia with VSD
 c. Pulmonary atresia without VSD
 d. Pulmonary atresia with VSD

163. Which of the following is *correct* regarding pulmonary arteriovenous fistulae?
 a. It occurs without associated congenital heart disease
 b. Cardiac failure is rare

c. Mucocutaneous telangiectasia is a common occurrence
d. All of the above

164. The occurrence of mucocutaneous telangiectasia with frequent episodes of epistaxis a feature of:
a. Pseudoxanthoma elasticum
b. Pulmonary arteriovenous fistulae
c. Thrombocytopenic pupura
d. Tetralogy of Fallot's

165. Pulmonary AV fistulae have predilection for
a. Both upper lobes of lungs
b. Both lower lobes of lungs
c. Left lobe
d. Lower lobes and right middle lobes

166. The most possible diagnosis in healthy young adult with abnormal density's on routine chest X-rays with mild cyanosis and hereditary hemorrhagic telangiectasia is:
a. Turner syndrome
b. Congenital pulmonary arteriovenous fistulae
c. Aortic atresia
d. Hypoplastic left heart syndrome

167. The combination of cyanosis and telangiectasia with a normal electrocardiogram and a normal cardiac silhouette on X-ray is characteristic feature of:
a. Hypoplastic left heart syndrome
b. Neonatal myocarditis
c. Congenital pulmonary arteriovenous fistulae
d. Ebstein's anomaly

168. A bounding arterial pulse in a mildly cyanotic infant with marked congestive heart failure indicates diagnosis of:
a. Large pulmonary AV fistulae
b. Persistence truncus arteriosus
c. Neonatal myocarditis
d. Large VSD with PAH

169. The left hilar comma is a useful radiologic sign of:
a. Tetralogy of Fallot
b. Truncus arteriosus
c. PDA
d. ASD with pulmonic stenosis

170. Which of the following is the commonest type of anatomic arrangement between truncus arteriosus and pulmonary circulation?
a. A short main pulmonary artery originating from the truncus and giving rise to right and left pulmonary arterial branches
b. The right and left pulmonary arterial branches arise independently but in close proximity to each other from the posterior wall of truncus
c. The two pulmonary arteries arising from truncus at some distance from each other
d. Complete pulmonary atresia with ventricular septal defect

171. Which of the following is *not* a component of Shone's complex?
a. Supraventricular stenosing ring
b. Parachute mitral valve
c. Subpulmonic stenosis with coarctation of aorta
d. Subaortic stenosis and coarctation of aorta

172. Which of the following 2-dimensional echocardiographic imaging with a feature of a single eccentrically located papillary muscle characterizes?
a. Parachute mitral valve
b. Congenital mitral stenosis
c. Mitral arcade
d. Rheumatic mitral stenosis

173. Two well-formed papillary muscle with a clearly defined but reduced interpapillary distance is a feature on echocardiography of:
a. Parachute mitral valve
b. Mitral arcade
c. Congenital mitral stenosis
d. Supramitral ring

174. Which of the following features forms the basis for the clinical diagnosis of Ebstein's anomaly?
a. The degree of abnormal attachment of the inferior tricuspid leaflet to the inlet trabecular ledge
b. The extent of atrializations of inflow portion of right ventricle
c. The electromechanical properties of the right atrium proper, the atrialized right ventricle and the functional right ventricle
d. Size of right ventricle

175. A 400-fold increase in the occurrence of which congenital anomaly is seen in mothers taking lithium carbonate:
a. Tetralogy of Fallot
b. Coarctation of aorta
c. Ebstein's anomaly
d. Single ventricle

176. Which of the following congenital cardiac malformation is consistently associated with the occurrence of WPW syndrome?
a. Single ventricle
b. Cor triatriatum
c. Ebstein's anomaly
d. Tetralogy of Fallot

177. Which is *correct* regarding electrophysiological properties of Ebstein's anomaly?
a. It is consistently associated with existence of right sided bypass tract leading to WPW (type B syndrome)
b. There is both intra-His and infra-His conduction delay in Ebstein's anomaly
c. Complete heart block is rarity despite prolonged HV intervals and markedly prolonged PR intervals
d. All of the above

178. Which of the following is the commonest QRS complex pattern found in patient with Ebstein's anomaly?
a. Right bundle branch block
b. Presence of second QRS complex attached to the preceding normal complex
c. Markedly inferiorly directed mean QRS axis
d. Presence of deep Q waves in lead II, III and avF

179. Which of the following conduction disturbances are *not* seen in Ebstein's anomaly?
a. Intra-His or Infra-His delay
b. Right bundle branch block
c. Bizarre second QRS attached to the preceding normal complex
d. Complete heart block

180. Normal or reduced caliber of both the aortic root and the pulmonary trunk associated with a box like cardiac silhouette is the distinctive radiological pattern of?
a. Single ventricle
b. Cardiomyopathy
c. Ebstein's anomaly
d. Ostium secundum ASD

181. Which of the following cardiac lesion is *not* associated with endocardial fibroelastosis?
a. Coarctation of aorta
b. Congenital mitral stenosis
c. Anomalous origin of the left coronary artery form the pulmonary trunk
d. Healing of myocardial infarction in adult CAD

182. The congenital cardiac defect resulting form rubella infection occurs in infant infected before:
a. Third week of pregnancy
b. Eight week of pregnancy
c. Eleventh week of pregnancy
d. Thirty-eight week of pregnancy

183. Which of the following clinical syndrome is associated with occurrence of pulmonic stenosis?
a. Congenital Rubella
b. Williams Syndrome
c. Arteriohepatic dysplasia
d. All of the above

184. The most frequent type of atrial septal defect is located in the region of:
a. Fossa ovalis
b. Ostium primum
c. Sinus venosus
d. Coronary sinus

185. Least common variety of atrial septal defect is:
a. Ostium secundum type
b. Ostium primum type
c. Sinus venosus type
d. Coronary sinus type

186. The spontaneous closure is not uncommon with:
a. Coronary sinus atrial septal defect
b. Sinus venosus type of ASD
c. Ostium secundum type of ASD
d. Ostium primum type of ASD

187. Which of the following variety of atrial septal defect is associated with high incidence of anomalous pulmonary venous drainage?
a. Ostium secundum type
b. Sinus venosus type
c. Ostium primum type
d. Coronary sinus ASD

188. Which is the commonest variety of partial anomalous pulmonary venous connection seen in cases of ASD?
a. Between the right upper or middle lobe pulmonary veins and right atrium or superior vena cava
b. The anomalous connection of left pulmonary vein to innominate vein
c. Connection between the right pulmonary vein to inferior vena cava
d. Bilateral partial anomalous pulmonary venous connection

189. Which is *not* correct regarding Scimitar syndrome?
a. There is partial anomalous pulmonary venous connection of entire right lung to inferior vena cava
b. The right lung and right pulmonary artery are hypoplastic
c. There is shifting of heart into the left hemithorax
d. The lower portion of the right lung is perfused by the systemic arteries arising form abdominal aorta

190. The commonest form of interatrial communication in patients with tricuspid atresia is:
a. Patent foramen ovale
b. Secundum ASD
c. Coronary sinus variety of ASD
d. Sinus venosus ASD

191. The commonest variety of tricuspid atresia is:
a. Tricuspid atresia without transposition, no pulmonic stenosis and large VSD
b. Tricuspid atresia without transposition, pulmonic stenosis, small VSD
c. Tricuspid atresia with transposition pulmonic stenosis large VSD
d. Tricuspid atresia with transposition no pulmonic stenosis

192. An abnormal left ward axis with counter clockwise depolarization is a feature of:
a. Tricuspid atresia with normally related great arteries and a small ventricular septal defect
b. Tricuspid atresia with transposition of great arteries and a small ventricular septal defect
c. Single ventricle with normally related great arteries
d. Single ventricle with transposition of great arteries

193. The term Holmes heart is used to describe which congenital malformation and it is associated arrangements
a. Tricuspid atresia with normally related great arteries and VSD
b. Single left ventricle with a rudimentary chamber, the aorta arising from rudimentary chamber and pulmonary trunk from the morphologic left ventricle.
c. Single ventricle with concordant arrangement whereas aorta arises from morphologic left ventricle and pulmonary trunk from rudimentary chamber
d. Tricuspid atresia with transposition of great arteries VSD and pulmonic stenosis

194. Precordial QRS complexes exhibiting a 'stereotyped' pattern is seen in which congenital heart disease?
a. Single ventricle with non inverted rudimentary chambers
b. Corrected transposition of great arteries
c. Tetralogy of Fallot with PDA
d. Tricuspid atresia

195. Which is *not* correct regarding Noonan syndrome?
a. The incidence of hypertrophic cardiomyopathy is approximately 20%
b. Cardiac involvement occurs in about two third of cases
c. Pulmonary artery stenosis is the commonest cardiac lesion
d. Pulmonic valve dysplasia is the commonest lesion

196. Which of the following is *not* found in coarctation of aorta?
a. Aneurysm of descending aorta
b. Aneurysm of abdominal aorta
c. Aneurysm of subclavian artery
d. Intracranial aneurysm of the circle of Willis

197. Which is *correct* regarding pregnancy and coarctation of aorta?
a. Blood pressure fluctuation are more in presence of pregnancy
b. Incidence of toxemia is higher in women with coarctation
c. Cardiac failure is quite common in pregnant women with coarctation of aorta
d. Pregnancy increases risk of aortic rupture and intracranial hemorrhage

198. A diminished or absent right brachial pulse in cases with coarctation of aorta implies:
a. Preductal coarctation
b. Postductal coarctation
c. Coarctation involving orifice of left subclavian artery
d. Anomalous origin of right subclavian artery distal to the coarctation

199. Bilateral rib notching in case of coarctation of aorta implies:
a. Narrowing distal to left subclavian artery
b. Narrowing of the orifice of left subclavian artery
c. Anomalous origin of right subclavian artery distal to the coarctation
d. Coexisting abdominal coarctation

200. Unilateral rib notching confining to left hemithorax is seen in:
a. Coarctation of aorta distal to left subclavian artery
b. Abdominal coarctation
c. Anomalous origin of right subclavian artery distal to the coarctation
d. Coarctation narrowing the orifice of left subclavian artery

201. Unilateral rib notching confining to right hemithorax is seen in:
a. Coarctation involving the orifice of left subclavian artery
b. Coarctation of aorta with anomalous origin of right subclavian artery distal to coarct segment
c. Coarctation located distal to left subclavian artery
d. Pseudocoarctation

202. Rib notching confined to lower ribs only is seen in
a. Pseudocoarctation
b. Neurofibromatosis
c. Abdominal coarctation
d. Coarctation of aorta distal to left subclavian artery

203. Which is *not* correct regarding rib notching and coarctation of aorta?
   a. Anterior ribs are spared
   b. Rib notching seldom appears before the age 6 years
   c. It usually seen between third and eight posterior ribs
   d. Pseudocoarctation produces similar rib notching pattern

204. Which of the following chromosomal abnormality is *not* associated with higher incidence of congenital cardiac defects?
   a. Trisomy 13
   b. Turner syndrome
   c. Edward syndrome
   d. Klinefelter syndrome

205. Which of the following is *not* correct regarding Down syndrome?
   a. Majority of patients have Trisomy 21
   b. The most characteristic cardiac anomaly in Down syndrome is defect of closure of endocardial cushions
   c. There is higher incidence of conotruncal and distal aortic arch abnormality in these patients
   d. All are correct

206. Which is *true* regarding Turner syndrome?
   a. 50–70% of patients have coarctation of aorta
   b. Blood pressure elevation is common even without coarctation
   c. There is high risk of dissection of aorta even in absence of coarctation
   d. All are true

207. Which of the following lesion is found in association with Turner syndrome?
   a. Bicuspid aortic valve
   b. Dilatation of ascending aorta
   c. Coarctation of aorta
   d. All of the above

208. Which of the following is a cardiovascular teratogens?
   a. Phenylalanine
   b. Vitamin D
   c. Hydantoin
   d. All of the above

209. Which of the following is *not* a cardiovascular teratogens?
   a. Valproic acid
   b. Trimethadione
   c. Warfarin
   d. Sodium cromoglycate

210. Which is the most common cardiovascular lesion in cases of Marfan syndrome?
   a. MVP
   b. Aortic regurgitation
   c. Dissection of aorta
   d. Aneurysm of aorta

211. Abnormality of which of the following chromosome is associated with occurrence of conotruncal malformations?
   a. Chromosome 13
   b. Chromosome 18
   c. Chromosome 21
   d. Chromosome 22

212. Genetic extracellular matrix abnormality leads to which type of congenital heart disease?
   a. Endocardial cushion defect
   b. Conotruncal malformation
   c. Left sided flow lesions
   d. Atrial septation

213. Which is *not* a feature of Kartagener's syndrome?
   a. Lateralisation of the heart
   b. Defect in ciliary motility
   c. Sperm hypermotility
   d. None of the above

214. Syndrome of CATCH-22 is associated with occurrence of which of the following congenital malformation?
   a. Secundum ASD
   b. VSD
   c. PDA
   d. Supravalvular AS

215. Which is the commonest cardiovascular lesion associated with Williams syndrome?
   a. Infantile hypercalcemia
   b. Bicuspid aortic valve
   c. Supravalvular AS
   d. Mitral valve prolapse

216. Which is a component of Williams syndrome?
   a. Supravalvular AS and peripheral pulmonic stenosis
   b. Diffuse vasculopathy
   c. Predisposition to cerebrovascular disease
   d. All of the above

217. Which of the following is most common teratogens to which human embryo and fetus are exposed?
   a. Hydantoin
   b. Warfarin
   c. Ethanol
   d. Retinoic acid

218. Which is *not* correct regarding fetal alcohol syndrome?
   a. The period of greatest vulnerability is first trimester
   b. Risk is not related to the amount of alcohol consumed
   c. Ventricular septal defects are more common
   d. None of the above

219. Cardiovascular defects, primarily of rotation (conotruncal malformation) are common with:
   a. Fetal alcohol syndrome
   b. Fetal hydantoin syndrome
   c. Retinoic acid embryopathy
   d. Hydantoin embryopathy

220. In fetal rubella effect, the *incorrect* statement is:
   a. Chances of fetal infection is more when mother is infected during last trimester
   b. It gives chronic viral illness in fetus, which can persist for years.
   c. PDA is the most common cardiovascular defect
   d. Peripheral pulmonary stenosis and fibromuscular proliferation of small and medium arteries often improve post nasally

221. The syndrome of Mulibrey nanism leads to:
   a. Familial heart block
   b. Familial hypertrophic cardiomyopathy
   c. Constrictive pericarditis
   d. Endocardial fibroelastosis

222. In which country hereditary cardiomyopathies (arrhythmogenic right ventricular dysplasia), causing familial dysrhythmia is common?
   a. Japan   b. Italy
   c. Philippines d. Taiwan

223. The association of familial syncope, sudden death and congenital deafness is:
   a. Ward–Romano syndrome
   b. Jervell and Lange-Nielsen syndrome
   c. Ellis-van Creveld syndrome
   d. Holt–Oram syndrome

ANSWERS WITH EXPLANATIONS

1. Ans. c. Ventricular septal defects

Braunwald 5th Ed; Page 878

Relative frequency of occurrence of cardiac malformations at birth

Disease	Percentage
Ventricular septal defect	30.5
Atrial septal defect	9.8
Patent ductus arteriosus	9.7
Pulmonic stenosis	6.9
Coarctation of the aorta	6.8
Aortic stenosis	6.1
Tetralogy of Fallot	5.8
Complete transposition of the great arteries	4.2
Persistent truncus arteriosus	2.2
Tricuspid atresia	1.3
All others	16.5

2. Ans. c. Hypoplastic left heart syndrome

Braunwald 5th Ed; Page 878

In general, children with congenital heart disease are predominantly male. Moreover, specific cardiac defect may show a definite gender preponderance. Patent ductus arteriosus, Ebstein's anomaly of tricuspid valve and atrial septal defect are more common in females where as valvular aortic stenosis, coarctation of the aorta, hypoplastic left heart, pulmonary and tricuspid atresia and transposition of great arteries are more common in males.

3. Ans. b. Ventricular septal defect

Braunwald 5th Ed; Page 878

The fetal alcohol syndrome consists of microcephaly, micrognathia, microphthalmia, prenatal growth retardation, developmental delay and cardiac defect. The most common cardiac defect is in the ventricular septum, i.e., VSD and it occurs in about 45% of affected infants.

4. Ans. d. All are true

Braunwald 5th Ed; Page 879

Genetics play important role in causation of congenital heart disease. A single gene mutation may be causative in the familial form of atrial septal defect with prolong AV conduction, mitral valve prolapse, VSD, congenital heart block, situs inversus, pulmonary hypertension and syndrome of Noonan, Leopard, Ellis-van Creveld and Kartagener syndrome. The <10% of all cardiac malformation can be accounted for bichromosomal aberrations or genetic mutations or transmission. In majority of the cases, it is only one of a pair of monozygotic twins is affected by congenital heart disease and it indicates that the vast majority of cardiovascular malformation are not inherited in a simple manner. Family studies have indicated a 2- to 10-fold increase in the incidence of congenital heart disease in siblings of affected patients or in offspring of affected parents. Malformation often are cordant or partially concordant within families.

5. Ans. d. All of the above

Braunwald 5th Ed; Page 880-881

Syndromes associated with cardiovascular involvement

Syndrome	Major cardiovascular manifestations	Major noncardiac abnormalities
Ellis-van Creveld	Single atrium or atrial septal defect	Chondrodystrophic dwarfism, nail dysplasia, polydactyly
TAR (thrombocytopenia-absent radius)	Atrial septal defect, tetralogy of Fallot	Radial aplasia or hypoplasia, thrombocytopnea
Holt–Oram	Atrial septal defect (other defects common)	Skeletal upper limb defect, hypoplasia of clavicles
Kartagener	Dextrocardia	Situs inversus, sinusitis, bronchiectasis
Laurence–Moon–Biedl–Bardet	Variable defects	Retinal pigmentation, obesity, polydactyly
Noonan	Pulmonic valve dysplasia, cardiomyopathy (usually hypertrophic)	Webbed neck, pectus, excavatum, cryptotchidism
Tuberous sclerosis	Rhabdomyoma, cardiomyopathy	Phakomatosis, bone lesions, hamartomatous skin lesions
Multiple lentigines (Leopard)	Pulmonic stenosis	Basal cell nevi, broad facies, rib anomalies, deafness
Rubinstein–Taybi	Patent ductus arteriosus (others)	Broad thumbs and toes, hypoplastic maxilla, slanted palpebral fissures
Familial deafness	Arrhythmias, sudden death	Sensorineural deafness
Weber–Osler–Rendu	Arteriovenous fistulas (lung, liver, mucous membranes)	Multiple telangiectasias
Apert	Ventricular septal defect	Craniosynostosis, midfacial hypoplasia, syndactyly
Crouzon's	Patent ductus arteriosus, aortic coarctation	Ptosis with shallow orbits, craniosynostosis, maxillary hypoplasia
Hypertrophic cardiomyopathy	Asymmetric septal hypertrophy	Family history of sudden death
Incontinentia pigment	Patent ductus arteriosus	Irregular pigmented skin lesions, patchy alopecia, hypodontia
Alagille (arteriohepatic dysplasia)	Peripheral pulmonic stenosis, pulmonic stenosis	Biliary hypoplasia, vertebral anomalies, prominent forehead, deep-set eyes
DiGeorge	Interrupted aortic arch, tetralogy of Fallot, truncus arteriosus	Thymic hypoplasia or aplasia, parathyroid aplasia or hypoplasia, ear anomalies
Friedreich's ataxia	Cardiomyopathy and conduction defects	Ataxia, speech defect, degeneration of spinal cord dorsal columns
Muscular dystrophy	Cardiomyopathy	Pseudohypertrophy of calf muscles, weakness of trunk and proximal limb muscles
Cystic fibrosis	Cor pulmonale	Pancreatic insufficiency, malabsorption, chronic lung disease
Sickle cell anemia	Cardiomyopathy, mitral regurgitation	Hemoglobin SS
Conradi–Hunermann	Ventricular septal defect, patent ductus arteriosus	Asymmetrical limb shortness, early punctate mineralization, large skin pores
Cockayne	Accelerated atherosclerosis	Cachectic dwarfism, retinal pigment abnormalities, photosensitivity dermatitis
Progeria	Accelerated atherosclerosis	Premature aging, alopecia, atrophy of subcutaneous fat, skeletal hypoplasia
Connective tissue disorders		
Cutis laxa	Peripheral pulmonic stenosis	Generalized disruption of elastic fibers, diminished skin resilience, hernias
Ehlers–Danlos	Arterial dilatation and rupture, mitral regurgitation	Hyperextensible joints, hyperelastic and friable

Continued

Continued

Syndrome	Major cardiovascular manifestations	Major noncardiac abnormalities
Marfan	Aortic dilatation, aortic and mitral incompetence	Gracile habitus, arachnodactyly with hyperextensibility, lens subluxation
Osteogenesis imperfect	Aortic incompetence	Fragile bones, blue sclera
Pseudoxanthoma elasticum	Peripheral and coronary arterial disease	Degeneration of elastic fibers in skin, retinal angioid streaks
Inborn errors of metabolism		
Pompe disease	Glycogen storage disease of heart	Acid maltase deficiency, muscular weakness
Homocystinuria	Aortic and pulmonary artery dilatation, intravascular thrombosis	Cystathionine synthetase deficiency, lens subluxation, osteoporosis
Mucopolysaccharidoses: Hurler, Hunter	Multivalvular and coronary and great artery disease; cardiomyopathy	*Hurler*: Deficiency of ∞-L-iduronidase, corneal clouding, coarse features, growth and mental retardation *Hunter*: Deficiency of L-idurano-sulfate sulfatase, coarse facies, clear cornea, growth and mental retardation
Morquio; Scheie; Maroteaux–Lamy	Aortic regurgitation	*Morquio*: Deficiency of N-acetylhexosamine sulfate sulfatase, cloudy cornea, severe bone changes involving vertebrae and epiphyses *Scheie*: Deficiency of ∞-L-iduronidase, cloudy cornea, normal intelligence, peculiar facies *Maroteaux–Lamy*: Deficiency of aryl-sulfatase B, cloudy cornea, osseous changes
Chromosomal abnormalities		
Trisomy 21 (Down syndrome)	Endocardial cushion defect, atrial or ventricular septal defect, tetralogy of Fallot	Hypotonia, hyperextensible joints, mongoloid facies, mental retardation
Trisomy 13 (D)	Ventricular septal defect, right ventricle patent ductus arteriosus, double-outlet right ventricle	Single midline intracerebral ventricle with midfacial defects, polydactyly, nail changes, mental retardation
Trisomy 18 (E)	Congenital polyvalvular dysplasia, ventricular septal defect, patent ductus	Clenched hand, short sternum, low arch dermal ridge pattern on fingertips, mental retardation
Cri du chat (short-arm deletion-5)	Ventricular septal defect	Cat cry, microcephaly, antimongoloid slant of palpebral fissures, mental retardation
XO (Turner)	Coarctation of the aorta, bicuspid aortic valve, aortic dilatation	Short female, broad chest, lymphedema, webbed neck
XXXY and XXXXX	Patent ductus arteriosus	*XXXY*: Hypogenitalism, mental retardation, radial-ulnar synostosis *XXXXX*: Small hands, incurving of fifth fingers, mental retardation
Sporadic disorders		
Vater association	Ventricular septal defect	Vertebral anomalies, anal atresia, tracheoesophageal fistula, radial and renal anomalies
Charge association	Tetralogy of Fallot (other defects common)	Colobomas, choanal atresia, mental and growth deficiency, genital and ear anomalies
Williams	Supravalvular aortic stenosis, peripheral pulmonic stenosis	Mental deficiency, Elfin facies, loquacious personality, hoarse voice
Cornelia de Lange	Ventricular septal defect	Micromelia, synophrys, mental and growth deficiency
Shprintzen (velocardiofacial)	Ventricular septal defect, tetralogy of Fallot, right aortic arch	Cleft palate, prominent nose, slender hands, learning disability
Long Q-T (Jervell and Lange–Nielsen, Romano–Ward)	Long Q-T interval, ventricular arrhythmias	Family history of sudden death, congenital deafness (not in Romano–Ward)

Continued

Continued

Syndrome	Major cardiovascular manifestations	Major noncardiac abnormalities
Teratogenic disorders		
Rubella	Patent ductus arteriosus, pulmonic valvular and/or arterial stenosis, atrial septal defect	Cataracts, deafness, microcephaly
Alcohol	Ventricular septal defect (other defects)	Microcephaly, growth and mental deficiency, short palpebral fissures, smooth philtrum, thin upper lip
Dilantin	Pulmonic stenosis, aortic stenosis, coarctation, patent ductus arteriosus	Hypertelorism, growth and mental deficiency, short phalanges, bowed upper lip
Thalidomide	Variable	Phocomelia
Lithium	Ebstein's anomaly, tricuspid atresia	None

6. Ans. c. Apert syndrome

Braunwald 5th Ed; Page 880-881

Refer to explanation for Q. No 5.

7. Ans. c. Both of the above

Braunwald 5th Ed; Page 880-881

Refer to explanation for Q. No 5.

8. Ans. c. Pseudoxanthoma elasticum

Braunwald 5th Ed; Page 880-881

Refer to explanation for Q. No 5.

9. Ans. d. Mucopolysaccharidoses

Braunwald 5th Ed; Page 880-881

Refer to explanation for Q. No 5.

10. Ans. b. Ventricular septal defect

Braunwald 5th Ed; Page 880-881

Refer to explanation for Q. No 5.

11. Ans. c. Dilantin

Braunwald 5th Ed; Page 880-881

Refer to explanation for Q. No 5.

12. Ans. a. 7-10%

Braunwald 5th Ed; Page 883-884

In fetal life, pulmonary arteries and arterioles are surrounded by a fluid medium, have relatively thick walls and small lumina, and resemble comparable arteries in the systemic circulation. The low pulmonary blood flow in the fetus (7-10% of the total cardiac output) is the result of high pulmonary vascular resistance. Fetal pulmonary vessels are highly reactive to changes in oxygen tension or in the pH of blood perfusing them as well as to a number of other physiological and pharmacological influences.

Although fetal somatic growth may be unimpaired, the hemodynamic effects in utero of many cardiac malformations may alter the development and structure of the fetal heart and circulation. Thus, total anomalous pulmonary venous connection in utero may result in underdevelopment of the left atrium and left ventricle and premature closure of the foramen ovale may result in hypoplasia of the left ventricle. Moreover, postnatally, the caliber of the aortic isthmus may be reduced in the presence of lesions in utero that create left ventricular hypertrophy and impede filling because of reduced compliance of that chamber. It may also be reduced in the presence of a lesion that interferes with left ventricular filling directly (e.g., mitral stenosis) or indirectly by diverting a proportion of left ventricular output away from the ascending aorta while increasing right ventricular output and ductus arteriosus flow (e.g., atrioventricular septal defect with left ventricular-right atrial shunt or aortic or subaortic stenosis with ventricular septal defect). Similarly, obstruction in utero to right ventricular outflow is associated with an increase in proximal aortic flow and diameter and almost never with aortic coarctation. In these and other examples, it is important to recognize that malformations compatible with fetal survival may nonetheless result in abnormal development of the circulation in utero and also affect circulatory adjustments after birth.

Compared with the adult heart the fetal and newborn heart is unique with respect to its ultra structural appearance, its mechanical and biochemical properties and its autonomic innervations.

During the late fetal and early neonatal development there is maturation of the excitation-contraction coupling process and the biochemical composition of the heart's energy-utilizing myofibrillar proteins and of adenosine triphosphate and creatinine phosphate energy-producing proteins. Moreover, fetal and neonatal myocardial cells are small in diameter and reduced in density, so that the young heart contains relatively more noncontractile mass (primarily mitochondria, nuclei, and surface membranes) than later in postnatal life. As a result, force generation and the extent and velocity of shortening are decreased, and stiffness and water content of ventricular myocardium are increased in the fetal and early newborn periods.

The diminished function of the young heart is reflected in its limited ability to increase cardiac output in the presence of either a volume load or a lesion that increases resistance to emptying. Although functional integrity exists of efferent and afferent cardiac autonomic pathways early in life, fetal and newborn myocardial lacks the complete development of sympathetic but not cholinergic innervations. Thus, adaptation to cardiocirculatory stress in fetal or early newborn life may be less effective than in adulthood.

13. Ans. b. The RV contributes about 45% and the left ventricle 55% to the total fetal cardiac output

Braunwald 5th Ed; Page 883-884

Refer to explanation for Q. No 12.

14. Ans. b. Reduction in systemic vascular resistance

Braunwald 5th Ed; Page 883-884

Refer to explanation for Q. No 12.

15. Ans. b. Within 72 hours

Braunwald 5th Ed; Page 883-884

Refer to explanation for Q. No 12.

16. Ans. d. Within four to twelve months of birth

Braunwald 5th Ed; Page 883-884

Refer to explanation for Q. No 12.

17. Ans. d. All of the above

Braunwald 5th Ed; Page 883-884

Refer to explanation for Q. No 12.

18. Ans. d. Increased fetal movements

Braunwald 5th Ed; Page 884

The development of fetal echocardiography has improved the diagnosis of intrauterine cardiac failure. The cardinal findings of fetal heart failure are scalp edema, ascites, pericardial effusion, and decreased fetal movements.

19. Ans. a. Patent ductus arteriosus

Braunwald 5th Ed; Page 884 & 889

In the preterm infant, especially under 1,500 g birth weight persistent patency of ductus arteriosus is the most common cause of cardiac decompensation and other form of structural heart diseases are rare. In the full-term newborn, the earliest important causes of heart failure are, the hypoplastic left heart and coarctation of aorta syndrome, sustained tachyarrhythmias, cerebral or hepatic arteriovenous fistula and myocarditis. Among the lesion commonly producing heart failure beyond age 1-2 weeks, when diminished pulmonary vascular resistance allows substantial left-to-right shunting are ventricular septal defect and atrioventricular septal defect, transposition of great arteries, truncus arteriosus and total anomalous venous connection often with pulmonary venous obstruction.

20. Ans. d. Ventricular septal defect

Braunwald 5th Ed; Page 884 & 889

Refer to explanation for Q. No 19.

21. Ans. c. Pleural and pericardial effusion

Braunwald 5th Ed; Page 884

The clinical expression of cardiac decompensation in the infant consist of distinctive sign of pulmonary and systemic venous congestion and altered cardio circulatory performance that resemble but often are not identical to those of older children or adult. These reflect the interplay between the hemodynamic burden and adaptive response. Common symptoms and signs are feeding difficulties, and failure to gain weight and grow, tachycardia, tachypnea, pulmonary rales and rhonchi, liver enlargement and cardiomegaly. Less frequent manifestations includes peripheral edema, ascites, pulsus alternans, gallop rhythm and inappropriate sweating. Pleural and pericardial effusions are exceedingly rare in these groups of patients.

22. Ans. d. All are correct

Braunwald 5th Ed: Page 884

Clinical manifestation of heart failure in infants varies comparison to their counterpart. Fatigue and dyspnea on exertion express themselves as a feeding problem in the infants. Characteristically, the respiratory rate in heart failure is rapid between 50 to 100 breaths/minutes. In the presence of left ventricular failure, interstitial pulmonary edema reduces pulmonary compliance and result into the tachypnea and intercostal retractions. Excessive pulmonary blood flow by way of significant left to right shunt may further decrease lung compliance. Moreover, upper airways obstruction may be produced by selective enlargement of cardiovascular structures. In patient with large left to right shunt and left atrial and main pulmonary artery enlargement, the left main bronchus may be compressed resulting in emphysematous expansion of left upper or lower lobe or left lower lobe collapse. Respiratory distress with grunting, flaring of the alae nasi and intercostal retraction observed when failure is severe and especially when pulmonary infection precipitate cardiac decompensation which often is the case. A resting heart rate with little variability is also characteristic of heart failure in infants. Hepatomegaly is regularly seen in infants in failure although liver tenderness is uncommon. Cardiomegaly may be assessed by X-ray but it must be recognized that in the normal newborn infant the cardiac diameter may be as much as 60% of thoracic diameter and the large thymus gland in infant occasionally interfere with evaluation of heart size. 2D-echocardiography and Doppler provide a good estimate of cardiac performance and chamber dimensions for diagnosis of heart failure in this subset of patients.

23. Ans. a. 3.9 mg/dL

Braunwald 5th Ed; Page 885

Cyanosis is produced by reduced hemoglobin in cutaneous vessels in excess of approximately 3 g/dL.

24. Ans. d. All are useful

Braunwald 5th Ed; Page 885

Hypercyanotic or hypoxemic spell commonly complicate the clinical course in younger children with certain type of cyanotic congenital heart disease especially tetralogy of Fallot. The spells are characterized by anxiety, hyperapnea and a sudden, marked increase in cyanosis. They are the result of abrupt reduction in pulmonary blood flow. Unless terminated the hypercyanotic episode may lead to the convulsion and may even prove fatal. The sudden reduction in the pulmonary blood flow may be precipitated by fluctuation in arterial pCO_2 and pH, a sudden fall in systemic or increase in the pulmonary vascular resistance or an acute increase in the severity of right ventricular outflow tract obstruction either by augmented contraction of the hypertrophied muscle in the right ventricular outflow tract or by a decrease in the right ventricular cavity volume owing to the tachycardia. The treatment of hypoxic spells consists of oxygen administration, placing the child in the knee chest position and administration of morphine sulfate. Additional medications that may prove to be of value include the intravenous administration of sodium bicarbonate to correct the accompanying acidosis, alpha adenoreceptor stimulant such as phenylephrine hydrochloride or methoxamine to raise peripheral resistance and diminish right to left shunting and beta adrenoreceptor blocking agents which reduces cardiac sympathetic tone and depresses cardiac contractility and increases the ventricular volume by reducing the heart rate.

25. Ans. d. All are correct

Braunwald 5th Ed; Page 886

Impaired growth and physical development and delayed onset of adolescence are common feature of many cyanotic and to a lesser extent acyanotic form of congenital heart disease. Mental development seldom is affected. The severity of growth disturbance depends on the anatomic lesions and its functional effect. Most children with mild defect grow normally. Weight gain is commonly slower than linear growth in acyanotic patient with large left to right shunts, whereas in cyanotic congenital heart disease height and weight is usually parallel each other. Boys appear to be more retarded in the growth than girls especially in the second decade. Skeletal maturity (i.e., bone age) is delayed in cyanotic children in relation to the severity of hypoxemia.

26. Ans. b. Cardiac catheterization

Braunwald 5th Ed; Page 887

There are standard methods of assessing the severity of pulmonary vascular obstructive disease. Clinical and electrocardiographic observations do not distinguish between reversible and irreversible elevation in pulmonary vascular resistance. Echocardiography and Doppler interrogation of heart may enable one to diagnose the presence of pulmonary hypertension but do not provide an accurate estimate of pressure or to a reliable calculation of pulmonary vascular resistance. The hemodynamic measurements at cardiac catheterization are the main stay in assessing the pulmonary vascular bed especially its reactivity. The premium on accuracy is high because the presence, degree, and reactivity of pulmonary vascular obstruction determine the feasibility and long-term outcome of surgery. Surgery must not be offered to the patient with severe, fixed pulmonary vascular obstruction even when the cardiac defect is anatomically correctable. Such patient either do not survive operation or if they do, are not benefited and more often than not are harmed.

27. Ans. d. Amoxycillin orally (3 g) before the procedure and repeated (1.5 g) after 6 hours

Braunwald 5th Ed; Page 888

Prophylactic antibiotics for protection from bacterial endocarditis:

I. **Standard prophylactic regimen for dental/oral/upper respiratory tract procedures**
   - Amoxicillin 3.0 g orally 1 hour before procedure, then 1.5 gm 6 hours after initial dose.
   - For amoxicillin/penicillin—allergic individuals: Erythromycin ethylsuccinate 800 mg or erythromycin stearate 1 g orally 2 hours before a procedure, then one-half the dose 6 hours after the initial administration.
   OR
   - Clindamycin 300 mg 1 hour before a procedure, and 150 mg 6 hours after initial dose.

II. **Alternative prophylactic regimens for dental/oral/upper respiratory tract procedures**
   - For patients unable to take oral medications: Ampicillin 2.0 g IV (or IM) 30 minutes before procedure, then 1.0 g ampicillin IV (or IM) or 1.5 g amoxicillin orally 6 hours after initial dose.

- For ampicillin/amoxicillin/penicillin—allergic patients unable to take oral medications: Clindamycin 300 mg IV 1 hour before a procedure and 150 mg IV (or orally) 6 hours after initial dose.
- Optional regimen for individuals considered to be at very high risk who are not candidates for the standard regimen: Ampicillin 2.0 g IV (or IM) plus gentamicin 1.5 mg/kg IV (or IM) (not to exceed 80 mg) one-half hour before procedure, followed by 1.5 g oral amoxicillin 6 hours after the initial dose. Alternatively, the parenteral regimen may be repeated 8 hours after the initial dose.
- Optional regimen for amoxicillin/ampicillin/penicillin—allergic patients: Vancomycin 1.0 g IV administered over 1 hour starting 1 hour before the procedure. No repeat dose is necessary.

III. **Regimens for Genitourinary/Gastrointestinal procedures**
- Standard Regimen: Ampicillin 2.0 g IV (or IM) plus gentamicin 1.5 mg/kg IV (or IM) (not to exceed 80 mg) one half hour before procedure, followed by 1.5 g oral amoxicillin 6 hours after the initial dose. Alternatively, the parenteral regimen may be repeated once 8 hours after the initial dose.
- For amoxicillin/ampicillin/penicillin—allergic patients: Vancomycin 1.0 g IV administered over 1 hour plus gentamicin 1.5 mg/kg IV (or IM) (not to exceed 80 mg) 1 hour before the procedure. May be repeated once 8 hours after initial dose.
- Alternative oral regimen in low-risk patients: Amoxicillin 3.0 g orally 1 hour before the procedure, then 1.5 g 6 hours after the initial dose.

Note: Initial pediatric dosages are listed below. Follow-up doses should be one-half the initial dose. Total pediatric dose should not exceed total adult dose.

Amoxicillin	50 mg/kg
Ampicillin	50 mg/kg
Clindamycin	10 mg/kg
Gentamicin	2.0 mg/kg
Vancomycin Erythromycin	20 mg/kg
Ethylsuccinate or stearate	20 mg/kg

28. Ans. d. All are correct

Braunwald 5th Ed; Page 889

It has long been recognized that there is unique fragility and liability of the neonatal circulation in response to diseases states and various physiological stimuli. It is often found that newborns may exhibit suboptimal therapeutic responses to drug such as digitalis which directly stimulate cardiac contractility. The age dependency of these observation have their basis in the reduce ability of the heart of premature and full-term newborns when compared with the heart and circulation of older children or adults to call on a functional reserve capacity to adapt to the stress. Studies have shown that there is a structural, functional, biochemical and pharmacological properties of the young heart defer considerably from those of its older counterpart. The young heart contains fewer myofilaments to generate force with shorten during contraction. In addition, the chamber is stiffness of young heart ventricle is greater than that seen in later in the life.

29. Ans. c. a + b

Braunwald 5th Ed; Page 890

Digoxin is the glycocyte used exclusively to treat pediatric patients for most of the cardiac illness because it is readily observed, available in convenient doses form and excreted rapidly from the body. Premature infants are more sensitive to digitalis than are full-term newborn, who in turn are more sensitive than the older infant. Infants absorb and excrete digoxin as well as adults do and the relative distribution of the glycocyte to different body tissue are also similar. The prevailing dose schedule for digoxin produces, higher serum concentration in infants than would be considered optimal for adults. The basis for the higher digitalis requirement in infancy is unclear although it may relate to an age dependent alteration in the sensitivity of myocardium per se to the glycocytes. Infants tolerate higher serum digoxin concentration than adults without developing signs of toxicity. In the adults, the usual therapeutic concentrations of digoxin are <2 ng/mL blood and toxicity commonly occurs above that level. In contrast in infants, therapeutic level of digoxin ranges from 1 to 5 ng/mL (mean 3.5) while toxicity is associated with concentration in excess of 3 ng/mL. Older children have therapeutic and toxic levels similar to those of adults.

30. Ans. c. 1–5 ng/mL

Braunwald 5th Ed; Page 890

Refer to explanation for Q. No 29.

31. Ans. b. Coarctation of aorta with PDA in transposition of great arteries

Braunwald 5th Ed; Page 891

Differential cyanosis indicates when one half of the body is pink and other half of the body is blue. Differential cyanosis always indicates the presence of congenital heart disease often with patency of ductus arteriosus and coarctation of aorta as component of abnormal anatomical complex. If the upper part of the body is pink, and lower part of the body is blue then coarctation of aorta or interruption of aortic arch is probable with oxygenated blood supplying the upper body and the desaturated blood supplying the lower body by way of right to left shunt through ductus arteriosus.

The latter also occur in patient with patent ductus arteriosus and markedly elevated pulmonary vascular resistance. A patient with transposition of great arteries and coarctation of aorta with retrograde flow through a patent ductus arteriosus demonstrate the reverse situation, i.e., the lower part of the body is pink and upper part of the body is blue. Simultaneous determination of oxygen saturation in the temporal or right brachial artery and femoral artery are helpful in confirming the presence of differential cyanosis.

32. Ans. c. Decreased or ineffective pulmonary blood flows

Braunwald 5th Ed; Page 893

Blood gas and pH patterns: Arterial blood gas analysis may be a reliable method of evaluating cyanosis, suggesting the type of altered physiology, and assessing responses to therapeutic maneuvers. Specimens for blood gas analysis should be obtained in room air and in 100% oxygen. Stick capillary samples from the patient's warmed heel may be used, although determinations obtained by arterial puncture are preferable for evaluation of oxygenation because they are less susceptible to alterations in regional blood flow in the critically ill infant. Sampling of right radial or temporal arterial blood is preferable because these sites are proximal to flow through a ductus arteriosus and do not reflect right-to-left ductal shunting, as would a sample from the descending aorta obtained by means of an umbilical artery catheter. A trial of continuous positive airway pressure may improve oxygenation in infants with either hyaline membrane disease or pulmonary edema.

Arterial blood gas patterns in various pathophysiological conditions are listed in the table below. Pattern 1 typically is observed in infants with ventilation–perfusion abnormalities resulting from primary respiratory disease, often associated with elevated pulmonary vascular resistance and venoarterial shunting across a patent foramen ovale or patent ductus arteriosus. Pulmonary hypoventilation with CO_2 retention produces pattern 2. In the presence of a lesion causing obligatory venous admixture, such as total anomalous pulmonary venous connection (pattern 3), the response to oxygen may reflect an increase in pulmonary venous return secondary to a fall in pulmonary vascular resistance. Pattern 4 typically is seen in infants with a cardiac malformation that results in reduced pulmonary blood flow. Oxygen administration in these infants does not alter the arterial pO_2. The alterations of pattern 5 are observed when systemic hypoperfusion is the principal hemodynamic problem. In these babies the arteriovenous oxygen difference is high, and the academia may be progressive and unrelenting.

Arterial blood gas patterns in various disorders causing cyanosis in infants

Pattern	pH	pO₂	pCO₂	Response to O₂	Venous pH	Suggested condition
1	↓	↓↓	↑	↑↑	↓	Hyaline membrane or other pulmonary parenchymal disease
2	↓	↓	↑↑↑	↑	↓	Hypoventilation
3	-	↓	-	↑	-	Venous admixture
4	↓	↓↓	-	-	↓	Decreased or ineffective pulmonary blood flow
5	↓↓↓	↓	-↑	-↑	↓↓↓	Systemic hypoperfusion

33. Ans. c. Tricuspid atresia

Braunwald 5th Ed; Page 894

Electrocardiogram is less helpful in suggesting a diagnosis of heart disease in the premature and newborn infant than in the older child. Right ventricular hypertrophy is a normal finding in the neonate. However, a specific observation may offer major clues to the presence of a cardiovascular anomaly. A counterclockwise superiorly oriented frontal QRS loop with absent or reduced right ventricular force suggest diagnosis of tricuspid atresia. When QRS axis is normal but left ventricular forces dominate, the diagnosis of pulmonary atresia must be considered. The counterclockwise superior QRS orientation is also observed in patient with endocardial cushion defect and in some patients with double outlet right ventricle. Right ventricular forces in these babies are found to be increased.

34. Ans. d. All of the above

Braunwald 5th Ed; Page 894

Chest radiography often is helpful in differentiating between respiratory and cardiac causes of cyanosis in the newborn period. Determination of a normal cardiac and abdominal situs aids in ruling out several kind of complex cyanotic cardiac malformation associated with asplenia, polysplenia with abdominal heterotaxy and dextrocardia. The evaluation of pulmonary vascular marking helps in categorizing congenital cardiac malformation in the newborn infants according to the function. In the presence of cyanosis, diminished pulmonary blood and diminished pulmonary vascular marking calls attention to the group of anomaly that includes tetralogy of Fallot, pulmonary stenosis with intact ventricular septum, pulmonary atresia, tricuspid atresia and Ebstein formation of tricuspid valve. Produce pulmonary blood flow is responsible for systemic arterial desaturation in these babies. Increase pulmonary vascular marking in the cyanotic infants are associated with lesion in which obligatory mixture of systemic venous and pulmonary venous blood occurs. The more common anomaly in this category include transposition of great arteries, hypoplastic left heart syndrome, truncus arteriosus and total anomalous venous drainage. A right sided aortic arch in X-ray chest suggests the presence of either TOF or persistent truncus arteriosus. An ovoid heart with a narrow base associated with increase pulmonary vascular marking is a typical of transposition of great arteries. A boot shaped heart with concavity of pulmonary vascular outflow tract suggests TOF, pulmonary atresia or tricuspid atresia.

35. Ans. c. 16 weeks of gestation

Braunwald 5th Ed; Page 894

Ultrasound technology allows the examination of human fetal cardiac development and function in uterus. Diagnostic quality of images of the fetus and fetal heart in utero can be obtained as early as 16th week of gestation.

36. Ans. c. Sinus venosus ASD

Braunwald 5th Ed; Page 900

Electrocardiogram often helps in diagnosing the different types of atrial septal defect. In patient with an ostium secundum defect, the electrocardiogram usually shows right axis deviation, right ventricular hypertrophy and r-s-R- patent in the right precordial lead with a normal QRS duration. Left axis deviation of the P wave in the frontal plane (manifested by a negative P wave in lead III), suggest the presence of a sinus venosus rather than an ostium secundum type of atrial septal defect. Left axis deviation and superior orientation and counterclockwise rotation of QRS loop in the frontal plane suggest the presence of either an ostium primum or a secundum atrial septal defect in association with mitral valve prolapse. Prolongation of PR interval may be seen with all type of atrial septal defects. The prolonged internodal conduction time may be related to the both the increase size of atrium and also an increase distance for internodal conduction produced by the defect itself. The diagnosis of ostium primum type of atrial septal defect is reliably established by selective left ventricular angiocardiography using rapid injection of relatively large quantities of contrast material. The finding includes an absence of AV septum and a deficiency of the inlet portion of ventricular septum with elongation of left ventricular outflow tract in relation to the inflow tract. The aortic valve is elevated and displaced anteriorly, relative to the atrioventricular valves changing the relation between the anterior components of the left AV valve and the aorta which produces a pathognomonic goose neck deformity seen angiographically in the diastole. It is best seen in anteroposterior projection in left ventricular angiography. This arrangement can also be defined in the subxiphoid long axis view of the left ventricular outflow tract in echocardiography.

37. Ans. b. Subcostal view

Braunwald 5th Ed; Page 900

Refer to explanation for Q. No 36.

38. Ans. d. Common AV canal defect

Braunwald 5th Ed; Page 900

Refer to explanation for Q. No 36.

39. Ans. b. It is visualized best in right anterior obligue left ventriculogram

Braunwald 5th Ed; Page 900

Refer to explanation for Q. No 36.

40. Ans. a. Membranous septum

Braunwald 5th Ed; Page 901

Ventricular septal defect: Among the most prevalent of cardiac malformations, defects of the ventricular septum occur commonly, both as isolated anomalies and in combination with other anomalies. The ventricular septum is made up of four comparements: The membraneous septum, the inlet septum, the trabecular septum and the outlet, or infundibular septum. Defects results from a deficiency of growth or a failure of alignment or fusion of component parts. Defects most commonly are classified as occurring in or adjacent to one or more of the septal components.

The most common defects occur in the region of the membraneous septum, and are referred to as paramembranous or perimembranous defects because they are larger than the membranous septum itself and are associated with a muscular defect at a portion of their perimeter. They are also known as infracristal, subaortic, or conoventricular defects. These perimembranous defects also can be defined by their adjacent areas as inlet, trabecular, or outlet. A second type of defect is one with an entirely muscular rim. Such muscular defects also can be defined as inlet, trabecular, vary greatly in size, shape and number. A third type of defect occurs when the outlet septum is deficient and commonly is referred to as supracristal, subpulmonary, outlet, infundibular, conoseptal. Because the aortic and pulmonary valves are in fibrous continuity, this type of defect also may be referred to as doubly committed subarterial. A septal deficiency of the site of the atrioventricular septum characterizes defects called atrioventricular septal, atrioventricular canal, or inlet septal defects.

The other feature of any defect may be a malalignment of the septal components. Either the inlet or the outlet septum can be malaligned. Malalignment of the inlet septum produces either mitral or tricuspid valve override and/or straddle. Malalignment of the outlet septum can be to the right or the left of the trabecular septum; when to the left of the trabecular septum, the ventricular septal defect is characteristic of tetralogy of Fallot, double-outlet ventricle, truncus arteriosus, and, in some cases, transposition of the great arteries.

41. Ans. d. Infundibular septum

Braunwald 5th Ed; Page 901

Refer to explanation for Q. No 41.

42. Ans. b. Appearance of pulmonary vascular obstructive disease

Braunwald 5th Ed; Page 903

Pulmonary hypertension is the serious complication of the presence of ventricular septal defect in a children which fail to close. It is of utmost importance to identify patients who develops irreversible pulmonary vascular obstructive disease (the Eisenmenger reaction). Retrospective analysis of children who developed this complication indicate that infants with systemic or near systemic pressures in the pulmonary artery at the time of initial hemodynamic study are most at-risk. If a child who previously had a louder murmur and a thrill associated with poor physical growth suddenly has a growth spurt, fewer respiratory infection and a diminution in the intensity of cardiac murmur and disappearance of the thrill, he or she may be developing severe obliterative changes in the pulmonary vascular bed. Increase in the intensity of pulmonary component of second heart sound, reduction in the heart size on chest X-ray and more pronounced right ventricular hypertrophy on electrocardiogram are often found and these changes occur because of the increase pulmonary vascular resistance cause a decrease in the left to right shunt. If these changes are suspected cardiac catheterization should be performed and if it is confirmed then prompt surgical repair is indicated before an inoperable predominate right to left shunt ensues in these patient. If operation is performed before age of 2 years, pulmonary vascular resistance may be expected to fall to normal level.

43. Ans. d. Aortic regurgitation

Braunwald 5th Ed; Page 903

Aortic regurgitation is a well-described complication of ventricular septal defect and it occurs in about 5% of the patients. It is usually noted after the age of 5 years when physician detects the early diastolic blowing murmur and wide pulse pressure of aortic regurgitation during examination of a patient with ventricular septal defect. The diagnosis is readily confirmed by Doppler echocardiography.

44. Ans. d. In most patients with VSD and aortic regurgitation, the ventricular septal defect is large

Braunwald 5th Ed; Page 903

In most patients with ventricular septal defect and aortic regurgitation, the ventricular septal defect is small to moderate in size and mild right ventricular outflow tract obstruction exist. The latter is caused by either subpulmonic infundibular stenosis or projection of herniated aortic cusp into the right ventricular outflow tract. The distinction between the types of ventricular septal defect with aortic regurgitation is usually made by 2D-echocardiography and Doppler and by selective left ventriculography to define the site of interventricular communication in combination with retrograde aortography to assess the anatomy and competence of aortic valve. The ventricular septal defect with aortic regurgitation is rare in Europe and in United States with the incidence of about 4% of all cases of isolated ventricular septal defect. Whereas in the Japan, the incidence is substantially higher about 10%. In the Japanese, in particular, aortic regurgitation is the result of herniation of aortic leaflet (usually the right coronary) through a subpulmonic supracristal ventricular septal defect.

45. Ans. d. All of the above

Braunwald 5th Ed; Page 905

The shift in oxygen dependence from placenta to the lungs, soon after the birth produces the sudden increase in the arterial blood oxygen tension, which along with alteration in the local prostaglandin milieu initiate constriction of the ductus arteriosus. Pulmonary pressure falls further as the ductus constrict. In healthy mature infant, the ductus arteriosus is profoundly constricted at 10–15 hours and is closed functionally by 72 hours with total anatomical closure following within a few weeks by a process of thrombosis, intimal proliferation and fibrosis. A high incidence exists in preterm infants of persistent patency of the ductus arteriosus because of an immaturity of these mechanism responsible for constriction. In surviving preterm infants, the ductus arteriosus is closed spontaneously within in 4–12 months of the birth.

46. Ans. d. Occurs mostly with other congenital anomalies

Braunwald 5th Ed; Page 905

There is a difference between patency of the ductus arteriosus in the preterm infant who lacks the normal mechanism for postnatal ductal closure because of immaturity and the full term newborn in whom patency of the ductus is a true congenital malformation, probably related to a primary anatomical defect of the elastic tissue within the wall of the ductus. In full-term infants and children, patency of the ductus arteriosus occurs particularly in females and in the offspring of pregnancy complicated by first trimester rubella. Although most frequent in isolated form, the anomaly may coexist with other malformations particularly coarctation of aorta, ventricular septal defect, pulmonic stenosis and aortic stenosis. Flow across the ductus is determined by pressure relation between the aorta and pulmonary artery and by the cross-sectional area and length of ductus itself. In aorticopulmonary septal defect, the usual defect consists of a communication between the aorta and pulmonary artery just above the semilunar valves. Persistent patency of ductus arteriosus is an associated lesion in 10–15% of the cases. Less common accompanying cardiovascular lesion includes VSD, aortic arch interruption, coarctation of aorta and right sided aortic arch.

47. Ans. b. PDA

Braunwald 5th Ed; Page 905

Refer to explanation for Q. No 46.

48. Ans. a. Before 3 months of age

Braunwald 5th Ed; Page 908

The early fatal course as well as early development of pulmonary vascular obstructive disease in patients of truncus arteriosus is responsible for poor prognosis associated with this lesion. In infants and young children with large left to right shunts surgical bending of one or both pulmonary arteries to reduce pulmonary flow has been used with little success. Corrective operation is indicated before age 3 months to avoid the development of severe pulmonary obstructive disease. Surgical treatment consists of closure of the ventricular septal defect, leaving the aorta arising from the left ventricle. The pulmonary arteries are detached from their truncus origin and a valve containing prosthetic conduit or aortic homograft valve conduit is used to establish continuity between right ventricle and pulmonary arteries. Important risk factors for perioperative deaths are severe truncal valve regurgitation, interrupted aortic arch, coronary artery anomalies and age at operation greater than 100 days. Patients with only one pulmonary artery are especially prone to early development of severe pulmonary vascular disease but otherwise are not at increase risk from surgery.

49. Ans. a. Right coronary artery

Perloff 3rd Ed; Page 511

Coronary arteriovenous fistula is an unusual anomaly that consists of communication between one of the coronary arteries and cardiac chamber or vein. The right coronary artery or its branches is the site of fistula in about 55% of cases. The left coronary artery is involved in 35% and both coronary arteries in 5% cases. Connection between coronary system and a cardiac chamber appear to represent persistent of embryonic intertrabecular phases and sinusoids. Most of these fistuals drain into the right ventricle, right atrium or coronary sinus. Fistulous communication to pulmonary artery, left atrium or left ventricle is much less frequent. Most often the shunt through the fistula is of a small magnitude and myocardial blood flow is not compromised. Rarely spontaneous closure may occur. Potential complication include pulmonary hypertension and congestive heart failure (if a large left to right shunt exists), bacterial endocarditis, rupture or thrombosis of fistula or an associated arterial aneurysm and myocardial ischemia distal to the fistula due to decrease coronary blood flow.

50. Ans. b. Right ventricle

Perloff 3rd Ed; Page 511

Refer to explanation for Q. No. 49.

51. Ans. a. Anomalous origin of left coronary artery from pulmonary trunk

Perloff 3rd Ed; Chapter 21, Page 504

The characteristic electrocardiographic pattern in patients with anomalous origin of coronary artery is in form of deep Q waves in association with ST segment alteration and T wave inversion in leads I, avL, V5 and V6. These finding greatly assist the distinction of this anomaly from myocarditis and dilated cardiomyopathy.

52. Ans. c. Aneurysm of circle of Wills

Braunwald 5th Ed; Page 911

Juxtaductal coarctation occurs 2–5 times more common in males than in females and there is high degree of association with gonadal dysgenesis (Turner syndrome) and bicuspid aortic valve. Other common associated anomalies include VSD and mitral stenosis or regurgitation. The most important extracardiac anomaly is aneurysm of circle of Willis. The cardiac anomalies that cause augmented ascending aortic blood flow (pulmonary atresia or stenosis, TOF), prevent development of a branch point and indeed are almost never seen in association with juxtaductal coarctation of aorta.

53. Ans. c. Tetralogy of Fallot

Braunwald 5th Ed; Page 911

Refer to explanation for Q. No 52.

54. Ans. a. Right ventricular hypertrophy and right axis deviation

Braunwald 5th Ed, Page 912

The characteristic electrocardiographic changes found in neonates and infant with coarctation of aorta is the right axis deviation and right ventricular hypertrophy. The electrocardiographic changes in children with coarctation of aorta reveals left ventricular hypertrophy of varying degree depending on the height of arterial pressure above the obstruction and the patient's age. Combined with right ventricular hypertrophy implies a complicated lesion.

55. Ans. c. Two D-echocardiography and Doppler assessment

Braunwald 5th Ed; Page 913

The diagnosis of aortic coarctation can be made by several non invasive and invasive modalities. The aortic coarctation may be visualized directly by 2 dimensional echocardiography from high parasternal or suprasternal notch views with short focus transducer and from the subxiphoid window with extended focal range transducers. Doppler examination reveals a flow disturbance and high velocity jet at the site of obstruction and provides a reasonable estimate of transcoarctation pressure gradient. Computed tomography, magnetic resonance imaging or cardiac catheterization and aortography also accurately localizes the site of obstruction, determines the length of coarctation and particularly identify associated malformation. Preoperative catheterization is avoided for selected patient with typical clinical and 2-D echocardiography and Doppler finding. Intravascular ultrasonography provides interesting morphological images suitable especially for comparison to postoperative status.

56. Ans. c. Paradoxical hypertension is noted more often following balloon angioplasty than the surgery

Braunwald 5th Ed; Page 913

Subclavian flap aortoplasty particularly in neonates and infants or surgical resection end to end anastomosis of uncomplicated juxtaductal coarctation of aorta can be accomplished with excellent result in most patients. In children, who are asymptomatic it is preferable to delay surgery until age 4-6 years at which time coarctation seldom recurs. Paradoxical hypertension of short duration often is noted in the immediate postoperative period, a phenomena much less common after balloon angioplasty. A resetting of carotid baroreceptor and increase catecholamines secretion appears to be responsible for the initial phase of postoperative systemic hypertension with latter, second phase of prolong elevation of systolic and particularly diastolic blood pressure related to activation of rennin angiotensin system. A necrotizing panarteritis of these small vessels of the gastrointestinal tract uncertain cause occasionally complicate the course of recovery. A 5-10% risk of recurrent narrowing exist after repair of coarctation in infancy such narrowing is best treated by magnetic resonance imaging or Doppler ultrasonography. This problem is treated most effectively by percutaneous balloon angioplasty which may be expected to markedly reduce the pressure difference across the site of coarctation.

57. Ans. d. All are correct

Braunwald 5th Ed; Page 913

The aortic isthmus, the portion of aorta between the left subclavian artery and ductus arteriosus, normally narrowed in the fetus and newborns. The lumen of aortic isthmus is about 2/3rd that of ascending and descending portion of aorta until age 6-9 months when the physiological narrowing disappeared. Pathological tubular hyperplasia of the aortic arch usually is noted in aortic isthmus and often is referred to as preductal or infantile coarctation of aorta. Associated major cardiac malformation occurs in virtually all such infants and includes large ventricular septal defect, atrioventricular septal defect, transposition of great arteries, the taussig-bing type of anomaly and double outlet right ventricle. The ventricular septal defect most often is subpulmonary lying within the substance of the infundibular septum.

58. Ans. d. All are correct

Braunwald 5th Ed; Page 913 - 914

The aortic arch interruption is rare and usually lethal anomaly. Unless treated surgically almost all infant die within the 1st month of life. Interruption distal to the left subclavian artery (type A) occurs with almost equal frequency to the interruptions distal to the left common carotid artery (type B). Interruption distal to the innominate artery (type C) is extremely uncommon. The right subclavian artery often is of variable origin frequently arising from the descending aortic segment distal to the interruption. Virtually all patients have associated intracardiac anomalies. A patent ductus arteriosus almost always connect the main pulmonary artery with descending aorta. With rare exception patient with interrupted aortic arch have either a VSD (80-90% of the cases) or an aorticopulmonary window (10-20%). There is a frequent association of this syndrome of aortic arch interruption with DiGeorge syndrome, a constellation of cardiac, parathyroid, thymic and facial anomalies attributed to the disruption of interaction of premigratory neural crest cells with endodermal pharyngeal pouch cells. In this syndrome, thymic hypoplasia or aplasia is accompanied by immunological and hypocalcemic problems.

59. Ans. c. 6 weeks

Braunwald 5th Ed; Page 878

The natural history of congenital heart disease begins before birth. The majority of congenital anomalies of the heart are present 6 weeks after conception and most anomalies compatible with 6 months of intrauterine life permits live offspring at term.

60. Ans. b. Congenital complete AV block

Perloff 3rd Ed; Chapter 1, Page 1

Congenital heart disease are not fixed anatomic defect that appear at birth but are instead a dynamic group of anomalies that originate in fetal life and change considerably during postnatal development. Certain defects are not anatomic in the gross morphological sense such as congenital complete heart block other such as Marfan syndrome and mitral valve prolapse are developmental disorders of connective tissue but by convention are not generally classified as congenital heart disease.

61. Ans. d. All of the above

Perloff 6th Ed; Page 1

A given congenital malformation may exist in relative harmony with the fetal circulation only to be modified considerably at least physiologically by the dramatic circulatory adjustment at birth. Weeks, months or years may elapse before the anomaly reveals itself as typical clinical picture. Physiologic and structural changes continue or conversely the malformation may vanish or witness spontaneous closure such as perimembranous ventricular septal defect. The ductus arteriosus in premature infant may remain widely patent for months, finally closing of its own accord and living the infant with a normal heart. A congenitally bicuspid aortic valve that is functionally normal at birth may take 2, 3 or more decades to stiffen, calcify and present as overt aortic stenosis.

62. Ans. d. All of the above

Braunwald 5th Ed; Page 884

The right and left ventricles do not function in series in the fetus. The fetal circulation is designed in such a way that blood with higher oxygen saturation preferencely reaches the myocardium and brain, whereas less saturated blood circulate preferencely to the placenta. The foramen ovale, the ductus venosus and the ductus arteriosus are intrinsic component of fetal circulation and normally close after birth.

63. Ans. c. Within 72 hours

Braunwald 5th Ed; Page 884

Profound circulatory changes occurs at birth. The lungs expand, pulmonary vascular resistance falls dramatically, pulmonary blood flow increases approximately 10-fold, the low resistance placenta circulation is removed and interruption of umbilical venous return is associated with closure of ductus venosus. Accordingly, gas exchange shift suddenly from the placenta to the lungs. The foramen ovale functionally closes because the 10-fold increase in the pulmonary arterial blood flow is translated into an increase in left atrial volume and pressure, whereas right atrial volume and pressure decline in response to interruption of umbilical venous return. The ductus arteriosus functionally closes within the first 48 hours of life in the majority of mature neonate.

64. Ans. c. Systolic mammary soufflé

Perloff 3rd Ed; Page 4

Murmur that occurs in the absence of either anatomic or physiologic abnormalities of the heart or circulation have been called functional, physiologic or benign murmur seven systolic and three continuous murmurs are found in normal children. Normal systolic murmurs include the vibratory systolic murmur of the still, the pulmonary systolic murmur, the peripheral pulmonary systolic murmur, the supraclavicular or brachiocephalic systolic murmur, the systolic mammary soufflé, the aortic systolic murmur and the cardiorespiratory systolic murmur. All normal systolic murmurs except the mammary soufflé are mid systolic, beginning after the first heart sound, and ending well before the second heart sound.

65. Ans. d. Its incidence increases towards adolescence

Perloff 6th Ed; Page 5

A common form of normal systolic murmur in children is vibratory murmur described by Still. Still's murmur is seldom heard in infancy but is prevalent after age 3 years with diminishing incidence towards adolescence. Normally, this Still's murmur intensity is grade II ranging from grades I to III. The murmur is maximal between the apex and lower left sternal age. The quality is distinctive, i.e., vibratory or buzzing with the uniform medium pure frequency requiring the stethoscope bell for its best appraisal.

66. Ans. d. All of the above

Perloff 6th Ed; Page 5–6

The venous hum is the most common type of normal continuous murmur. It is universal in children and occurs but much less frequently in healthy young adults even in absence of thyrotoxicosis, anemia or pregnancy. The maximal intensity of the venous hum is in the supraclavicular fossa just lateral to the sternocleidomastoid muscles. The hum may radiate widely and is often bilateral. It is usually more prominent on the right side. Loud venous hum in the children radiate below the clavicle where they are sometime mistaken for a patent ductus arteriosus murmur. The intensity of venous hum varies from faint to grade VI and an occasional patient is subjectively and unpleasantly aware of a loud hum which is sometime sensed as audible pulsatile tinnitus. The venous hums are best elicited with the patient sitting upright.

67. Ans. d. All of the above

Perloff 6th Ed; Page 7

A less common form of normal continuous murmur which is sometime heard during late pregnancy and in the early postpartum period of lactating women is the mammary soufflé. The continuation of systolic murmur beyond the second heart sound into the diastole results in a continuous mammary soufflé. Maximal intensity can be anywhere over either breast but there is a tendency for murmur to be louder in the second or third right or left intercostal space on either side or bilaterally. A distinct gap is usually present between the first heart sound and the onset of murmur. The continuous murmur is typically louder in systole with the diastolic portion often fading completely before the subsequent first heart sound. The pitch may be relatively high but the murmur is not musical. It is best heard with the patient supine and may vanish all together in upright position. The Valsalva maneuver does not affect intensity, however it is characteristically influenced by local compression. Light pressure with the stethoscope tend to augment the murmur and to bring out its continuous features. Conversely, the firm pressure with the stethoscope or digital pressure adjacent to the site of auscultation can completely abolish the murmur. The loudness of the murmur may vary spontaneously from day-to-day, from hour-to-hour or from beat-to-beat.

68. Ans. a. Peaking at second heart sound

Perloff 6th Ed; Page 13

The location of a continuous mammary soufflé may arouse suspicion of patent ductus arteriosus or an arteriovenous fistula. The typical ductus murmur peaks at the second heart sound, whereas the mammary soufflé generally peaks much earlier. Obliteration by local compression excludes patent ductus arteriosus. An arteriovenous fistula may generate a continuous murmur, i.e., maximal in systole and that attenuates with the pressure. However, the day-to-day (or cycle-to-cycle) variation of the mammary soufflé and its invariable disappearance after termination of lactation are the features suggesting that it is a mammary soufflé.

69. Ans. a. Rate dependent

Perloff 6th Ed; Page 41

Two important of sequale of congenital complete heart block are complete dissociation between atrial and ventricular contraction and decrease in the ventricular rate in response to the subsidiary (junctional) pacemaker. The slow heart rate, the long diastolic filling period and the large end diastolic volume results in augmented myocardial contractile force and increase in stroke volume. Resting cardiac output is maintained at normal level by increased end diastolic volume (stroke volume) rather than by a decrease in end systolic volume (ejection fraction). In congenital complete heart block, an increase in cardiac output with the exercises is chiefly rate dependent. Moderate isotonic exercise general provoke and increases the ventricular rate and cardiac output.

70. Ans. d. Systemic lupus erythematosus

Perloff 6th Ed; Page 43

Mothers with systemic lupus erythematosus who have had one child with neonatal heart block are at greater risk of having subsequent offspring with the heart block. Children of mother with lupus may not only have congenital heart block but may subsequently develop the overt connective tissue disease. Conversely, maternal lupus may not become manifest for years after the birth of an infant with congenital complete heart block.

71. Ans. a. Fetal echocardiography

Perloff 6th Ed; Page 41

The history of congenital complete heart block begins in utero. Fetal echocardiography helps not only in a establishing the diagnosis of congenital complete heart block but determines whether the heart block is or is not associated with structural heart disease, an important distinction in light of the difference in etiology and in the natural history.

72. Ans. d. All are correct

Perloff 6th Ed; Page 43

Refer to explanation for Q. No 70.

73. Ans. d. All are correct

Perloff 6th Ed; Page 42

When intrauterine complete heart block is associated with structural cardiac defect like left isomerism or ventricular inversion, only 14% of fetus survived the neonatal period. Conversely 85% of fetus with isolated intrauterine complete heart block live beyond the neonatal period, a survival rate similar to that in isolated congenital complete heart block diagnosed after birth. In these cases, approximately 90% of infants and children were alive at long-term follow-up. Nonimmune fetal hydrops indicate profound cardiac failure but isolated intrauterine complete heart block is rarely accompanied by congestive heart failure.

74. Ans. d. All are correct

Perloff 6th Ed; Page 47

A definite diagnosis of complete heart block can be made by electrocardiogram. The P wave (atrial activity) and the QRS complex (ventricular activity) are completely independent with no arithmetical relationship between the two. In acquired complete heart block period of synchronization (accrochage) sometime occurs but this phenomenon is uncommon in congenital complete heart block. Impulses originating in sinus node or atrium do not activate the ventricle, but examples of changes from partial to complete heart block or from complete to partial heart block are occasionally encountered. The atrial rate is rapid relative to the ventricular rate and tends to decrease with age after infancy the ventricular rate remains relatively constant until well into the adulthood. Rarely congenital atrial flutter coexists with congenital complete heart block.

75. Ans. b. Absent left precardial Q waves

Perloff 6th Ed; Page 47

In electrocardiogram, there is voltage criteria for left ventricular hypertrophy (volume over load) are sometime present together with prominent left precardial Q wave. In contrast, left precardial Q waves are conspicuously absent when complete heart block accompanies congenitally corrected transposition of great arteries in situs solitus with left sided heart. Right ventricular hypertrophy or biventricular hypertrophy has been also seen though rarely. These features helps in differentiating isolated complete heart block from that of congenitally corrected transposition of great arteries associated with complete heart block.

76. Ans. c. Atrioventricular valve regurgitation

Perloff 6th Ed; Page 60

The longevity pattern in uncomplicated congenitally corrected transposition are good but not normal because of the potential vulnerability of a morphologic right ventricle in the systemic location. After the initial mortality related to congestive heart failure in infancy, survival is relatively constant at a rate of approximately 1-2% per year. The major variable that relates to decrease long-term survival is the presence and degree of left atrioventricular valve regurgitation.

77. Ans. a. VSD

Perloff 6th Ed; Page 59

The ventricular septal defect, pulmonary stenosis and abnormalities of left atrioventricular valve and of conduction tissue are quite prevalent to be considered as integral part of basic malformation of corrected transposition of great arteries. A ventricular septal defect is the most prevalent anomaly and is present in almost 78% of cases at necropsy.

78. Ans. b. VSD

Perloff 6th Ed; Page 492

Truncus arteriosus is characterized by a single great artery that lives the base of heart and give arise to coronary, pulmonary and systemic arteries. The truncus is equipped with a single semilunar valve. A second semilunar valve is neither present nor implied. Because the single arterial trunk receive the output of both ventricle, a VSD is a obligatory defect in patients with truncus arteriosus.

79. Ans. a. Truncus with short main pulmonary artery and giving right and left pulmonary arteries

Perloff 6th Ed; Page 492

The truncus arteriosus is classified by Collets and Edwards and subsequently modified by Van Praagh in 1965. Type 1 is the commonest variety and is characterized by a short main pulmonary artery that originates from the truncus and give rise to right and left pulmonary arterial branches. Type 1 and 2 of the Collets and Edwards were characterized by right and left pulmonary arterial branches that arose directly from the truncus arteriosus by separate ostia. These two types are now considered as a single category and referred as Type 2. In about 15% of cases, one pulmonary arterial branch is absent or hypoplastic so that truncus give rise to a single pulmonary arterial branch this is type 3 of Van Praagh. The absence of hypoplastic pulmonary arterial branch is usually on the site of aortic arch in contrast to absent pulmonary artery in patients with TOF. Type 4 truncus arteriosus is now designated as pulmonary atresia with ventricular septal defect, so Type 1 is the commonest variety of truncus arteriosus.

80. Ans. d. All of the above

Perloff 6th Ed; Page 492

The truncal valve is equipped with three leaflets (tricuspid) in 50-60% of cases and a quadricuspid in most of the rest. Bicuspid in a distinct minority and very rarely pantacuspid or hexacuspid. The truncal and mitral valve are in fibrous continuity. A three leaflets truncal valve differ from a normal trileaflet aortic valve owing to the presence of raphe and because of the significant cuspal inequality in the patient with truncus arteriosus. A tricuspid truncal valve with raphe and cusp in excess of three (generally quadricuspid) is believe to represent morphogenetic combination of aortic and pulmonary valves. Trileaflet truncal valve are thicker than normal aortic valve in the patient with similar age. In addition to the abnormality of the size and number, the truncal cusp are often focally or diffusely thickened or poorly supported.

81. Ans. d. All of the above

Perloff 6th Ed; Page 495

Bounding arterial pulse in a mildly cyanotic infant with congestive heart failure can be seen in patient with TOF with aortic regurgitation, in patient with truncus arteriosus and in patient with absent pulmonary valve.

82. Ans. c. a and b

Perloff 6th Ed; Page 496

When a bounding arterial pulse occurs in a mildly cyanotic infant with congestive heart failure consideration of truncus arteriosus is warranted. The pulse pressure is wide because a low pulmonary vascular resistance permits diastolic flow from truncus into pulmonary bed so the systemic diastolic pressure falls. The rate of rise of the arterial pulse is brisk because of rapid ejection of a large left ventricular stroke volume. Truncal valve regurgitation is another cause of bounding arterial pulse in these patients. The effect on pulse is the same as that of aortic regurgitation.

83. Ans. c. Truncus arteriosus

Perloff 6th Ed; Page 500

Truncus arteriosus give us to the characteristic radiological appearance. The combination of increased pulmonary arterial blood flow and mild cyanosis is diagnostically important in the clinical recognition of truncus arteriosus. The pulmonary vascular pattern shows evidence of venous congestion due to the left ventricular failure. The main pulmonary artery segment is flat or concave when separate pulmonary arterial branches arise directly from the truncus. The concavity is especially apparent in right anterior/projection. A dilated left pulmonary artery may occupy this area of concavity but it shadow is usually recognized as such. A prominent left pulmonary artery sometimes assumes a distinctive appearance, costing a relatively high shadow as it emerges from cardiac silhouette and curves upward and to the left. This left hilar comma is a useful radiologic sign of truncus arteriosus. A left hilar comma is especially evident when the aortic arch is right sided.

84. Ans. d. None of the above

Perloff 3rd Ed; Chapter 8, Page 165

Auscultation: The first heart sound may be increased but not as consistently as in acquired mitral stenosis. A loud first heart sound, as well as an opening snap, requires abrupt movement of the mobile belly of the anterior mitral leaflet, so it is not surprising that these auscultatory signs are infrequent in congenital mitral stenosis because the morphologies do not provide the necessary preconditions. Systolic murmurs are sometimes heard between the apex and lower left sterna edge, even in isolated congenital mitral stenosis. Such murmurs, if holosystolic, are due either to mitral regurgitation (incompetent parachute mitral valve) or to tricuspid regurgitation caused by pulmonary hypertension. On one occasion, an isolated supravalvular ring caused mitral regurgitation for unclear reasons. Opening snaps are uncommon but not unknown, for the reasons just mentioned. Mid diastolic rumbling murmurs with presystolic accentuation are sometimes heard at the apex.

However, these murmurs are often subtle or entirely absent, and there are good reasons why this is so. Mitral stenotic murmurs are not well heard at the fast heart rates that prevail in sick infants with congenital mitral valve obstruction and heart failure. In addition, an enlarged, hypertensive right ventricle occupies the cardiac apex so that the stethoscope cannot be placed over the left ventricular impulse, where the murmur is ordinarily maximal. The second heart sound reflects pulmonary hypertension. Inspiratory splitting is close, and the pulmonic component is loud.

85. Ans. d. All of the above

Braunwald 5th Ed; Page 1013

Frequent premature atrial contractions often presage atrial fibrillation and administration of antiarrhythmic drugs may be effective in preventing these complications. However, once atrial fibrillation has developed these agents may be ineffective in restoring sinus rhythm or even in maintaining sinus rhythm following electrical cardioversion because of the pathological changes that occurs in the atrium secondary to the arrhythmia itself. After electrical cardioversion, sinus rhythm can often be maintained with antiarrhythmic drugs in young patients with mild mitral stenosis without marked left atrial enlargement who have been in atrial fibrillation less than 6 months and who are maintained by adequate doses of quinidine. If elective cardioversion is to be attempted in the patient with mitral stenosis and atrial fibrillation, a preparatory three weeks course of anticoagulation should be given to minimize the risk of systemic embolism when the sinus rhythm resume.

86. Ans. a. Ehlers–Danlos syndrome

Braunwald 5th Ed; Page 1030

Mitral valve prolapse occurs as a primary condition unassociated with other disease more frequently. However, it has been reported in association with many conditions. Mitral valve prolapse occurs quite commonly in heritable disorders of connective tissue that increases the size of the mitral leaflet and apparatus including the Marfan syndrome, Ehlers–Danlos syndrome, osteogenesis imperfecta, pseudoxanthoma elasticum and periarteritis nodosa as well as with myotonic dystrophy. It is also seen in association with congenital malformation such as Ebstein anomaly of tricuspid valve, atrial septal defect of ostium secundum variety and Holt–Oram syndrome.

87. Ans. a. MVP

Braunwald 5th Ed; Page 1030-1032

The mitral valve prolapse (MVP) syndrome has been given many names, including the systolic click murmur syndrome, Barlow syndrome, billowing mitral cusp syndrome, myxomatous mitral valve, floppy valve syndrome, and redundant cusp syndrome. It is a common but variable clinical syndrome that results from diverse pathogenic mechanisms of one or more portions of the mitral valve apparatus, the valve leaflets, chordate tendineae, papillary muscle, and valve annulus. The MVP syndrome has become recognized as one of the most prevalent cardiac valvular abnormalities, affecting as much as 3–5% of the population. It is twice as frequent in females as in males. In 1963 Barlow et al. demonstrated that midsystolic clicks and late systolic murmurs, the auscultatory hallmarks of this syndrome, are frequently associated with prolapse of the mitral valve, often associated with regurgitation.

The auscultatory findings are best elicited with the diaphragm of the stethoscope. The patient should be examined in the supine, left decubitus, and sitting positions. The physical findings unique to the MVP syndrome are detected by auscultation and can be corroborated by phonocardiography. The most important is a systolic click at least 0.14 sec after S1. This can be differentiated from a systolic ejection click because it occurs distinctly after the beginning of the upstroke of the carotid pulse. Occasionally, multiple mid- and late systolic clicks are audible most readily along the lower left sterna border and are believed to be produced by sudden tensing of the elongated chordate tendineae and of the prolapsing leaflets. The click is often, although not invariably, followed by a mid- to late-crescendo systolic murmur that continues to A2. This murmur is similar to that produced by papillary muscle dysfunction, which is readily understandable because both result from mid-to late-systolic MR. In general, the duration of the murmur is a function of the severity of the MR, and when the murmur is confined to the latter portion of systole, MR usually is not severe. However, as MR becomes more severe, the murmur commences earlier and becomes holosystolic.

It is important to emphasize the variability of the physical findings in the MVP syndrome. Some patients exhibit both a midsystolic click and a mid-late systolic murmur; others present with one or the other of these two findings; still others have only a click on one occasion and only a murmur on another, both on a third examination and no abnormality at all on a fourth. MVP may also cause an early diastolic sound or murmur, best heard at the apex or left sterna border 70–110 msec following A2 at a time when the prolapsed posterior leaflet descends into the left ventricle. Conditions other than MVP cause mid systolic clicks; these include tricuspid valve clicks; atrial septal aneurysms, and extracardiac causes.

Dynamic auscultation: The auscultatory and phonocardiographic findings are exquisitely sensitive to physiological and pharmacological interventions, and recognition of the changes induced by these interventions is of great value in the diagnosis of the MVP syndrome. The mitral valve begins to prolapse when the reduction of left ventricular volume during systole reaches a critical point at which the valve leaflets no longer coapt; at that instant, the click occurs and the murmur commences. Any maneuver that decreases left ventricular volume, such as reduction of impedance to left ventricular outflow, a reduction in venous return, or an augmentation of contractility, results in an earlier occurrence of prolapse during systole. As a consequence, the click and onset of the murmur move closer to S1. When prolapse is severe or left ventricular size is markedly reduced or both, prolapse may begin with the onset of systole, and as a consequence the click may not be audible and the murmur may be holosystolic. On the other hand, when left ventricular volume is augmented by an increase in venous return, a reduction of myocardial contractility, bradycardia, or an increase in the impedance to left ventricular emptying, both the click and the onset of the murmur will be delayed. Indeed, if the left ventricle becomes extremely large, prolapse may not occur at all, and the abnormal auscultatory features may disappear entirely.

During the straining phaseo of the Valsalva maneuver, upon sudden standing, and early during the inhalation of amyl nitrite, cardiac size decreases, and both the click and the onset of the murmur occur earlier in systole. In contrast, a sudden change from the standing to the supine position, leg-raising, squatting, maximal isometric exercise, and to a lesser extent, expiration will delay the click and the onset of the murmur. During the overshoot phase of the Valsalva maneuver (i.e., 6–8 cycles following release) and with prolongation of the R-R interval, either following a premature contraction or in atrial fibrillation, the click and onset of the murmur are usually delayed, and the intensity of the murmur is reduced. Maneuvers that elevate arterial pressure, such as isometric exercise, increase the intensity of the click and murmur.

In general, when the onset of the murmur is delayed, both its duration and intensity are diminished, reflecting a reduction in the severity of MR. With some maneuvers, however, there is a discrepancy between changes in the intensity and duration of the murmur. Following amyl nitrite inhalation, e.g., the reduced left ventricular size results in an earlier click and longer murmur, but the lower left ventricular systolic pressure diminishes the severity of regurgitation and the intensity of the murmur. Conversely, phenylephrine and methoxamine delay the click and the onset of the murmur, but the larger volume of regurgitation consequent to the elevated left ventricular systolic pressure increases regurgitation and the intensity of the murmur.

88. **Ans. d. All are true**

Braunwald 5th Ed; Page 1030–1032

Refer to explanation for Q. No 87.

89. **Ans. b. Amylnitrite inhalation**

Braunwald 5th Ed; Page 1030–1032

Refer to explanation for Q. No 87.

90. Ans. d. Bicuspid aortic valve

Perloff, 3rd Ed; Chapter 7, Page 132

Infective endocarditis or endarteritis is a potential serious complication in the natural history of coarctation of aorta. Infection tend to occur between ages 10 and 40 years. Although this complication is unlikely in infants and young children, it is not only observed in this age group but has been responsible for saccular mycotic aneurysm. The most common location of infection is not at the site of coarctation but on the particularly susceptible bicuspid aortic valve.

91. Ans. b. Hypertension is necessary precondition

Perloff, 3rd Ed; Chapter 7, Page 132

Cerebrovascular accident is another major complication in patient with coarctation of aorta. An aneurysm of the circle of Willis is usually responsible for hemorrhage much less commonly. Importantly aneurysm may occur in other cerebral arteries also. Intracranial bleeding is occasionally caused by perforation of a mycotic cerebral aneurysm. Rarely a thrombus or embolus lodges in intracranial vessel. The majority of patients who succumb to cerebral hemorrhage do so in the second or third decade. Hypertension is not a necessary precondition because cerebral complication can occur in normotensive patient, long after successful repair of coarctation.

92. Ans. a. The incidence of toxemia is high in women with coarctation

Perloff, 3rd Ed; Chapter 7, Page 132

The risk of pregnancy in patient with coarctation is less than one's thought. Blood pressure fluctuations are similar in direction to those in uncomplicated pregnancy but form a higher base line. The incidence of toxemia is lower in women with coarctation than in pregnant women with other form of hypertension and rarely cardiac failure develops. Pregnancy increases the risk of aortic rupture and intracranial hemorrhage because gestational changes occurs in connective tissues edge to the abnormalities inherent in the arterial valves. Infective endocarditis is a threat because of potential bacteremia during delivery.

93. Ans. d. All are correct

Perloff, 3rd Ed; Chapter 7, Page 144

Notching of the ribs, a classic radiologic sign of coarctation of aorta results from collateral flow through dilated, tortuous, pulsatile posterior intercostal arteries. The notches originate in the costal groove rather than on the most inferior rib margins. Notching varies from rib to rib and from patient to patient and may be single, multiple, shallow, deep, broad or narrow. The notches typically appears as a regular scalloped areas on the under surfaces of posterior ribs. Anterior ribs are spared because the anterior intercostal arteries do not run in costal grooves. Rarely, the superior margin of a rib is notched by a tortuous overhanging intercostal artery that makes contact with the rib below. Rib notching seldom appears below age of 6 years but exceptional example have been described as earliest as at age of 2 years. When coarctation is located distal to the left subclavian arteries, which is a usual site, bilateral notching is seen between the 3rd and 8th posterior rib. Notching is rarely found either above the 3rd or below the 9th rib. Anatomic variations in the site of coarctation are accompanied by important modification of these radiologic patterns. The development of arterial collaterals depends upon patency of the origin of two subclavian arteries. When coarctation narrows the orifice of left subclavian artery collateral fail to develop on that side, an unilateral rib notching is seen only on the contralateral right posterior ribs. When there is anomalous origin of the right subclavian artery distal to the coarctation, collaterals fails to developed in right hemithorax so unilateral rib notching is confined to the left side. The retroesophageal aberrant right subclavian artery is sometime identified as posterior indentation on the barium esophagogram. When the coarctation is in abdominal aorta notching if present at all is confined to the lower ribs.

94. Ans. d. Abdominal coarctation

Perloff, 3rd Ed; Chapter 7, Page 144

Refer to explanation for Q. No 93.

95. Ans. d. Tortuous internal mammary artery

Perloff, 3rd Ed; Chapter 7, Page 146

In older children and adults with coarctation of aorta lateral X-ray may show retrosternal notching or scalloping caused by dilated tortuous internal mammary arteries.

96. Ans. c. Rib notching

Perloff, 3rd Ed; Chapter 7, Page 146

The kinked aorta in pseudocoarctation has an arch and descending portion that resemble those in true coarctation. The transverse arch and descending aorta form a three sign above and below the kink. Pseudocoarctation is quite evident in the X-ray chest but rib notching is conspicuously absent.

97. Ans. d. Complete interruption of aortic arch

Perloff, 3rd Ed; Chapter 7, Page 148

Complete interruption of the aortic arch was first described in 18th century by Raffle Steidele's. The eponym Steidele's complex is sometime applied to this rare malformation. Which is characterized by complete anatomic discontinuity or less commonly by an atretic fibrous remanant between the arch or isthmus and descending aorta.

98. Ans. d. All are equally common

Perloff, 3rd Ed; Chapter 7, Page 148

The classification of Celoria and Pattsons remains in current use to classify the site of interruption. Interruption between the left common carotid and left subclavian artery is slightly commoner than isthmic interruption distal to the left subclavian artery (type A), whereas the less common site between the innominate and left carotid artery (i.e., type C), subtypes are based upon on anomalous origin of the right subclavian artery.

99. Ans. b. Type B interrupted aortic arch

Perloff, 3rd Ed; Chapter 7, Page 151

The DiGeorge syndrome (Thymic aplasia) is associated with interruption between left carotid and left subclavian arteries (type B interrupted aortic arch). Hypoplastic mandible, defective ears and short philtrum are features of the physical appearance of this syndrome, which includes aplasia or hypoplasia of the thymus and parathyroid glands.

100. Ans. b. Infundibular pulmonic stenosis

Perloff; 3rd Ed; Chapter 18, Page 405

Subvalvular pulmonary stenosis is either infundibular or subinfundibular. Infundibular pulmonary stenosis is caused by anterior and rightward malalignment of infundibular septum and it occurs with ventricular septal defect.

101. Ans. b. Williams syndrome

Perloff, 3rd Ed; Chapter 10, Page 191

Bilateral stenosis of pulmonary arterial branches with supravalvular aortic stenosis is a component of Williams syndrome and is associated with peculiar facies, abnormal dentition, mental retardation and infantile hypercalcemia.

102. Ans. b. Maternal Viremia is not a prerequisite for placental and fetal rubella infections

Perloff, 3rd Ed; Chapter 10, Page 191

There is association between stenosis of pulmonary artery and its branches and maternal rubella. Maternal viremia is a prerequisite for placental and fetal rubella infection. Most cases occur following primary rather than rubella reinfection. When maternal rubella occurs later than 16th week of gestation, the risk of fetal damage appears to be very small. Maternal rubella can have devastating nonteratogenic effects on fetal development including a spontaneous abortion and still birth. Cardiac defects and deafness consistently occur in infant infected during the first 10th week of gestation. Patent ductus arteriosus and pulmonary artery stenosis usually coexist with the patent ductus arteriosus the more prevalent of the two lesions.

103. Ans. a. Patent ductus arteriosus

Perloff, 3rd Ed; Chapter 10, Page 191

Refer to explanation for Q. No 102.

104. Ans. d. All of the above

Perloff, 3rd Ed; Chapter 20, Page 468

Interrupted aortic arch, pulmonary atresia with VSD, hypoplastic left heart syndrome, all the three are ductus dependent lesions.

105. Ans. d. Atrial septal defect

Braunwald 5th Ed; Page 878

The true incidence of congenital cardiovascular malformation is difficult to determine accurately. About 0.8% of live births are complicated by a cardiovascular malformation. This figure does not take into account, the two most common cardiac anomalies, i.e., the congenital non stenotic bicuspid aortic valve and leaflet abnormality associated with mitral valve prolapse. Moreover, the widely quoted 0.8% incidence figure fail to include small preterm infants almost all of whom have persistent patent ductus arteriosus. Cardiac malformation occurs 10 times more often in stillborn than in live born babies and many early spontaneous abortion are associated with chromosomal defects. Taken in general, children with congenital heart disease are predominately male. Moreover is specific defect may show a definite gender preponderance. Patent ductus arteriosus, Ebsteins anomaly of tricuspid valve and atrial septal defect are more common in female whereas valvular aortic stenosis, coarctation of aorta, hypoplastic left heart, pulmonary and tricuspid atresia and transposition of great arteries are more common in male. Extracardiac anomalies occurs in about 25% of infants with significant cardiac disease and their presence may significantly increase mortality. The extra cardiac anomalies often are multiple, in part involving the musculoskeletal system. One-third of infants with both cardiac and extracardiac anomalies have some established syndrome.

106. Ans. c. Extracardiac anomalies occurs in approximately 50% of infants

Braunwald 5th Ed; Page 878

Refer to explanation for Q. No 105.

107. Ans. c. Amiodarone

Braunwald 5th Ed; Page 878

Teratogenic disorders		
Rubella	Patent ductus arteriosus, pulmonic valvular and/or arterial stenosis, atrial septal defect	Cataracts, deafness, microcephaly
Alcohol	Ventricular septal defect (other defects)	Microcephaly, growth and mental deficiency, short palpebral fissures, smooth philtrum, thin upper lip
Dilantin	Pulmonic stenosis, aortic stenosis, coarctation, patent ductus arteriosus	Hypertelorism, growth and mental deficiency, short phalanges, bowed upper lip
Thalidomide	Variable	Phocomelia
Lithium	Ebstein's anomaly, tricuspid atresia	None

108. Ans. d. 8th week

Braunwald 5th Ed; Page 879

During normal cardiac development in the 1st month of gestation, the primitive straight cardiac tube is formed comprising the sinoatrium, the primitive ventricles, the bulbus cardis and truncus arteriosus in the series from cephalad to caudad. In the second month of gestation, this tube doubles over on itself to form two parallel pumping system, each with two chambers and a great arteries. The two atria develop from sinoatrium. The atrioventricular canal is divided by endocardial cushion into the tricuspid and mitral orifices and the right and left ventricles develop from the primitive ventricle and bulbus cardis. Differential growth of myocardium cell causes the straight cardiac tube to bear to the right and bulboventricular portion of tube doubles over on itself bringing the ventricles side by side. Migration of atrioventricular canal to the right and of the ventricular septum to the left sub to align each ventricle with its appropriate atrioventricular valve. At the distal end of cardiac tube, the bulbus cardis divide into subaortic muscular conus and subpulmonic muscular conus. The sub-pulmonic conus elongate and subaortic conus resorbs allowing the aorta to move posteriorly and connect to the left ventricle.

109. Ans. b. 1, 2 and 5

Braunwald 5th Ed; Page 882-883

The truncus arteriosus, the primitive truncus arteriosus is connected to the dorsal aorta in embryo by six pairs of aortic arches. Although six aortic arches appears sequentially, portion of the aortic arch system and dorsal aorta disappear at different times during the embryogenesis. The first, second and fifth sets of paired arches regresses completely. The proximal portion of sixth arches becomes the right and left pulmonary arteries and distal left sixth arch becomes the ductus arteriosus. The third aortic arch forms the connection between internal and external carotid arteries while the left fourth arch becomes the arterial segment between the left carotid and subclavian arteries. The proximal portion of right subclavian artery forms from the right fourth arch. An abnormality in the regression of arch system in number or site can produce a wide variety of arch anomalies whereas a failure of regression usually results in a double aortic arch malformation.

110. Ans. d. Distal half of left 6th aortic arch

Braunwald 5th Ed; Page 882-883

Refer to explanation for Q. No 109.

111. Ans. c. 55%

Braunwald 5th Ed; Page 883

The oxygenated blood in fetus returns from the placenta through the umbilical vein and enters the portal venous system. A variable amount of this stream bypasses the hepatic microcirculation and enters the inferior vena cava by way of ductus venosus. Inferior vena cava blood is composed to flow from ductus venosus, hepatic vein and lower body venous drainage which is deflected to a significant extent across the foreman ovale into the left atrium. All superior vena cava blood passes directly to the tricuspid valve entering the right ventricle. Most of the blood that reaches the right ventricle bypasses the high resistance, unexpanded lungs and pass through the ductus arteriosus into the descending aorta. The right ventricle contributes about 55% and left ventricle 45% to the total fetal cardiac output. The major portion of blood ejected from the left ventricle supplies the brain and upper part of the body while the lesser portion flows to the coronary arteries. The balance, passes across the aortic isthmus to the descending aorta where it joins with the large stream from the ductus arteriosus before flowing into the lower part of the body and placenta. In the fetal life, pulmonary arteries and arterioles are surrounded by a fluid medium and have relatively thick valves and a small lumina and resembles comparable arteries in the systemic circulation. The low pulmonary blood flow in the fetus (7-10% of the total cardiac output) is the result of high pulmonary vascular resistance. Fetal pulmonary vessels are highly reactive to changes in oxygen tension or in the pH of the blood perfusing them as well as to a number of other physiological and pharmacological inferences.

112. Ans. b. 10% of total cardiac output

Braunwald 5th Ed; Page 883

Refer to explanation for Q. No 111.

113. **Ans. d. 48-72 hours after birth**

Braunwald 5th Ed; Page 883

The fundamental change that normally occurs at birth is a division of the single, parallel fetal circulation into separate independent circulation. Inflation of the lung at the first inspiration produces a marked reduction in pulmonary vascular resistance. Pulmonary pressure falls further as the ductus constrict in healthy mature infant. The ductus arteriosus is profoundly constricted at 10-15 hours and is closed functionally by 72 hours with total anatomical closure following within a few weeks by a process of thrombosis, intimal proliferation and fibrosis. A high incidence in preterm infants are of persistent patency of ductus arteriosus because of an immaturity of the mechanism responsible for the constriction of the ductus. In surviving preterm infants the ductus arteriosus spontaneously closes within 4-12 months of the birth.

114. **Ans. d. 4-12 months of birth**

Braunwald 5th Ed; Page 883

Refer to explanation for Q. No 113.

115. **Ans. d. Patent ductus arteriosus**

Braunwald 5th Ed; Page 884

In the preterm infant especially under 1500 g birth weight, persistent patency of the ductus arteriosus is the most common causes of cardiac decompensation.

116. **Ans. c. Gallop rhythm**

Braunwald 5th Ed; Page 884

The common symptom and sign of congestive heart failure in fetus or in infants are feeding difficulties and failure to gain weight and grow, tachypnea, tachycardia, pulmonary rales and ronchi, liver enlargement and cardiomegaly. Less frequent manifestation includes peripheral edema, ascites, pulsus alternans, gallop rhythm and inappropriate sweating. Pleural and pericardial effusion are exceedingly rare.

117. **Ans. a. Cerebral thrombosis**

Braunwald 5th Ed; Page 885

Common complications noted in patient with cyanotic congenital heart disease are cerebral abscess, cerebrovascular accident, cerebral thrombosis, paradoxical embolism, retinopathy and hemoptysis. Cerebrovascular accident and brain abscess occurs particularly in cyanotic patient with substantial arterial desaturation. Cerebral thrombosis is most common under age two years in severely cyanotic children even in presence of relatively low hematocrit and occurs especially in clinical setting in which oxygen requirements are raised by fever or blood viscosity increases as in dehydration. Brain abscess is an important complication of cyanotic congenital heart disease. Such abscess are rare under 18 months of age and commonly are of insidious onset marked by headache, low grade fever, vomiting and change in personality. Seizure or paralysis less frequently seen at the onset of brain abscess. Abscess must be suspected in any cyanotic child with focal neurological signs. Morbidity and mortality are related inversely to the oxygen saturation level. Brain abscess is thought to occur in about 2% of the population with cyanotic congenital heart disease with mortality rate of 30-40% and is often related to the delay in diagnosis and treatment. Paradoxical embolism is a rare complication of cyanotic congenital heart disease, usually observed at necropsy. Emboli arising in systemic vein may pass directly into the systemic circulation because right to left intracardiac shunt allow venous blood to bypass the normal filtering action of lung. Retinopathy occurs due to the dilated tortuous vessels progressing to the papilledema and retinal edema and it is occasionally observed in cyanotic patients and it appears to be related to the decreased arterial oxygen saturation and/or to the erythrocytosis but is not due to the hypercapnia. Hemoptysis is an another uncommon but major complication seen in cyanotic patient with congenital heart disease and occur most often in the presence of pulmonary vascular obstructive disease or in patient with an extensive bronchial collaterals circulation or pulmonary venous congestion. Massive hemoptysis almost always represent rupture of a dilated bronchial artery.

118. **Ans. d. Alpha-adrenoceptor blockers**

Braunwald 5th Ed; Page 885

Hypercyanotic or hypoxemic spells commonly complicate the clinical course in young children with certain type of cyanotic heart disease especially TOF. The spells are characterized by a anxiety, hyperpnea and intense increase in cyanosis. They are the result of an abrupt reduction in pulmonary blood flow. Unless terminated the hypercyanotic episode may lead to convulsion and may prove fatal. Sudden reduction in pulmonary blood flow may be precipitated by fluctuation in arterial pCO_2 and pH, a sudden fall in systemic or increase in pulmonary vascular resistance or an acute increase in the severity of right ventricular outflow tract obstruction either by augmented contraction of the hypertrophied muscle in the right ventricle outflow tract or by a decrease in right ventricular cavity volume owing to the tachycardia. The treatment of hypoxic spell consists of oxygen administration, placing the child in knee chest position and administration of morphine sulfate. Additional medications that may prove to be of value includes the intravenous administration of sodium bicarbonate to correct the accompanying acidosis, alpha adreno receptor stimulant such as phenylephrine hydrochloride or methoxamine to raise peripheral resistance and diminish right to left shunting and beta adreno-receptor blocking agent which reduces cardiac sympathetic tone and depresses cardiac contractility and in directly increases the ventricular volume by reducing the heart rate.

119. Ans. c. Seizures and paralysis frequently heralds the onset of a brain abscess

Braunwald 5th Ed; Page 885

Refer to explanation for Q. No 117.

120. Ans. c. Hypercapnia

Braunwald 5th Ed; Page 885

Refer to explanation for Q. No 117.

121. Ans. a. Preload reserve

Braunwald 5th Ed; Page 889

In the neonatal heart, the preload or diastolic reserve is limited while the systolic reserved is available to some extent to adopt to acute or chronic stress such as pressure or volume load. While the heart rate reserve is reduce in newborn.

122. Ans. c. 1–5 ng/mL

Braunwald 5th Ed; Page 890

In infant's therapeutic level of digoxin ranges from 1–5 ng/mL (mean 3.5) while toxicity is associated with concentration in excess of 3 ng/mL.

123. Ans. d. All of the above are used

Braunwald 5th Ed; Page 890

The treatment of congestive heart failure in infant involves uses of digitalis and diuretics. Other pharmacological agents can be used in certain subset of the patients, in situation in which cardiac decompensation is not the result of obstructive lesion, catecholamine may be used temporarily to alleviate cardiac failure while the patient is awaiting more definitive operative treatment. In infants with coarctation of aorta syndrome in whom ductal constriction and marks the aortic branch point producing aortic narrowing or with aortic arch interruption, heart failure may be reserved dramatically by the intravenous infusion of prostaglandin E1 (0.03–0.1 mg/kg/min) which results in dilatation of the ductus arteriosus and may bring relief of obstruction. Conversely, in preterm infants in whom the patent ductus arteriosus is responsible for profound cardiopulmonary deterioration constriction of ductus arteriosus may be accomplished by inhibition of prostaglandin synthesis with the non steroidal anti-inflammatory agents, i.e., indomethazine at a dose of 0.2 mg/kg intravenous. Vasodilator therapy also is used in infants or children with heart disease in whom preload or afterload alteration may be expected to improve cardiac performance.

124. Ans. d. All of the above

Perloff, 3rd Ed; Chapter 20, Page 473/601

Differential cyanosis virtually always indicates the presence of congenital heart disease often with the patency of the ductus arteriosus and coarctation of aorta as component of abnormal anatomical complex. If the upper part of the body is pink and lower part of body is blue, coarctation of aorta or interruption of aortic arch is probable with oxygenated blood supplying the upper part of the body and desaturated blood supplying the lower part of body by way of right to left flow through the ductus arteriosus. This situation also occur in patient with patent ductus arteriosus and markedly elevated pulmonary vascular resistance. A patient with transposition of great arteries and coarctation of aorta with retrograde flow through the patent ductus arteriosus demonstrates reverse situation, i.e., the lower part of body is pink and upper part is blue.

125. Ans. c. Both of the above

Perloff, 3rd Ed; Chapter 20, Page 473/601

Refer to explanation for Q. No 125.

126. Ans. a. Tricuspid atresia

Perloff, 3rd Ed; Chapter 25, Page 564

In a newborn with cyanotic CHD, counterclockwise superiorly oriented frontal QRS loop with absent or reduce right ventricular forces suggest diagnosis of tricuspid atresia.

127. Ans. d. Radiographic examination

Braunwald 5th Ed; Page 893

Chest radiography often is useful and differentiating between the respiratory and cardiac causes of cyanosis in newborn period.

128. Ans. d. All of the above

Braunwald 5th Ed; Page 894

Chest radiography often is useful in differentiating between respiratory and cardiac causes of cyanosis in the newborn period. Determination of a normal cardiac and abdominal situs aids in ruling out several kinds of complex cyanotic cardiac malformations associated with asplenia or polysplenia with abdominal heterotaxy and dextrocardia. The distinct appearance of pulmonary parenchymal disease, such as the classic reticulogranular pattern of hyaline membrane disease, may allow a specific radiological diagnosis. In those premature infants with a large ductus arteriosus the radiographic appearance often evolves from the typical findings of hyaline membrane disease to increased pulmonary vascular markings and finally to perihilar and generalized pulmonary edema.

In the presence of cyanosis diminished pulmonary vascular markings call attention to the group of anomalies that includes tetralogy of Fallot, pulmonic stenosis with intact ventricular septum, pulmonic atresia, tricuspid atresia, and Ebstein's malformation of the tricuspid valve. Reduced pulmonary blood flow is responsible for the systemic arterial desaturation in these babies. Increased pulmonary vascular markings in the cyanotic infant are associated with lesions in which an obligatory admixture of systemic venous and pulmonary venous blood occurs. The more common anomalies in this category include transposition of the great arteries, hypoplastic left heart syndrome, truncus arteriosus, and total anomalous pulmonary venous drainage.

As mentioned earlier, overall heart size in the normal newborn infant is greater than in the older child, and cardiothoracic ratios up to 0.60 are within normal limits. The thymus shadow occasionally obscures the cardiac silhouette and prohibits accurate estimation of heart size. An enlarged heart on X-ray examination suggests a cardiac disorder. However, in the presence of severe respiratory difficulties with an increase in carbon dioxide tension and a decrease in both pH and arterial oxygen tension, cardiomegaly may be only moderate. A right aortic arch suggests the presence of either tetralogy of Fallot or persistent truncus arteriosus. An ovoid heart with a narrow base associated with increased pulmonary vascular marking is typical of transposition of the great arteries. A boot-shaped heart with concavity of the pulmonary outflow tract suggests tetralogy of Fallot, pulmonary atresia, or tricuspid atresia.

129. Ans. a. Transposition of great arteries

Braunwald 5th Ed; Page 894

Refer to explanation for Q. No 128.

130. Ans. c. 16th week of gestation

Braunwald 5th Ed; Page 894

Fetal echocardiography: Ultrasound technology now allows examination of human fetal cardiac development and function in utero. Diagnostic-quality images of the fetal heart in utero can be obtained as early as 16 weeks of gestation. Cardiac structures are imaged primarily by cross-sectional echocardiography and augmented by a combination of range-gaged pulse Doppler ultrasonography and M-mode echocardiography. The analysis of the structure and function of the fetal heart during the second and third trimesters of pregnancy has allowed cardiologists to counsel prospective parents, and in a number of instances to formulate management plans for pregnancy, delivery, and the immediate postnatal period. Using fetal echocardiography, major forms of congenital heart disease have been diagnosed in utero, and cardiac rhythm abnormalities have been detected, permitting direct efforts at transplacental therapy. In particular, it has been established that a high incidence exists of cardiac pathology in the presence of nonimmune fetal hydrops. It appears clear that hydrops fetalis often represents end-stage fetal cardiac decompensation. Atrioventricular valve insufficiency often causes fetal right ventricular volume overload and systemic venous hypertension leading to hydrops fetalis.

Pulsed Doppler ultrasound examination of the fetus importantly supplements the echocardiographic findings in identifying the responsible defects, such as Ebstein's malformation of the tricuspid valve, atrial isomerism with atrioventricular septal defects, and the absent pulmonary valve and hypoplastic left heart syndrome.

131. Ans. c. 10–20%

Braunwald 5th Ed; Page 896

About 10–20% of patients with ostium secundum atrial septal defect have prolapse of mitral valve as an associated anomaly. Lutembacher's syndrome is a condition where there is a combination of secundum atrial septal defect and mitral stenosis which is almost invariably the result of acquired rheumatic valvulitis.

132. Ans. d. All of the above

Braunwald 5th Ed; Page 896

The magnitude of left to right shunt through an atrial septal defect depends on the size of the defect and the relative compliance of the ventricle and the relative resistance in both the pulmonary and systemic circulation. In patient with a small atrial septal defect the left atrial pressure makes it is the right by several mm Hg where as the mean pressure in both the atria are nearly identical when the defect is large. Left to right shunt occurs predominately in late ventricular systole and early diastole with some augmentation during atrial contraction. The shunt results in diastolic overloading of the right ventricle and increase in pulmonary blood flow. During the first few days and weeks of life, pulmonary resistance fall and systemic resistance rise facilitates right ventricular emptying and impeding left ventricular emptying and therefore, the left to right shunt increases. Early in infancy, left to right flow through even a large interarterial communication, commonly is limited by both reduced chamber compliance of the thick neonatal right ventricle and elevated pulmonary and low systemic vascular resistance of the neonate circulatory system.

133. Ans. b. Late ventricular systole and early diastole

Braunwald 5th Ed; Page 896

Refer to explanation for Q. No 132.

134. Ans. c. Sinus venosus type of ASD

Braunwald 5th Ed; Page 897

Left axis deviation of P wave in the frontal plane (manifested by negative P wave in lead III) suggest the diagnosis of sinus venosus type of atrial septal defect.

135. Ans. b. Ostium primum ASD

Braunwald 5th Ed; Page 897

Left axis deviation and superior orientation and counterclockwise rotation of QRS loop in the frontal plane suggest the presence of either an ostium primum defect or a secundum atrial septal defect in association with mitral valve prolapse.

136. Ans. d. Complete AV canal defect

Braunwald 5th Ed; Page 900

Goose neck deformity as evident angiographically suggest that the diagnosis of complete AV canal defect. **Also see the answers of Q. No 36 to 39.**

137. Ans. c. 40%

Braunwald 5th Ed; Page 902

A wide spectrum exists in the natural history of ventricular septal defect ranging from spontaneous closure to congestive heart failure and death in early infancy. Within this spectrum are possible development of pulmonary vascular obstruction, right ventricular outflow tract obstruction, aortic regurgitation and infective endocarditis. It is unusual for a ventricular septal defect to cause difficulty in the immediate postnatal period, although congestive heart failure during the first six months of life is a frequent occurrence. A ventricular septal defect that either decreases in size or closes completely during the 1st year of life present no problem. A spontaneous closure occurs by age of 3 years in about 45% of patients born with VSD. Occasional patients, however do not experiences spontaneous closure until age 8–10 years or even later. Closure is more common in patients born with a small VSD. Nonetheless about 7% of the infants with a large defects and congestive heart failure early in the life also may experience spontaneous closure. Partial rather than complete closure is common in patients with both large and small ventricular septal defect. Anatomically reduction of the ventricular septal defect often is based on adherence of tricuspid valve to the defect, hypertrophy of septal muscles or ingrowth of the fibrous tissue. Rarely, the closure of ventricular septal defect is the result of the prolapse of an aortic cusp or infective endocarditis. Some defects close when an aneurysm forms in ventricular septum.

138. Ans. d. 7–8%

Braunwald 5th Ed; Page 902

Refer to explanation for Q. No 138.

139. Ans. d. 12% of cases

Braunwald 5th Ed; Page 929

An atrial septal defect coexists with the tetralogy of Fallot in about 15% of cases, the term 'Pentalogy of Fallot' has been applied to this combination.

140. Ans. c. Formation of septal aneurysm

Braunwald 5th Ed; Page 902

Rarely the closure of VSD is the result of an aneurysm which forms on ventricular septum. On auscultation, a click may be heard in early systole as the aneurysm tenses towards the right. The septal aneurysm may be detected by echocardiography as an anterior systolic bulge in right ventricular outflow tract.

141. Ans. d. It is rare complication in Japanese

Braunwald 5th Ed; Page 903

Ventricular septal defect with aortic regurgitation: This well-described complication of ventricular septal defect occurs in about 5% of patients. It usually is noted after age 5 years when a physician detects the early diastolic blowing murmur and wide pulse pressure of aortic regurgitation while following a patient with a ventricular septal defect. The diagnosis is readily confirmed by Doppler echocardiography. In such patients aortic regurgitation may become the predominant hemodynamic abnormality. It is of interest that ventricular setpal defect with aortic regurgitation is rare in Europe and the United States. With an incidence of about 4% of all cases of isolated ventricular septal defect, whereas in Japan the incidence is substantially higher (about 10%). In the Japanese, in particular, aortic regurgitation is the result of herniation of an aortic leaflet (usually the right coronary) through a subpulmonic supracristal ventricular septal defect.

142. Ans. a. PDA

Braunwald 5th Ed; Page 906

Aorticopulmonary window or fenestration is an anomaly where the usual defect consist of a communication between the aorta and pulmonary artery just above the semilunar valves. Persistent patency of ductus arteriosus is an associated lesion in 10–15% of the cases. Less common accompanying cardiovascular lesions includes VSD, aortic origin of the right pulmonary artery, aortic arch interruption, coarctation of aorta and right sided aortic arch.

143. Ans. a. VSD

Braunwald 5th Ed; Page 907

Persistent truncus arteriosus is a rare but serious anomaly in which a single vessel forms the outlet of both ventricles and give rise to the systemic pulmonary and coronary arteries. The defect results from failure of septation of the embryonic truncus by the infundibular truncal septum. It is always accompanied by a VSD, frequently with a right sided aortic arch. The VSD is due to the absence or underdevelopment of distal portion of pulmonary infundibulum. The truncal valve is usually tricuspid but is quadricuspid in about 1/3rd of patients and rarely it can be bicuspid. Truncal valve regurgitation and truncal valve stenosis are seen in 10-15% of the patients. There may be a single coronary artery, displacement of coronary ostia or a single posterior descending coronary artery arises from the right coronary artery or less often from the left circumflex artery especially in patient with single coronary artery.

144. Ans. c. Unruptured aneurysm is always asymptomatic

Braunwald 5th Ed; Page 910

Congenital aneurysm of an aortic sinus of Valsalva particularly the right coronary sinus is an uncommon anomaly that occurs 3 times more often in the males than in females. The malformation consists of a separation or lack of fusion between the media of aorta and the annulus fibrosis of the aortic valve. The receiving chamber of the aorticocardiac fistula usually is the right ventricle but occasionally when the noncoronary cusp is involved the fistula drains into the right atrium. About 5-15% of aneurysm originates in posterior or noncoronary sinus. Seldom is the left aortic sinus involve. Associated anomalies are common and include bicuspid aortic valve, VSD and coarctation of aorta. The unruptured aneurysm usually does not produce a hemodynamic abnormality although pressure on the intracardiac conduction system by an unruptured aneurysm may be the rare cause of complete atrioventricular block. Rarely myocardial ischemia may be caused by coronary arterial compression. Rupture is often of abrupt onset, causes chest pain and create continuous arteriovenous shunting and volume overloading of both right and left heart chambers, which result in heart failure and additional complication is IE which may originate either on the edge of aneurysm or on those areas in the right side of the heart, which are traumatized by the jet like stream of blood flowing through the fistula.

145. Ans. d. All of the above

Braunwald 5th Ed; Page 911

The coarctation of aorta lesion consists of a localized shelf like thickening and infolding of media of the posterolateral aortic wall opposite that the ductus arteriosus. The wall of aorta into which the ductus or ligamentum arteriosum inserts is not involved. Juxtaductal coarctation occurs 2-5 times more common in males than in females and there is high degree of association with gonadal dysgenesis, i.e., Turner syndrome, and bicuspid aortic valve. Other common associated anomalies include VSD and mitral stenosis or regurgitation. The most important extracardiac anomaly is the aneurysm of circle of Willis. The cardiac anomalies that cause augmented ascending aortic blood flow, e.g., pulmonary atresia or stenosis, TOF which prevent development of a branch point are almost never seen in association with juxtaductal coarctation of aorta.

146. Ans. c. Aneurysm of circle of Willis

Braunwald 5th Ed; Page 911

Refer to explanation for Q. No 145.

147. Ans. b. Type B

Braunwald 5th Ed; Page 913

Aortic arch interruption is rare and usually lethal anomaly. Unless treated surgically almost all infant die within the 1st month of life. Interruption distal to the left subclavian artery (type A) occurs with almost equal frequency to interruption distal to the left common carotid artery (type B). Interruption distal to the innominate artery (type C) are extremely uncommon. The right subclavian artery often is of variable origin frequently arising from the descending aortic segment distal to the interruption.

148. Ans. b. 5-10%

Braunwald 5th Ed; Page 913

The management of coarctation of aorta consists of balloon angioplasty and surgical treatment in form of subclavian flap aortoplasty. Controversy exists concerning the role of balloon angioplasty in the treatment of native coarctation especially in neonate. There is concern about residual pressure gradient, aneurysm formation, aortic dissection, rupture and femoral arterial complication especially late after angioplasty. Subclavian flap aortoplasty particularly in neonate and infants is the surgical resection and end to end anastomosis of uncomplicated juxtaductal coarctation of aorta and it can be accomplished with excellent result in most patients. A 5-10% of risk of recurrence of narrowing exists after the repair of coarctation in infancy. Such narrowing is best detected by MRI or Doppler.

149. Ans. d. Patent ductus arteriosus

Braunwald 5th Ed; Page 914

DiGeorge syndrome is a constellation of cardiac parathyroid, thymic and facial anomalies attributed to the disruption of the interaction of premigratory neural crest cells with endodermal pharyngeal pouch cells. In these syndrome, thymic hypoplasia or aplasia is accompanied by immunological and hypocalcemic problem. Major clinical problem is severe congestive heart failure as a consequence of volume overload of the left ventricle resulting from an associated intracardiac left to right shunt and of pressure overload imposed by systemic hypertension. Virtually all patients have patent ductus arteriosus which leads to the congestive heart failure.

150. Ans. a. Thickening of aortic valve and impaired mobility of cusps secondary to trauma of jet

Braunwald 5th Ed; Page 918

Discrete subaortic stenosis accounts for 8-10% of all cases of congenital aortic stenosis and occurs twice as frequently in males as in females. The lesion consists of a membranous diaphragm or fibrous ring encircling the left ventricular outflow tract or a long fibromuscular narrowing just beneath the base of aortic valve. The sub aortic stenosis is usually the result of a malalignment VSD with deviation posteriorly of the outlet septum into the left ventricular outflow tract. It is often associated with coarctation of aorta or interruption of aortic arch. Mild degree of aortic valvular regurgitation commonly are observed in patients with discrete subaortic stenosis and appears to be caused by thickening of the valve and impaired mobility of the cusp, secondary to the trauma created by the high velocity jet passing through the subaortic diaphragm. Further deformation of these abnormal valve cusp by the vegetation following endocarditis often result in severe aortic regurgitation.

151. Ans. a. Distal to left subclavian artery

Braunwald 5th Ed; Page 914

Aortic arch interruption: It is a rare and usually lethal anomaly; unless treated surgically almost all infants die within the first month of life. Interruptions distal to the left subclavian artery (Type A) occur with almost equal frequency to interruptions distal to the left common carotid artery (Type B); interruptions distal to the innominate artery (Type C) are extremely uncommon. The right subclavian artery often is of variable origin, frequently arising from the descending aortic segment distal to the interruption. The clinical presentation resembles that seen in tubular hypoplasia or severe juxtaductal coarctation of the aorta with a patent ductus arteriosus.

152. Ans. b. Cor triatriatum

Braunwald 5th Ed; Page 923

Cor triatriatum is the malformation resulting from failure of resorption of the common pulmonary vein resulting into a left atrium divided by an abnormal fibromuscular diaphragm into posterosuperior chamber receiving the pulmonary veins and in anteroinferior chamber giving rise to left atrial appendage and leading to the mitral orifice. The communication between the divided atrial chambers may be large, small or absent depending on the size of the opening in the dividing diaphragm which remain the degree of obstruction to the pulmonary venous return. The diagnosis of this condition is established by 2D echocardiography or TEE. Cardiac catheterization and angiography are necessary only if major associated cardiac anomalies are suspected. The diagnosis should be suspected at cardiac catheterization if the pulmonary arterial wedge pressure is higher than a simultaneous left atrial pressure. The diagnosis also may be established by visualizing the obstructing lesion angiographically.

153. Ans. a. Infundibular

Braunwald 5th Ed; Page 929

The overall incidence of this anomaly approaches 10% of all forms of congenital heart disease, and it is the most common cardiac malformation responsible for cyanosis after one year of age. The four components of this malformation are: (1) ventricular septal defect; (2) obstruction to right ventricular outflow; (3) overriding of the aorta; and (4) right ventricular hypertrophy. TRhe basic anomaly is the result of an anterior deviation of the septal insertion of the infundibular ventricular septum from its usual location in the normal heart between the limbs of the trabecular septum. The interventricular malalignment defect usually is large, approximating the aortic orifice in size, and is located high in the septum just below the right cusp of the aortic valve, separated from the pulmonic valve by the crista supraventricularis. The aortic root may be displaced anteriorly and straddle or override the septal defect, but as in the normal heart, it lies to the right of the origin of the pulmonary artery. In most cases no dextroposition of the aorta exists, overriding of the aorta is a phenomenon secondary to the subaortic location of the ventricular septal defect.

Hemodynamics: The degree of obstruction to pulmonary blood flow is the principal determinant of the clinical presentation. The site of obstruction is variable, infundibular stenosis is the only major obstruction in about 50% of patients and coexists with valvular obstruction in another 20-25%. Supravalvular and peripheral pulmonary arterial narrowing may be observed, and unilateral absence of a pulmonary artery (usually the left) is found in a small number of patients. Circulation to the abnormal lung is accomplished by bronchial and other collateral arteries. Atresia of the pulmonic valve, infundibulum, or main pulmonary artery occasionally is referred to as pseudotruncus arteriosus. True truncus arteriosus with absent pulmonary arteries (Type 4) differs from Fallot's tetralogy, in which pulmonary artery branches are present but are fed by a patent ductus arteriosus and/or bronchial arteries. A right sided aortic knob, aortic arch, and descending aorta occur in about 25% of patients with tetralogy of Fallot. The coronary arteries may have surgically important variations: The anterior descending artery may originate from the right coronary artery; a single right coronary artery may give off a left branch that courses anterior to the pulmonary trunk; a single left coronary artery may give off a right branch that crosses the infundibulum of the right ventricle. Enlargement of the infundibulum branch of the right coronary artery often presents a problem with respect to a right ventriculotomy.

Associated cardiac anomalies exist in about 40% of patients. Major associated cardiac anomalies include patient ductus arteriosus, multiple (usually muscular) ventricular septal defects, and complete atrioventricular septal defects. Localized single or multiple peripheral pulmonary arterial stenotic lesions are common; rarely, the right or left pulmonary artery may arise anomalously from the ascending aorta. Infrequently, aortic valve regurgitation results from aortic cusp prolapse. Associated extracardiac anomalies are present in 20-30% of patients.

When right ventricular outflow tract obstruction is severe, the pulmonary blood flow is markedly reduced, and a large volume of unsaturated systemic venous blood is shunted from right to left across the ventricular septal defect. At the opposite end of the spectrum, the term acyanotic or pink tetralogy of Fallot often is used to describe an interventricular communication and a milder degree of obstruction to right ventricular outflow with little or no venoarterial shunting.

154. Ans. a. Severity of RVOT obstruction

Braunwald 5th Ed; Page 929

Refer to explanation for Q. No 153.

155. Ans. d. All of the above

Braunwald 5th Ed; Page 929

During cardiac catheterization, catheter from right ventricle may enter into aorta in condition like large VSD. Transposition of great arteries, single ventricle, TOF, and truncus arteriosus.

156. Ans. c. Somatic tremor effect

Hurst's 8th Ed; Page 346

Characteristic ECG changes develop when the body temperature drops to approximately 30°C. The QT interval becomes prolonged. In addition, a deflection, called an "Osborn wave", appears in a place said to be located between the end of the QRS complex and the beginning of the ST segment. This deflection has been attributed to delayed depolarization, to a current of injury, or to 'early' repolarization. In leads facing the left ventricle, the deflection is positive, and its size is inversely related to body temperature. The role played by the intramyocardial M cells in its genesis has been discussed previously.

Muscle tremor and alternating current interference are thought to be the most common artifacts. But in clinical practice, worldwide experience in ECG has shown that recordings of precordial electrodes are made with astonishingly marked neglect as to the employment of the proper chest landmarks. Simonson found that in a controlled study, placemen tof the V2 electrode varied 10 cm vertically and 8 cm horizontally in 103 healthy subjects. Moreover, Kerwin et al found a rather large error in placement of chest electrodes (2-3 cm in both the horizontal and vertical directions) in repeated trials in the same patients by the same technicians. A more recent study found that there was a superior displacement of >0.625 in V1 and V2 and inferior and upward displacement of >0.625 in V4, V5 and V6. Such a variability creates severe problems for computer interpretation of serial ECGs and considerable difficulties for the diagnosis of MI in the presence of LBBB. The most frequent cause of "poor R wave progression in the anteroseptal leads" is misplacement of the corresponding electrodes. Improper limb lead placement has gone beyond switching of right arm left arm cables. The method depicted based on the analysis of extremity leads only, is simpler than those incorporating the analysis of bipolar standard leads. Not frequently recognized in ECG textbooks is the incontrovertible fact that, in some centers, even the sanctity of the attachment of the right leg (ground) cable to the right leg has been violated. Finally, overshooting, overdamping, the indiscriminate use of filters, the running down of standardization battery, the range and changing size as well as polarity of large unipolar pacemaker spikes, and the almost microscopic size of some bipolar spikes should be taken into consideration.

Somatic tremor effect is due to shivering of patient and is most specific EKG finding of hypothermia.

157. Ans. a. Ostium secundum ASD

Perloff 3rd Ed; Chapter 13 Page 239

In patient with Ebstein's anomaly an interarterial communication consisting of a patent foramen ovale or an ostium secundum ASD is present in more than half of the cases. The most common important associated defect is pulmonic stenosis or atresia. Other coexisting anomaly may include the ostium primum type of ASD and VSD alone or in combination with other lesions. The Ebstein lesion commonly is observed in association with congenital corrected transposition of great arteries in which tricuspid valve is in the left atrioventricular orifice.

158. Ans. c. Ebstein anomaly

Perloff, 3rd Ed; Chapter 13, Page 239

In an occasional patient with Ebstein's anomaly, it is often seen that there is a transient neonatal cyanosis with recurrence a decade or more later. A right to left interarterial shunt disappears as neonatal pulmonary vascular resistance normalizes and recurs later as the filling pressure rises in the functionally abnormal right ventricle. This is a characteristic feature of Ebstein anomaly.

159. Ans. c. 'Second QRS' complex

Perloff, 3rd Ed; Chapter 13, Page 247

Major electrophysiologic abnormalities in Ebstein's anomaly:
1. Intra-atrial conduction disturbance—"right atrial P wave abnormalities," PR interval prolongation
2. Atrioventricular nodal conduction disturbance—PR interval prolongation
3. Infranodal conduction disturbances
   a. Intra- or infra-His disturbances
   b. Right bundle branch block
   c. Bizarre 'second' QRS attached to preceding 'normal' complex
4. Type B Wolff–Parkinson–White
5. Supraventricular tachycardia
6. Atrial fibrillation or flutter
7. Electromechanical dissociation in atrialized right ventricle
8. Irritability of atrialized right ventricle
9. Q waves in leads V1–V4

The QRS complex in patient with Ebstein anomaly is typically prolonged and exhibits a right ventricular conduction defect of right bundle branch block type in 75–90% of the cases. There is also a distinctive pattern of Bizarre 'second' QRS complex attached to the preceding normal complex. Intracardiac electrical mapping confirm that atrialize right ventricle produces the second QRS. QRS prolongation occurs in infant.

160. Ans. b. Left bundle branch block pattern

Perloff 3rd Ed; Chapter 13, Page 247

Refer to explanation for Q. No 159.

161. Ans. d. Hemodynamic study with intracardiac electrogram

Braunwald 5th Ed; Page 935

The diagnosis of Ebstein anomaly can be made with reasonable accuracy with the help of echocardiography. Invasive study is rarely necessary. The principle echocardiographic findings observed in patient with this anomaly as well as in those with other form of right ventricular volume overload or an increase in the right ventricular dimension, paradoxical ventricular septal motion, an increase in tricuspid valve excursion and an abnormal closing velocity of tricuspid valve. More specific findings for Ebstein anomaly include a delay in the tricuspid valve closure relative to the mitral closure and a decrease in the EF slope of the tricuspid valve, an abnormal anterior position of the tricuspid valve during the diastole. 2 dimensional echocardiographic techniques are superior for observation of the inferior and leftward displacement of the tricuspid valve and simultaneously demonstrate the abnormal positional relation between the tricuspid and mitral valves. Specific diagnosis requires identification usually from an apical four chamber view of displacement of the septal tricuspid leaflet. Tricuspid regurgitation if present is detected by Doppler examination. Invasive studies is rarely necessary. When cardiac catheterization is performed, the intracavitary electrogram recorded just proximal to the tricuspid valve shows the right ventricular type of complex while the pressure recorded is that of the right atrium. A right to left atrial shunt anomaly is present. The hemodynamic findings depend on degree of tricuspid regurgitation. The cardiac muscle is unusually irritable and high incidence of significant arrhythmias during catheterization has been noted. Selective right ventricular angiocardiography shows the position of the displaced tricuspid valve, the size of right ventricle and configuration of the outflow portion of the right ventricle.

162. Ans. a. Aortic atresia without VSD

Perloff 6th Ed; Chapter 31, Page 522

In hypoplastic left heart syndrome variants of aortic atresia without ventricular septal defect, there is relative infrequency of left ventricular hypertrophy in electrocardiogram despite a thick walled left ventricle and it is a point of clinical importance and theoretical interest. The reasons lie in the small volume of the ventricular cavity. Variation in the end diastolic volume affects the magnitude of QRS forces which are generated at the end diastole. An increase in the end diastolic volume increases the amplitude of early portion of QRS where decrease has the opposing effect. Consistent with these observations are the greater left ventricular forces that results when aortic atresia is associated with a ventricular septal defect and an adequately develop left ventricular chamber.

163. Ans. d. All of the above

Perloff, 3rd Ed; Chapter 30, Page 644

Pulmonary arteriovenous fistula typically occurs without associated congenital heart disease but coexistence of atrial septal defect have been described. An occasional patient may have mild to moderate pulmonary hypertension. The arteriovenous fistula of the lungs are regarded as the pulmonary manifestation of the generalized congenital vascular disorders. The telangiectatic lesion themselves are tiny localized arteriovenous fistula composed of dilated fragile vessel with a single layer of endothelium and no muscular or elastic recoils. Rupture in these telangiectasia occurs readily because of the fragility of thin dilated vascular membranes. Telangiectasias are found on the skin, lips and nasal or oral mucous membrane, beneath the nails and in gastrointestinal tract, liver, central nervous system and kidney. Epistaxis are frequent and recurrent bleeding from the mouth or lips is common. Telangiectases in the tracheobronchial tree contribute to the hemoptysis. Inappropriately placed lesions may cause malena, hematuria, intraocular hemorrhage, vaginal bleeding and cerebrovascular accidents.

164. Ans. b. Pulmonary arteriovenous fistulae

Perloff, 3rd Ed; Chapter 30, Page 644

Refer to explanation for Q. No 163.

165. Ans. d. Lower lobes and right middle lobes

Perloff, 3rd Ed; Chapter 30, Page 641

The congenital pulmonary arteriovenous fistula is caused by abnormal development of pulmonary arteries and veins from a common vascular complex. The lesion can be either solitary or multiple, unilateral or bilateral or minute and diffuse throughout both the lungs. The majority of pulmonary arteriovenous fistula involves the lower lobes or right middle lobe. The incidence of localization at these sites have been estimated at 75%.

166. Ans. b. Congenital pulmonary arteriovenous fistulae

Perloff, 3rd Ed; Chapter 30, Page 648

Pulmonary arteriovenous fistula are usually discovered in healthy, young adults with abnormal density on routine chest X-ray or with cyanosis and hereditary hemorrhagic telangiectasia. Dyspnea and fatigue are mild, even in the presence of conspicuous cyanosis. Intermittent epistaxis and hemoptysis punctuate the history. Recurrent bleeding also occurs from the mouth, lips or gastrointestinal tract. Members of the family often have similar affliction. More often, pulmonary arteriovenous fistula is a cause of cyanosis with normal pulmonary arterial blood flow and pressure and clinically normal ventricle. The combination of cyanosis and telangiectasia with a normal electrocardiogram and a normal cardiac silhouette on X-ray is characteristic and diagnosis is virtually conclusive when fistula cast distinctive shadow in the chest film.

167. Ans. c. Congenital pulmonary arteriovenous fistulae

Perloff, 3rd Ed; Chapter 30, Page 648

Refer to explanation for Q. No 166.

168. Ans. b. Persistence truncus arteriosus

Perloff, 3rd Ed; Page 492, 495, 496 & 500

It is already given with the answers for of Q. No 79 to 83.

169. Ans. b. Truncus arteriosus

Perloff, 3rd Ed; Page 492, 495, 496 & 500

It is already given with the answers for of Q. No 79 to 83.

170. Ans. a. A short main pulmonary artery originating from the truncus and giving rise to right and left pulmonary arterial branches

Perloff, 3rd Ed; Page 492, 495, 496 & 500

It is already given with the answers for of Q. No 79 to 83.

171. Ans. c. Subpulmonic stenosis with coarctation of aorta

Perloff, 3rd Ed; Chapter 8, Page 164

Shone-s' complex is a developmental complex consisting of four obstructions in series, i.e. supravalvular stenosing ring, parachute mitral valve, subaortic stenosis and coarctation of the aorta. Not all four obstructive lesions are necessarily significant or even present in the cases and other major anomaly may coexist in patient with Shone-s' complex.

172. Ans. a. Parachute mitral valve

Perloff, 3rd Ed; Chapter 8, Page 167

Two-dimensional echocardiography with Doppler interrogation and color flow mapping helps in establishing the diagnosis of congenital mitral stenosis, delineates the morphologic type and determines the degree of obstruction. Real time imaging identifies the presence and movement of stenotic leaflets and of supravalvular membranes and establishes papillary muscles architecture. Two dimensional imaging establishes the number of papillary muscles and the interpapillary distance and also whether or not a single papillary muscle is present. A single eccentrically located papillary muscle characterizes the parachute mitral valve. Two well-defined or two well-formed papillary muscles with a clearly defined but reduced interpapillary distance are a feature of typical congenital mitral stenosis. A supravalvular ring is more readily identified on two-dimensional imaging when the membrane is sufficiently about the mitral valve so as to be distinguishable from it. When the membrane is adherent to mitral valve which is often the case, it is difficult to image and may be apparent only in diastole. An anomalous mitral arcade can be identified with either two papillary muscle or multiple papillary muscles and the functional state of mechanism can be established with color flow imaging and spectral Doppler interrogation. The diagnosis of double orifice mitral valve can be made along with the relative sizes of orifice is determined and the cordal insertion can be identified and the functional state (functionally normal, stenotic or incompetent) can be established by 2D-echocardiogram.

173. Ans. b. Mitral arcade

Perloff, 3rd Ed; Chapter 8, Page 167

Refer to explanation for Q. No 172.

174. Ans. c. The electromechanical properties of the right atrium proper, the atrialized right ventricle and the functional right ventricle

Perloff, 3rd Ed; Chapter 13, Page 237

The electromechanical properties of the right atrium proper, the atrialized right ventricle and functional right ventricle are important features of Ebstein anomaly and it provided the first sound basis for clinical diagnosis. The right atrium proper generates a right atrial pressure pulse and intracavitary atrial electrogram. The right ventricle proper, i.e., functional right ventricle generates a right ventricular pressure pulse and a right ventricular intracavitary electrocardiogram. The intervening atrialized right ventricle generates an intracavitary right ventricular electrogram but an atrial pressure pulse because the atrialized right ventricle contains right ventricular muscle fiber. Mechanical stimulation provoke a right ventricular electrogram but risk inducing ventricular tachycardia and fibrillation remains high.

175. Ans. c. Ebstein's anomaly

Perloff, 3rd Ed; Chapter 13, Page 239

The Ebstein anomaly of the tricuspid valve has a consistent association with the maternal use of lithium carbonate, a drug employed for the treatment of bipolar disorders. Data suggest that lithium carbonate may be teratogenic in humans. The Danish Registry estimated that the relative risk of Ebstein anomaly in offspring was increased by 500-fold. The probability of occurrence of Ebstein anomaly in general population is one in 20,000 so that likelihood of the malformation occurring spontaneously in a pregnant woman taking lithium is one in 20 millions. Current estimates show that the increase risk is around 28-fold considerably less than the estimates from the Danish Registry.

176. Ans. c. Ebstein's anomaly

Perloff, 3rd Ed; Chapter 13, Page 244

Ebstein anomaly of the tricuspid valve is the only congenital cardiac malformation consistently associated with preexcitation, i.e., type B Wolf–Parkinson–White (WPW syndrome) and therefore the combination of palpitations (paroxysmal rapid heart action) with type B WPW pre-excitation and cyanosis constitute presumptive diagnostic evidence of Ebstein anomaly. Anomalous conduction can be either permanent or intermittent and delta waves with normal PR interval are sometime present. Bypass conduction is typically associated with left superior QRS axis. Electrophysiological studies have identify both intra-His and infra-His delay in Ebstein anomaly. Prolong HV intervals are ascribed to impaired conduction or to a long route of conduction within the atrialized right ventricle. These conclusions are consistent with the observations that despite prolong HV interval and marked prolongation of PR interval, complete heart block is a rarity in patient with Ebstein anomaly.

Please refer the answer of Q. No 159 also.

177. Ans. d. All of the above

Perloff, 3rd Ed; Chapter 13, Page 244

Refer to explanation for Q. No 176.

178. Ans. a. Right bundle branch block

Perloff, 3rd Ed; Chapter 13, Page 244

Refer to explanation for Q. No 176.

179. Ans. d. Complete heart block

Perloff, 3rd Ed; Chapter 13, Page 244

Refer to explanation for Q. No 176.

180. Ans. c. Ebstein's anomaly

Perloff, 3rd Ed; Chapter 13, Page 247

The X-ray picture in the patient with Ebstein's anomaly is quiet distinctive. Pulmonary vasculature is either normal or reduced but for all practical purposes is never increased. Normal pulmonary blood flow accompanies acyanotic Ebstein anomaly with mild tricuspid deformity, whereas reduced pulmonary vascularity is feature of cyanotic Ebstein anomaly with severe deformity. The pulmonary trunk is uniformly inconsequential and is not to be mistaken for infundibular shadow with either straightened left cardiac border or forms a conspicuous convex shoulder at the left basal aspect of the heart. The most consistent and dramatic feature of the X-rays is right atrial silhouette which is seldom normal even when the overall heart size is. The right atrial shadow is almost invariably conspicuous sometimes dramatically show. Rightward convexity of right atrium in conjunction with the leftward shoulder of the dilated infundibulum accounts for a box like cardiac shadow. Ebstein anomaly is the only form of cyanotic congenital heart disease in which both the aortic root and pulmonary trunk are likely to be reduced in caliber.

181. Ans. b. Congenital mitral stenosis

Perloff, 3rd Ed; Chapter 9, Page 180

Primary endocardial fibroelastosis is classified clinically as two types; a dilated form and a contracted form. The disorder is characterized by diffuse, opaque, pearly white thickening of the left ventricular endocardium due to the proliferation of collagen and especially of elastic tissue. In primary form of endocardial fibroelastosis coexisting congenital anomalies are absent. Another form of endocardial fibroelastosis is the variety associated with congenital malformation of the heart especially aortic stenosis, Coarctation of aorta, anomalous origin of left coronary artery from pulmonary trunk and hypoplastic left heart. Fibroelastosis has been described in infants with myocardial infarction due to thrombosis of coronary arteries and it has also been seen in adult as, a healing myocardial infarction may be accompanied by endocardial fibroelastosis in the area of the infarct.

182. Ans. c. Eleventh week of pregnancy

Perloff, 3rd Ed; Chapter 10, Page 191

There is association between the stenosis of pulmonary artery and its branches and maternal rubella infection. Maternal viremia is a prerequisite for placental and fetal rubella infection. Most cases occur following primary disease rather than rubella reinfection. When maternal rubella occurs later than 16th week of gestation, the risk of fetal damage appears to be very small. Maternal rubella can have devastating non teratogenic effects on the fetal development including its spontaneous abortion and still birth. Cardiac defects and deafness consistently occurs in infants infected during the first 10 weeks of gestation. Patent ductus arteriosus and pulmonary artery stenosis usually coexist with patent ductus arteriosus the more prevalent of the two lesions.

183. Ans. d. All of the above

Perloff, 3rd Ed; Chapter 10, Page 196

Noonan syndrome, Rubella syndrome, Williams syndrome and arteriohepatic dysplasia (Alagille syndrome) are the common syndrome associated with occurrence of pulmonary stenosis.

184. Ans. a. Fossa ovalis

Perloff, 3rd Ed; Chapter 15, Page 272

The most frequent type of ASD is in the ostium secundum (fossa ovalis) location. Sinus venosus atrial septal defect constitute 2-3% of interarterial communications. A coronary sinus arterial septal defect is the least common variety and as the navue implies is located in the site normally occupied by right atrial ostium of the coronary sinus.

185. Ans. d. Coronary sinus type

Perloff, 3rd Ed; Chapter 15, Page 272

Refer to explanation for Q. No 184.

186. Ans. c. Ostium secundum type of ASD

Perloff, 3rd Ed; Chapter 15, Page 274

Ostium secundum ASD seldom manifest themselves as symptomatic congenital heart disease in infants and young children but when they do approximately 33% are believe to close spontaneously between ages 1 year and 2 years. Spontaneous closure can occur up to age of 30 months. The responsible mechanism remains to be established but atrial septal aneurysm have been assigned a role in spontaneous closure of an associated atrial septal defect.

187. Ans. b. Sinus venosus type

Perloff, 3rd Ed; Chapter 15, Page 275

When one or more, but not all, of all the pulmonary veins connect to the right atrium, the term 'partial anomalous pulmonary venous connection' is used. Total anomalous pulmonary venous connection signifies that all pulmonary veins connect anomalously. Approximately 10-15% of patients with ostium secundum atrial septal defect have partial anomalous pulmonary venous connection. Sinus venosus defects of the superior vena cava type are associated with anomalous connection of right superior pulmonary vein to the right atrium or superior vena cava in 80-90% of the cases. The commonest variety of partial anomalous pulmonary venous connection (about 90%) is between their right upper or middle lobe pulmonary veins and the right atrium or superior vena cava. Partial anomalous pulmonary venous connection of the right lung is usually associated with an atrial septal defect. An intact atrial septum is exceptional. Anomalous connection of left pulmonary veins occurs only 10% as often as anomalous connection of right pulmonary veins. An atrial septal defect is usually coexists. Anomalous connection left pulmonary vein is generally to the innominate vein or to a persistent left superior vena cava that attaches to an innominate vein. Bilateral partial anomalous pulmonary venous connections are rare.

188. Ans. a. Between the right upper or middle lobe pulmonary veins and right atrium or superior vena cava

Perloff, 3rd Ed; Chapter 15, Page 275

Refer to explanation for Q. No 187.

189. Ans. c. There is shifting of heart into the left hemithorax

Perloff, 3rd Ed; Chapter 15, Page 275

The scimitar syndrome is a rare but well-described constellation of cardiopulmonary anomalies. The syndrome consists of total or partial anomalous pulmonary venous connection of the right lung to the inferior vena cava and is usually but not invariably associated with hypoplasia of ipsilateral lung and pulmonary artery. The term 'scimitar' was applied because the shadow on the X-ray resembles a scimitar or Turkish sword. The lower portion of the right lung is perfused by systemic arteries that arise from the abdominal aorta. The scimitar syndrome rarely involved the left lung. The scimitar syndrome is often diagnosed with confidence from plane film of chest X-ray. The confluence of right pulmonary veins forms a distinctive shadow parallel to or behind the right cardiac border as the venous channel courses downwards to join the inferior vena cava. Hypoplasia of right lung and right pulmonary artery causes a shift of the heart into the right hemithorax but the anomalous venous channel sometime remains apparent. The left lung may exhibit an increase in the pulmonary vascularity because of the left to right shunt.

190. Ans. a. Patent foramen ovale

Perloff, 3rd Ed; Chapter 25, Page 554

The interarterial communication in tricuspid atresia takes the form of a patent foreman ovale in about 3 quarter of cases and is therefore restrictive. Atrial septal defect is much less common and when present is always in form of ostium secundum defect. Aneurysmal dilatation of foreman ovale and/or atrium septum occasionally occurs. The aneurysmal bulges sometime large enough to obstruct left atrial flow.

191. Ans. b. Tricuspid atresia without transposition, pulmonic stenosis, small VSD

Perloff, 3rd Ed; Chapter 25, Page 555

Anatomic variation beyond the mitral valve and left ventricles set the stage for clinical classification of tricuspid atresia based on the origin of the aortic root and pulmonary trunk and upon the absence or presence of degree of obstruction to pulmonary blood flow as suggested by Edward and Tondan. In about 90% of the cases, the great arteries are normally related and in virtually all the rest the two great arteries are completely transposed. The tricuspid atresia without transposition can exist with pulmonary atresia and no VSD, it can exist with pulmonary stenosis and a small VSD and it can exist with no pulmonary stenosis and large VSD. Similarly tricuspid atresia with transposition can exist with pulmonary atresia, with pulmonary stenosis and with no pulmonary stenosis. The commonest variety of tricuspid atresia is normally related great arteries, pulmonic stenosis and a small VSD.

192. Ans. a. Tricuspid atresia with normally related great arteries and a small ventricular septal defect

Perloff, 3rd Ed; Chapter 25, Page 565

The direction of the QRS axis in the frontal plane is a considerable diagnostic importance in the clinical recognition of tricuspid atresia. An abnormal leftwards axis with counterclockwise depolarization is a feature of common variety of tricuspid atresia with normally related great arteries and a small ventricular septal defect. The electrical axis seem to depend largely upon the relative mass of the right and left ventricle. Left axis deviation is a characteristic features of tricuspid atresia with small left ventricular septal defect and rudimentary right ventricle but not of tricuspid atresia with large VSD and well-developed right ventricle.

193. Ans. c. Single ventricle with concordant arrangement whereas aorta arises from morphologic left ventricle and pulmonary trunk from rudimentary chamber

Perloff 3rd Ed; Chapter 26, Page 575

In single ventricle or univentricular heart, the great arterial connection can be either discordant or concordant. In the usual variety of univentricular heart with left ventricular morphology, the aorta arises from the outlet chamber and the pulmonary trunk arise from the main ventricular compartment which is morphologic left ventricle. The term transposition is appropriate because the ventriculoarterial connections are discordant. The distinctly less common concordant arrangement in which aorta arise from morphologic left ventricle and pulmonary trunk from outlet chambers has been called the Holmes heart.

194. Ans. a. Single ventricle with noninverted rudimentary chambers

Perloff 3rd Ed; Chapter 26, Page 582

Precordial QRS complex exhibiting a stereotype pattern is suggestive of single ventricle with noninverted rudimentary chamber.

195. Ans. c. Pulmonary artery stenosis is the commonest cardiac lesion

Perloff 3rd Ed; Page 144

The Noonan syndrome is characterized by short stature, neck abnormalities (short or webbed neck), eye abnormalities (Ptosis and Hypertelorism), low set ears, low posterior hairline, thoracic abnormalities, high arched palate, abnormalities of skin, micrognathia and penile abnormalities. Mental retardation occurs in a proximately one-third of patients and congenital heart disease is present in as many as two third. The commonest cardiac lesions are dysplastic pulmonary valve stenosis in approximately 60% cases and hypertrophic cardiomyopathy in approximately 20% of the cases.

196. Ans. b. Aneurysm of abdominal aorta

Perloff 3rd Ed; Chapter 7; Page 128

A variety of aneurysm develops in patient with coarctation of aorta. Dilatation of aortic root and of the descending aorta just distal to the coarctation is the rule. Dissecting aneurysm with hemopericardium has been described. The relationship between the bicuspid aortic valve and ascending aortic aneurysm or dissection is common. The segment of aorta immediately distal to the coarctation often exhibit cystic medial necrosis, an abnormality that provides a pathological basis for aneurysm formation. Among the most dangerous aneurysm are those involving the circle of Willis that set the stage for fatal intracranial hemorrhage. In addition, aneurysm occasionally develops in the distal aortic arch and in the intercostal artery.

197. Ans. d. Pregnancy increases risk of aortic rupture and intracranial hemorrhage

Perloff 3rd Ed; Page 147

The risk of pregnancy in patient with coarctation is marginal. Blood pressure fluctuations are similar in direction to those in uncomplicated pregnancy, but from a higher baseline. The incidence of toxemia is lower in women with coarctation than in pregnant women with other form of hypertension and cardiac failure seldom develops. Nevertheless, pregnancy increases in the risk of aortic rupture and intracranial hemorrhage because gestational changes in connective tissue adds to the abnormalities inherent in the arterial walls. Infective endocarditis is the threat because of potential bacteremia during delivery.

198. Ans. d. Anomalous origin of right subclavian artery distal to the coarctation

Perloff 3rd Ed; Page 148

Abnormal differences in the upper and lower extremity arterial pulses and blood pressure are clinical hallmark of coarctation of aorta. The radiofemoral delay is the hallmark for clinical diagnosis of coarctation of aorta. However, presence of bicuspid aortic valve and its stenosis and presence of aortic regurgitation have variable effect on character of the pulse. In simple term, coarctation of aorta amplifies the brachial arterial pulse and obscure the sign of aortic stenosis, whereas aortic regurgitation amplify the femoral pulse and occur the signs of coarctation. Important variation in the anatomic arrangement of coarctation can be inferred from comparative analysis of arterial pulsation. The right and left brachial artery should be compared by palpation and by blood pressure determination. Absence or diminution of left brachial pulse means that coarctation has compromised the orifice of left subclavian artery. A diminished or absent right brachial pulse implies anomalous origin of right subclavian artery distal to the coarctation. Absence of both brachial arterial pulses signifies that the coarctation is obstructing the orifice of left subclavian artery while the right subclavian arises anomalously below the coarctation. In typical isthmic coarctation the abdominal aorta is seldom palpable. When the coarctation is in the abdomen however, the abdominal aorta proximal to the constriction is readily palpable. In pseudocoarctation arterial pulses are normal because there is no obstruction in aortic lumen.

199. Ans. a. Narrowing distal to left subclavian artery

Perloff, 3rd Ed; Chapter 7, Page 144

Notching of the ribs, a classic radiologic sign of coarctation of aorta result from collateral flow through dilated tortuous pulsatile posterior intercostal arteries. The notches originate in the costal groove rather than on the most inferior rib margin. Notching vary from rib to rib and from patient to patient and may be single, multiple, shallow, deep, broad or narrow. The notches typically appears as irregular scalloped areas on the under surfaces of posterior ribs. Anterior ribs are spared because anterior intercostals arteries do not run in costal groove. Rarely, the superior margin of ribs is notched by a tortuous, overhanging intercostals artery that make contact with the rib below. Rib notching seldom appear before age 6 years but it has been described as earlier 2 years of age. When coarctation is distal to the left subclavian artery which is usual site, bilateral notching is seen between the third and eighth posterior ribs. Notching is rarely found either above the third or below the ninth ribs. Anatomic variations in the site of coarctation are accompanied by the important modifications of these radiologic patterns. The development of arterial collateral depend upon patency of the origin of the two subclavian arteries. When coarctation narrows the orifice of left subclavian artery collateral circulation fail to develop on that side and unilateral rib notching is seen only in the contralateral right posterior rib. When there is anomalous origin of right subclavian artery distal to the coarctation, collateral fail to develop in the right hemithorax so unilateral notching is confine to the left side. The retroesophageal aberrant right subclavian artery sometime identified as a posterior indentation on barium esophagram. When coarctation is in the abdominal aorta, notching if present at all is confine to the lower rib. In older children and adults, lateral X-ray may show retrosternal notching or scalloping caused by dilated tortuous internal mammary artery.

200. Ans. c. Anomalous origin of right subclavian artery distal to the coarctation

Perloff, 3rd Ed; Chapter 7, Page 144

Refer to explanation for Q. No 199.

201. Ans. a. Coarctation involving the orifice of left subclavian artery

Perloff, 3rd Ed; Chapter 7, Page 144

Refer to explanation for Q. No 199.

202. Ans. c. Abdominal coarctation

Perloff, 3rd Ed; Chapter 7, Page 144

Refer to explanation for Q. No 199.

203. **Ans. d. Pseudocoarctation produces similar rib notching pattern**

Perloff, 3rd Ed; Chapter 7, Page 144

Refer to explanation for Q. No 199.

204. **Ans. d. Klinefelter syndrome**

Braunwald 5th Ed; Page 1656

Most forms of aneuploidy and most duplications and deletion of more than a chromosome band are associated with defects of cardiovascular system. Exception are 47,XXX, 47,XYY, an 47,XXY (Klinefelter syndrome) in which the incidence of congenital heart disease is probably not elevated over the population baseline.

205. **Ans. c. There is higher incidence of conotruncal and distal aortic arch abnormality in these patients**

Hurst's 8th Ed; Chapter 96; Page 1728

Down syndrome is the most common phenotype due to human chromosomal aberration and occurs in about once in every 600 births. Most patients have trisomy 21 and risk of this aberration is exponentially related to maternal age. The risk is lowest for young women and rises steeply after the age of 35 reaching to 4% for women over age of 45. The most common cause of morbidity and mortality in Down syndrome patients are congenital heart defect present in 40-50% of cases, hematological malignant disease and duodenal atresia. The most characteristic cardiac anomaly in Downs' syndrome is the defect of closure of endocardial cushions. Complicating the clinical problem in such patient and those with simple septal defect is higher predisposition to pulmonary hypertension in the face of elevated pulmonary blood flow. About 1/3rd of congenital heart defects are complex and these patients tend to be most ill. Mitral valve prolapse is found with the frequency exceeding that in age and gender match control. The aortic and pulmonary valve cusps are predisposed to fenestration in adulthood.

206. **Ans. d. All are true**

Braunwald 5th Ed; Page 1657

Among the patient with 45X karyotype syndrome reported frequency of congenital CV defect vary from 20-50% depending on how patients were ascertained. 50-70% of those with CV defect have clinically important aortic coarctation usually of the postductal type. A variety of other cardiac malformation may occur either singly and in combination with coarctation. There is a strong tendency for left sided flow abnormalities as a major pathogenetic mechanism. Bicuspid aortic valve and dilatation of ascending aorta (with the risk of dissection and histopathology showing elastic fiber abruption occurs even in absence of coarctation) and hypoplastic left heart has been reported. Partial anomalous pulmonary venous drainage without an ASD is fairly common and should be suspected when right ventricular overload is detected in these patients on echocardiography. Blood pressure elevation is common even without coarctation or after its repair. There is a high frequency renal anomalies in these patients which could be cause of hypertension and it may account for high prevalence of hypertension in these patients.

207. **Ans. d. All of the above**

Braunwald 5th Ed; Page 1657

Refer to explanation for Q. No 206.

208. **Ans. d. All of the above**

Braunwald 5th Ed; Page 1663

Cardiovascular defects associated with prenatal exposure to teratogens

Teratogen	Cardiovascular abnormalities
Ethanol	~50% have CHD: VSD (~50% close spontaneously), TOF, ASD, ECD, absence of a pulmonary artery
Hydantoin	~10% have CHD: VSD, ASD, PS
Lithium	<3% have Ebstein anomaly
Phenylalanine	~20% have CHD: TOF
Retinoic acid	>50% have CHD: TGA, TOF, VSD, IAA
Rubella	>50% have CHD: PDA with or without ASD, VSD, PPS, IAA
Trimethadione	~50% have CHD: Complex combinations most frequent (involving VSD, ASD, PDA, AS, PS), VSD, TOF
Valproic acid	>50% have CHD: Left- and right-sided flow lesions: CoA, HLH, ASD, VSD, pulmonary atresia
Vitamin D	Supravalvular aortic stenosis is the cardinal manifestations; PPS
Warfarin	~10% have CHD: PDA, PS; rarely, intracranial hemorrhage

209. **Ans. d. Sodium cromoglycate**

Braunwald 5th Ed; Page 1663

Refer to explanation for Q. No 208.

210. **Ans. a. MVP**

Braunwald 5th Ed; Page 1656

In patients with Marfan syndrome, the most common cardiovascular features are mitral valve prolapse and dilatation of the sinus of Valsalva. Associated clinical problems of mitral regurgitation, aortic regurgitation and aortic dissection account if untreated for most of the early mortality that results in an average age of death in the fourth and fifth decades. Children tend to be more severely affected by mitral valve disease, whereas aortic problems are progressive and more likely in adolescence and beyond. Mitral valve prolapse is age dependent and more common in women with the Marfan syndrome the incidence reaches 60-80% when patients are studied by 2D echocardiography and generally the valve leaflets have an elongated and redundant appearance. Progression of severity as judge by the appearance or worsening of mitral regurgitation by clinical and echocardiographic criteria occurs in at least one quarter of patient.

211. Ans. d. Chromosome 22

Braunwald 5th Ed; Page 1658

Conotruncal malformation is as a result of defect in a region of chromosome 22 which plays a major role in the development of conotruncus, branchial arches and the face. It was first detected for the patients with DiGeorge syndrome, where small deletions involving chromosome 22q11 was found to be responsible. This condition includes developmental anomalies of the 4th brachial arch and derivative of the 3rd and 4th pharyngeal pouches. Hypoplasia of the thymus and parathyroid causes immune deficiency and hypocalcemia. The cardiac defect ranges from TOF to ventricular septal defect, truncus arteriosus, interrupted aortic arch type B and right sided aortic arch and are often lethal.

212. Ans. a. Endocardial cushion defect

Braunwald 5th Ed; Page 1658

Extracellular matrix abnormality may lead to the defects related to endocardial cushions. There is a high frequency of endocardial cushions defect and atrioventricular septal defect in patients with Down syndrome. The distinctiveness of endocardial cushion defect in patient with normal chromosome and in those with trisomy 21 has been suggested because of difference in the associated cardiovascular malformation.

213. Ans. c. Sperm hypermotility

Braunwald 5th Ed; Page 1658

The situs and looping defects are categorized under the title of heterotaxy. Several Mendelian phenotypes points to single gene that have a major effect on determining laterality. Kartagener syndrome is an autosomal recessive condition leading to lateralization of the heart (situs solitus and situs universus are equally likely in homozygotes) coexists with defect in ciliary mobility which leads to sinusitis bronchiectasis and sperm immotility.

214. Ans. a. Secundum ASD

Braunwald 5th Ed; Page 1658

The acronym Catch-22 is used for cardiac anomaly, abnormal facies, thymic hypoplasia, cleft palate and hypocalcemia is a form of conotruncal malformation and ventricular septal defect is the commonest abnormality noted in these patients.

215. Ans. c. Supravalvular AS

Braunwald 5th Ed; Page 1662

Williams syndrome is a sporadic but in and more often is a highly variable autosomal dominant condition. The full spectrum of Williams syndrome includes infantile hypercalcemia, abnormal ("Elfin") facies, mental deficiency, short statured, multiple peripheral pulmonary stenosis and supravalvular aortic stenosis. Occasional, cardiovascular manifestations are mitral valve prolapse, bicuspid aortic valve and hypertension. Although patient usually survive the problems of infancy and so catch up growth, progressive problems of joint contractures, genitourinary and gastrointestinal dysfunction and psychosocial adjustments defines the long-term prognosis in these patients. Supravalvular aortic stenosis is due to heterozygosity for a mutation in tropoelastin. Because elastic fibers are intrinsic to the media of elastic and muscular arteries, a diffuse progressive arteriopathy develops with thickening of the wall and reduction of the lumen. The natural history of the arterial disease is just emerging as patient with Williams syndrome live longer and or followed prospectively. A predisposition to cerebrovascular disease seems certain in these cases of Williams syndrome.

216. Ans. d. All of the above

Braunwald 5th Ed; Page 1662

Refer to explanation for Q. No 215.

217. Ans. c. Ethanol

Braunwald 5th Ed; Page 1663

Please refer the Answer of Q. No 208 and 209.

218. Ans. b. Risk is not related to the amount of alcohol consumed

Braunwald 5th Ed; Page 1664

Fetal alcohol syndrome: Ethanol is the most common teratogen to which the human embryo and fetus are exposed. The period of greatest vulnerability is the first trimester and the risks are clearly related to the amount of alcohol consumed. The risk of fetal alcohol syndrome occurring in an offspring of a chronic alcoholic woman is 30-50%. The features are highly variable and include growth retardation, mild-to-moderate mental retardation, hyperactivity, short palpebral fissures, a smooth philtrum with a thin upper lip and small distal phalanges. Congenital heart defects occurs in more than one half of the children with a full spectrum of phenotypes. VSD are most common and often insignificant but ASD, TOF and aortic coarctation can occur.

219. Ans. c. Retinoic acid embryopathy

Braunwald 5th Ed; Page 1664

Retinoic acid embryopathy: Isotretinoin was not recognized as a teratogen until after it was licensed for the treatment of acne. The vulnerable period extends from 1st week through the 4th month of gestation. The risk of miscarriage and still birth are elevated. The phenotype includes anomalies of craniofacies and gross neuroanatomical disruption. Cardiovascular defects are common and emphasize a variety of conotruncal malformation. Live born infants often succumb to the cardiac and brain anomalies. Vitamin "A" derivatives such as retinoic acid function as morphogens during embryogenesis serving as signals for cell migration. The cardiovascular defects primarily those of rotation and folding occurs in this syndrome and it is suggestive of disruption of normal developmental homeostatic system.

220. Ans. a. Chances of fetal infection is more when mother is infected during last trimester

Braunwald 5th Ed; Page 1664

Fetal rubella effects: About 50% of fetus become infected with the rubella virus when the mother is infected during the first trimester. Not only does the infected fetus suffer varied and severe interference with development and organogenesis but it acquires a chronic viral illness that can persist for years. The most common features of the embryopathy are mental deficiency, deafness, cataract and cardiovascular defects. Patent ductus arteriosus is common as are septal defect. Peripheral pulmonary artery stenosis and fibromuscular proliferation of medium and small arteries often improve postnatally in these patients.

221. Ans. c. Constrictive pericarditis

Braunwald 5th Ed; Page 1665

The syndrome of mulibrey Nanism is a combination of a mnemonic for muscles, liver, brain and eye and an archaic word for DWAFISM (nanism). This syndrome was described in Finland. Growth failure from an early age is common and there is a occurrence of sign and symptoms of constrictive pericarditis, which develops insidiously and treatment by pericardiectomy is life saving in these patients.

222. Ans. b. Italy

Braunwald 5th Ed; Page 1666

Hereditary cardiomyopathy are causes of familial dysrhythmia and notable example is arrhythmogenic right ventricular dysplasia (ARVD). ARVD is an autosomal dominant condition with variable expression. Although ARVD is uncommon, the familial forms shows cluster of high incidence in some region of italy and is an underappreciated cause of life-threatening arrhythmia. The right ventricle is involved primarily in most cases with thinning and replacement of myocardium by fat and fibrosis. Dysrhythmia, usually ventricular but occasionally supraventricular may precede signs of right ventricular dysfunction. About 1/3rd of cases are familial, generally in an autosomal dominant pattern. Whether the primary process is homogeneous or not and whether true dysplasia, degeneration (due to a metabolic defect or muscular dystrophy) or inflammation plays the leading roles are unclear. The association of familial syncope, sudden death and congenital defects are known as Jervell and Lange-Nielsen syndrome. This is an autosomal recessive condition and the parents of affected children are more likely than average to be consanguineous. Although heterozygotes have normal hearing and no overt primary rhythm disturbances, the QTC interval may be slightly prolonged. The frequency of long QTC among deaf children is about one in 100 so routine electrocardiographic screening of anyone with congenital deafness is warranted to rule out this syndrome.

223. Ans. d. Holt-Oram syndrome

Braunwald 5th Ed; Page 880-881 & 1667

Please refer the answer of Q. No 5 to 11.

Chapter 17: Acquired Disease of Infants and Childhood

1. **Commonest etiological organism causing myocarditis in utero is:**
   a. Coxsackie virus
   b. Rubella virus
   c. Adenovirus
   d. Influenza virus

2. **The most common causative virus for infective myocarditis in childhood beyond infancy is:**
   a. Rubella virus
   b. Coxsackie A and B
   c. Adeno virus
   d. Echo virus

3. **Which of the following investigation is specific in diagnosis of active myocarditis?**
   a. Technetium labeled leukocyte imaging
   b. Radionuclide gallium 67 scanning
   c. MRI
   d. Echocardiography

4. **Which of the following therapeutic agent use is associated with better survival and improved recovery of left ventricular function in children with acute viral myocarditis?**
   a. Antiviral drugs
   b. Immunosuppressant drugs
   c. Steroid and other anti-inflammatory drugs
   d. High dose intravenous gamma globulin

5. **Which of the following is *not* correct regarding diphtheric myocarditis?**
   a. It occurs in 10% of affected patients with diphtheria
   b. It is due to direct invasion of myocardium by the bacillus
   c. It is due to bacterial endotoxins
   d. There is marked depletion of myocardial carnitine

6. **Which of the following therapeutic agent is known to reverse the diphtheric cardiac dysfunction and reduces the risk of cardiac death?**
   a. IV penicillin
   b. IV corticosteroids
   c. Diphtheric antitoxins
   d. Parenteral carnitine

7. **Which of the following EKG abnormalities is associated with high mortality in diphtheric myocarditis?**
   a. ST-T Changes
   b. EKG pattern of myocardial infarction
   c. Ventricular arrhythmias
   d. Complete heart block

8. **Late developing chronic myocarditis is a feature of infection with:**
   a. Coxsackie B virus
   b. C-diphtheria
   c. *Trypanosoma cruzi*
   d. Human immunodeficiency virus

9. **The cardiac involvement is often in which variety of glycogen storage disease:**
   a. Type II (Pompe's disease)
   b. Type III
   c. Type IV
   d. Type VI

10. **The electrocardiographic patterns of extremely tall, broad QRS complexes with short PR interval is found in:**
    a. Infantile Beriberi
    b. Pompe's disease
    c. Chagas disease
    d. Idiopathic dilated cardiomyopathy

11. **The most probable diagnosis in an edematous, irritable infant with prominent signs of systematic venous congestion and right ventricular dilatation is:**
    a. Protein calorie malnutrition
    b. Infantile Beriberi
    c. Tropical endomyocardial fibrosis
    d. Kawasaki disease

12. **Which is *not* correct regarding cardiac involvement in Kawasaki disease?**
    a. Coronary arterial involvement is seen approximately 20% of cases
    b. Majority of children with coronary artery aneurysm diagnosed in acute phase have persistence of a aneurysm at later age
    c. Use of corticosteroid is detrimental in acute phase of disease
    d. Multiple doses of immunoglobulin is beneficial

CHAPTER 17 | Acquired Disease of Infants and Childhood

13. All the following are *correct* regarding coronary artery involvement in Kawasaki disease *except*?
   a. In > 50% cases with coronary aneurysm diagnosed in acute phase of disease, have normal vessel on angiography after 1-2 years
   b. Intravenous gamma globulin reduces likelihood of developing giant coronary aneurysm
   c. In patient with acute coronary thrombosis, intracoronary thrombolytic therapy has proved fatal
   d. When required bypass, patency rate of saphenous vein graft is poor

14. Which is *not* a cause of systemic hypertension in children?
   a. Coarctation of aorta
   b. Gonadal dysgenesis
   c. Kawasaki disease
   d. Solitary renal cyst

15. Which level of serum cholesterol and triglycerides needs treatment in children?
   a. 50th percentile for their age
   b. 75th percentile for their age
   c. 95th percentile for their age
   d. Children do not require treatment

ANSWERS WITH EXPLANATIONS

1. Ans. b. Rubella virus

Braunwald 5th Ed; Page 988-989

Infectious process that cause inflammatory disease of heart may occur at any age, including fetal life. Causative agents include viruses, Rickettsiae, bacteria, spirochetes, fungi, protozoa and helminths. Coxsackie B and rubella viruses are the most common causative agents in infective myocarditis of the newborn. Active rubella myocarditis occurs in utero and may cause variable degree of myocardial damage. Invariably other cardiovascular manifestation of rubella syndrome dominates the clinical picture. Coxsackie B typically causes outbreak of epidemic myocarditis but may occur in the isolated infant in the newborn nursery commonly with a fatal outcome. The illness is of sudden onset and it is characterized by fever, tachycardia, signs of systemic hypoperfusion, cyanosis and occasionally cardiac failure. In some infants, signs and symptoms of encephalomyelitis and hepatitis predominate. The diagnosis is suggested by electrocardiographic findings of atrial and/or ventricular arrhythmias, generalized ST segment and T wave changes and low voltage QRS complexes, accompanied by the appearance of marked generalized cardiomegaly and pulmonary vascular congestion on chest X-ray. Echocardiography reveals dilatation of both ventricles and depressed indices of cardiac performance. The diagnosis is strongly suggested or confirmed when the virus can be isolated from pericardial fluid, pharyngeal secretion, facies and when elevation occurs in type specific neutralizing hemagglutination—inhibiting or compliment fixing antibody. Numerous viral agents have been identified as a cause of myocarditis in childhood beyond infancy. The most common are coxsackie A and B, influenza, adeno virus and ECHO virus. Myocarditis usually of mild degree may be associated with the common viral infection disease of the childhood including mumps, measles, infectious mononucleosis, Varicella and Variola. Diagnosis is suggested by the presence of sustained tachycardia out of proportion to fever, cardiomegaly, without significant murmurs, poor quality heart sounds, a gallop rhythm, and unexplained arrhythmias and electrocardiographic findings. Radionuclide gallium 67 scanning of the heart showing intense gallium uptake provide suggestive evidence of acute myocarditis. Technetium—labeled leukocyte scanning may also prove useful in evaluation. Magnetic resonance imaging holds promise for the noninvasive diagnosis of acute myocarditis showing consistently greater than the normal myocardial/skeletal muscle signal intensity ratios. The vast majority of these children recover from the acute episode of myocarditis with few or no sequela. The result of treating patient with antiviral therapy or with immunosuppressant and anti-inflammatory drugs have been inconclusive or disappointing. In some cases, high doses IV gamma globulin is administered, and recent studies suggested that this approach results in better survival and improved recovery of left ventricular function. Cardiac transplantation has been successful in some of these children with cardiomyopathy and a chronic refractory heart failure, however cardiac transplantation in children especially in infant or very young children is complicated by growth suppression related to the required steroid doses and complexity and severity of the immunosuppression in this infection prone age groups.

2. Ans. b. Coxsackie A and B

Braunwald 5th Ed; Page 988-989

Refer to explanation for Q. No 1.

3. Ans. a. Technetium labeled leukocyte imaging

Braunwald 5th Ed; Page 988-989

Refer to explanation for Q. No 1.

4. Ans. d. High dose intravenous gamma globulin

Braunwald 5th Ed; Page 988-989

Refer to explanation for Q. No 1.

5. Ans. b. It is due to direct invasion of myocardium by the bacillus

Braunwald 5th Ed; Page 989

Diphtheritic cardiomyopathy: Diphtheria usually occurs in unimmunized children. Cardiac involvement is the result of bacterial endotoxin rather than cardiac invasion by the bacillus. Cardiac dysfunction appears to be related to abnormal fat metabolism because diphtheria toxin causes marked depletion of myocardial carnitine, a cofactor required for the β-oxidation of the fats. Cardiac involvement occurs in about 10% of affected patients and is the most common cause of death from this disease. Heart disease is most reliably indicated by electrocardiographic changes which range from ST segment and T wave changes to arrhythmias and conduction disturbance including complete heart block.

Occasionally electrocardiographic pattern of myocardial infarction may emerge. The electrocardiogram is a fair indicator of the extent of the myocardial involvement and of prognosis. The prognosis is favorable if only ST segment and T wave changes are observed in the absence of conduction system disturbances. Right or left bundle branch block and complete atrioventricular block are associated with mortality rates of 50-80%. The electrocardiographic findings may be accompanied by evidence of myocardial dysfunction and ventricular chamber dilatation on cardiac ultrasound. The treatment of diphtheritic cardiomyopathy usually is unsatisfactory. All patients should receive diphtheria antitoxin and intravenous penicillin after appropriate skin testing. Corticosteroid therapy is of no value. Digitalis should be administered cautiously because it may increase atrioventricular block. Diuretics and antiarrhythmic drugs are usually indicated. Transvenous pacemaker is instituted for complete AV block. Parenteral administration of carnitine (100 mL/kg/day) has been found to partially reverse diphtheritic cardiac dysfunction and reduce the risk of cardiac death. If the child recovers from the acute episode of diphtheritic cardiomyopathy, the prognosis is quite good.

6. Ans. d. Parenteral carnitine

Braunwald 5th Ed; Page 989

Refer to explanation for Q. No 5.

7. Ans. d. Complete heart block

Braunwald 5th Ed; Page 989

Refer to explanation for Q. No 5.

8. Ans. c. *Trypanosoma cruzi*

Braunwald 5th Ed; Page 989

Chagas disease is a chronic parasitosis caused by *Trypanosoma cruzi*. Its most important clinical manifestation is a late developing, chronic myocarditis and much less frequently an early acute myocarditis and it is fatal in up to 10% of cases. In approximately 30% of patients, who survived the acute state, cardiomyopathy may occur after an interval of 10-30 years. The cardiac findings are often accompanied by digestive and autonomic disorders. The diagnosis is usually made by endomyocardial biopsy. There is no satisfactory treatment. Administration of mixed gangliosides intramuscularly may be beneficial in reducing arrhythmias.

9. Ans. a. Type II (Pompe's disease)

Braunwald 5th Ed; Page 992

Glycogen storage disease is the result of a deficiency of one or more of the enzymes involved in the biosynthesis and degradation of glycogen. Cardiomyopathy is rare but may be observed in Type III, Type IV and Type VI of this disease. The heart is importantly involved in Type II (Pompe's disease), which results from a deficiency of α-1 4-glucosidase (acid maltase). This disease is a hereditary error of metabolism transmitted through a single recessive gene. Generalized glycogenesis takes place, occurring especially in the heart, the skeletal muscle and the liver. As a result, the heart enlarges often to a marked degree and congestive heart failure supervenes. Clinical signs of type II glycogen storage disease usually become prominent in the early neonatal period. Glycogen deposits within myocardium usually is of uniform variety, although occasionally the interventricular septum involvement produces subpulmonic obstruction or a constellation of features indistinguishable from hypertrophic obstructive cardiomyopathy. Characteristic clinical symptoms includes failure to thrive, progressive hypotonia, lethargy and a weak cry. Prominent early features include non specific cardiac murmur, cardiomegaly, signs of congestive heart failure, poor skeletal muscle tone and weakness. The electrocardiogram shows extremely tall broad QRS complex with short PR interval. The PR interval may be result of the facilitated atrioventricular conduction due to myocardial glycogen deposition. Chest X-ray shows enlarged globular heart associated with pulmonary vascular congestion. Cardiac glycogenosis leads to progressive impairment of myocardial function. Pompe's disease is uniformly fatal usually within the first year of life. Death quite often is the result of either cardiac failure or complication of respiratory management such as pneumonia or aspiration.

10. **Ans. b. Pompe's disease**

Braunwald 5th Ed; Page 992

Refer to explanation for Q. No 9.

11. **Ans. b. Infantile Beriberi**

Braunwald 5th Ed; Page 994

Thiamine (vitamin B1) deficiency mainly occurs in the region of South East Asia, India, Brazil and Africa in which the staple diet is polystrides or cassava. Thiamine functions as a coenzyme in decarboxylation of alpha ketoacid and in the utilization of pentose in the hexose monophosphate shunt. A reduction in the myocardial energy production causes symptom in infants usually between one and four months of age, who is breastfed by a thiamine deficient mother. Rarely improper and ill advise parental feeding practices lead to the vitamin deficiency. Such infants are usually edematous, irritable, pale and anorectic. Hoarseness or aphonia is common owing to the involvement of the recurrent laryngeal nerve. Typically cardiac involvement manifest as dilatation of right ventricle and prominent signs of systemic venous congestion. Electrocardiographic findings are non specific and radiological findings principally consist of right ventricular dilatation. Infantile Beriberi may be rapidly fatal but respond quickly and well to the administration of thiamine (20–50 mg intravenous) initially with the reduction of dose to 10 mg/day for several days and then orally for several weeks. Dramatic amelioration occurs within a few days of the cardiac findings. Cure is risk complete with known sequally.

12. **Ans. b. Majority of children with coronary artery aneurysm diagnosed in acute phase have persistence of a aneurysm at later age**

Braunwald 5th Ed; Page 997

13. **Ans. c. In patient with acute coronary thrombosis, intracoronary thrombolytic therapy has proved fatal**

Braunwald 5th Ed; Page 997

Kawasaki disease (mucocutaneous lymph node syndrome): Kawasaki disease is a generalized vasculitis of unknown etiology. Up to 80% of the cases occurs in children < 5 years of age and most are under age of 2 years. Fewer than 2% of patients have recurrence. The syndrome present with fever, and ocular and oral manifestations followed in 5 days by a rash and endurative edema of the hands and feet with palmer and plantar erythema. Finally, after about 2 weeks cutaneous desquamation occurs. Infants and children with this syndrome should be closely watched for signs of cardiac involvement. A significant number of patients show evidence of myocarditis or pericarditis or both in the early stage of the disease. Pericardial effusion is detected by echocardiography in approximately 30% of the patients. It rarely progress to tamponade and usually resolves without specific therapy. Electrocardiographic evidence of myocarditis with low voltage and non specific ST-T changes are seen in about 45% of the patients. Echocardiographic evidence of poor left ventricular function is seen in 25% cases, cardiomegaly on chest X-ray radiograph in 25% and gallop rhythm in 12%. Coronary arterial abnormality develop in approximately 20% of untreated patients and are the most common cause of short and long term morbidity and mortality. In these children, aneurysm of coronary artery with narrowing, tortuosity and obstruction are detected by 2D echocardiography, aortography and coronary angiography. The appearance > 6 weeks after the illness is uncommon. About half of the children with coronary aneurysm diagnosed shortly after the acute phase of the disease subsides, have normal appearing vessel by angiography 1 to 2 years later. Patient with giant aneurysm (internal diameter > 8 mm) have the worst prognosis and greater chance of developing coronary thrombosis, stenosis or myocardial infarction. In those patients with residual cardiac abnormality after recovery from the acute illness phase, a variety of findings have been described. These include impairment of left ventricular function, secondary to coronary arterial involvement, papillary muscles dysfunction with mitral regurgitation, impaired left ventricular function and abnormalities of the distensibility of the coronary artery. The initial management during the acute phase for Kawasaki disease is directed at reducing inflammation, especially in the coronary arterial tree and myocardium. Later, the treatment is directed towards preventing coronary thrombosis by inhibiting platelet aggregation. Specific treatment awaits discovery of the etiological agent. Corticosteroid is detrimental during the acute illness. Salicylates in a higher doses (80–100 mg/kg/day) until the patient is afebrile is a basic treatment followed by 3–5 mg/kg orally once daily for up to 6–8 weeks. All children diagnosed with Kawasaki disease within 10 days of onset of fever should receive intravenous gamma globulin and high dose aspirin as early as possible. In some patients with acute coronary thrombosis, especially those with giant coronary aneurysm intracoronary thrombolytic therapy may prevent total occlusion of the artery. The prognosis of children with vascular involvement is guarded. All candidates for PTCA, bypass grafting and cardiac transplant. The patency rate of saphenous vein graft is generally unsatisfactory. Bypasses using the internal mammary artery and gastroepiploic artery grafts appear to offer better long-term patency and growth in caliber than saphenous vein graft.

14. Ans. c. Kawasaki disease

Braunwald 5th Ed; Page 998

Conditions and drugs associated with hypertension in infants and children

Congenital	Acquired renal
• Coarctation of the aorta • Gonadal dysgenesis (Turner syndrome) • Rubella syndrome • Pseudoxanthoma elasticum • (Ehlers–Danlos syndrome) • Ask-Upmark syndrome (Segmental renal artery dysplasia) • Renal arterial abnormalities • Multiple systemic and pulmonary artery stenoses • Solitary renal cyst • Hydronephrosis	• Unilateral hydronephrosis • Unilateral pyelonephritis • Renal trauma • Renal tumors • Unilateral multicystic kidney • Unilateral ureteral occlusion • Renal artery stenosis • Renal arteritis • Fibromuscular dysplasia of the renal artery • Renal fistula • Renal artery aneurysm • Chronic pyelonephritis superimposed on abnormal kidneys • Nephritis: Shunt nephritis, acute poststreptococcal disease, anaphylactoid purpura, disseminated lupus erythematosus • Renal tuberculosis • Renal cortical necrosis: Hemolytic uremic syndrome; sepsis • Renal vein thrombosis • Radiation nephritis • Post renal transplantation

Genetic
- Diabetes mellitus
- Neurofibromatosis (von Recklinghausen's disease)
- Adrenogenital syndrome
- Pheochromocytoma
- Polycystic kidney disease (Infantile and adult forms)
- Familial nephritis (Alport syndrome)
- Little syndrome
- Fabry's disease (angiokeratoma corporis diffusum)
- Familial dysautonomia (Riley–Day syndrome)
- Essential hypertension
- Tuberous sclerosis with angiolipomas
- Primary hyperparathyroidism
- Porphyria

Pharmacological
- Sympathomimetics: Ephedrine, epinephrine, isoproterenol
- Adrenal steroids
- Heavy metals: Mercury, lead
- Licorice

Acquired, other than renal
- Hyperthyroidism
- Retrosternal goiter
- Guillain–Barré syndrome or poliomyelitis
- Cerebral edema
- Stevens–Johnson syndrome
- Neuroblastoma
- Hypercalcemia or hypernatremia
- Adrenal adenoma or hyperplasia: Primary aldosteronism or Cushing's syndrome
- Hyperuricemic nephropathy
- Burns

15. Ans. c. 95th percentile for their age

Braunwald 5th Ed; Page 1002–1003

The importance of prevention of arteriosclerosis in childhood is widely accepted. Hyperlipidemic children are at high-risk of becoming hyperlipidemic adults and or therefore a greater risk of future atherosclerotic disease. Although opinion vary about the feasibility of maintaining low serum lipid level in normal children by dietary modification, there is consensus that children whose serum cholesterol or triglyceride level are beyond the 95th percentile for their age and gender should be treated. The guidelines for abnormal level in the first-two decades of life are as follow:

Fasting lipid and lipoprotein levels (mg/dl) in children by age

	Males			Females		
	5%	50%	95%	5%	50%	95%
Cholesterol						
0–4 years	114	155	203	112	156	200
5–9 years	121	160	203	126	164	205
10–14 years	119	158	202	124	160	201
15–19 years	113	150	197	120	158	203
Triglycerides						
0–4 years	29	56	98	34	64	112
5–9 years	30	56	101	32	60	105
10–14 years	32	66	125	37	75	131
15–19 years	37	78	148	39	75	132
HDL cholesterol						
5–9 years	38	56	74	36	53	73
10–14 years	37	55	74	37	52	70
15–19 years	30	46	63	35	52	74
LDL cholesterol						
5–9 years	63	93	129	68	100	140
10–14 years	64	100	140	68	97	132
15–19 years	62	94	130	59	96	137

Cardiomyopathies

1. Which is *not* correct regarding dilated cardiomyopathy?
   a. The natural history of clinical syndrome of heart failure is dependent on the course of myocardial failure
   b. Most powerful predictor of outcome is LV ejection fraction
   c. The treatment which improves the intrinsic ventricular function improves the natural history of heart failure
   d. The treatment with positive Inotropes is associated with a favorable outcome

2. Which of the following is *not* a component of adjunctive therapy for ischemic cardiomyopathy?
   a. Anticoagulation
   b. Amiodarone
   c. Maintenance of potassium level to high normal range
   d. AICD

3. Within the WHO classification hypertensive heart disease is classified in which category:
   a. Dilated CMP
   b. Restrictive CMP
   c. Unclassified category
   d. Any of the above

4. Valvular cardiomyopathy is never seen with:
   a. Mitral regurgitation
   b. Aortic regurgitation
   c. Aortic stenosis
   d. Pure mitral stenosis

5. Which of the following category of drugs has been shown to prolong the time of surgery in patients with aortic regurgitation and normal LV function?
   a. Digitalis
   b. ACE inhibitors
   c. Calcium channel blockers
   d. Nitrates

6. Which of the following is *not* correct regarding idiopathic dilated CMP?
   a. Incidence of IDC increases with age
   b. Males are afflicted at a higher rate
   c. It may be familial in > 50% of cases
   d. All of the above

7. All the following statements are correct regarding anthracycline cardiomyopathy *except*:
   a. Incidence of heart failure increases with total cumulative dose to 450 mg/m^2 of BSA
   b. Pre- and postchemotherapy radiation increases the risk
   c. There is relative absence of dilatation and hypertrophy with a higher heart rate than usually encountered in ambulatory heart failure
   d. Beta blockers has no effective role

8. Sudden cardiac death in HCM is mostly seen with all *except*:
   a. Children and young adults
   b. Previously asymptomatic patients
   c. While sedentary or during mild exertion
   d. Patients with marked LVOT gradient

9. All the following features are seen in chest radiogram in patients with restrictive cardiomyopathy *except*:
   a. Absence of ventricular enlargement
   b. Left or biatrial enlargement
   c. Presence of pulmonary venous hypertension
   d. Calcification in cardiac silhouette

10. The most characteristic pathophysiologic abnormality in hypertrophic cardiomyopathy is:
    a. Systolic dysfunction
    b. Diastolic dysfunction
    c. Outflow tract gradient
    d. All of the above

11. The most common symptom in hypertrophic cardiomyopathy is:
    a. Angina pectoris
    b. Palpitation
    c. Dyspnea
    d. Syncope

12. A triple apical beat is *not* an uncommon physical sign in cases with:
    a. LV aneurysm
    b. Hypertrophic cardiomyopathy
    c. Arrhythmogenic right ventricular dysplasia
    d. Restrictive cardiomyopathy

13. The arterial pressure tracing demonstrating spike and dome pattern is characteristic of:
    a. Cardiac tamponade
    b. Hypertrophic cardiomyopathy
    c. Constrictive pericarditis
    d. Restrictive cardiomyopathy

14. Which of the following hemodynamic finding is *not* seen in hypertrophic cardiomyopathy?
    a. Elevated left ventricular end diastolic pressure
    b. Elevated systemic vascular resistance
    c. Elevated pulmonary artery pressure
    d. A pressure gradient in right ventricular out flow tract

15. Square root sign in ventricular pressure recording suggests diagnosis of:
    a. Dilated cardiomyopathy
    b. Restrictive cardiomyopathy
    c. Hypertrophic cardiomyopathy
    d. Arrhythmogenic right ventricular dysplasia

16. All the following variety of cardiomyopathy has preserved systolic function *except*:
    a. Ischemic cardiomyopathy
    b. Restrictive cardiomyopathy
    c. Hypertrophic cardiomyopathy
    d. Arrhythmogenic right ventricular dysplasia

17. Which of the following clinical condition forms specific indication for endomyocardial biopsy?
    a. Monitoring of cardiac allograft rejection
    b. Detection and monitoring of myocarditis
    c. Differentiation between restrictive and constrictive heart disease
    d. Unexplained life-threatening ventricular tachyarrhythmias

18. AV conduction defects characterizes which variety of cardiomyopathy:
    a. Dilated cardiomyopathy
    b. Restrictive cardiomyopathy
    c. Hypertrophic cardiomyopathy
    d. Arrhythmogenic right ventricular dysplasia

19. The presence of which of the following marker is associated with occurrence of idiopathic dilated cardiomyopathy:
    a. Angiotensin converting enzymes DD genotype
    b. HLA antigens DR4 and DQW 4
    c. Antimyocardial antibodies
    d. All of the above

20. Which of the following pharmacological agent has been found to reduce mortality in dilated cardiomyopathy?
    a. Amiodarone   b. Metoprolol
    c. Carvedilol   d. Digoxin

21. Which of the following is major cause of nonischemic dilated cardiomyopathy:
    a. Viral infection
    b. Alcohol
    c. Cocaine abuse
    d. Anthracycline toxicity

22. Which of the following is *correct* regarding alcoholic cardiomyopathy?
    a. Mild depression of cardiac function in chronic alcoholics are seen even before clinical manifestation
    b. Overt alcoholic liver disease and cardiac involvement usually do not occur together
    c. A concomitant skeletal myopathy involving the shoulder and pelvic girdle is a frequent finding
    d. All of the above

23. Holiday heart syndrome in a chronic alcoholic is characterize by all the following arrhythmia occurrence *except*:
    a. Atrial fibrillation
    b. Atrial flutter
    c. Frequent ventricular premature contraction
    d. High grade AV block

24. Recurrent ventricular tachyarrhythmias of left bundle branch block configuration of QRS complex is seen in which type of cardiomyopathy:
    a. Restrictive cardiomyopathy
    b. Hypertrophic cardiomyopathy
    c. Arrhythmogenic right ventricular dysplasia
    d. Dilated cardiomyopathy

25. Which of the following antiarrhythmic drug has been shown to be effective in controlling the arrhythmias in arrhythmogenic right ventricular dysplasia?
    a. Quinidine   b. Amiodarone
    c. β-adrenoceptor blockers   d. Procainamide

26. The most characteristic pathophysiological abnormality in hypertrophic cardiomyopathy is:
    a. Systolic dysfunction
    b. An outflow tract gradient
    c. Diastolic dysfunction
    d. All of the above

27. Restrictive cardiomyopathies are characterized by all *except*:
    a. Normal or reduced diastolic volume of ventricles
    b. Normal or reduced systolic volume of ventricles
    c. Increased ventricular wall thickness
    d. Normal ventricular wall thickness

28. Cardiovascular involvement in pseudoxanthoma elasticum includes all *except*:
    a. Arterial calcification
    b. Premature coronary artery disease

c. Peripheral vascular disease
d. Dilated cardiomyopathy

29. The classical triad of cirrhosis, bronze skin and diabetes such as diagnosis of:
a. Pseudoxanthoma elasticum
b. Cystinosis
c. Hemochromatosis
d. Wilson's disease

30. Which of the following right sided structure is spared in endomyocardial fibrosis?
a. Right atrium
b. Right ventricle
c. Tricuspid valve
d. Pulmonary valve leaflets and artery

31. Which is the causative organism of lyme disease?
a. *Trypanosoma Cruzi*
b. *Borrelia Burgdorferi*
c. *Toxoplasma gondii*
d. Epstein-Barr virus

32. Erythema migrans is a feature of:
a. Chaga's disease
b. Sarcoidosis
c. Lyme disease
d. Hypereosinophilic syndrome

33. Cardiac involvement in lyme disease predominately manifest as:
a. Myocarditis
b. Pericarditis
c. DCMP
d. Conduction abnormality

34. Lyme disease can be treated with:
a. Course of steroids
b. Methotrexate
c. Course of doxycycline or amoxicillin
d. Plasmapheresis

35. A combination of deafness, maternally inherited diabetes, and heart failure in a relatively young patient suggest diagnosis of:
a. Fabry's disease
b. Gaucher's disease
c. Amyloid heart disease
d. Mitochondrial cardiomyopathy

36. The predominant site of cardiac involvement, known as the triangle of dysplasia, is seen in:
a. Alcoholic cardiomyopathy
b. Diabetic cardiomyopathy
c. Arrhythmogenic right ventricular cardiomyopathy
d. Takotsubo cardiomyopathy

37. All the statement are correct regarding ventricular tachycardia in arrhythmogenic right ventricular dysplasia "*except*":
a. Ventricular tachycardia is generally well tolerated even at rapid rate
b. Antiarrhythmic drugs suppress symptomatic arrhythmia and prevent sudden death
c. Beta-blocking agent slows progression of ventricular dysfunction in ARVC
d. All are correct

38. Which of the following drug has been shown to prevent disease progression in arrhythmogenic right ventricular dysplasia?
a. Amiodarone
b. ARNI
c. ACE inhibitor
d. Beta blockers

39. Which of the following statement is *incorrect* regarding Takotsubo cardiomyopathy?
a. Often there is a stressful trigger
b. The regional wall motion abnormality in single epicardial vascular territory is seen.
c. There is an absence of culprit atherosclerotic coronary artery disease
d. Malignant ventricular arrhythmia with QT prolongation may occur

40. Which of the following arrhythmia is common in Takotsubo cardiomyopathy?
a. Complete heart block
b. Monomorphic ventricular tachycardia
c. Atrial fibrillation and flatter
d. Torsades de pointes associated with QT prolongation

41. Cardiac magnetic resonance (CMR) in a patient with heart failure and preserved ejection fraction without wall thickening suggest diagnosis of:
a. Infiltrative cardiomyopathy
b. Cardiac amyloidosis
c. Cardiac sarcoidosis
d. Constrictive pericarditis

42. Which of the following infiltrative disorder present predominantly as dilated cardiomyopathy?
a. Cardiac amyloidosis
b. Fabry's disease
c. Cardiac sarcoidosis
d. Glycogen storage disease

43. Sarcoid granulomas have a predilection for which of the following cardiac structure?
a. Pericardium
b. Myocardium
c. Cardiac valves
d. Conduction system of the heart

44. Noncaseating granulomas in myocardium is a feature of:
   a. Cardiac amyloidosis
   b. Sarcoid cardiomyopathy
   c. Lyme disease
   d. Fabry's disease

45. Which of the following parameter is used for defining left ventricular noncompaction?
   a. LV size and function
   b. Ratio of compacted to noncompacted myocardium
   c. The thickness of trabeculation
   d. All of the above

46. The "purest form" of tachycardia induced cardiomyopathy is caused by:
   a. Paroxysmal supraventricular tachycardia
   b. Atrial fibrillation
   c. Sinus tachycardia
   d. Permanent reciprocating junctional tachycardia

47. Which of the following is *incorrect* regarding tachycardia induced cardiomyopathy?
   a. Duration of arrhythmia more than heart rate is critical factor in causation
   b. It improves within 3–6 months after correction
   c. Tachycardia induced LV diastolic dysfunction is not reported
   d. All are correct

48. Which of the following is the investigation of choice for diagnosis of catecholaminergic polymorphic ventricular tachycardia (CPVT)?
   a. Holter monitoring
   b. EP study
   c. Endomyocardial biopsy
   d. Exercise stress test

49. CPVT is characterized by all the following *except*:
   a. Baseline long QT syndrome
   b. Bidirectional ventricular tachycardia
   c. Exercise induced syncope
   d. Sinus bradycardia and prominent U wave

50. Which of the following should *not* be used for treatment of CPVT?
   a. Betablocker
   b. Flecainide
   c. Left cardiac sympathetic denervation
   d. Amiodarone

51. Which of the following electrophysiologic function is affected in Brugada syndrome?
   a. Cardiac sodium current
   b. The calcium current
   c. Transient outward potassium current
   d. All of the above

52. Decrease in heart rate variability (HRV) is a marker of:
   a. Increase of sympathetic and parasympathetic tone
   b. Decrease of sympathetic and parasympathetic tone
   c. Increase of sympathetic and decrease of parasympathetic tone
   d. Decrease of sympathetic and increase of parasympathetic tone

53. All the following statement are correct regarding arrhythmogenic cardiomyopathy *except*:
   a. Clinically present as ventricular tachycardia
   b. Onset is in young, adult age
   c. There is increased right ventricular diastolic dimension
   d. Left ventricle is spared

54. Which of the following is a major criteria for diagnosis of arrhythmogenic cardiomyopathy?
   a. Regional RV akinesia or dyskinesia
   b. Residual myocytes 60–75% by morphometric analysis
   c. Inverted T wave in leads V_1 and V_2
   d. Nonsustained or sustained ventricular tachycardia of LBBB morphology with superior axis

55. All the following are major criteria for diagnosis of arrhythmogenic right ventricular dysplasia *except*:
   a. Inverted T waves in right precordial leads
   b. Epsilon wave
   c. Nonsustained or sustained ventricular tachycardia of LBBB morphology with superior axis
   d. Nonsustained and sustained ventricular tachycardia, LBBB morphology with inferior axis

56. Which of the following is preferred imaging modality for arrhythmogenic cardiomyopathy?
   a. Echocardiography
   b. MDCT
   c. Cardiac MRI
   d. Endomyocardial biopsy

57. Which of the following drug is used to inhibit the secretion of vasoactive substance in patients with carcinoid syndrome?
   a. Histamine antagonist
   b. Somatostatin analogue
   c. Phosphodiesterase inhibitors
   d. Hydroxylase inhibitor

58. What is the dangerous complication of valve replacement in carcinoid heart disease?
   a. Intractable cardiac failure
   b. Infective endocarditis
   c. Valve dehiscence
   d. Acute carcinoid crisis

59. Subaortic gradient and associated systolic murmur in HOCM can reduce with which of the following?
   a. Phenylephrine
   b. Nitroglycerin
   c. Isoproterenol
   d. Dobutamine

60. Which of the following is the most useful technique for assessment of microvascular function in patients with hypertrophic cardiomyopathy?
   a. Echocardiography
   b. Cardiac CT
   c. Cardiac MRI (CMRI)
   d. Positron emission tomography (PET)

61. What is expected LV outflow gradient in patients of HCM with loud murmur of at least grade III/VI?
   a. >20 mm
   b. >30 mm
   c. >50 mm
   d. >80 mm

62. The common ECG abnormality in patients with hypertrophic cardiomyopathy includes all *except*:
   a. Increased voltage consistent with LV hypertrophy
   b. ST-T changes
   c. Diminished R wave in lateral precordial leads
   d. All above changes can be seen

63. Which statement is *not* correct regarding ECG in hypertrophic cardiomyopathy (HCM)?
   a. Normal ECG exclude the possibility of future sudden death
   b. Increased voltage (tall R waves or deep S waves) are weakly correlated with magnitude of LV hypertrophy
   c. Increased voltage do not reliably distinguish obstructive from nonobstructive HCM
   d. All are incorrect

64. The most reliable marker for evolution to end stage disease in hypertrophic cardiomyopathy (HCM) is:
   a. Septal LV wall thickness >20 mm
   b. Nonsustained ventricular tachycardia demonstrated on ambulatory ECG
   c. Recurrent syncope
   d. Family history of HCM with systolic dysfunction

65. Which of the following statement is *correct* regarding hypertrophic cardiomyopathy and sudden cardiac death?
   a. It occurs most commonly in adolescents and adults younger than 30 years of age
   b. Most sudden cardiac death occurs during sedentary or modest physical activity
   c. Risk of sudden death is unrelated to the pattern or location of LV hypertrophy
   d. All are correct

66. Which of the following finding in HOCM, in absence of conventional risk marker calls for prophylactic ICD?
   a. T wave alternans in ECG
   b. Myocardial bridging of left anterior descending coronary artery
   c. Extensive late gadolinium enhancement on contrast enhanced CMR
   d. All of the above

67. Which of the following is a drug of choice for improving symptoms and exercise capacity in patients with HCM without outflow tract obstruction?
   a. Beta blockers
   b. Disopyramide
   c. Verapamil
   d. Allosteric myosin inhibitors

68. "Morrow" procedure is a:
   a. Transapical aortic valve replacement
   b. Transapical mitral commissurotomy
   c. Transaortic ventricular septal myectomy
   d. Apical mitral valve replacement

69. Which of the following is most effective drug in reducing atrial fibrillation recurrences in HCM?
   a. Beta blockers
   b. Verapamil
   c. Disopyramide
   d. Amiodarone

70. The most common arrhythmia following alcohol consumption is:
   a. Supraventricular tachycardia
   b. Atrial fibrillation
   c. Atrial flutter
   d. Ventricular tachycardia

71. Which of the following is *not* reported with cocaine abuse?
   a. Takotsubo cardiomyopathy
   b. Acute myocardial infarction
   c. Brugada pattern in ECG
   d. All can be seen

72. Which of the following group of drugs increases the risk for atherosclerosis?
   a. Ergotamine
   b. Triptans
   c. Bromocriptine
   d. Highly active antiretroviral therapy (HAART)

73. Which of the following group of drugs are known to be associated with acute myocardial infarction?
   a. Methysergide
   b. Pergolide
   c. Triptans
   d. Fenfluramine

74. Which of the following features differentiate atherosclerosis in HIV patients compared to atherosclerosis seen in general population?
   a. Localized vessel involvement
   b. More calcified plaques
   c. More noncalcified plaques which are lipid laden and prone to rupture
   d. Very few high risk plaques

75. Which of the following is *incorrect* regarding acute coronary syndrome in HIV patients?
   a. HIV patients are usually older age group
   b. They often have multi vessel coronary artery disease
   c. They have poor outcomes
   d. All are incorrect

76. All the following are correct regarding acute coronary syndrome in HIV patients *except*:
   a. These patients are usually young male
   b. They often have single vessel disease
   c. In hospitalized patients have excellent immediate outcomes
   d. Restenosis rate following drug eluting stent are higher in HIV patients

77. The incidence of which of following cardiac involvement has declined dramatically following ART?
   a. Coronary artery disease
   b. Pulmonary hypertension
   c. Cardiomyopathy
   d. All of the above

78. Dilated form of cardiomyopathy are characterized by all *except*:
   a. Ventricular chamber enlargement
   b. Atrial chamber enlargement
   c. Systolic dysfunction
   d. Normal LV wall thickness

79. Which of the following medicine used in treatment of autoimmune disease can produce iatrogenic cardiomyopathy?
   a. Hydroxychloroquine
   b. Etanercept
   c. Infliximab
   d. All

80. What level of alcohol consumption may lead to alcoholic cardiomyopathy?
   a. <2 standard size drink or <40 g/day
   b. <3 standard size drink or <80 g/day
   c. 3 standard size drink or alcohol consumption over 80 g/day
   d. 4 standard size drink or alcohol consumption over 100 g/day

81. Premature ventricular contraction induced cardiomyopathy is seen with the PVCs frequency of:
   a. >5,000 PVCs in 24 hours
   b. >10,000 PVCs in 24 hours
   c. >20,000 PVCs in 24 hours
   d. >40,000 PVCs in 24 hours

82. Which of the following chemotherapeutic agents produces nonreversible injury (Type I) leading to cardiomyopathy?
   a. Anthracycline
   b. Trastuzumab
   c. Sunitinib
   d. Lapatinib

83. Mid cavitary obstruction in hypertrophic cardiomyopathy is due to:
   a. Disproportionate thickening of interventricular septum
   b. Disproportionate thickening of interventricular septum and LV free wall
   c. Hypertrophied papillary muscle abutting against the septum
   d. Elongated mitral leaflet

84. Which of the following characterizes mitral regurgitation in hypertrophic obstructive cardiomyopathy?
   a. Jet of mitral regurgitation is directed laterally and posteriorly
   b. It predominates during mid and late systole
   c. The severity of mitral regurgitation is proportional to the severity of LVOT obstruction
   d. All of the above

85. Which is the mechanism of syncope in patient with hypertrophied cardiomyopathy?
   a. LVOT obstruction
   b. Activation of LV baroreceptor resulting in reflex vasodilatation
   c. Atrial and ventricular arrhythmia
   d. All contributes

86. All the following statement increases intensity of systolic murmur in HOCM during dynamic auscultation *except*:
   a. From squatting to standing position
   b. Inhalation of a amyl nitrite
   c. After a premature ventricular beat
   d. Standing to squat position

CHAPTER 18 | Cardiomyopathies

87. "Dagger Shaped" signal on continuous wave Doppler is seen in:
a. Valvular aortic stenosis
b. Hypertrophic obstructive cardiomyopathy
c. Pulmonary stenosis
d. Mitral regurgitation

88. In HOCM, while inducing "Brockenbrough" phenomenon, which of the following does *not* occur?
a. Increased in contractility
b. Increased in the dynamic obstruction
c. Increased in the outflow tract gradient
d. Increased in the aortic pulse pressure

89. Which of the following is a calcium channel blocker of choice in treatment of hypertrophic cardiomyopathy?
a. Diltiazem   b. Nifedipine
c. Verapamil   d. Amlodipine

90. Which of the following drug is *not* used in treatment of atrial fibrillation in HOCM?
a. Verapamil   b. Diltiazem
c. Digoxin   d. Amiodarone

91. Which is the most common complication of alcohol septal ablation in treatment of HOCM?
a. Myocardial infarction
b. Ventricular septal defect and myocardial perforation
c. Coronary artery dissection
d. Complete heart block

92. In dual chamber pacing for HOCM what should be the location of RV lead to have maximum reduction in outflow tract gradient?
a. HIS bundle   b. Basal septum
c. Mid septum   d. RV apex

ANSWERS WITH EXPLANATIONS

1. Ans. d. The treatment with positive inotropes is associated with a favorable outcome

Hurst's 10th Ed; Page 2039

The vast majority of cases of heart failure are caused by heart muscle disease (cardiomyopathy). Within the WHO categorization of cardiomyopathy, the most common cause of clinical syndrome of heart failure is a secondary (ischemic, valvular, hypertensive, etc.,) or a primary (e.g., idiopathic or familial) dilated cardiomyopathy defined as a ventricular chamber exhibiting increased diastolic and systolic volumes and a low (<40%) ejection fraction. The natural history of the clinical syndrome of heart failure depends on the course of myocardial failure since: (1) the most powerful single predictor of outcome is the degree of left ventricular dysfunction as assessed by the LV ejection fraction; (2) the treatment that improves intrinsic ventricular function, improves the natural history of heart failure; (3) use of positive inotropic agents is associated with an adverse effect on outcome.

2. Ans. d. AICD

Hurst's 10th Ed; Page 2044

The treatment of ischemic dilated cardiomyopathy in general consists of use of: (i) ACE inhibitors in asymptomatic or symptomatic patients; (ii) β-blockers in symptomatic patients; (iii) Diuretics in volume overloaded patients; (iv) Spironolactone in advance patients; (v) Digoxin in symptomatic patients. Recent data have demonstrated the effectiveness of devices in treating ischemic dilated cardiomyopathies, including implantable cardioverters/defibrillators for patients without intraventricular conduction defects, and biventricular pacing plus ICD for patients with intraventricular conduction defects. Additionally adjunctive therapy includes anticoagulation in subjects with lower LV ejection fraction to prevent thromboembolic complications, amiodarone to treat symptomatic arrhythmias, maintenance of potassium level in high normal range to prevents sudden death, keeping serum digoxin level <1.0 ng/mL, frequent clinic visit to adjust medication and an aggressive approach to treating ischemia including revascularization.

3. Ans. d. Any of the above

Hurst's 10th Ed; Page 2045

A hypertensive dilated cardiomyopathy is diagnosed when myocardial systolic function is depressed out of proportion to the increase in wall stress. A subject presenting in heart failure with a hypertensive crisis would not carry this diagnosis unless ventricular dilatation and depressed systolic function remained after correction of hypertension. In addition to producing a pure form of hypertensive cardiomyopathy, hypertension is a major risk factor for heart failure from any cause. Within the WHO/IFSC classification over the 'hypertensive heart disease' may present in the dilated, restrictive or unclassified categories.

4. Ans. d. Pure mitral stenosis

Hurst's 10th Ed; Page 2045

A valvular cardiomyopathy occurs when a valvular abnormalities is present and myocardial systolic function is depressed out of proportion to the increase in wall stress. This most commonly occurs with left sided regurgitant lesion (mitral regurgitation and aortic regurgitation), less commonly with aortic stenosis and never as a consequence of pure mitral stenosis.

5. Ans. c. Calcium channel blockers

Hurst's 10th Ed; Page 2046

The treatment of a valvular dilated cardiomyopathy is surgical valve replacement or repair as soon as the cardiomyopathy is detected. Catheter valvuloplasty may be an option for patients with severe aortic stenosis, who are not good surgical candidate for reasons other than heart failure. Medical treatment may be the only option in subjects with aortic insufficiency or mitral regurgitation whose LV function is severely impaired. The medical treatment of either disorder should be similar to the treatment of ischemic cardiomyopathy plus aggressive afterload reduction usually with hydralazine/nitrate on top of ACE inhibitors. The calcium channel blockers amlodipine is another option for afterload reduction, particularly for aortic insufficiency where calcium blocker therapy has been shown to improve survival.

6. Ans. d. All of the above

Hurst's 10th Ed; Page 2046

Idiopathic dilated cardiomyopathy is diagnosed by excluding significant coronary artery disease, valvular abnormalities and other causes. Idiopathic dilated cardiomyopathy is a relatively common cause of heart failure with an estimated prevalence rate of 0.04% and incidence rate vary from 0.005 to 0.006%. The true incidence of idiopathic dilated cardiomyopathy is undoubtably higher owing to the fact that subjects may remain asymptomatic until marked ventricular dysfunction has occurred. The incidence of idiopathic dilated cardiomyopathy increases with age and males are affected at a higher rate than females. Idiopathic dilated cardiomyopathy may be familial in as many as 35–50% of cases when first degree relatives are carefully screened.

7. Ans. d. Beta blockers has no effective role

Hurst's 10th Ed; Page 2049

Anthracycline cardiomyopathy: The commonly used and highly efficacious anthracycline antibiotic anticancerous agents, doxorubicin and daunorubicin produce a dose related cardiomyopathy that may limit their clinical application. Within the WHO/ISFC classification, an anthracycline cardiomyopathy would most likely be in the dilated category but because the extent of dilatation may initially be minimal it could also be in the unclassified category. The cardiomyopathy produced by these agents depends on total cumulative dose. For the more widely used compound doxorubicin (adriamycin), the incidence of heart failure due to cardiomyopathy dramatically increases above total cumulative dose of 450 mg/m^2 in subjects without underlying cardiac problem or other risk factors. Prior mediastinal radiation involving the heart is powerful risk factors for anthracycline cardiomyopathy and the risk is also evident if radiation treatment follows chemotherapy. In subjects with risk factors, anthracycline cardiomyopathy can present at lower cumulative dose than 450 mg/m^2. Although the diagnosis of anthracycline cardiomyopathy can be made clinically the definitive diagnosis depends on demonstration of substantial number of cardiac myocytes exhibiting the characteristic anthracycline effect. Tissue sampling is best done by endomyocardial biopsy. There are some distinguishing clinical features of anthracycline cardiomyopathy that may relate to its pathophysiology. These include a relative absence of hypertrophy and dilatation and a higher heart rate (110 to 130 bpm) than is usually encountered in ambulatory heart failure. The reason for this features are that the onset of symptom may be relative acute (remodeling takes time to develop) and the anthracycline inhibits contractile protein synthesis thus reducing time for compensatory dilatation and remodeling. In this situation, the only option for stabilizing cardiac output is increasing the heart rate since increasing stroke volume via a large end-diastolic volume has been precluded. The increase heart rate is produced by greater than expected hyperadrenergic state and therefore this subject may be exceptionally depended on adrenergic support.

Subject who develop anthracycline or anthracycline cardiomyopathy should be aggressively treated with conventional heart failure treatment since some degree of reversibility is likely. Conventional treatment consists of ACE inhibitors, digoxin and diuretics. β-adrenergic blockade has been used successfully in some subjects but because of the high adrenergic drive it may be difficult to administer. On the other hand, the heightened adrenergic mechanism may be producing a commensurate amount of adverse effect on the myocardium and show the potential for a favorable response may be even greater than in other kind of cardiomyopathy.

8. Ans. d. Patients with marked LVOT gradient

Hurst's 10th Ed; Page 2066

Sudden death is the most devastating complication of hypertrophic cardiomyopathy. Sudden death occurs most frequently in the asymptomatic or mildly symptomatic patients and mainly in the young population. There are several clinical features associated with a high-risk for sudden death in patient with hypertrophic cardiomyopathy. Those patients who have had a prior cardiac arrest or spontaneous sustained ventricular tachycardia are at highest risk. A family history of premature sudden death in a patient with hypertrophic cardiomyopathy potent a high-risk particularly if there are multiple occurrences. Other less predictive parameters include unexplained syncope, non sustained ventricular tachycardia, abnormal blood pressure response to exercise and extreme left ventricular hypertrophy (wall thickness > 30 mm).

9. Ans. d. Calcification in cardiac silhouette

Hurst's 10th Ed; Page 2076

The chest radiograph in a patient with restrictive cardiomyopathy usually reveals normal sized ventricles, although atrial enlargement and pericardial effusion may produce and an enlarged cardiac silhouette. Pleural effusion and signs of pulmonary congestion may also be present.

10. Ans. b. Diastolic dysfunction

Braunwald 5th Ed; Page 1414 & 1419

The condition hypertrophic cardiomyopathy is characterized by inappropriate myocardial hypertrophy that occurred in the absence of an obvious cause for the hypertrophy (such as aortic stenosis or systemic hypertension) often predominately involving the interventricular septum of a nondilated left ventricle that showed hyperdynamic ventricular function. In some patients with hypertrophic cardiomyopathy, a dynamic pressure gradient in the subaortic area that divided the left ventricle into a high pressure apical region and a low pressure subaortic region is seen and this state of the patients are labeled as hypertrophic subaortic stenosis (IHSS). The most characteristic pathophysiological abnormality in hypertrophic cardiomyopathy is diastolic rather than systolic dysfunction and therefore HCM is characterized by abnormal stiffness of the left ventricle with result in impaired ventricular filling. This abnormality in diastolic relaxation produces increased left ventricular and diastolic pressure with resulting pulmonary congestion and dyspnea, the most common symptom in HCM, despite typically hyperdynamic left ventricular systolic function.

11. Ans. c. Dyspnea

Braunwald 5th Ed; Page 1414 & 1419

Refer to explanation for Q. No 10.

12. Ans. b. Hypertrophic cardiomyopathy

Braunwald 5th Ed; Page 1419 & 1420

The majority of patient with hypertrophic cardiomyopathy are asymptomatic or only mildly symptomatic and often are identified during screening of relatives of the patients with hypertrophic cardiomyopathy. The first clinical manifestation of disease in some individual may be sudden death. The disease is identified most often in adults in their 30s and 40s and it occurs more often than commonly suspected in elderly patients.

The most common clinical symptom is dyspnea occurring in up to 90% of symptomatic patients which is largely a consequence of elevated left ventricular diastolic and therefore left atrial and pulmonary venous pressure which results principally from impaired ventricular filling owing to diastolic dysfunction. Angina pectoris (found in about third-fourth of symptomatic patients), fatigue, presyncope and syncope are also common. Palpitation, paroxysmal nocturnal dyspnea, overt congestive failure and dizziness are found less frequently although severe congestive heart failure culminating into death may be seen. Exertion tends to exacerbate many of the symptoms.

Physical examination may be normal in asymptomatic patients without gradient, particularly those with the apical variant of hypertrophic cardiomyopathy, save for a left ventricular lift and a loud fourth heart sound, but finding are usually prominent in patient with left ventricular outflow tract pressure gradient. The apical precordial impulse is often displaced laterally and is usually abnormally forceful and enlarge. Because of decrease left ventricular compliance, a prominent presystolic apical impulse that results from forceful atrial systole often is present. This may results in a double apical impulse as a result of the prominent "A" wave. A more characteristic but less frequently recognize abnormality is a triple apical beat, the third impulse is being a late systolic bulge that occurs when the heart is almost empty and is performing near isometric contraction.

13. Ans. b. Hypertrophic cardiomyopathy

Braunwald 5th Ed; Page 1419 & 1420

Refer to explanation for Q. No 12.

14. Ans. b. Elevated systemic vascular resistance

Braunwald 5th Ed; Page 1422

The hemodynamic features during cardiac catheterization in patient with hypertrophic cardiomyopathy demonstrates diminished diastolic left ventricular compliance and in some patient is systolic pressure gradient within the body of the left ventricle, which is separated from a subaortic chamber by the thickened septum and the anterior leaflet of mitral valve that abets the septum. The pressure gradient may be quite labile and may vary between 0–175 mm Hg in same patient under different conditions, because of the same patient under different condition, because of the liability of the gradient. The arterial pressure tracing may demonstrate a "spike and dome" configuration similar to the carotid pulse recording. As a consequence of diminish left ventricular compliance, the mean and particularly the A wave in the left atrial pressure pulse and the left ventricular and diastolic pressure are usually elevated. Cardiac out put may be depressed in patient with long-standing severe gradient. In the majority of patient it is normal, occasionally it is elevated. Hemodynamic abnormalities in hypertrophic cardiomyopathy are not limited in the left heart. Approximately one-fourth of patients demonstrate pulmonary hypertension which is usually mild but in some cases may be moderate-to-severe. This is due to elevated mean left atrial pressure as a consequence of diminished left ventricular compliance. A pressure gradient in the right ventricular outflow tract occurs in approximately 15% of patients who have obstruction to left ventricular outflow and appears to results from markedly hypertrophied right ventricular tissue. Right atrial and right ventricular and diastolic pressure may be slightly elevated. The systemic vascular resistance is often normal.

15. Ans. b. Restrictive cardiomyopathy

Braunwald 5th Ed; Page 1406

Functional classification of the cardiomyopathies

	Dilated	Restrictive	Hypertrophic
Symptoms	Congestive heart failure, particularly left sided	Dyspnea, fatigue	Dyspnea, angina pectoris
	Fatigue and weakness Systemic or pulmonary emboli	Right sided congestive heart failure Signs and symptoms of systemic disease: amyloidosis, iron storage disease, etc.	Fatigue, syncope, palpitations
Physical examination	Moderate to severe cardiomegaly; S3 and S4 Atrioventricular valve regurgitation, especially mitral	Mild to moderate cardiomegaly: S2 or S4 Atrioventricular valve regurgitation; inspiratory increase in venous pressure (Kussmaul's sign)	Mild cardiomegaly apical systolic thrill and heave; brisk carotid upstroke S4 common systolic murmur that increases with Valsalva maneuver
Chest roentgenogram	Moderate to marked cardiac enlargement, especially left ventricular	Mild cardiac enlargement	Mild to moderate cardiac enlargement
	Pulmonary venous hypertension	Pulmonary venous hypertension	Left atrial enlargement
Electrocardiogram	Sinus tachycardia Atrial and ventricular arrhythmias	Low voltage Intraventricular conduction defects	Left ventricular hypertrophy ST-segment and T wave abnormalities
	ST segment and T wave abnormalities Intraventricular conduction defects	AV conduction defects	Abnormal Q waves Atrial and ventricular arrhythmias
Echocardiogram	Left ventricular dilatation and dysfunction	Increased left ventricular wall thickness and mass	Asymmetrical septal hypertrophy (ASH)
	Abnormal diastolic mitral valve motion secondary to abnormal compliance and filling pressure	Small or normal-sized left ventricular cavity Normal systolic function	Narrow left ventricular outflow tract Systolic anterior motion (SAM) of the mitral valve
		Pericardial effusion	Small or normal-sized left ventricle
Radionuclide studies	Left ventricular dilatation and dysfunction (RVG)	Infiltration of myocardium (201 TI)	Small or normal-sized left ventricle (RVG)
		Small or normal-sized left ventricle (RVG)	Vigorous systolic function (RVG)
		Normal systolic function (RVG)	Asymmetrical septal hypertrophy (RVG or 201 TI)
Cardiac catheterization	Left ventricular enlargement and dysfunction	Diminished left ventricular compliance	Diminished left ventricular compliance
	Mitral and/or tricuspid regurgitation	"Square root sign" in ventricular pressure recordings	Mitral regurgitation Vigorous systolic function
	Elevated left- and often right-sided filling pressures Diminished cardiac output	Preserved systolic function Elevated left- and right-sided filling pressures	Dynamic left ventricular outflow gradient

16. **Ans. a. Ischemic cardiomyopathy**

Braunwald 5th Ed; Page 1406

Refer to explanation for Q. No 15.

17. **Ans. a. Monitoring of cardiac allograft rejection**

Braunwald 5th Ed; Page 1406

Clinical Indications for Endomyocardial Biopsy
Definite
- Monitoring of cardiac allograft rejection
- Monitoring of anthracycline cardiotoxicity

Possible
- Detection and monitoring of myocarditis
- Diagnosis of secondary cardiomyopathies
- Differentiation between restrictive and constrictive heart disease

Uncertain
Unexplained, life threatening ventricular tachyarrhythmias

AIDS
Formulation of prognosis in idiopathic dilated cardiomyopathy.

18. **Ans. b. Restrictive cardiomyopathy**

Braunwald 5th Ed; Page 1406

Refer to explanation for Q. No 15.

19. **Ans. d. All of the above**

Braunwald 5th Ed; Page 1409

The idiopathic dilated cardiomyopathy represents a common expression of myocardial damage that has been produced by a variety of unidentified myocardial insults. Although the cause (remains unclear), interest has centered on three possible basic mechanisms of damage, i.e., familial and genetic factors, viral myocarditis and other cytotoxic insults and immunological abnormalities. Familial linkage of the dilated cardiomyopathy occurs more commonly than often appreciated. In 20% of patients, a first degree relative also shows evidence of dilated cardiomyopathy suggesting that familial transmission is relatively frequent. Most familial cases demonstrate autosomal dominant transmission but the disease is genetically quite heterogeneous and autosomal recessive and sex-linked inheritance has been found. There is great interest in using molecular genetic technique to identify markers of disease susceptibility in asymptomatic carriers at-risk for the eventual development of overt clinical dilated cardiomyopathy. An example of such a marker may be the angiotensin-converting enzyme DD genotype, i.e., found with increase frequency in dilated cardiomyopathy patient.

One intriguing familial metabolic deficiency is that of carnitine with improvement occurring in myopathy with carnitine repletion.

There has been wide speculation that an episode of subclinical viral myocarditis initiate an autoimmune reaction that culminate in the development of full blown dilated cardiomyopathy. About 15% of patients with myocarditis progresses to dilated cardiomyopathy. In some patients who exhibit the clinical feature of dilated cardiomyopathy, endomyocardial biopsy reveals evidence of an inflammatory myocarditis. Other evidence favoring the concept that dilated cardiomyopathy is a post viral disorder includes the presence of high antibody viral titer, viral specific RNA sequences in an apparent viral particle in patients with idiopathic dilated cardiomyopathy. Abnormalities of both humoral and cellular immunity has been found in patients with dilated cardiomyopathy. There is speculation that antibodies might be result of myocardial damage rather than the cause. There appears to be an association with specific HLA class II antigens such as DR IV and DQW IV suggesting that abnormalities of immunoregulation may play a role in causation of dilated cardiomyopathy. Circulating antimyocardial antibodies to variety of antigens have been identified.

20. **Ans. c. Carvedilol**

Braunwald 5th Ed; Page 1411

Because of evidence that activation of the sympathetic nervous system may have deleterious cardiac effects β-adrenoreceptor blockade (usually with metoprolol) has been suggested as treatment for dilated cardiomyopathy. Results have been generally very favorable with evidence of improved symptoms, exercise capacity and left ventricular function and a suggestion that survival has been improved. β-blockers are well tolerated with infrequent aggravation of heart failure. The mechanism of beneficial action of β-adrenoreceptor blockers is unknown but may relate to: (a) negative chronotropic effect with reduce myocardial oxygen demand; (b) reduced myocardial damage due to catecholamines; (c) improved diastolic relaxation; (d) inhibition of sympathetically mediated vasoconstriction; (e) increase in myocardial β-adrenoreceptor density and (f) improved calcium handling ex-lower rates. Despite the encouraging data, the use of β-blockers in dilated cardiomyopathy is still considered investigational. Recent data indicate that Carvadilol (a β-adrenoreceptor blocker with α-adrenoreceptor blocking and an antioxidant effect) substantially reduces mortality in dilated cardiomyopathy.

21. **Ans. b. Alcohol**

Braunwald 5th Ed; Page 1412

Chronic excessive consumption of alcohol may be associated with congestive heart failure, hypertension, cerebrovascular accidents, arrhythmias and sudden death. It is the major cause of secondary nonischemic dilated cardiomyopathy in the Western world and accounts for upward of one-third of all cases of dilated cardiomyopathy.

22. **Ans. d. All of the above**

Braunwald 5th Ed; Page 1412

Alcoholic cardiomyopathy most commonly occurs in man 30-55 years of age, who have been heavy consumer of alcohol for more than 10 years. It is frequently possible to demonstrate mild depression of cardiac function in chronic alcoholic even before cardiac dysfunction becomes clinically manifest. Abnormalities of both systolic function (reduced ejection fraction) and diastolic function (increased myocardial wall stiffness) have been demonstrated in alcoholic patients without cardiac symptoms by variety of invasive and noninvasive techniques. Although overt alcoholic liver disease and cardiac involvement usually do not occur together even cirrhotic patients without signs or symptoms of heart disease have demonstrable evidence of asymptomatic myocardial disease. A concomitant skeletal muscle myopathy involving the shoulder and pelvic girdle is a frequent finding and degree of muscle weakness and histological abnormality in skeletal muscles parallels that in the heart.

23. **Ans. d. High grade AV block**

Braunwald 5th Ed; Page 1413

Electrocardiographic abnormalities are common in patient with dilated cardiomyopathy and frequently are the only the indication of alcoholic heart disease during the preclinical phase. Alcoholic patients without other evidence of heart disease often are seen after developing palpitation, chest discomfort or syncope, typically following a binge of alcohol consumption on a weekend, particularly during the year end holidays' season. This is called as the 'holiday heart syndrome'. The most common arrhythmias observed is atrial fibrillation, followed by atrial flutter and frequent ventricular premature contraction. Alcohol consumption may predispose to atrial flutter or fibrillation even in non-alcoholics. Hypokalemia may play a role in the genesis of some of these arrhythmias. Supraventricular arrhythmias are also frequently observed in patients with overt alcoholic cardiomyopathy. Sudden unexpected death is not uncommon in young adult alcoholic and is likely that ventricular fibrillation is responsible.

24. **Ans. c. Arrhythmogenic right ventricular dysplasia**

Braunwald 5th Ed; Page 1413 & 1415

Arrhythmogenic right ventricular dysplasia is a unique cardiomyopathy and is marked by partial or total replacement of right ventricular muscles by adipose and fibrous tissue and may be associated with reentrant ventricular tachyarrhythmias of right ventricular origin (left bundle branch configuration of the QRS complex).

The cause of myocardial changes is unclear but in about one-third of cases there is autosomal dominant inheritance of the disease. It is distinct from the 'Uhls' disease which is marked by extreme thinning of ventricular wall. The diagnosis of arrhythmogenic right ventricular dysplasia is based on a constellation of clinical, electrocardiographic, histological and echocardiographic findings. Typical clinical features include male preponderance, normal physical examination, inverted T waves in right precordial electrocardiographic leads, symptom of palpitation and syncope and a risk of sudden death. In some patient with ventricular arrhythmias of no evident cause, clinically subtle right ventricular dysplasia may be etiologic. Noninvasive and invasive evaluation demonstrates a dilated, poorly contractile right ventricle usually with a normal left ventricle, although some degree of ventricular dysfunction has been seen. Magnetic resonance imaging (MRI) shows promise for identifying patient with this condition. Antiarrhythmic therapy especially with β-adrenoreceptor blockers often is effective in controlling the arrhythmias. The arrhythmias appear to be related to the abnormalities of regional right ventricular sympathetic innervations as demonstrated by noninvasive scintigraphy. Cryoablation of the presumed arrhythmogenic focus has been successful in resolving the ventricular arrhythmias in some patients.

25. **Ans. c. β-adrenoreceptor blockers**

Braunwald 5th Ed; Page 1413 & 1415

Refer to explanation for Q. No 24.

26. **Ans. c. Diastolic dysfunction**

Braunwald 5th Ed; Page 1415

The most characteristic pathophysiological abnormalities in hypertrophic cardiomyopathy is diastolic rather than systolic dysfunction.

27. **Ans. c. Increased ventricular wall thickness**

Hurst's 14th Ed; Page 1482

According to definition of European Society of Cardiology "Restrictive cardiomyopathies are defined as restrictive ventricular physiology in the presence of normal or reduced diastolic volume of one or both ventricles, normal or reduced systolic volumes and normal ventricular wall thickness".

28. **Ans. d. Dilated cardiomyopathy**

Hurst's 14th Ed; Page 1489

Pseudoxanthoma elasticum is a rare autosomal recessive systemic disease of the connective tissue that affects the extracellular matrix of multiple organs. The cardiovascular manifestations are characterized by the development of arterial calcifications, premature coronary artery and peripheral vascular disease, and

29. Ans. c. Hemochromatosis

Hurst's 14th Ed; Page 1491

The iron overload cardiomyopathy can result from a primary genetic disease caused by defects in genes coding proteins active in iron metabolism, typically hereditary hemochromatosis, or from secondary causes of iron overload such as acquired hematologic diseases. The clinical diagnosis is by presence of a classical triad of cirrhosis, bronze skin and diabetes.

30. Ans. d. Pulmonary valve leaflets and artery

Hurst's 14th Ed; Page 1496

Endomyocardial fibrosis typically involves only the heart and spares other organs and tissues. The heart appears enlarged mostly as a result of atrial dilatation. The endocardium is thickened from fibrosis that is prominent in the right ventricle at the apical level. Endomyocardial fibrosis embeds the right ventricular trabeculae, obliterates the apex of the right ventricle, and fixes the tricuspid valve apparatus. The pulmonary valve leaflets and arteries are not involved. The coronary arteries and small intramural vessels are also usually spared.

31. Ans. b. *Borrelia Burgdorferi*

Hurst's 14th Ed; Page 1549

Lyme disease is a tick-borne disease caused by *B burgdorferi*. From 60 to 80% of cases of lyme disease demonstrate characteristic rashes (erythema migrans) typically accompanied by fever, headache, and fatigue. Untreated Lyme disease can evolve to chronic arthritis and neurologic and cardiac manifestations. Cardiac involvement occurs in minority of patients and predominantly manifests with conduction abnormality, followed by arrhythmias, myocarditis, pericarditis, and DCM.

32. Ans. c. Lyme disease

Hurst's 14th Ed; Page 1549

Refer to explanation for Q. No 31.

33. Ans. d. Conduction abnormality

Hurst's 14th Ed; Page 1549

Refer to explanation for Q. No 31.

34. Ans. c. Course of doxycycline or amoxicillin

Hurst's 14th Ed; Page 1550

Lyme disease is treated with a 10-21-day course of doxycycline or amoxicillin orally. Intravenous ceftriaxone (2 g every 24 hours for 2-3 weeks) may be indicated when the infection is not detected in the early stages or is refractory to initial treatments.

35. Ans. d. Mitochondrial cardiomyopathy

Hurst's 14th Ed; Page 1551

Combination of deafness, maternally inherited diabetes and heat failure in a relatively young patient is typically seen in mitochondrial cardiomyopathy.

36. Ans. c. Arrhythmogenic right ventricular cardiomyopathy

Braunwald 11th Ed; Page 1586

Arrhythmogenic right ventricular dysplasia is a genetically determined cardiomyopathy characterized by fibrofatty replacement of the myocardium. The right ventricle is commonly involved, however biventricular involvement occurs in 50% of cases. The predominant site of cardiac involvement, known as the triangle of dysplasia, includes involvement of RV outflow tract, an area below the tricuspid valve, and the RV apex. This disorder is conceptualized as having three stages – an early subclinical phase in which imaging studies are negative but during which sudden cardiac death can still occur; a phase in which RV abnormalities are obvious without any clinical manifestation of RV dysfunction but with the development of a symptomatic ventricular arrhythmia; and finally, progressive fibrofatty replacement and infiltration of the myocardium leading to severe RV dilation and aneurysm formation and associated right sided heart failure.

37. Ans. b. Antiarrhythmic drugs suppress symptomatic arrhythmia and prevent sudden death

Braunwald 11th Ed; Page 1588

The mainstay of therapy for arrhythmogenic right ventricular dysplasia is suppression and prevention of ventricular arrhythmias and risk for sudden cardiac death, and prevention of disease progression. The intense physical exertion is known to be associated with earlier onset of symptoms and an increased risk of sustained ventricular tachycardia and sudden death and therefore patients with a definite diagnosis of ARVC should be advised not to participate in athletic activity. The classical monomorphic VT in ARVC with predominant right ventricular involvement is generally well tolerated, even at a rapid rate, possibly because of preserved LV function in most patients. However, ventricular tachycardia of a different morphology may occur and sudden death is not uncommon. Antiarrhythmic drugs may suppress a symptomatic arrhythmia but have not been shown to prevent sudden death. Beta-blocking agents may suppress catecholamine-triggered arrhythmia and slow progression of ventricular dysfunction and have been recommended as potentially valuable in all patients with ARVC. An implantable defibrillator (ICD) is recommended in patients with aborted sudden death, syncope, or decreased LV function. Catheter ablation has not been shown to reduce sudden death but is valuable in a patient with an ICD and frequent arrhythmias or in occasional patients with very well tolerated single-morphology ventricular tachycardia (VT). Beta-blocking drugs may suppress catecholamine triggered arrhythmia and slow progression of ventricular dysfunction in ARVC.

38. Ans. d. Beta blockers

Braunwald 11th Ed; Page 1588

Refer to explanation for Q. No 37

39. Ans. b. The regional wall motion abnormality in single epicardial vascular territory is seen

Braunwald 11th Ed; Page 1590

Definition of Takotsubo syndrome/cardiomyopathy according to the position statement from the Taskforce on Takotsubo syndrome of the Heart Failure Association of the European Society of Cardiology
- Transient regional wall motion abnormalities of LV or RV myocardium occur and are frequently, but not always, preceded by a stressful trigger (emotional or physical).
- The regional wall motion abnormalities usually extend beyond a single epicardial vascular distribution and often result in circumferential dysfunction of the ventricular segments involved.
- There is an absence of culprit atherosclerotic coronary artery disease, including acute plaque rupture, thrombus formation, and coronary dissection or other pathologic conditions, to explain the pattern of temporary LV dysfunction observed (e.g., hypertrophic cardiomyopathy, viral myocarditis).
- New and reversible electrocardiography (ECG) abnormalities (ST segment elevation, ST depression, LBBB, T-wave inversion and/or QTc prolongation) are seen during the acute phase (first 3 months).
- Significantly elevated levels of serum natriuretic peptide (BNP or NT-pro BNP) are seen during the acute phase.
- A positive but relatively small elevation in cardiac troponin can be measured with a conventional assay, (i.e., disparity between the troponin level and the amount of dysfunctional myocardium present).
- Recovery of ventricular systolic function is apparent on cardiac imaging at follow-up (3–6 months).

40. Ans. d. Torsades de pointes associated with QT prolongation

Braunwald 11th Ed; Page 1590

Malignant ventricular arrhythmia particularly Torsades de pointes associated with Takotsubo-related QT prolongation, may occur, and rarely complete heart block.

41. Ans. d. Constrictive pericarditis

Braunwald 11th Ed; Page 1591

The differential diagnosis of idiopathic restrictive cardiomyopathy includes infiltrative cardiomyopathies, such as amyloidosis, or constrictive pericarditis. Amyloidosis is associated with increased LV wall thickness and subtle abnormalities in LV systolic function, with specific findings on cardiac biopsy. A thickened pericardium noted on echocardiography, CT, or CMR in a patient with heart failure and a preserved ejection fraction without wall thickening suggests constrictive pericarditis.

42. Ans. c. Cardiac sarcoidosis

Braunwald 11th Ed; Page 1591

Restrictive cardiomyopathies are a heterogeneous group of diseases characterized by a nondilated left ventricle, often with a well-preserved ejection fraction. The predominant manifestation is diastolic dysfunction as a result of myocardial disease. Some infiltrative cardiac diseases such as amyloidosis produce an restrictive cardiomyopathy, whereas others, such as sarcoidosis, have an infiltrative component but are predominantly manifested as dilated cardiomyopathy. Sarcoidosis is a multisystem disorder of unknown cause characterized histologically by noncaseating granulomas. Noncaseating granulomas, the hallmark of the disease, are patchily distributed even in severe disease. Granulomatous lesions are associated with edema and inflammation, and widespread myocardial fibrosis is seen late in the disease.

43. Ans. d. Conduction system of the heart

Braunwald 11th Ed; Page 1594

The most common clinical feature of cardiac sarcoidosis is biventricular heart failure. Mitral regurgitation is caused by papillary muscle involvement in addition to LV dilation, and it may be severe. Sarcoid granulomas have a predilection for the cardiac conduction system, and high-degree AV block may occur, either as an initial manifestation of cardiac sarcoidosis or later in the course of disease. Both atrial and ventricular arrhythmias are common.

44. Ans. b. Sarcoid cardiomyopathy

Braunwald 11th Ed; Page 1591

Refer to explanation for Q. No 42

45. Ans. b. Ratio of compacted to noncompacted myocardium

Braunwald 11th Ed; Page 1588

The left ventricular noncompaction is defined either by echocardiography or CMR approaches. The criteria used to define LVNC use ratios of compacted to noncompacted myocardium. The LV size and function are not components of the diagnosis.

46. Ans. d. Permanent reciprocating junctional tachycardia

Braunwald 11th Ed; Page 1589

Tachycardia for a prolonged period can result in diastolic and systolic ventricular dysfunction, even in the absence of other cardiac diseases. This condition is known as tachycardia-induced cardiomyopathy. The diagnosis of tachycardia induced cardiomyopathy can be made only retrospectively when correction of an arrhythmia is associated with improved ventricular function. The duration of the arrhythmia, more than the heart rate, is probably a critical factor in tachycardia induced cardiomyopathy. The 'purest' form of tachycardia induced cardiomyopathy is caused by incessant or extremely frequent atrial tachycardia or permanent reciprocating junctional tachycardia, often in a child or young patients with systolic dysfunction. Most cases of tachycardia-induced cardiomyopathy improve within 3–6 months after correction of the arrhythmia, but occasional patients have seen improvement, as late as 1 year. Tachycardia-induced LV diastolic dysfunction may occur in humans in the presence of normal ejection fraction, and it may be responsible for the symptoms of heart failure in many patients with arrhythmia and a preserved LV ejection fraction.

47. Ans. c. Tachycardia induced LV diastolic dysfunction is not reported

Braunwald 11th Ed; Page 1589

Refer to explanation for Q. No 46.

48. Ans. d. Exercise stress test

Hurst's 14th Ed; Page 1916

Catecholaminergic polymorphic ventricular tachycardia patients often present with exercise induced syncope. These patients often have normal resting ECG with occasional cases demonstrating sinus bradycardia and a prominent U wave. A distinctive pattern of arrhythmia is observed during exercise or acute emotion. An alternating 180° QRS axis on a beat-to-beat basis, the so-called bidirectional ventricular tachycardia, supraventricular tachycardia are often seen. The exercise stress test is the most important diagnostic test for suspected CPVT (patients with normal ECG and syncope, presyncope or dizziness triggered by exercise or acute emotion). Beta blockers, Flecainide, left cardiac sympathetic denervation and ICD for prevention of sudden death is included as strategy of treatment.

49. Ans. a. Baseline long QT syndrome

Hurst's 14th Ed; Page 1916

Refer to explanation for Q. No 48.

50. Ans. d. Amiodarone

Hurst's 14th Ed; Page 1916

Refer to explanation for Q. No 48.

51. Ans. d. All of the above

Hurst's 14th Ed; Page 1917

Several genes besides *SCN-5A* gene (variant named as Brs1) have been causally linked to the Brugada syndrome. In these patients, all the three main electrophysiologic functions are affected, i.e., the cardiac sodium current, the calcium current and transient outward potassium current.

52. Ans. c. Increase of sympathetic and decrease of parasympathetic tone

Braunwald 11th Ed; Page 549

Heart rate variability (HRV) reflects the balance between sympathetic and parasympathetic nervous system activity in the heart. A decrease in heart rate variability is a marker of increased sympathetic and decreased parasympathetic tone. It has been found that HRV fell in days to weeks leading to hospitalization for heart failure.

53. Ans. d. Left ventricle is spared

Hurst's 14th Ed; Page 1509

Arrhythmogenic cardiomyopathy is a rare primary myocardial disease that is clinically characterized by life-threatening ventricular arrhythmias secondary to fibrofatty replacement of ventricular myocytes. In the first systematic description of 24 adult cases in 1982, Marcus outlined the profile of right ventricular (RV) dysplasia as a pathologic condition primarily affecting the right ventricle and characterized by partial or total absence of RV musculature due to substitution by fatty and fibrous tissue. However, in 2002 task force criteria incorporated new knowledge on the genetic basis of the disease, improving diagnostic sensitivity and maintaining diagnostic specificity. The structural, histological, ECG, arrhythmic, and genetic features were structured in major and minor criteria. The task force document formally introduced the biventricular variant and of left dominant variant. The latter criteria support the broader new term of *arrhythmogenic cardiomyopathy*. Therefore, the disease is currently called arrhythmogenic cardiomyopathy, ARVC/D, ARVC, or ARVD. The involvement of the left ventricle in ACM had been originally described by Marcus and confirmed in several additional studies.

54. Ans. d. Nonsustained or sustained ventricular tachycardia of LBBB morphology with superior axis

Hurst's 14th Ed; Page 1510

Criteria for diagnosis of arrhythmogenic cardiomyopathy

Definite diagnosis: 2 major or 1 major and 2 minor criteria or 4 minor criteria from different categories
Borderline diagnosis: 1 major and 1 minor or 3 minor criteria from different categories
Possible diagnosis: 1 major or 2 minor criteria from different categories

Type 1 criteria	Type II criteria	Type III criteria	Type IV criteria	Type V criteria	Type VI criteria
Global or regional dysfunction and structural alterations	Tissue characterization of wall	Repolarization abnormalities	Depolarization/Conduction abnormalities	Arrhythmias	Family history

Major

By 2D echo: • Regional RV akinesia, dyskinesia, or aneurysm and one of the following (end diastole): – PLAX RVOT ≥ 32 mm [corrected for body size (PLAX/BSA) ≥ 19 mm/m²] – PSAX RVOT ≥ 36 mm [corrected for body size (PSAX/BSA) ≥ 21 mm/m²] – Fractional area change ≤ 33% **By MRI:** • Regional RV akinesia or dyskinesia or dyssynchronous RV contraction and one of the following: – Ratio of RV end-diastolic volume to BSA ≥ 110 mL/m² (male) or 100 mL/m² (female) – RV ejection fraction ≤ 40% **By RV angiography:** Regional RV akinesia, dyskinesia, or aneurysm	Residual myocytes < 60% by morphometric analysis (or < 50% if estimated), with fibrous replacement of the RV free wall myocardium in ≥ 1 sample, with or without fatty replacement of tissue on endomyocardial biopsy	Inverted T waves in right precordial leads (V₁, V₂, and V₃) or beyond in individuals > 14 years of age (in the absence of complete right bundle branch block QRS ≥ 120 ms)	Epsilon wave (reproducible low-amplitude signals between end of QRS complex to onset of the T wave) in the right precordial leads (V₁ to V₃)	Nonsustained or sustained ventricular tachycardia of left bundle branch morphology with superior axis (negative or indeterminate QRS in leads II, III, and aVF and positive in lead aVL)	• ACM confirmed in a first-degree relative who meets current Task Force criteria • ACM confirmed pathologically at autopsy or surgery in a first-degree relative • Identification of a pathogenic mutation categorized as associated or probably associated with ACM in the patient under evaluation

Minor

By 2D echo: • Regional RV akinesia or dyskinesia and one of the following (end diastole): – PLAX RVOT ≥ 29 to < 32 mm [connected for body size (PLAX/BSA) ≥ 16 to < 19 mm/m²] – PSAX RVOT ≥ 32 to < 36 mm [conected for body size (PSAX/BSA) ≥ 18 to < 21 mm/m²] – Fractional area change > 33 to ≤ 40% **By MRI:** • Regional RV akinesia or dyskinesia or dyssynchronous RV contraction and one of the following: – Ratio of RV end-diastolic volume to BSA ≥ 100 to < 110 mL/m² (male) or ≥ 90 to < 100 mL/m² (female) – RV ejection fraction > 40 to ≤ 45%	Residual myocytes 60% to 75% by morphometric analysis (or 50% to 65% if estimated), with fibrous replacement of the RV free wall myocardium in ≥ 1 sample, with or without fatty replacement of tissue on endomyocardial biopsy	• Inverted T waves in leads V₁, and V₂ in individuals > 14 years of age (in the absence of complete right bundle branch block) or in V₄, V₅ or V₆ • Inverted T waves in leads V₁, V₂, V₃, and V₄ in individuals > 14 years of age in the presence of complete right bundle branch block	• Late potentials by SAECG in ≥ 1 of 3 parameters in the absence of a QRS duration of ≥ 110 ms on the standard ECG • Filtered QRS duration (fQRS) ≥ 114 ms • Duration of terminal QRS < 40 µV (low-amplitude signal duration) ≥ 38 ms • Root-mean-square voltage of terminal 40 ms ≤ 20 µV • Terminal activation duration of QRS ≥ 55 ms measured from the nadir of the S wave to the end of the QRS, including r' in V₁, V₂ or V₃, in the absence of complete right bundle branch block	• Nonsustained or sustained ventricular tachycardia of RV outflow configuration, left bundle branch block morphology with inferior axis (positive QRS in leads II, III, and aVF and negative in lead aVL), or unknown axis • > 500 ventricular extrasystoles per 24 hours (Holter)	• History of ACM in a first-degree relative in whom it is not possible or practical to determine whether the family member meets current Task Force criteria • Premature sudden death (< 35 years of age) as a result of suspected ACM in a first-degree relative • ACM confirmed pathologically or by current Task Force criteria in second-degree relative

55. Ans. d. Non-sustained and sustained ventricular tachycardia, LBBB morphology with inferior axis.

Hurst's 14th Ed; Page 1510

Refer to explanation for Q. No 54.

56. Ans. c. Cardiac MRI

Hurst's 14th Ed; Page 1518-1519

RV angiography, transthoracic echocardiography, and cardiac MRI can be used to evaluate for structural and functional abnormalities of the RV. RV angiography is rarely performed, and it demonstrate regional RV wall abnormalities including dyskinesia, akinesia, or aneurysm formation. Transthoracic echocardiography is more commonly used, and besides providing information on regional wall abnormalities, it can provide information regarding RV dimensions and function. Echocardiography however has a limited assessment of RV structure and function as a result of the inherent limitation in assessing a complex three-dimensional chamber with limited two-dimensional views. Cardiac MRI provides a superior assessment of regional and global function as well as provide information on tissue characteristics, (i.e., fibrosis and intramyocardial fat).

57. Ans. b. Somatostatin analogue

Braunwald 11th Ed; Page 1598

The therapy for carcinoid syndrome are generally not curative and includes debulking the hepatic metastases by embolization or by partial resection and by the use of octreotide, a somatostatin analogue that binds to somatostatin receptors on the surface of carcinoid tumor cells and inhibits the secretion of vasoactive substances. Although the development and progression of carcinoid heart disease are associated with increasing 5-hydroxyindoleacetic acid level, a decrease in 5-HIAA levels afterward does not appear to cause a change in the cardiac valvular lesions, and they may even progress.

58. Ans. d. Acute carcinoid crisis

Braunwald 11th Ed; Page 1598

Valve replacement in carcinoid heart disease can be performed whenever indicated. Valve replacement carries a unique complex problem in form of development of an acute carcinoid crisis characterized by profound hypotension, severe flushing, bronchospasm, and arrhythmias.

59. Ans. a. Phenylephrine

Braunwald 11th Ed; Page 1606

Subaortic gradient and associated ejection systolic murmur can be spontaneously variables, reduced or abolished by intervention, which decrease myocardial contractility, (e.g., beta-adrenergic blocking drugs) or increase ventricular volume or arterial pressure (e.g., squatting, isometric handgrip, and phenylephrine). Alternatively, gradient can be augmented by circumstances in which arterial pressure or ventricular volume is reduced (Valsalva maneuver, administration of nitroglycerin or amyl nitrite, blood loss, dehydration) or when LV contractility is increased (premature ventricular contractions, infusion of isoproterenol or dobutamine, or physiologic exercise).

60. Ans. d. Positron emission tomography (PET)

Braunwald 11th Ed; Page 1606

Myocardial ischemia due to microvascular dysfunction is an important pathophysiological component of HCM disease process, promoting adverse LV remodeling and ultimately affecting the clinical course. Positron emission tomography (PET) is the technique most useful in the assessment of microvascular function. A marked reduction in coronary reserve demonstrated with PET early in the clinical course has been reported to be a determinant of the prognosis.

61. Ans. b. > 30 mm

Braunwald 11th Ed; Page 1607

The physical finding in patients with HCM vary largely due to the hemodynamic state. Patients with LVOT obstruction characteristically have a medium pitch systolic ejection murmur at the lower left sternal border and apex that varies in intensity with the magnitude of the subaortic gradient. It increases with the Valsalva maneuver, during or immediately after exercise, or on standing. Such variability, along with the characteristic lack of radiation of the murmur to the neck, helps in differentiating dynamic subaortic obstruction from fixed aortic stenosis. Most HCM patients with loud murmurs of at least grade 3/6 are likely to have LV outflow gradients of >30 mm Hg. Arterial pulses may rise rapidly with the bisferiens pulse contour.

62. Ans. d. All above changes can be seen

Braunwald 11th Ed; Page 1609

Normal ECG patterns are more commonly associated with mild LV hypertrophy and has a favorable clinical course, but do not exclude the possibility of future sudden cardiac death. Increased voltages (tall R waves or deep S waves) are only weakly correlated with the magnitude of LV hypertrophy and do not reliably distinguish obstructive from nonobstructive HCM.

63. Ans. a. Normal ECG exclude the possibility of future sudden death

Braunwald 11th Ed; Page 1609

Refer to explanation for Q. No 62.

64. Ans. d. Family history of HCM with systolic dysfunction

Braunwald 11th Ed; Page 1609

About 2 to 3% of patients with HCM develop advanced (end-stage) heart failure, usually associated with systolic LV dysfunction (ejection fraction < 50%), a consequence of small vessel mediated myocardial ischemia and diffuse transmural scarring. The most reliable marker for evolution to end-stage disease appears to be a family history of HCM with systolic dysfunction.

65. Ans. d. All are correct

Braunwald 11th Ed; Page 1610

Sudden cardiac death in HCM may occur at any age, most commonly in adolescents and adults younger than 30 years of age. Although the risk of sudden cardiac death can extend into midlife, it is significantly less common in patients over the age of 60 years. The potential for lethal ventricular tachyarrhythmias is mitigated at the more advanced ages. Whereas most sudden cardiac death during sedentary or modest physical activities, sometimes it is seen with vigorous exertion.

Patient with one or more of the following markers are more prone for sudden cardiac death and for whom primary prevention with ICD is recommended:

- Family history of one or more premature HCM related death
- Unexplained syncope especially if it was recent and in young patients
- Hypotensive or attenuated blood pressure response to exercise
- Multiple, repetitive or prolonged, nonsustained bursts of VT on serial ambulatory ECGs
- Massive LV apical aneurysm

The risk for sudden death is unrelated to the pattern or location of the LV hypertrophy.

66. Ans. c. Extensive late gadolinium enhancement on contrast enhanced CMR

Braunwald 11th Ed; Page 1611

Few patients with HOCM without any of the conventional primary prevention risk factors remains susceptible to sudden cardiac death. Extensive late LGE on contrast enhanced CMR (particularly when it is present in 15% or more of the LV mass) has been shown to be associated with an increased sudden death risk. It is a new marker and independent predictor of sudden cardiac death, even in the absence of conventional risk factors, and calls for implantation of prophylactic ICD. There is no evidence that particular ECG patterns like T-wave alternans, or myocardial bridging of the left anterior descending coronary artery which is more frequently seen in patients with HCM than the general population, predict risk in HCM.

67. Ans. c. Verapamil

Braunwald 11th Ed; Page 1612

Verapamil improves the symptoms and exercise capacity in patients with HOCM without LVOT obstruction. This is because of it can control heart rate and improved ventricular relaxation and filling and also serve as a potential treatment for chest pain by increasing the myocardial blood flow.

68. Ans. c. Transaortic ventricular septal myectomy

Braunwald 11th Ed; Page 1614

Morrow procedure is a transaortic ventricular septal myectomy which involves resection of a small portion of muscle (usually 3–10 g) from the basal septum to relieve obstruction in HOCM.

69. Ans. d. Amiodarone

Braunwald 11th Ed; Page 1615

Symptomatic atrial fibrillation is the most common sustained arrhythmia in HCM. Atrial fibrillation is not associated with increased HCM related mortality or a promoter of progressive heart failure symptoms. Paroxysmal, persistent, or permanent atrial fibrillation occurs in 20-25% of HCM patients, increasing in incidence with age and related to left atrial enlargement and dysfunction. Symptomatic paroxysmal AF can adversely impact the quality of life. Although data specifically in HCM are limited, amiodarone is regarded as the most effective drug in reducing AF recurrences. Beta blockers and verapamil are usually administered to control the heart rate in patients with persistent or permanent AF.

70. Ans. b. Atrial fibrillation

Braunwald 11th Ed; Page 1633

Ethanol consumption is associated with a variety of atrial and ventricular arrhythmias, most commonly: (1) atrial or ventricular premature beats, (2) supraventricular tachycardia, (3) atrial flutter, (4) atrial fibrillation, (5) ventricular tachycardia, or (6) ventricular fibrillation. The most common ethanol-induced arrhythmia is atrial fibrillation. Ethanol is of causal importance in about a third of subjects with new-onset atrial fibrillation. Most episodes occur after binge drinking, usually on weekends or holidays—hence the term "holiday heart" syndrome. Ethanol enhances vulnerability to the induction of atrial flutter and fibrillation. Treatment of these ethanol-induced arrhythmias is abstinence.

71. Ans. d. All can be seen

Braunwald 11th Ed; Page 1636

Cocaine abuse is associated with number of cocaine related cardiovascular complications including angina pectoris, acute myocardial infarction, cardiomyopathy including stress cardiomyopathy (Takotsubo syndrome), aortic dissection and sudden cardiac death. Cocaine abuse is associated with many cardiac arrhythmias and conduction disturbances like sinus tachycardia, sinus bradycardia, supraventricular tachycardia, bundle branch block, complete heart block, ventricular fibrillation and flutter. Cocaine inhibits action potential generation and conduction and therefore it prolonged QRS and QT intervals, as a result of its sodium channel blocking effect. Due to this, it may produce Brugada type electrocardiographic features and torsades pointes.

72. Ans. d. Highly active antiretroviral therapy (HAART)

Braunwald 11th Ed; Page 1638

Subjects treated with highly active antiretroviral therapy (HAART) have been observed to have severe hypertriglyceridemia, marked elevations in lipoprotein(a) and hypercholesterolemia, increased LDL and decreased HDL cholesterol levels, and insulin resistance and therefore they have an increased risk for atherosclerosis. The medicinal use of serotonin agonists, such as ergotamine and methysergide (migraine therapy), bromocriptine, cabergoline, and pergolide (Parkinson disease therapy), and fenfluramine and dexfenfluramine (appetite suppressants) has been associated with left- and right-sided valvular disease. Two medications used to treat subjects with migraine headaches, ergotamine and triptans, have been associated with acute MI. Ergotamine causes vasoconstriction of the intracerebral and extracranial arteries; rarely, its use has been associated with coronary arterial vasospasm and acute MI. Similarly, triptans also exert their therapeutic effects by inducing cerebral arterial vasoconstriction.

73. Ans. c. Triptans

Braunwald 11th Ed; Page 1638

Refer to explanation for Q. No 72.

74. Ans. c. More noncalcified plaques which are lipid laden and prone to rupture

Braunwald 11th Ed; Page 1654

Atherosclerosis in HIV patients is a distinctive pathological entity compared to atherosclerosis seen in the general population. Autopsy studies have proved that coronary atherosclerosis in HIV patients resembles transplant vasculopathy. It is characterized by diffuse, circumferential vessel involvement with proliferation of smooth muscle cells mixed with abundant elastic tissue. In addition, calcification of the internal elastic media has been described in HIV patients.

Cardiac computed tomography has shown that the prevalence of coronary artery calcification are similar in HIV patients as the normal population. However, CT angiographic studies reveal that noncalcified plaques are almost three times more commonly present in HIV patients compared to the normal population. Noncalcified plaques are more likely to be lipid laden, inflammatory, and prone to rupture. High-risk features of plaque have also been reported in the setting of HIV.

75. Ans. d. All are incorrect

Braunwald 11th Ed; Page 1655

The clinical presentation of acute coronary syndrome differs in HIV patients compared with uninfected individuals. HIV patients are on average more than a decade younger than uninfected persons and are more likely to be men, to be current smokers, and to have low HDL cholesterol levels. Their risk scores tend to be lower and they are more likely to have single-vessel than multiple-vessel coronary artery disease. In general, HIV patients hospitalized with acute coronary syndrome have excellent immediate outcomes.

76. Ans. d. Restenosis rate following drug eluting stent are higher in HIV patients

Braunwald 11th Ed; Page 1655

In earlier studies, HIV patients had higher rates of restenosis after PCI with bare metal stents, compared with uninfected patients. Recent studies, in which most patients received drug-eluting stents, have shown similar medium-term outcomes between HIV patients and matched controls.

77. Ans. c. Cardiomyopathy

Braunwald 11th Ed; Page 1655–1656

The impact of early ART on CVD and CV risk in HIV remains unknown. However, ART accelerate atherosclerosis by inducing hyperlipidemia especially hypertriglyceridemia, hypercholesterolemia, and reduction of HDL. Many of the antiviral especially abacavir is associated with increased risk of myocardial infarction. The treatment of HIV with ART has not resulted in reduction in pulmonary arterial hypertension. However, the incidence of cardiomyopathy has declined dramatically since the introduction of ART. Whether ART can reverse establish cardiomyopathy is also not known.

78. Ans. b. Atrial chamber enlargement

Hurst's 14th; Page 1408

According to American Heart Association classification, dilated form of cardiomyopathy are characterized by ventricular chamber enlargement and systolic dysfunction with normal LV wall thickness.

79. Ans. d. All

Hurst's 14th Ed; Page 1421

The iatrogenic cardiomyopathy can result from common medication use for autoimmune diseases, the cardiac phenotypes are restrictive/dilated in case of hydroxychloroquine toxicity and dilated in case of tumor necrosis factor (TNF)-α inhibitors, (e.g., etanercept, infliximab, adalimumab).

80. Ans. c. 3 standard size drink or alcohol consumption over 80 g/day

Braunwald 11th Ed; Page 1632

Light to moderate alcohol intake is beneficial for cardiovascular health, whereas habitual heavy alcohol consumption is associated with increased risk of LV dilatation and dysfunction (alcoholic cardiomyopathy), arrhythmias, systemic hypertension, ischemic heart disease, stroke, and skeletal muscle abnormalities. Heavy alcohol consumption corresponds to daily ingestion of at least three standard-size drinks or alcohol consumption over 80 g. Light-moderate alcohol intake corresponds to less than three standard-sized drinks or < 80 g/day. A standard-sized portions of wine, liquor, or beer contain approximately the same amount of alcohol, the daily amount of ethanol is usually measured per number of standard drinks.

The toxic effect of alcohol is expected for daily alcohol consumption over 80 g (3 or more standard size drink per day) lasting 5 years or more before the onset of diagnosis.

81. Ans. c. More than 20,000 PVCs in 24 hours

Hurst's 14th Ed; Page 1430

Premature ventricular contraction induced cardiomyopathy is characterized by LV dilatation and/or dysfunction, diastolic dysfunction and ventricular strain by speckle tracking imaging. A dose-response relation has been demonstrated in serial evaluations of LV function among 239 consecutive patients with frequent PVCs and no obvious cardiac disease. > 20,000 PVCs per 24 hours were associated with subclinical deterioration in LVEF, whereas > 10,000 PVCs per 24 hours showed LV dilation without a change in LVEF.

82. Ans. a. Anthracycline

Hurst's 14th Ed; Page 1432

Heart muscle toxicity as a result of chemotherapeutic agents is generally characterized by nonreversible injury (type I) as a result of the presence of structural damage (e.g., anthracycline or high dose cyclophosphamide DCM) and type II, i.e., potentially reversible on cessation of therapy in absence of structural abnormality it is seen with targeted therapy, (i.e., Trastuzumab, Sunitinib, Lapatinib). In patients who are first treated with drugs causing type I injury and then with drug causing type II injury, the damage may be cumulative.

83. Ans. c. Hypertrophied papillary muscle abutting against the septum

Hurst's 14th Ed; Page 1446

Dynamic LVOT obstruction caused by contact between the mitral valve leaflets during ventricular systole is present in one-third of patients at rest and one-third patients during exercise or physical maneuvers that reduce ventricular volume or increase contractility in HOCM. The obstruction to the LV outflow typically varies with loading conditions and contractility of the ventricle. Obstruction can also be present in the mid cavity as a result of hypertrophied papillary muscles abutting against the septum. Mitral regurgitation is common in patients with LVOT tract obstruction and is an important cause of dyspnea. Mitral regurgitation is caused by the distortion of the mitral valve apparatus from systolic anterior motion secondary to LVOT tract obstruction. The jet of mitral regurgitation is directed laterally and posteriorly, predominates during mid and late systole, and is proportional to the severity of LVOT tract obstruction.

84. Ans. d. All of the above

Hurst's 14th Ed; Page 1446

Refer to explanation for Q. No 83.

85. Ans. d. All contributes

Hurst's 14th Ed; Page 1448

The hypertrophic cardiomyopathy has three predominate symptoms, dyspnea, angina and syncope. Dyspnea is usually caused by a combination of LVOT tract obstruction, mitral regurgitation, and LV diastolic dysfunction. Angina, usually in the absence of epicardial coronary disease, is caused by a number of mechanisms, including small-artery narrowing, intramural compression of small arteries from myocardial hypertrophy, abnormal diastolic filling, oxygen supply-demand mismatch, and abnormal coronary flow reserve. Transient loss of consciousness occurs in approximately 20% of HCM patients. In most cases, it is a result of syncope caused by LVOT tract obstruction, activation of LV baroreceptors resulting in reflex vasodilatation, and atrial and ventricular arrhythmia.

86. Ans. d. Standing to squat position

Hurst's 14th Ed; Page 1448

Dynamic auscultation in HCM helps to differentiate the murmur of HCM from that of valvular aortic stenosis and mitral regurgitation. Maneuvers that decrease preload will increase the dynamic gradient and increase the intensity of the murmur.

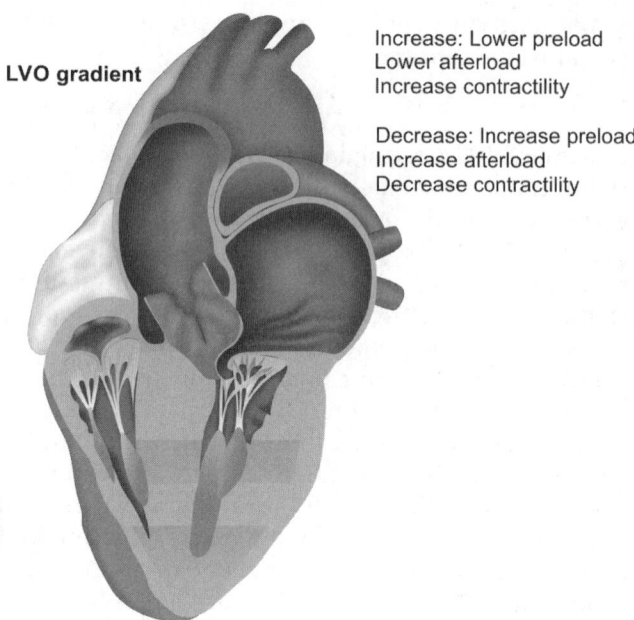

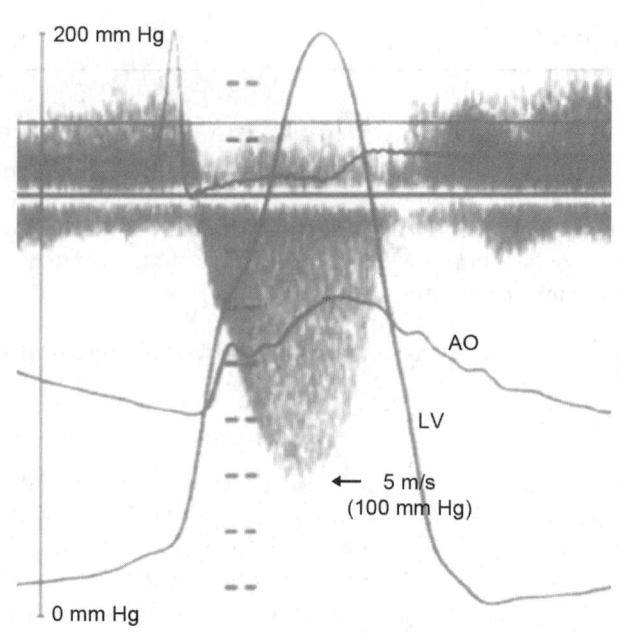

The most reliable method of diagnosing the dynamic LVOT tract obstruction is the response of the murmur to the standing-squat-stand position. From the standing position to a prompt squat, the murmur will markedly decrease in intensity, as a result of increases in afterload and preload. From the squatting to standing position, there will be an increase in intensity of the murmur immediately as afterload is reduced. A progressive increase in intensity of the murmur will continue for the next 4-5 beats as preload to the left side of the heart is reduced. Exercise like walking or climbing stairs, can be used to provoke the murmur. Other maneuvers that are used to change the intensity of the murmur include leg-raising to increase preload (and thereby decrease the intensity of the murmur) and the inhalation of amyl nitrite to decrease afterload, increase heart rate, and increase the intensity of the murmur. There is also an increase in intensity of the systolic murmur after a premature ventricular beat.

87. **Ans. b. Hypertrophic obstructive cardiomyopathy**

Hurst's 14th Ed; Page 1452

In HOCM, dynamic LVOT obstruction is characterized by systolic anterior motion of the mitral valve apparatus and an open ventricular chamber. The dynamic LVOT obstruction is characterized by a high-velocity, "dagger shaped" signal on continuous wave Doppler. LVOT obstruction is defined as an instantaneous peak Doppler LVOT pressure gradient of >30 mm Hg at rest or during physiologic provocation such as Valsalva maneuver, standing, or exercise. A gradient of > 50 mm Hg is usually considered to be the threshold at which LVOT obstruction becomes hemodynamically important.

88. **Ans. d. Increased in the aortic pulse pressure**

Hurst's 14th Ed; Page 1455

In patients with HOCM, when there is little resting obstruction, provocation using the Valsalva maneuver or infusion of isoproterenol can be performed in the catheterization laboratory. The Brockenbrough phenomenon—the hallmark of latent obstruction refers to the phenomenon after a premature contraction, in which an increase in the contractility of the ventricle results in a marked increase in the degree of dynamic obstruction.

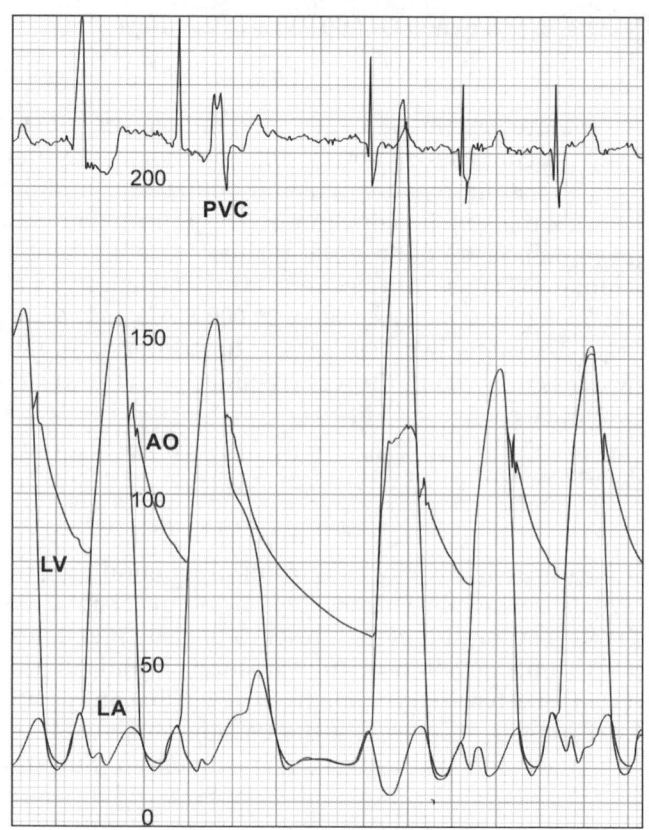

This is seen as an increase in the outflow gradient and a decrease in the aortic pulse pressure after the pause. This is in contradistinction to a fixed obstruction in which there is an increase in gradient from the increase in stroke volume but also an increase in aortic pulse pressure.

89. Ans. c. Verapamil

Hurst's 14th Ed; Page 1457

Nondihydropyrine calcium channel blockers—specifically, verapamil and diltiazem are of value in the treatment of HCM, particularly if β-blockers are contraindicated or ineffective. By preventing calcium influx, they not only decrease inotropy and chronotropy, but also improve abnormal diastolic relaxation. Verapamil is used most frequently because of its minimal effect on afterload. Clinical studies have shown a decrease in both basal and provoked gradients during acute drug intervention with verapamil. Verapamil has been shown to improve exercise tolerance by 20-30%. Calcium channel blockers may improve angina to a greater degree than β-blockers. The dose of verapamil should be titrated up to 480 mg/day to obtain a resting heart rate of 60 bpm. Dihydropyridine calcium channel blockers should be avoided in patients with LVOT obstruction, because these pure vasodilators can increase the severity of the outflow tract by reducing afterload. Digoxin should be avoided in HOCM for control of rate in AF.

90. Ans. c. Digoxin

Hurst's 14th Ed; Page 1457

Refer to explanation for Q. No 89.

91. Ans. d. Complete heart block

Hurst's 14th Ed; Page 1458

Alcohol septal ablation is a procedure in which alcohol is infused in the septal perforator arteries in order to cause necrosis and scarring of the proximal interventricular septum. The subsequent wall thinning and remodeling of the basal septum results in reduction of the outflow tract obstruction. The major complication of alcohol septal ablation is complete heart block, which, with small doses of alcohol which occurs in about 7-20% of patients. Patients are more likely to experience complete heart block if left bundle branch block is present prior to the ablation procedure. Other complications of septal ablation include coronary artery dissection, excessive myocardial infarction from leakage of the alcohol into coronary arteries, ventricular septal defects, and myocardial perforation. A maximum LV wall thickness < 16 mm at the point of leaflet-septal contact is a risk factor for ventriculo-septal defects in both alcohol septal ablation or myectomy.

92. Ans. d. RV apex

Hurst's 14th Ed; Page 1459

Dual chamber pacing from right ventricular apex can decrease the outflow tract gradient as a result of alteration of ventricular contraction and decrease in systolic projection of the basal septum into the LVOT. There are some technical considerations when using pacemaker therapy for treatment of patients with HCM. Pacing or sensing the atrium, in addition to pacing the ventricle, is necessary to maintain the hemodynamic contribution of atrial contraction. There should be an optimal AV delay for maximizing hemodynamic performance. If the paced AV interval is too short, it may increase left atrial pressure and reduce preload, whereas an overly long AV delay can result in incomplete pre-excitation of the right ventricle with suboptimal reduction in gradient. It is essential to have the pacemaker tip placed in the apex of the right ventricle to achieve the maximum reduction in gradient, and pacing parameters need to be optimized to achieve maximum pre-excitation of the right ventricular apex with minimal compromise of LV filling.

CHAPTER 19

Cor Pulmonale and Pulmonary Embolism

COR PULMONALE/DVT

1. Which of the following conditions produces acute pulmonary arterial hypertension?
   a. Acute LVF
   b. Mitral stenosis
   c. Adult respiratory distress syndrome
   d. Fibrosing mediastinitis

2. The mean pulmonary arterial pressure immediately before birth is:
   a. 20 mm Hg
   b. 40 mm Hg
   c. 50 mm Hg
   d. 80 mm Hg

3. The gold standard method for the diagnosis of pulmonary hypertension is:
   a. Lung scans
   b. Echocardiography
   c. Right heart catheterization
   d. Lung biopsy

4. Which of the following hemodynamic parameter is always normal in cases of primary pulmonary hypertension?
   a. Pulmonary artery pressure
   b. Pulmonary vascular resistance
   c. Pulmonary capillary wedge pressure
   d. Cardiac output

5. Which of the following drugs selectively relaxes the pulmonary vessels without affecting systemic arterial pressure?
   a. Nifedipine
   b. Verapamil
   c. Nitric oxide
   d. Arachidonic acid metabolites

6. The most common connective tissue disorder complicated by pulmonary hypertension is:
   a. Scleroderma
   b. Systemic lupus erythematosus
   c. Polyarteritis nodosa
   d. Mixed connective tissue disease

7. Which of the following does *not* cause global alveolar hypoventilation?
   a. Encephalitis
   b. Sleep apnea syndrome
   c. Asbestosis
   d. COPD

8. The mortality of untreated pulmonary embolism is:
   a. <10%
   b. 10–15%
   c. >50%
   d. >90%

9. The common sources of symptomatic pulmonary embolism is:
   a. Thrombi in the thigh
   b. Thrombi in calf veins
   c. Pelvic vein thrombosis
   d. Thrombi in the right heart

10. Which of the following has *not* been shown to be effective in preventing DVT?
    a. Low molecular weight heparin
    b. Low dose oral warfarin
    c. Aspirin
    d. Intravenous dextran

11. The most sensitive and specific test for recognition of DVT is:
    a. Doppler technique
    b. Impedance plethysmography
    c. Venography
    d. Fibrinogen scanning

12. The most sensitive test to diagnose DVT in high-risk patients for DVT intra- or postoperatively is:
    a. Plethysmography
    b. Fibrinogen labeled iodine scanning
    c. Venography
    d. Peripheral venous Doppler

13. In what percentage of untreated case of proximal DVT have pulmonary embolism?
    a. 20%
    b. 20–30%
    c. >50%
    d. 70–80%

14. What is the probability of pulmonary embolism in patients with DVT limited to the distal lower extremity?
   a. <10%
   b. 30–40%
   c. >60%
   d. None of them

15. Which is the most frequent cause of chronic cor pulmonale?
   a. Chronic bronchitis
   b. Interstitial fibrosis
   c. Alveolar hypoventilation
   d. Adult respiratory distress syndrome

16. Which of the following is *not* correct regarding right ventricle?
   a. It is the dominant chamber for the first three months of life
   b. It is more compliant than LV
   c. It is better able to handle an increase in pressure than volume
   d. None of the above

17. In patients with chronic cor-pulmonale which of the following is first electrocardiographic changes to suggest right ventricular hypertrophy?
   a. Clockwise rotation
   b. Right axis deviation
   c. qR pattern in aVR
   d. P-pulmonale

18. Which of the following statement is *correct*?
   a. Pulse wave Doppler is more sensitive than continuous wave Doppler for detecting tricuspid regurgitation
   b. Echocardiography measured RV wall thickness correlates poorly with RV weight determined at autopsy
   c. Radionuclide ventriculography is better than echocardiography to show changes in RV function
   d. All of the above

19. Which of the following is gold standard technique for measuring right ventricular volume?
   a. Echocardiography
   b. Radionuclide ventriculography
   c. MRI
   d. Thallium imaging

20. The diagnosis of sleep apnea is established by:
   a. Clinical history and examination
   b. Pulmonary function test
   c. MRI
   d. Polysomnography

21. Which of the following statements regarding sleep apnea syndrome is *not* correct?
   a. Affected patients are usually not obese
   b. Only 20% of patients have coexisting COPD
   c. Oxygen therapy should be used liberally
   d. Continuous positive airway pressure (CPAP) is to be used for treating obstructive apnea

22. All are correct regarding digitalis and COPD, *except*:
   a. Digitalis increases contractility of RV myocardium and also produce pulmonary vasoconstriction
   b. Digitalis should be used only in cases of COPD with LV failure
   c. Digoxin is not indicated in the routine management of cor pulmonale
   d. All of the above

23. Cardiovascular effects of theophylline includes all, *except*:
   a. Increase in heart rate
   b. Increase in pulmonary artery pressure
   c. Increase in RVEF
   d. Increase in LVEF

24. Cardiovascular effects of theophylline includes all, *except*:
   a. Reduction in pulmonary artery pressure
   b. Increase in biventricular pump function
   c. Enhanced myocardial contractility and reduction in afterload
   d. All of the above

25. Which of the following statement is *not* correct regarding use of beta-adrenergic agonist in CopD?
   a. It causes pulmonary vasodilatation
   b. It has direct inotropic action on myocardium and increases RVEF and LVEF
   c. These benefits are not sustained during chronic administration
   d. All are correct

ANSWERS WITH EXPLANATIONS

1. Ans. c. Adult respiratory distress syndrome

Hurst's 14th Ed, Page 1785–86

Pulmonary hypertension is a hemodynamic abnormality common to a variety of conditions characterized by increased right ventricular after load and work. The clinical manifestation, natural history and reversibility of pulmonary hypertension depends on the nature of pulmonary vascular lesion and the etiology and severity of hemodynamic disorder. Pulmonary arterial hypertension can be either acute or chronic. The acute form is usually a result of either pulmonary embolism or the adult respiratory distress syndrome. Cor pulmonale signifies the presence of pulmonary hypertension and cardiac dysfunction in the setting of disease affecting the structure or functioning of the lung. Pulmonary hypertension in patients with chronic lung disease tends to be less severe than in connective tissue disease, chronic thromboembolic disease or idiopathic pulmonary arterial hypertension. Pulmonary hypertension may be severe in some patient with interstitial lung disease.

2. Ans. c. 50 mm Hg

Hurst's 14th Ed, Page 1786

Immediately before birth pulmonary and systemic arterial blood pressure are nearly equal and about 70/40 mm Hg with a mean of 50 mm Hg. Immediately after birth with closure of the ductus arteriosus and initiation of ventilation, pulmonary arterial pressure falls rapidly to about one half of the systemic level. Thereafter pulmonary arterial pressure gradually decreases over several weeks to reach adulthood.

3. Ans. c. Right heart catheterization

Hurst's 14th Ed, Page 1789

The gold standard for the diagnosis of pulmonary hypertension is right heart catheterization. This technique enables the direct determination of right atrial and ventricular pressure, pulmonary arterial pressure, pulmonary artery wedge pressure, pulmonary blood flow (cardiac output) and the response of these parameter to interventions like use of vasodilators, oxygen, exercise. The measurement and samples obtained during cardiac catheterization may help in calculating pulmonary vascular resistance. Noninvasive methods are less reliable and less informative in diagnosis of pulmonary arterial hypertension.

4. Ans. c. Pulmonary capillary wedge pressure

Hurst's 14th Ed, Page 1795-1797

The diagnosis of primary pulmonary arterial hypertension depends on three different types of evidence: (1) clinical, radiographic and ECG manifestation of pulmonary hypertension; (2) hemodynamic features consisting of abnormally high pulmonary arterial pressure and pulmonary vascular resistance in association with normal left sided filling pressure and a normal or low cardiac output; and (3) exclusion of the causes of secondary pulmonary hypertension. Hemodynamic features of idiopathic pulmonary arterial hypertension is a combination of a high pulmonary arterial pressure, a normal or low cardiac output and a normal left atrial or pulmonary arterial wedge pressure. Calculated pulmonary vascular resistance is high, generally leading to the logical conclusion that the resistance vessels, i.e., the small muscular artery and arteriole are the predominate site of vascular obstruction. During exercise, as cardiac output increases, pulmonary arterial pressure increases further. The increment in the pressure in the pulmonary hypertensive circuit are much more striking than in the normotensive pulmonary arterial circulation owing to the inability of existing vasculature to dilate or recruit unused vessel to accommodate the rise in pulmonary blood flow.

5. Ans. c. Nitric oxide

Hurst's 14th Ed, Page 1802

Treatment of idiopathic pulmonary arterial hypertension focuses on use of vasodilator because there is an increase in the pulmonary vascular tone, which contribute to high pulmonary arterial pressure in the patients with idiopathic pulmonary arterial hypertension. The bulk of pulmonary vascular obstruction is clearly anatomic. Vasodilators offers the prospects of decreasing pulmonary arterial pressure and therefore hemodynamic burden on the right ventricle is reduced and it also brings reversibility of the anatomic lesion. Nitric oxide is used in the treatment of idiopathic pulmonary arterial hypertension. Nitric oxide is synthesized in endothelial cells and it is proved that the endothelial derived relaxing factor that contributes to the low initial tone of pulmonary circulation. It has the advantage of other vasodilators of selectively relaxing pulmonary vessels without affecting systemic arterial pressure. It is currently being used as a test of vasoreactivity in a wide variety of pulmonary hypertensive state and also has been used to control pulmonary hypertension in the syndrome of persistent pulmonary hypertension in the newborn. Sildenafil which enhances nitric oxide activity by inhibiting phosphodiesterase Type V, the enzyme responsible for catabolism of cyclic guanosine monophosphate, also was recently approved for the treatment of pulmonary arterial hypertension.

6. Ans. b. Systemic lupus erythematosus

Hurst's 14th Ed, Page 1792

Pulmonary vascular disease is an important component of certain connective tissue diseases, most commonly systemic lupus erythematosus (SLE), scleroderma, and the dermatomyositis. Although pulmonary hypertension can complicate many connective tissue diseases, it has been documented most often in SLE and progressive systemic sclerosis and its variant syndrome. The possibility has been raised that idiopathic pulmonary arterial hypertension is an inflammatory or autoimmune disease. The high frequency of both collagen vascular disease and idiopathic pulmonary arterial hypertension in women and the occurrence of Raynaud phenomena in up to 20% of patients with idiopathic pulmonary arterial hypertension has been used as additional evidence. Finally, there is high incidence of positive serological tests for antibodies particularly in women with idiopathic pulmonary arterial hypertension.

7. Ans. d. COPD

Hurst's 14th Ed, Page 1794-95

In patients who hypoventilate despite normal lungs (alveolar hypoventilation) the primary pathogenetic mechanism is alveolar hypoxia potentiated by respiratory acidosis. These abnormal alveolar and arterial blood gases play the same role in eliciting pulmonary hypertension in patients with alveolar hypoventilation as in those in whom the abnormal alveolar and blood gases are the result of ventilation perfusion abnormality. In individuals with normal lungs, the alveolar hypoventilation generally originates from an inadequate ventilatory drive (e.g., after encephalitis or in central sleep apnea), covert obstruction of upper airways (e.g., in obstructive sleep apnea), an ineffective chest bellows (e.g., after poliomyelitis or polymyositis), lungs entrapped by neoplasm or fibrosis (e.g., asbestosis) or in the cases of morbid obesity.

8. Ans. b. 10-15%

Hurst's 14th Ed, Page 1809

Approximately 100 thousand patients in the United States die each other directly as a consequence of acute pulmonary embolism. Three months mortality in unselected patients with acute pulmonary embolism is as high as 15%. Although a number of patients die of comorbidities that predispose them to the thromboembolic events, a substantial number of patients die from pulmonary embolism within hour of presentation before the diagnosis can be confirmed and therapy initiated or because the diagnosis was overlook.

9. Ans. b. Thrombi in calf veins

Hurst's 14th Ed, Page 1809

Virchow proposed the triad of factors leading to intravascular coagulation including stasis, vessel wall injury and hypercoagulability. Risk factor for deep vein thrombosis are based on these processes.

The overwhelming majority of emboli originate from the deep veins of the lower extremities although any venous bed can be involved. Although thrombi may form at any point along the vein wall most originate in the valve pocket. The veins of the calf are the most common site of origin with subsequent extension of clot prior to the embolization. Eventually, the thrombus may expand to fill the vessel entirely with both retrograde and proximal extension. Embolization does not occur if the thrombus can partially or completely resolved by three mechanism, i.e., recanalization, organization and lysis.

10. Ans. c. Aspirin

Hurst's 14th Ed, Page 1827

Aspirin has not been shown to be effective in preventing deep vein thrombosis.

11. Ans. c. Venography

Hurst's 14th Ed, Page 1816

A number of diagnostic techniques can be used to evaluate the patients with suspected deep vein thrombosis (DVT). Duplex ultrasonography is the most common technique used in the many part of the world. Impedance plethysmography is used at some centers and a number of important trials have been performed. Magnetic resonance imaging (MRI) appears to have some important advantages but it has not generally been used as a first line test because of cost and lack of availability. CT venography used alone or in conjunction with CT angiography appears to have a sensitivity and specificity equivalent to that of Duplex ultrasonography but exposes the patient to additional radiation. Contrast venography remains the gold standard but it is performed infrequently in view of accuracy of ultrasound. Each diagnostic technique has advantages and limitations. Although diagnostic algorithm may be suggested for suspected DVT, these are institution specific, depending on resources and available expertise with certain techniques.

12. Ans. b. Fibrinogen labeled iodine scanning

Hurst's 11th Ed; Page 1601

The most sensitive test to diagnose DVT in high-risk patients for DVT intra or postoperatively is fibrinogen labeled iodine scanning.

13. Ans. c. >50%

Hurst's 14th Ed, Page 1810

Trauma particularly of the lower extremity and pelvis increases the risk of DVT. Pulmonary embolism has been identified at autopsy in as many as 60% of patients with lower extremity fractures and mortality has been attributed to pulmonary embolism in as many as 50% of patients dying after hip fracture. The incidence of venous thromboembolism increases with time after traumatic event. Autopsy confirmed pulmonary embolism in patients surviving for less than 24 hours after trauma has been demonstrated in 3.3%, increasing to 5.5% in patients surviving up to 7 days. Pulmonary emboli occurred in 18.6% of patients surviving for a longer time.

14. Ans. a. <10%

Hurst's 14th Ed, Page 1810

Prior venous thromboembolism (VTE) forecasts increase the risk of recurrence. Surgical patients with a previous history of VTE who do not receive prophylaxis develop postoperative DVT in >50% of cases. Surgery itself significantly enhances the risk. Surgery patients without additional risk factors develop DVT in nearly 20% of cases if neither pharmacologic nor mechanical prophylaxis is applied.

15. Ans. a. Chronic bronchitis

Hurst's 11th Ed; Chapter 64; Page 1617-1625

Acute cor pulmonale is defined as right heart strain or overload secondary to acute pulmonary hypertension often due to massive pulmonary embolism. Chronic cor pulmonale is characterized by hypertrophy and dilatation of right ventricle secondary to the pulmonary hypertension caused by the disease of pulmonary parenchyma and/or pulmonary vascular system between the origin of main pulmonary artery and the entry of the pulmonary veins into the left atrium. The most frequent cause of chronic cor pulmonale is chronic obstructive pulmonary disease (COPD) resulting from chronic obstructive bronchitis or emphysema, whereas the most important cause of acute cor pulmonale is pulmonary thromboembolism. In addition to COPD, thromboembolic disease, a number of other disorders may cause cor pulmonale such as:

- Diseases affecting the pulmonary vasculature:
  - Primary diseases of the arterial wall:
    - Primary pulmonary hypertension
    - Granulomatous pulmonary arteritis
    - Toxin-induced pulmonary hypertension:
      a. Aminorex fumarate
      b. Intravenous drug abuse
    - Chronic liver disease
    - Peripheral pulmonic stenosis.
  - Thrombotic disorders:
    - Sickle cell diseases
    - Pulmonary microthrombi.
  - Embolic disorders:
    - Thromboembolism
    - Tumor embolism
    - Other embolism (amniotic fluid, air)
    - Schistosomiasis and other parasitic diseases.
- Pressures on pulmonary arteries by mediastinal tumors, aneurysms, granulomata, or fibrosis.
- Diseases of the neuromuscular apparatus and chest wall:
  - Neuromuscular weakness
  - Kyphoscoliosis
  - Thoracoplasty
  - Pleural fibrosis
  - Sleep apnea syndromes
  - Idiopathic hypoventilation.
- Diseases affecting air passages of the lung and alveoli:
  - Chronic obstructive pulmonary diseases
  - Cystic fibrosis
  - Congenital developmental defects
  - Infiltrative or granulomatous diseases:
    - Idiopathic pulmonary fibrosis
    - Sarcoidosis
    - Pneumoconiosis
    - Scleroderma
    - Mixed connective tissue disease
    - Systemic lupus erythematosus
    - Rheumatoid arthritis
    - Polymyositis
    - Eosinophilic granuloma
    - Malignant infiltration
    - Radiation
  - Upper airways obstruction
  - Pulmonary resection
  - High-altitude disease.

16. Ans. c. It is better able to handle an increase in pressure than volume

Hurst's 11th Ed; Chapter 64; Page 1617-1625

In humans born at or near sea level, the right ventricle is dominant chamber for the first three months of life. During this time, the right ventricle is larger and heavier and has a greater end-diastolic volume than the left ventricle. The left ventricle, however gradually becomes dominant and in adults the right ventricle is relatively thin walled and crescent shaped. The structure and the pumping function of two ventricles are essentially the same before birth and therefore the difference in the adults is attributed to the flow resistance in respective circulation. In the normal adult, right ventricle is thin walled and crescent shaped and its pumping action is similar to that of a bellows working in series with a low pressure circuit in contrast to the concentric contraction of the left ventricle. The thin walled right ventricle is more compliant than the left ventricle and compared with the left ventricle, it is better suited to handle the increase in the volume than the pressure.

17. Ans. a. Clockwise rotation

Hurst's 11th Ed; Chapter 64; Page 1617-1625

Electrocardiography is highly specific but rather insensitive for detecting right ventricular hypertrophy. Classic electrocardiographic criteria for cor pulmonale is mentioned as below:

ECG criteria for cor pulmonale without obstructive disease of the airways:

- Right-axis deviation with a mean QRS axis to the right of +110°
- R/S amplitude ratio in V1 > 1
- R/S amplitude ratio in V6 < 1
- Clockwise rotation of the electrical axis
- P-pulmonale pattern
- S1Q3 or S1 S2 S3 pattern
- Normal voltage QRS.

ECG changes in chronic cor pulmonale with obstructive disease of the airways:

- Isoelectric P waves in lead I or right axis deviation of the P vector.
- P-pulmonale pattern (an increase in P-wave amplitude in II, III, AVf).
- Tendency for right axis deviation of the QRS.
- R/S amplitude ratio in V6 < 1.
- Low voltage QRS.
- S1 Q3 or S1 S2 S3 pattern.

- Incomplete (and rarely complete) right bundle branch block.
- R/S amplitude ratio in V1 > 1.
- Marked clockwise rotation of the electrical axis.
- Occasional large Q wave or QS in the inferior or mid precordial leads, suggesting healed myocardial infarction.

These were derived from patients with congenital heart disease and have not been sensitive in patient with chronic obstructive pulmonary disease, apparently because moderate right ventricular hypertrophy is a late event in cor pulmonale occurring only after prolonged dilatation of the right ventricle. Right ventricular hypertrophy is suggested by clockwise rotation, right axis deviation, a qR pattern in lead aVR, an electrocardiographic evidence of right atrial enlargement (P-pulmonale) in that order. In patient with chronic obstructive pulmonary disease, the mean QRS axis is directed posteriorly, superiorly and to the right with an apparent left axis deviation in a standard limb leads. This pattern along with low voltage is associated most often with emphysema. Electrocardiography is less accurate for detecting right ventricular hypertrophy in patients with COPD than in patient with primary pulmonary arterial hypertension. This is because COPD causes flattening of the diaphragm and hyperinflation of the lung.

18. Ans. d. All of the above

Hurst's 11th Ed; Chapter 64; Page 1617-1625

Doppler echocardiography has improved the assessment of pulmonary artery pressure in patients with chronic obstructive lung disease or cor pulmonale. The mean right atrial pressure and the peak systolic pressure gradient between the right ventricle and right atrium must be measured and the result added so as to estimate peak systolic pulmonary artery pressure. The height of the jugular venous pulse is used to estimate the right atrial pressure. The tricuspid valve regurgitant jet can be assessed by Doppler echocardiography to measure the right ventricular—atrial gradient. Tricuspid regurgitation occurs in normal subjects and in patient with COPD. By augmenting the signals with an intravenous infusion of saline the quality of signal to detect tricuspid regurgitation using continuous wave Doppler can be improved. Although continuous wave Doppler echocardiography fails to produce an adequate assessment in 35% of patients, even with intravenous saline contrast, pulse wave Doppler is more sensitive for detecting tricuspid insufficiency. The difficulty in differentiating the right ventricular wall from its surrounding structures limit the use of echocardiography for detecting right ventricular hypertrophy. Echocardiographically measured right ventricular wall thickness has correlated poorly with right ventricular weight determined at autopsy. Unlike radionuclide ventriculography, echocardiographic can not readily show changes in right ventricular function in patients with COPD and pulmonary arterial hypertension.

19. Ans. c. MRI

Hurst's 8th Ed; Chapter 101; Page 1895-1903

MRI produces the best images of the right ventricle and is therefore considered to with the gold standards for measuring right ventricular dimension.

20. Ans. d. Polysomnography

Hurst's 8th Ed; Chapter 101; Page 1895-1903

Sleep apnea syndromes are classified into three general types:
- *Central apnea*: In which air flow is stopped in conjunction with cessation of all respiratory muscles effort;
- *Obstructive apnea*: In which upper airway obstruction causes cessation of air flow despite continuing effort of the respiratory muscles;
- *Mixed apnea*: In which air flow obstruction and respiratory effort both is stopped initially in the episode followed first by resumption of unsuccessful respiratory effort. Patient with sleep apnea rarely reach deep sleep and therefore are chronically sleep deprived. Common clinical manifestations are loud snoring, somnambulism, tremors, myoclonus, altered state of consciousness, nocturnal enuresis, morning headache, dump day time, hypersomnolence, hallucination and systemic hypertension. Patient with sleep apnea also often have severe bradyarrhythmia which occurs during apneic episodes and tachyarrhythmia which occurs when breathing resumes. The arrhythmias consist of sinus bradycardia, sinus arrest, long asystolic period, sinoatrial block, premature atrial contraction, atrial fibrillation, ventricular premature beats bigeminy, trigeminy, multifocal premature beats and ventricular tachycardia. Clinical effect of apnea differs with the type, frequency and intensity of abnormal respiratory pattern. The affected patients are usually not obese and breathe normally when awake. The diagnosis of sleep apnea is established by polysomnography. About 25% of patients with sleep apnea have COPD and most of these eventually develop pulmonary hypertension. Diagnosis of coexisting sleep apnea and COPD can be difficult and both disorders must be treated to control symptom. The management of obstructive sleep apnea varies. In patients with sleep apnea, sedative and antihistaminic should be avoided or withdrawn and oxygen therapy should be used cautiously. Narcoleptics and uncontrolled oxygen therapy have resulted in death in some patients. Central apnea is treated with respiratory stimulant or nocturnal ventilatory support with respirators. Phrenic nerve or diaphragmatic pacing has also been recommended. Obstructive apnea is most often treated with nasal continuous positive airway pressure (CPAP) and far less commonly by tracheostomy.

21. Ans. c. Oxygen therapy should be used liberally

Hurst's 8th Ed; Chapter 101; Page 1895-1903

Please refer to the answer of Q. No 20.

22. Ans. d. All of the above

Hurst's 8th Ed; Chapter 101; Page 1895-1903

The effect of digitalis on right ventricular function is complex. Digitalis increases the contractility of the right ventricular myocardium but also produces pulmonary vasoconstriction. Digitalis is known to reduce venous return and may adversely effect the cardiac output. Digitalis therapy should be used only in patient with acute cor pulmonale and coexistent left ventricular failure. In patients with obstructive lung disease, digitalis causes an increase incidence of adverse side effect (e.g., cardiac arrhythmias) due to the effect of hypoxia. Digoxin is not indicated in routine hemodynamic management of cor pulmonale but it has been found that intravenous digoxin improved diaphragm strength and blood flow in patients with chronic obstructive lung disease who had acute respiratory failure and therefore there is a role for digoxin in the management of acutely decompensated patients with COPD.

23. Ans. b. Increase in pulmonary artery pressure

Hurst's 8th Ed; Chapter 101; Page 1895-1903

Theophylline is widely used drug as for its bronchodilator activity. Theophylline appears to have beneficial cardiovascular effect in patients with chronic obstructive lung disease with and without cor pulmonale. Intravenous aminophylline acutely decreases pulmonary artery pressure and increases both right ventricular and left ventricular ejection fraction. The long-term consequences of oral theophylline therapy on right ventricular function in patients with COPD are also favorable. A combination of reduced after load (lower pulmonary and systemic vascular resistance) and enhance myocardial contractility probably accounts for improved biventricular function with theophylline therapy. Theophylline acts directly to lower vascular resistance.

24. Ans. d. All of the above

Hurst's 8th Ed; Chapter 101; Page 1895-1903

Please refer to the explanation of Q. No 23.

25. Ans. d. All are correct

Hurst's 8th Ed; Chapter 101; Page 1895-1903

The selective beta-adrenergic receptor agonist have salutary effect in cor pulmonale by causing pulmonary vasodilatation and they also have direct ionotropic action on myocardium. In short-term studies, these drugs have been shown to lower pulmonary vascular resistance, increase cardiac output and increase right and left ventricular ejection fraction in most patient with chronic obstructive lung disease and cor pulmonale. However, these benefits are not sustained during chronic administration especially if patient is also receiving concomitant supplemental oxygen therapy.

INFECTIVE ENDOCARDITIS

1. **Which of the following is the most common causative organism for endocarditis on native valves in nonintravenous drug abusers?**
   a. Streptococci
   b. Staphylococci
   c. Enterococci
   d. Fungi

2. **Which is *not* correct regarding viridans streptococci?**
   a. This is the normal inhabitant of the oropharynx
   b. These are the most common cause of endocarditis in nonintravenous drug abusers
   c. They are resistant to penicillin
   d. They cause infections primarily on abnormal heart valves

3. ***Streptococcus bovis* endocarditis occurs in patients of:**
   a. Old age
   b. Colonic polyps
   c. Colonic malignancies
   d. All

4. **Which is *not* correct regarding endocarditis due to *Streptococcus pneumoniae*?**
   a. It has predilection for tricuspid valve
   b. Alcoholism is a recognized risk factor
   c. The course is fulminant
   d. All of the above

5. **Which is *not* correct regarding right sided endocarditis in drug abusers:**
   a. *Staphylococcus aureus* is most common organism
   b. Majority have pneumonia of multiple septic emboli
   c. The murmur of tricuspid regurgitation is frequently present
   d. All are correct

6. **Which of the following hematological parameters is almost always altered in SaBe?**
   a. Total leukocyte count
   b. Total differential count
   c. Platelet count
   d. ESR

7. Which of the following hematological parameters is frequently normal in SaBe?
   a. Total leukocyte count
   b. Differential leukocyte count
   c. Platelet count
   d. Total RBC count

8. What is the sensitivity of 2D echocardiography in diagnosing the vegetation of SABE?
   a. >90%   b. 80%
   c. 60%   d. <50%

9. What is the minimum time required for vegetation to be seen by echocardiography?
   a. 6 weeks   b. 4 weeks
   c. 3 weeks   d. 2 weeks

10. Which of the following technique helps in evaluating the non tissue PVE?
    a. Serial phonocardiography
    b. Cine radiography
    c. Doppler echocardiography
    d. All the three in combination

11. Which of the following is *not* an absolute indication for surgery in SABE?
    a. Refractory heart failure
    b. Unstable prosthesis
    c. Myocardial abscess
    d. Multiple embolic episodes

12. Multiple septic emboli is a feature of endocarditis involving:
    a. Prosthetic valve   b. Tricuspid valve
    c. Chordae tendineae   d. Pulmonary valve

13. Which is the most common organism causing infective endocarditis in intravenous drug abuser:
    a. *Staphylococcus aureus*   b. Streptococci
    c. Enterococci   d. Fungi

14. Which of the most common organism involved in nosocomial infective endocarditis:
    a. *Staphylococcus aureus*   b. Enterococci
    c. Streptococci   d. Chlamydia

15. Which of the following is commonest organism involved in both early and late prosthetic valve endocarditis?
    a. Streptococci
    b. Pneumococci
    c. Fungi
    d. *Staphylococcus epidermidis*

16. The commonest organism causing infective endocarditis over an arteriosclerotic aneurysm is:
    a. *Staphylococcus aureus*
    b. Fungi
    c. Streptococci
    d. *Salmonella*

17. Which of the etiological agent is rarely recovered from blood during the course of endocarditis?
    a. Chlamydia   b. Mycoplasma
    c. Aspergillus d. Legionella

18. Which of the following is the cause of loss of vision during the course of endocarditis?
    a. Embolization to brain or retinal artery
    b. Optic neuritis
    c. Endophthalmitis
    d. Any of the above

19. Which is the most common site of embolization during SaBe?
    a. CNS   b. Lungs
    c. Coronary artery d. Spleen

20. The higher frequency of bacteremia is seen with all of the following procedure, *except*:
    a. Extraction of teeth
    b. Periodontal surgery
    c. Brushing teeth or irrigation
    d. Tonsillectomy

21. Which of the following gastrointestinal procedure is *not* associated with high rate of bacteremia?
    a. Upper GI endoscopy
    b. Sclerotherapy for varices
    c. Esophageal dilatation
    d. ERCP

22. Which is the most frequent major complication of infective endocarditis?
    a. Embolization   b. Heart failure
    c. Periannular abscess d. Mycotic aneurysm

23. Heart failure is most commonly associated with infective endocarditis of?
    a. Mitral valve   b. Aortic valve
    c. Pulmonary valve d. Tricuspid valve

24. Mycotic aneurysm in infective endocarditis occurs most commonly in:
    a. Anterior cerebral artery and its branches
    b. Posterior cerebral artery and its branches
    c. Middle cerebral artery and its branches
    d. Cortical branches

25. Which of the following has high positive predictive value for the presence of perivalvular abscess formation during course of IE?
   a. Persistent fever
   b. Persistent bacteremia despite antibiotic therapy
   c. Heart failure
   d. New conduction block

26. Which of the following statement is *true* regarding periannular extension of infection in IE?
   a. It is more often seen in aortic valve IE
   b. It is more common with prosthetic valve IE
   c. Development of new AV block in setting of aortic valve IE has a high positive predictive value for presence of perivalvular abscess formation
   d. All are true

27. Commonest organism implicated in causation of IE over tricuspid valve is:
   a. Streptococci
   b. *Staphylococcus aureus*
   c. Gram-negative bacilli
   d. Coagulase negative staphylococci

28. The common predisposing lesion for infective endocarditis in older men (>60 years) is:
   a. Patent ductus arteriosus
   b. Ventricular septal defect
   c. Bicuspid aortic valve
   d. Coronary artery bypass graft

29. Which of the following is a *correct* statement?
   a. The incidence of IE is less among patients with MVP with no murmur compared to those with mitral valve prolapsed and murmur
   b. Infection with human immune deficient virus (HIV) is not a significant risk factor for IE, unless associated with IV drug abuse
   c. In cases with IE affecting tricuspid valve in drug abusers, the murmur of tricuspid regurgitation is uncommon
   d. All are correct

30. The predominant organism implicated in early prosthetic valve endocarditis is:
   a. Staphylococcus epidermidis
   b. *Staphylococcus aureus*
   c. Gram-negative bacilli
   d. *Candida*

31. The mortality is highest with pVe due to:
   a. *Staphylococcus aureus*
   b. *Streptococcus viridans*
   c. *Staphylococcus epidermidis*
   d. *Candida*

32. *Staphylococcus aureus* endocarditis is associated with:
   a. Urinary catheter
   b. Central venous lines
   c. Tunnelled lines
   d. Hemodialysis catheter

33. *Streptococcus bovis* endocarditis is frequently associated with:
   a. Hemodialysis catheter
   b. Prosthetic valves
   c. Transvenous pacemakers
   d. Polyps or malignancy of colon

34. Nonbacterial thrombotic endocarditis (nBTe) is common in patients with:
   a. Malignancy
   b. Disseminated intravascular coagulation
   c. Valvular heart disease
   d. All of the above

35. The constitutional symptoms of infections of SaBe are mediated by:
   a. Fibronectin
   b. Tissue factor production
   c. Cytokines
   d. Antibody—complement interaction

36. Fever is absent or minimal in cases of SaBe in:
   a. Elderly age group
   b. CHF
   c. Chronic renal failure
   d. All

37. The classical peripheral manifestations of IE are virtually absent in IE involving:
   a. Mitral valve
   b. Pulmonary valve
   c. Aortic valve
   d. Tricuspid valve

38. Risk of embolization in cases of IE is more with:
   a. Vegetation ≥ 10 mm
   b. Mitral regurgitation
   c. *Staphylococcus aureus*
   d. All

39. Neurological symptoms and signs are more frequent when IE is caused by:
   a. *Streptococcus viridians*
   b. *Staphylococcus aureus*
   c. Fungi
   d. All of the above

40. The *correct* statement regarding treatment of *Staphylococcus aureus* and coagulase negative staphylococcal pVe is:
   a. It should be treated with three antibiotics in combination
   b. Rifampicin provides unique anti-staphylococcal activity when infection involves foreign bodies
   c. Rifampicin resistant staphylococci rapidly emerges when rifampicin is used alone
   d. All are correct

41. Periannular abscess due to IE, suspected but not detected by initial and repeated TEE may be detected by:
   a. CT scan
   b. Cardiac magnetic resonance
   c. Cardiac catheterization and angiography
   d. Nuclear scan

42. Prophylaxis against IE is *not* recommended for which of the following category of cardiac conditions?
   a. Prosthetic cardiac valves
   b. Previous infective endocarditis
   c. Unrepaired cyanotic congenital heart disease
   d. Mitral valve prolapse

43. Acute fulminating course with high grade bacteremia is seen in infective endocarditis due to which of the following organism:
   a. *E-faecalis*
   b. *Staphylococcus aureus*
   c. *Pseudomonas*
   d. *Streptococcus viridans*

44. All are true statement about risk of embolization in cases with infective endocarditis, *except*:
   a. It is higher for mitral than for aortic valve endocarditis
   b. Right sided vegetations that are >1 cm have higher embolic rates
   c. Static vegetations size on antimicrobial therapy seen on serial echocardiogram may be associated with higher embolic rates
   d. Risk is higher with *S. aureus* infection

45. Which is the most common causative organism in the cardiac device related infective endocarditis?
   a. *Streptococcus viridans*
   b. Fungi
   c. *Staphylococcus aureus*
   d. Enterococci

ANSWERS WITH EXPLANATIONS

1. Ans. b. Staphylococci

Hurst's 14th Ed; Page 1622 & 1625

Viridans group streptococci are alpha, hemolytic streptococci are frequent cause of community acquired native valve endocarditis. Viridans streptococci are responsible for 30-65% of cases of native valve endocarditis in older children and adults. They are normal resident of oropharynx and gain easy access to the circulation following dental or gingival trauma. The viridians streptococci are usually highly sensitive to penicillin and thus can often be eradicated with penicillin monotherapy. These organism cause infection in abnormal/disease valve.

Also refer to the answer of Q. No 5.

2. Ans. c. They are resistant to penicillin

Hurst's 14th Ed; Page 1622 & 1625

Please refer to the explanations of Q. No 1 and 5.

3. Ans. d. All

Hurst's 14th Ed; Page 1625

Streptococcus bovis, a normal inhabitant of human gastrointestinal tract is noteworthy as IE caused by this organism is strongly suggestive of gastrointestinal malignancy, colonic polyp formation or diverticular disease when meticulously investigated gastrointestinal pathologists discovered it in as many as 60% of patients with *Streptococcus bovis* IE.

4. Ans. d. All of the above

Hurst's 14th Ed; Page 1625

Streptococcus pneumoniae is responsible for infective endocarditis (IE) in about 10% of cases. *Streptococcus pneumoniae* bacteremia often begins with respiratory infection and nearly half of patients with pneumococcal IE suffer from chronic alcoholism as *S. pneumoniae* can infect normal valve tissue and usually results in acute fulminant illness often associated with severe valve damage, perivalvular extension, embolic complications, pericarditis, meningitis, high mortality (25-50%).

5. Ans. d. All are correct

Hurst's 14th Ed; Page 1622

IE is one of the most severe complication of injection (i.e., IE or subcutaneous) drug abuse. The incidence of IE among intravenous drug users is approximately 2-5% per year. The incidence of IE and causative agents in this population are mostly related to contaminated injection techniques (example sharing of hypodermic needles, the injection of unsterile particulate material, i.e., Talc) and the high prevalence of HIV infection. *Staphylococcus aureus* is the most common etiological agent and causes >60% of IE in intravenous drug abusers. The distinctive feature of IE in intravenous drug user is that it is a predominantly a disease of right heart with 60-70% of cases involving the tricuspid valve. The tricuspid valve may be particularly susceptible to bacterial infection because of chronic degenerative changes caused by the repetitive injection of irritant (e.g., Talc) into peripheral veins. Septic pulmonary emboli has common, clinical manifestation as pleuritic chest pain, shortness of breath, cough and hemoptysis. In 65-75% of patients, chest X-ray reveals abnormalities related to septic pulmonary emboli. Murmurs of tricuspid regurgitation are noted less than one half of these patients.

6. Ans. d. ESR

Braunwald 6th Ed; Page 1723

In patient with IE, anemia with normochromic, normocytic red blood cells indices, a low serum iron level and low serum iron binding capacity is found in 70-90% of patients. In subacute IE, the white blood cells count is usually normal. In contrast, a leukocytosis with increased segmented granulocytes is common in acute IE. Thrombocytopenia occurs only rarely. The ESR elevated in almost all patients with IE, except those with CHF, renal failure or disseminated intravascular coagulation.

7. Ans. c. Platelet count

Braunwald 6th Ed; Page 1723

Please refer to the explanation of Q. No 6.

8. Ans. c. 60%

Braunwald 5th Ed; Page 1088

The 2D echocardiography with color Doppler, especially a biplane or multiplaner, TEE helps in diagnosis and follow-up of the patient with IE. The sensitivity of TTE for the detection of vegetation in patients with native valve endocarditis is approximately 60-65% whereas that of TEE is about 85-95%. TEE is preferred approach in patient in whom TTE technically suboptimal and is the procedure of choice for imaging pulmonary valve and suspected prosthetic valve endocarditis. The vegetation can be seen by echocardiography as early as two weeks from the onset of symptoms.

9. Ans. d. 2 weeks

Braunwald 5th Ed; Page 1088

Please refer to the explanation of Q. No 8.

10. Ans. d. All the three in combination

Braunwald 5th Ed; Page 1088

Please refer to the explanation of Q. No 8.

11. Ans. c. Myocardial abscess

Braunwald 5th Ed; Page 1094

The indication for cardiac surgery in patients with IE.

Absolute indication:
- Moderate-to-severe CHF caused by valve dysfunction
- Unstable prosthesis, prosthesis orifice obstructed
- Uncontrolled infection despite optimal antimicrobial therapy
- *Unavailable effective antimicrobial therapy*: Endocarditis caused by *fungi, brucellae, Pseudomonas aeruginosa* (aortic or mitral valves)
- *Staphylococcus aureus* PVE with an intracardiac complication
- Relapse of PVE after optimal therapy
- Fistula to pericardial sac.

Relative indication:
- Perivalvular extension of infection, intracardiac fistula, myocardial abscess with persistent fever
- Poorly responsive *S. aureus* NVE (aortic or mitral valves)
- Relapse of NVE after optimal antimicrobial therapy
- Culture—negative NVE or PVE with persistent fever (≥10 d)
- Large (>10 mm diameter) hypermobile vegetation (with or without prior arterial embolus)
- Endocarditis caused by highly antibiotic—resistant enterococci.

12. Ans. b. Tricuspid valve

Braunwald 6th Ed; Page 1723

Please refer to the explanation of Q. No 6.

13. Ans. a. *Staphyococcus aureus*

Braunwald 6th Ed; Page 1723

Please refer to the explanation of Q. No 6.

14. Ans. a. *Staphyococcus aureus*

Braunwald 5th Ed; Page 1080

Healthcare associated endocarditis includes true nosocomial IE as well as IE arising in the community after a recent hospitalization or as a direct consequence of long-term indwelling devices such as central venous lines and hemodialysis catheters. Healthcare associated endocarditis may involve normal or abnormal native valves including the tricuspid, transvenous pacemakers, defibrillators and prosthetic valves. Hemodialysis is independently associated with *S. aureus* IE. Gram-positive cocci, i.e., *Staphylococcus aureus* are the predominant cause of nosocomial IE.

15. Ans. d. *Staphylococcus epidermidis*

Hurst's 14th Ed; Page 1626

Coagulase negative *Staphylococcus epidermidis* are a major cause of prosthetic valve endocarditis, particularly during the initial year after valve surgery, an important cause of nosocomial IE and the cause of 3-8% of nonvalvular endocarditis usually in the setting of prior valve abnormality.

16. Ans. d. *Salmonella*

Hurst's 14th Ed; Page 1626

IE caused by gram-negative bacilli is an uncommon and tend to occur in intravenous drug users, immunocompromised patients, patients with advanced liver disease and prosthetic heart valve recipients. *Salmonellae species* have a particular predilection for atherosclerotic plaque and may infect arterial aneurysm.

17. Ans. c. *Aspergillus*

Hurst's 14th Ed; Page 1626

Fungal endocarditis is a relatively new syndrome and is associated with an exceeding high mortality (survival rate <20%). *Candida* and *Aspergillus species* are the most common causes of fungal IE and are associated with large bulky vegetation that can obstruct native or prosthetic valve orifices and it can embolize to large vessel (e.g., the femoral artery). Blood cultures are usually positive in cases of candida IE where they are rarely positive with aspergillus. Fungal endocarditis is an indication for surgical replacement of an infected valve.

18. Ans. d. Any of the above

Hurst's 14th Ed; Page 1627

Conjunctival petechiae are small, bright-red hemorrhages that are easily seen with eyelid eversion. They are not specific for endocarditis, being found sometimes after cardiac surgery and with septicemia. Nevertheless, the discovery of conjunctival hemorrhages in a patient with unexplained fever and a heart murmur makes the diagnosis of IE highly likely. Retinal hemorrhages are found in 10–25% of both SBE and ABE. Their appearance is quite variable. Roth's spots appear to represent cytoid bodies and associated hemorrhage caused by microinfarction of retinal vessels. Roth's spots are not foci of infection and are nonspecific to IE. Loss of vision during IE may be caused by embolization to the brain or retinal artery or from optic neuritis or ophthalmitis. Endophthalmitis may occur in patients with candida IE and/or candidemia. The typical retinal lesions are rounded, white, cotton-like exudates.

Also refer to the explanation of Q. No 19.

19. Ans. a. CNS

Hurst's 14th Ed; Page 1634

Embolization is a dreaded complication of IE. Central nervous system involvement is most common. Stroke comprises up to 65% of embolic events and may be the presenting signs of IE in up to 14% of cases.

20. Ans. c. Brushing teeth or irrigation

Hurst's 14th Ed; Page 1644

The dental procedure like extraction, periodontal procedure, dental implants, root canal and initial placement of bands, intraligamentary local anesthesia are associated with and respiratory procedure like tonsillectomy, adenoidectomy are associated with high-risk of bacteremia and therefore prophylaxis is recommended.

21. Ans. a. Upper GI endoscopy

Hurst's 14th Ed; Page 1633

The gastrointestinal procedure associated with high rate of bacteremia are: (a) sclerotherapy for varices; (b) esophageal stricture dilatation; (c) biliary tract surgery or ERCP; (d) any surgery involving intestinal mucosa. However, endoscopy even with biopsy is associated with very low-risk of bacteremia and prophylaxis is not recommended.

22. Ans. b. Heart failure

Hurst's 14th Ed; Page 1633

Complication rates with IE have remained relatively unchanged despite advances in diagnosis and antimicrobial therapy. Usual complications are heart failure, embolization, mycotic aneurysm, periannular extension of infection and renal dysfunction. Heart failure is the most frequent major complications of IE. Its development potentiates adverse outcomes with medical therapy alone and is an indication for surgical intervention in most cases. Heart failure is most commonly associated with aortic valve IE (29%), followed by mitral valve (20%) and then tricuspid valve (8%) involvement.

23. Ans. b. Aortic valve

Hurst's 14th Ed; Page 1633

Please refer to the explanation of Q. No 22.

24. Ans. c. Middle cerebral artery and its branches

Hurst's 14th Ed; Page 1635

Mycotic aneurysm represents a small but extremely dangerous subset of embolic complications. They occur most frequently in the intracranial arteries and have a particular predilection for middle cerebral artery and its branches. They result from septic embolization to arterial vasa vasorum, with subsequent spread of infection and weakening of the vessel valve.

25. Ans. d. New conduction block

Hurst's 14th Ed; Page 1635

Extension or spread of infection beyond the valve annulus is a serious development during the course of IE and usually produces the need for surgical therapy. Persistent fever and bacteremia despite antibiotic therapy, heart failure or new conduction block should raise suspicion for this complication. Although relatively insensitive sign, the development of new AV block in the setting of aortic valve IE has a high positive predictive value for the presence of perivalvular abscess formation. Periannular extension may occur in 10-40% of all native valve IE and complicates aortic valve IE more commonly than either mitral or tricuspid valve IE. Periannular extension is more common with prosthetic valve IE (occurring in >50% of patients), as the prosthetic sewing ring is often the primary site of infection. Perivalvular extension set the stage for abscess formation, perforation, fistula development and hemodynamic deterioration.

26. Ans. d. All are true

Hurst's 14th Ed; Page 1635

Please refer to the explanation of Q. No 25.

27. Ans. b. *Staphylococcus aureus*

Hurst's 14th Ed; Page 1622

Please refer to the explanation of Q. No 5.

28. Ans. c. Bicuspid aortic valve

Braunwald 6th Ed; Page 1724

Congenital heart disease is the substrate for IE in 10-20% of young adults and 8% of older adults. Among adults, the common predisposing lesions are patent ductus arteriosus, ventricular septal defect and bicuspid aortic valve, the latter particularly found among older men above age of 60 years.

29. Ans. d. All are correct

Braunwald 5th Ed; Page 1078

Mitral valve prolapse is a predominant predisposing structural cardiac abnormality in adults accounting for 7-13% of native valve endocarditis not related to drug abuse or nosocomial infection. The increase risk of endocarditis is largely confined to patients with prolapse, thick valve leaflet (>5 mm) and mitral regurgitation murmur especially among men and patients older than 45 years. Among patients with MVP and systolic murmur, the incidence of IE is 52 per 100 thousand persons year compared with a rate of 4.6 per 100 thousand person year among those with prolapse and no murmur.

Infection with human immunodeficiency virus (HIV) unless associated with IV drug abuse is not a significant risk factors for IE.

Also refer to the explanation of Q. No 5.

30. Ans. a. *Stephylococcal epidermidis*

Braunwald 5th Ed; Page 1079

Epidemiological studies suggest that prosthetic valve endocarditis constitute 10-30% of all cases of IE in developed countries. The prosthetic valve endocarditis has been called early when symptoms begin within 60 days of valve surgery and late with onset thereafter. These terms were established to distinguish prosthetic valve endocarditis that occurs early as a complication of valve surgery from later infection that was likely to be community acquired. The microbiology of prosthetic valve endocarditis when considered by time of onset reflects in part the presumed nosocomial or community acquisition of infection. Coagulase negative staphylococci, primarily *Streptococcus epidermidis* are a prominent cause of early prosthetic valve endocarditis. *S. aureus*, gram negative bacilli, enterococci and fungi (particularly candida species) are also common causes prosthetic valve endocarditis during this period. The microbiology of late prosthetic valve endocarditis resembles that of community acquired native valve endocarditis. Streptococci, *S. aureus*, enterococci and coagulase-negative, staphylococci are the major causes.

31. Ans. a. *Staphylococcus aureus*

Braunwald 5th Ed; Page 1079-1080

Among patients with prosthetic valve endocarditis, the in hospital mortality ranges from 14-41% and that for early and late infection from 30-46% and 19-34%, respectively. Mortality for *S. aureus* PVE regardless of time of onset remains high, i.e., 36-47%.

32. Ans. d. Hemodialysis catheter

Braunwald 5th Ed; Page 1080

Healthcare associated endocarditis includes true nosocomial IE as well as IE arising in the community after a recent hospitalization or as a direct consequences of long-term indwelling devices, such as central venous lines, tunnelled lines, and hemodialysis catheters. Healthcare associated endocarditis, unrelated to concurrent cardiac surgery, makes up 5-29% of all cases of IE in various series and may involve normal or abnormal native valves, including the tricuspid, transvenous pacemakers and defibrillators, and prosthetic valves. Hemodialysis is independently associated with *S. aureus* IE.

33. Ans. d. Polyps or malignancy of colon

Braunwald 5th Ed; Page 1080

Streptococcus bovis, part of gastrointestinal tract normal flora cause 20-40% of episodes of streptococcal native valve endocarditis. *Streptococcus bovis* are highly penicillin susceptible in contrast to relative penicillin resistance of enterococci. *Streptococcus bovis* endocarditis is frequently associated with coexisting polyps or malignancy in the colon and therefore colonoscopy is warranted in these patients.

34. Ans. d. All of the above

Braunwald 5th Ed; Page 1082

The nonbacterial thrombotic endocarditis (NBTE) is a result of endothelial injury and hypercoagulable state. NBTE is more common with increasing age and in patients with malignancy, disseminated intravascular coagulation, uremia, burns, systemic lupus erythematosus, valvular disease and intracardiac catheters.

35. Ans. c. Cytokines

Braunwald 5th Ed; Page 1083

The constitutional symptoms of infections of SABE are mediated by cytokines.

36. Ans. d. All

Braunwald 5th Ed; Page 1084

Fever is almost universal symptoms in patients with IE. However, it may be absent or minimal in elderly persons or in those with CHF, severe debility or chronic renal failure and occasionally in patients with native valve endocarditis caused by coagulase negative staphylococci.

37. Ans. d. Tricuspid valve

Hurst's 14th Ed; Page 1627

The classic peripheral manifestations of IE are petechiae, splinter hemorrhage, Osler's nodes, Janeway lesions and Roth spots. These classic peripheral manifestation are encountered less frequently these days and are virtually absent in IE restricted to tricuspid valve.

38. Ans. d. All

Braunwald 5th Ed; Page 1085

Symptomatic systemic emboli are relatively common and frequently precede or coincide with diagnosis of IE. The incidence decreases promptly during administration of effective antibiotic therapy. Embolic events are infrequent after two weeks of therapy. The risk of emboli generally increases with large vegetation (>10 mm), mitral vegetation, *S. aureus*, IE and increasing vegetation size during therapy.

39. Ans. b. *Staphylococcus aureus*

Braunwald 5th Ed; Page 1085–1086

Neurological symptoms and signs are caused most commonly by embolic stroke and more frequent when infective endocarditis is caused by *Staphylococcus aureus* and are associated with increased mortality rate.

40. Ans. d. All are correct

Braunwald 6th Ed; Page 1738

S aureus and coagulase-negative staphylococcal PVE should be treated with three antibiotics in combination. Rifampicin provides unique antistaphylococcal activity when infection involves foreign bodies. However, Rifampicin-resistant staphylococci rapidly emerge when Rifampicin is used alone or in combination with only vancomycin or a beta-lactam antibiotic or staphylococcal PVE. Consequently, staphylococcal PVE is treated with two antimicrobials plus Rifampicin.

41. Ans. b. Cardiac magnetic resonance

Braunwald 5th Ed; Page 1088

TEE is superior to TTE for detecting invasive infection in patients with native and prosthetic valve endocarditis. Doppler and color flow imaging and contrast echocardiography defines fistulas. Abscess suspected but not detected by initial or repeated TEE may be detected by cardiac magnetic resonance including magnetic resonance angiography. Cardiac catheterization add little to these imaging studies and is not recommended unless coronary angiography is needed.

42. Ans. d. Mitral valve prolapse

Hurst's 14th Ed; Page 1636

The American Heart Association has issued new and dramatically restricted recommendation for hemoprophylaxis of IE. The prophylaxis should be restricted to those patients whose cardiac abnormalities places them at highest risk for morbid outcome from IE viz. (a) prosthetic cardiac valves; (b) previous IE; (c) congenital heart disease—unrepaired cyanotic congenital heart disease, including those with palliative shunts and conduits, completely repaired congenital heart disease with prosthetic material or device either by surgery or catheter intervention during the first 6 months after the procedure, repaired congenital heart disease with residual defects at the site or adjacent to the site of a prosthetic patch or prosthetic device (which inhibit endothelialization) and cardiac transplantation recipients who develop cardiac valvulopathy.

Prophylaxis is no longer recommended for patients with mitral valve prolapsed or for cardiac conditions other than those noted.

43. Ans. b. *Staphylococcus aureus*

Hurst's 14th Ed; Page 1626

S. aureus is respected as a highly virulent organism and has the capacity to infect and destroy normal endocardial surfaces. *S. aureus* IE is frequently fulminant when it involves left-sided cardiac valves and often results in major complications such as heart failure, perivalvular extension with conduction disturbances, embolization and metastatic infection. *S. aureus* as a causative organism is an independent predictor of poor prognosis in IE and is associated with a 25–30% mortality.

44. Ans. b. Right sided vegetations that are >1 cm have higher embolic rates

Hurst's 14th Ed; Page 1635

In varies series, systemic embolization occurred in 22–50% of IE cases. However, the prediction of individual patient risk for embolization has proven difficult. Embolization risk appears to decrease precipitously following 2 weeks of appropriate antibiotic therapy from 13 to < 1.2

embolic events per 1000 patient—days. In many series, the risk of embolization appeared to be higher for mitral than for aortic valve endocarditis (approximately 25% vs 10% respectively), particularly with anterior leaflet involvement. A number of echocardiographic studies demonstrated a trend toward higher embolic rates with left sided vegetations that are >1 cm in diameter and more recent work suggests that vegetation size >1.5 cm is a predictor of IE related mortality. Increasing or static vegetation size with antimicrobial therapy seen on serial TEE is associated with higher embolic rates. One interesting report suggested an interaction between vegetation size and the presence of patient-specific antiphospholipid antibodies. The risk of embolization may also derive from microbial-specific features and is consistently higher with *S. aureus, S. lugdunensis*, certain streptococcal strains, *Haemophilus influenzae*, and fungi.

45. Ans. c. ***Staphylococcus aureus***

Hurst's 14th Ed; Page 1644

The rate of pacemaker and intracardiac cardioverter-defibrillator placement has dramatically increased in the past 10 years. Staphylococcal species are the causative organisms in >70% of device infections. The large majority of cardiac device infections are likely caused by pocket site contamination at the time of device placement. Hematogenous seeding from a distant focus of infection, particularly one caused by *S. aureus* can cause late-onset infection.

PULMONARY EMBOLISM

1. Which is *not* a component of Virchow triad?
   a. Inflammation
   b. Stasis
   c. Vessel wall injury
   d. Hypercoagulability

2. Which of the following is a risk factor for VTE during automobile or airplane trip?
   a. Use of oral contraceptive
   b. Flight distance of >5000 km
   c. Flight duration longer than 8 hours
   d. All of the above

3. During the episode of acute pulmonary embolism, what is the degree of pulmonary artery obstruction to give rise to acute hemodynamic compromise and right heart failure?
   a. 25%
   b. 30–40%
   c. 40–50%
   d. 50–60%

4. Which of the following symptoms is suggestive of massive life-threatening pulmonary embolism?
   a. Dyspnea
   b. Chest pain
   c. Hemoptysis
   d. Syncope

5. D-Dimer level may be elevated in all, *except*:
   a. Cancer
   b. Pulmonary embolism
   c. Second and third time of trimester of pregnancy
   d. All of the above

6. All the following are ECG findings in acute pulmonary embolism, *except*:
   a. T wave changes and ST segment abnormality
   b. Incomplete or complete RBBB
   c. Clockwise rotation of QRS vector
   d. Anti-clockwise rotation of QRS vector

7. Most frequent ECG sign of massive pulmonary embolism is:
   a. Sinus tachycardia
   b. Right bundle branch block
   c. T wave inversion in V2 or V3
   d. Clockwise rotation of QRS vector

8. Which of the following ECG finding is predictor of RV dysfunction and adverse clinical outcomes in acute pulmonary embolism?
   a. T wave inversion in V2
   b. Pseudo infarction pattern (Qr in V1)
   c. Right bundle branch block
   d. a + b

9. Which of the following is *not* a part of Wells score for clinical prediction of pulmonary embolism?
   a. Surgery or immobilization within past 4 weeks
   b. Active cancer
   c. Unilateral lower limb pain
   d. Previous pulmonary embolism or DVT

10. Which of the following is *not* the part of Wells score for clinical prediction of pulmonary embolism?
   a. Hemoptysis
   b. Heart rate >100/min
   c. Active cancer
   d. Pain on lower limb deep venous palpation

11. In patients with acute pulmonary embolism, severe hypokinesis of the RV free wall combined with preserved systolic contraction of RV apex is known as:
   a. Hampton hump
   b. Westermark sign
   c. Moe's sign
   d. McConnell's sign

12. A disturbed RV ejection pattern (60/60 sign) consisting of an RV acceleration time <60 milliseconds in the presence of a tricuspid insufficiency pressure gradient <60 mm Hg suggest:
   a. Low pressure tricuspid regurgitation
   b. Acute pulmonary embolism
   c. Ebstein anomaly
   d. Right sided cardiomyopathy

13. Which of the following is the gold standard test for diagnosing deep vein thrombosis?
   a. Compression ultrasonography
   b. Magnetic resonance imaging
   c. CT venography
   d. Contrast venography

14. Which of the following is a "high weight" parameters in clinical prediction rules for 30 days mortality (pulmonary embolism severity index)?
   a. Pulse rate > 110/min
   b. Systolic blood pressure < 100 mm Hg
   c. Respiratory rate > 30/min
   d. Arterial oxygen saturation < 90%

15. Which of the following clinical finding has been assigned highest point in clinical prediction for 30 days mortality (pulmonary embolism severity index)?
   a. Pulse rate > 110/min
   b. Systolic blood pressure <100 mm Hg
   c. Respiratory rate > 30/min
   d. Altered mental status

16. Which of the following is *not* the part of simplified Pulmonary Embolism in Severity Index (sPESI)?
   a. Pulse > 110/min
   b. Systolic pressure < 90 mm Hg
   c. Arterial oxygen saturation < 90%
   d. Respiratory rate > 30/min

17. All the following comorbidity illness increases the 30-day mortality in patients with pulmonary embolism, *except*:
   a. Cancer
   b. Chronic heart failure
   c. Chronic lung disease
   d. Chronic renal failure

18. Which of the following combination of vasopressor is helpful in supporting hemodynamic in patients with hypotensive pulmonary embolism?
   a. Dopamine + Dobutamine
   b. Dopamine + Norepinephrine
   c. Dobutamine + Epinephrine
   d. Dobutamine + Norepinephrine

19. Which of the following is *incorrect* regarding heparin induced thrombocytopenia?
   a. HIT typically develop 48 hours after initiation of heparin therapy
   b. Risk of HIT is lower with LMWH
   c. Fondaparinux does not cause HIT
   d. All of the above

20. In management of venous thromboembolism, VKA (vitamin K-antagonist) therapy should be initiated with concomitant UFH or LMWH because:
   a. Combination of these two improves anticoagulation
   b. VKA administration may lead to prothrombotic state
   c. Heparin alone administration can lead to prothrombotic state
   d. All of the above

21. "Purple toes syndrome" is a complication associated with which of the following drug?
   a. NOAC
   b. Vitamin K antagonists (VKA)
   c. Thrombolytic therapy
   d. Antiplatelet drugs

22. Which level of INR has the highest benefit-to-risk ratio with the VKA therapy for venous thromboembolism?
   a. INR 1.5 to 2.0
   b. INR 2.2 to 2.3
   c. INR 2.5 to 3.0
   d. INR 3.0 to 3.5

23. Initial parenteral anticoagulation is not needed with which of the following NOACs in treatment of venous thromboembolism?
   a. Rivaroxaban and Apixaban
   b. Dabigatran and Edoxaban
   c. Rivaroxaban and Dabigatran
   d. Apixaban and Edoxaban

24. Which of the following is *not* an indication for use of vena cava filters in treatment of pulmonary embolism?
   a. Contraindication to anticoagulation
   b. Recurrent embolism while on adequate therapy
   c. Bleeding complication during anticoagulation in acute phase
   d. All patients with submassive pulmonary embolism

25. Which of the following drug do *not* offers significant benefit in prophylaxis against venous thromboembolism (VTE)?
   a. Unfractionated heparin
   b. LMWA
   c. New oral anticoagulants (NOAC)
   d. Antiplatelet drug

26. Which of the following is the safest drug to be used as an anticoagulant in patients with pulmonary embolism in pregnancy?
   a. Unfractionated heparin
   b. Fondaparinux
   c. Vitamin K antagonist
   d. NOAC's

ANSWERS WITH EXPLANATIONS

1. Ans. a. Inflammation

Hurst's 14th Ed; Page 1809

Virchow triad is for intravascular coagulation, it includes triad of stasis, vessel wall injury, and hypercoagulability. Risk factors for venous thromboembolism (VTE) are based on these processes.

2. Ans. d. All of the above

Hurst's 14th Ed; Page 1810

Long automobile or airplane trips appear to be risk factors for VTE. The proportion of subjects who develop acute pulmonary embolism (PE) during or after airplane travel appears to be associated with other thrombotic risk factors, such as the presence of the factor V Leiden mutation or the use of oral contraceptive agents and correlates with the flight distance. The risk of PE significantly increases with a flight distance of >3107 miles (5000 km) or a duration longer than 8 hours.

3. Ans. d. 50–60%

Hurst's 14th Ed; Page 1812

The hemodynamic effects of embolism is related to three factors, i.e., the degree of reduction of the cross-sectional area of pulmonary vascular bed, the pre-existing status of the cardiopulmonary system, and the physiological consequences of both hypoxic and neuro-humorally mediated vasoconstriction. Obstruction of the pulmonary vascular bed by embolism acutely increases the workload on the right ventricle. In patients without pre-existing cardiopulmonary disease, obstruction of <20% of the pulmonary vascular bed results in a number of compensatory events that minimizes adverse hemodynamic consequences. Recruitment and distension of pulmonary vessels occur, resulting in a normal or near normal pulmonary artery pressure and pulmonary vascular resistance. Cardiac output is maintained by increases in the RV stroke volume and increases in the heart rate. As the degree of pulmonary vascular obstruction exceeds 30 to 40%, increases in pulmonary artery pressure and modest increases in right atrial pressure occur. The Frank-Starling mechanism maintains right ventricular stroke work and cardiac output. When the degree of pulmonary artery obstruction exceeds 50 to 60%, compensatory mechanisms are overcome, cardiac output begins to decrease, and right atrial pressure increases dramatically. With acute obstruction beyond this point, the right heart dilates, RV wall tension increases, RV ischemia may develop, the cardiac output decreases, and systemic hypotension develops.

4. Ans. d. Syncope

Hurst's 14th Ed; Page 1812

Pulmonary embolism must always be considered when unexplained dyspnea is present. Pleuritic chest pain and hemoptysis are common in patients with pulmonary embolism. Cough may be present. Anxiety and light headedness are symptoms that may be caused by pulmonary embolism. Severe dyspnea and syncope are the principal symptoms that may suggest massive, life-threatening pulmonary embolism.

5. Ans. d. All of the above

Hurst's 14th Ed; Page 1812

The plasma d-dimer is a specific derivative of cross-linked fibrin. Increased levels of cross-linked fibrin degradation products are an indirect but suggestive marker of intravascular thrombosis, indicating endogenous fibrinolysis. An increased d-dimer level is nonspecific for pulmonary embolism and may be seen with advancing age and in patients with various conditions, including infections and other inflammatory states, cancer, myocardial infarction, the postoperative state, and the second and third trimesters of pregnancy. The specificity of d-dimer in suspected pulmonary embolism decreases with the age.

6. Ans. d. Anti-clockwise rotation of QRS vector

Hurst's 14th Ed; Page 1813

Electrocardiography (ECG) findings in acute pulmonary embolism are generally nonspecific and include T-wave changes, ST-segment abnormalities, incomplete or complete right bundle branch block, right-axis deviation in the extremity leads, and clockwise rotation of the QRS vector in the precordial leads. These changes are due to right-heart dilation. In milder cases, only anomaly may be sinus tachycardia, present in approximately 40% of patients. Atrial arrhythmias, particularly atrial fibrillation, may be associated with pulmonary embolism. Approximately 20% of patients with pulmonary embolism have no ECG changes. The "classic" S1Q3T3 pattern is present only in 10% of pulmonary embolism cases. Patients with massive pulmonary embolism, ECG changes of acute cor pulmonale such as the S1Q3T3 pattern, right bundle branch block, a P-wave pulmonale, or right-axis deviation may be found.

ECG may be helpful in predicting adverse clinical outcomes in patients with pulmonary embolism. It has been found that a T-wave inversion in V2 or V3 is the most frequent ECG sign of massive pulmonary embolism. In one of the pulmonary embolism studies, both the pseudo-infarction pattern (Qr in V1) and T-wave inversion in V2 were closely related to the presence of RV dysfunction and were found to be independent predictors of adverse clinical outcome.

7. Ans. c. T wave inversion in V2 or V3

Hurst's 14th Ed; Page 1813

Please refer to the answer of Q. No 6.

8. Ans. d. a + b

Hurst's 14th Ed; Page 1813

Please refer to the answer of Q. No 6.

9. Ans. c. Unilateral lower limb pain

Hurst's 14th Ed; Page 1813

Clinical prediction rules for pulmonary embolism (Well's score)

Items	Points assigned	
	Original version	Simplified version
Wells score		
Previous PE or DVT	1.5	1
Heart rate ≥ 100 bpm	1.5	1
Surgery or immobilization within the past 4 weeks	1.5	1
Hemoptysis	1	1
Active cancer	1	1
Clinical signs of DVT	3	1
Alternative diagnosis less likely than PE	3	1
Clinical probability		
Three-level score		
Low	0–1	N/A
Intermediate	2–6	N/A
High	≥7	N/A
Two-level score		
PE unlikely	0–4	0–1
PE likely	≥5	≥2
Revised Geneva score	**Original version**	**Simplified version**
Previous PE or DVT	3	1
Heart rate ≥ 100 bpm:		
• 75–94 bpm	3	1
• ≥95 bpm	5	2
Surgery or fracture within the past month	2	1
Hemoptysis	2	1
Active cancer	2	1
Unilateral lower limb pain	3	1

Continued

Continued

Items	Points assigned	
	Original version	Simplified version
Pain on lower limb deep venous palpation and unilateral edema	4	1
Age ≥ 65 years	1	1
Clinical probability		
Three-level score		
Low	0–3	0–1
Intermediate	4–10	2–4
High	≥11	≥5
Two-level score		
PE unlikely	0–5	0–2
PE likely	≥6	≥3

10. Ans. d. Pain on lower limb deep venous palpation

Hurst's 14th Ed; Page 1813

Please refer to the answer of Q. No 9.

11. Ans. d. McConnell's sign

Hurst's 14th Ed; Page 1816

The imaging plays an important role in diagnosis of pulmonary embolism. Common mode of imaging applied for diagnosis of pulmonary embolism includes chest radiography, CT of chest, pulmonary angiography, VQ scan, compression ultrasonography of the limbs and echocardiography. Chest radiography is abnormal in majority of patients with pulmonary embolism, but findings are nonspecific and subtle. Classic radiographic evidence of pulmonary infarction (Hampton hump) or decreased vascularity (Westermark sign) is suggestive but uncommon. A normal chest radiograph in the presence of significant dyspnea and hypoxemia without evidence of bronchospasm or anatomic cardiac shunt is strongly suggestive of pulmonary embolism. The echocardiography is a simple portable and readily available tool for risk assessment and treatment guidance in patient with acute pulmonary embolism. Acute pulmonary embolism may lead to right ventricular pressure overload and dysfunction which can be detected by echocardiography. Because the negative predictive value of echocardiography is 40–50%, a normal result can not exclude pulmonary embolism.

Patient with severe RV dysfunction due to pulmonary embolism may demonstrate McConnell's sign which is severe hypokinesia of RV free wall combined with preserved systolic contraction of RV apex. A disturbed RV ejection pattern ("60/60" sign) consists of an RV acceleration time <60 milliseconds in the presence of a tricuspid insufficiency pressure gradient <60 mm Hg may suggest pulmonary embolism but is not highly sensitive or specific. When combined these two signs were 94% specific and 36% sensitive in diagnosing acute pulmonary embolism even in the presence of pre-existing cardiopulmonary disease. Approximately 40% of normotensive patients with symptomatic pulmonary embolism have echocardiographic evidence of RV dysfunction.

In the majority of cases, pulmonary embolism originates from lower extremity DVT. Compression ultrasonography (Duplex ultrasonography) is the most commonly used technique to diagnose deep vein thrombosis.

Magnetic resonance imaging appears to be very accurate, but it is not a first-line test because of cost and inconvenience. CT venography used alone or in conjunction with CT angiography appears to have a sensitivity and specificity equivalent to that of duplex ultrasonography but exposes the patient to additional radiation. Contrast venography remains the gold standard but is rarely used.

12. Ans. b. Acute pulmonary embolism

Hurst's 14th Ed; Page 1816

Please refer to the answer of Q. No 11.

13. Ans. d. Contrast venography

Hurst's 14th Ed; Page 1816

Please refer to the answer of Q. No 11.

14. Ans. b. Systolic blood pressure < 100 mm Hg

Hurst's 14th Ed; Page 1819

Clinical prediction rule for 30-day mortality (Pulmonary embolism severity index)

Predictor	Points assigned
Demographic characteristics	
Age	Age, in years
Male gender	+10
Comorbid illness	
Cancer	+30
Chronic heart failure	+10
Chronic lung disease	+10
Clinical findings	
Pulse rate ≥ 110/min	+20
Systolic blood pressure < 100 mm Hg	+30
Respiratory rate ≥ 30/min	+20
Temperature < 36°C	+20
Altered mental status	+60
Arterial oxygen saturation < 90%	+20

15. Ans. d. Altered mental status

Hurst's 14th Ed; Page 1819

Please refer to the answer of Q. No 14.

16. Ans. d. Respiratory rate > 30/min

Hurst's 14th Ed; Page 1819

Clinical prediction rule for 30-day mortality (Simplified pulmonary embolism severity index)

Predictor	Points assigned
Demographic characteristics	
Age	+1 (if age > 80 y)
Comorbid illness	
Cancer	+1
Chronic heart failure or lung disease	+1
Clinical finding	
Pulse ≥ 110/min	+1
Systolic blood pressure < 100 mm Hg	+1
Arterial oxygen saturation < 90%	+1

17. Ans. d. Chronic renal failure

Hurst's 14th Ed; Page 1819

Please refer to the answer of Q. No 14.

18. Ans. d. Dobutamine + Norepinephrine

Hurst's 14th Ed; Page 1821

When massive pulmonary embolism associated with hypotension or severe hypoxemia is suspected, supportive treatment should be immediately initiated. Intravenous (IV) saline can be infused rapidly, but caution is recommended as excessive fluid may result in further RV dilatation, increased RV wall tension, and a decreased cardiac output that may result in right ventricular ischemia. Death from massive pulmonary embolism results from right ventricular failure, and dobutamine is known to augment right ventricular output. A vasopressor, such as norepinephrine, combined with dobutamine might offer optimal results. However, there is a lack of large randomized data evaluating the use of various vasopressors in the setting of massive pulmonary embolism.

19. Ans. a. HIT typically develop 48 hours after initiation of heparin therapy

Hurst's 14th Ed; Page 1822

HIT typically develops 5 or more days after the initiation of heparin therapy and occurs in 5 to 10% of patients. If a patient is placed on heparin and the platelet count progressively decreases either by 50% or to 100,000/μL or less, heparin therapy should be discontinued. Although the risk of HIT appears to be lower with LMWH, clinician should be aware that HIT can occur with the use of either form of heparin. In contrast to heparin compounds, fondaparinux does not cause heparin-induced thrombocytopenia (HIT).

20. Ans. b. VKA administration may lead to prothrombotic state

Hurst's 14th Ed; Page 1822

VKA therapy should be initiated with concomitant UFH or LMWH. The first few days of VKA administration may lead to prothrombotic state because of rapid depletion of anticoagulants protein C and S. The procoagulant effect of VKA can be prevented by overlapping heparin with warfarin for at least 5 days.

21. Ans. b. Vitamin K antagonists (VKA)

Hurst's 14th Ed; Page 1823

VKAs have a narrow therapeutic window, and risk of bleeding increases with increasing INR. The optimal INR value of 2.2 to 2.3 has the highest benefit-to-risk ratio. VKA related bleeding is seen in patients with hepatic disease, renal dysfunction, alcoholism, drug interactions, trauma, cancer, and a history of gastrointestinal bleeding. The risk of bleeding is greatest in the first month after initiation of anticoagulation. Rare complication of VKA are skin necrosis and cholesterol microembolization causing "purple toes" syndrome by enhancing crystal release from ulcerated plaques.

22. Ans. b. INR 2.2 to 2.3

Hurst's 14th Ed; Page 1823

Please refer to the answer of Q. No 21.

23. Ans. a. Rivaroxaban and Apixaban

Hurst's 14th Ed; Page 1823

The newer generation of oral anticoagulants called as novel oral anticoagulants, or NOACs have been found to be noninferior in terms of efficacy and possibly safer in terms of major bleeding than the standard parenteral/VKA regimen. It is an alternative to standard treatment. Four NOACs have been approved for the treatment of VTE: rivaroxaban, dabigatran, apixaban, and edoxaban. Rivaroxaban and apixaban allow for single-drug therapy, eliminating the need for initial parenteral anticoagulation, whereas dabigatran and edoxaban are initiated after a short course of parenteral anticoagulation regimen.

24. Ans. d. All patients with submassive pulmonary embolism

Hurst's 14th Ed; Page 1825

Routine use of vena cava filters in patients with pulmonary embolism is not recommended. The indications for filter placement include contraindications to anticoagulation, recurrent embolism while on adequate therapy, and significant bleeding complications during anticoagulation in the acute phase.

25. Ans. d. Antiplatelet drug

Hurst's 14th Ed; Page 1827

Prophylaxis for venous thromboembolism can be pharmacologic or nonpharmacologic. Pharmacologic prophylaxis options include low-dose UFH, LMWH, fondaparinux, warfarin, and new oral anticoagulants. LMWHs are used in clinical practice for both the prevention and treatment of established VTE. The LMWH preparations are advantageous because the dose-response relationship is more predictable and can be administered subcutaneously once or twice daily (without monitoring). Aspirin has a slight benefit but not enough to be used alone as a standard therapy to prevent VTE.

26. Ans. a. Unfractionated heparin

Hurst's 14th Ed; Page 1829

The treatment of pulmonary embolism in pregnancy is based on heparin anticoagulation, because heparin does not cross the placenta and is not found in breast milk in significant amounts. Weight-adjusted LMWH is the preferred treatment because of its safety profile. Fondaparinux should not be used in pregnancy because of lack of data. Vitamin K antagonist should not be administered throughout pregnancy, especially during the first and third trimesters. NOACs are not approved for used during pregnancy. Thrombolytic treatment during pregnancy and peripartum period should be used only in life threatening situation.

CHAPTER 20: Cardiac Arrhythmia, Pacing and Electrophysiology

CARDIAC ARRHYTHMIA

1. Palpitation or awareness of the heartbeat is caused by which of the following mechanisms?
   a. Rapid heart rate
   b. Irregularity in heart rhythm
   c. Increase in force of cardiac contraction
   d. Any of the above

2. An episode of tachycardia terminated by Valsalva maneuver or carotid sinus massage suggests presumptive diagnosis of:
   a. Sinus node re-entry
   b. Atrioventricular re-entrant tachycardia
   c. Atrioventricular nodal re-entrant tachycardia
   d. Any of the above

3. Which of the following feature distinguishes syncope of neurological origin from cardiac cause?
   a. There is no postictal confusional state
   b. Tongue biting or incontinence is uncommon
   c. Early seizure activity
   d. All of the above

4. Which of the following is responsible for "autopsy negative" sudden cardiac death?
   a. Long QT syndrome
   b. Brugada syndrome
   c. Catecholaminergic polymorphic ventricular tachycardia (CPVT)
   d. All of the above

5. Sudden cardiac death more likely to occur at rest or with sleep is seen in:
   a. Arrhythmogenic right ventricular dysplasia
   b. Long QT syndrome (type I and II)
   c. Structural heart diseases
   d. Brugada syndrome

6. Sudden cardiac death occurring at rest or with sleep is seen in:
   a. Brugada syndrome
   b. Long QT S3 (LQTS3) variety
   c. Both of the above
   d. None of the above

7. Intermittent canon 'a' wave, variable intensity of first heart sound and variable peak systolic blood pressure suggests diagnosis of:
   a. AV nodal re-entrant tachycardia
   b. Atrioventricular re-entrant tachycardia
   c. Junctional tachycardia
   d. Ventricular tachycardia

8. Transient termination of tachycardia on carotid sinus massage which restarts when carotid sinus massage ceases suggest diagnosis of:
   a. AV nodal re-entrant tachycardia
   b. Atrioventricular re-entrant tachycardia
   c. Permanent form of AV junctional reciprocating tachycardia
   d. Ventricular tachycardia

9. Which of the following tachycardia *cannot* be terminated with carotid sinus massage:
   a. AVRT
   b. AVNRT
   c. Adenosine sensitive atrial tachycardia
   d. Junctional tachycardia

10. Which of the following is investigation of choice for evaluation of suspected serious arrhythmia that occurs infrequently and cannot be provoked at diagnostic electrophysiologic study?
   a. Holter monitoring
   b. Event recording
   c. Implantable loop recorders
   d. Head up tilt table testing

11. Which of the following statement is *not* correct?
   a. Individual without heart disease may have ventricular ectopic associated with exercise
   b. Multiform PVCs or complex ventricular arrhythmias are uncommon response to exercise in healthy individuals
   c. PVCs at rest suppressed by exercise rules out coronary artery disease
   d. All are correct

12. Premature ventricular complex with variable coupling can be caused by:
   a. Parasystole
   b. Changing conduction in a re-entrant circuit
   c. Changing discharge rates of triggered activity
   d. All of the above

13. Which of the following morphological features of premature ventricular complexes are predictor of developing cardiomyopathy?
   a. Frequent PVCs greater than 24% of all beats during 24 hours Holter monitoring
   b. Very wide QRS PVCs
   c. PVCs of epicardial origin
   d. All of the above

14. Ventricular tachycardia originating from which of the following location exhibit narrower QRS complex?
   a. Left ventricular free wall
   b. Right ventricle free wall
   c. Apical origin VT
   d. Septal origin VT

15. Negative precordial lead concordance is feature of ventricular tachycardia arising from which location?
   a. Free wall of left ventricle
   b. Free wall of right ventricle
   c. Apical origin VT
   d. Septal origin VT

16. Ventricular tachycardia with positive precordial lead concordance indicates site of origin of ventricular tachycardia in:
   a. Left ventricular free wall
   b. Right ventricular free wall
   c. Basal portion of ventricle
   d. Apical portion of ventricle

17. Ventricular tachycardia in which predominately positive QRS complexes are seen in inferior leads (II, III, aVF), suggests site of origin of VT is in:
   a. Posterior left ventricle
   b. Posterior right ventricle
   c. Left ventricular free wall
   d. Outflow tract ventricular tachycardia

18. If there are predominantly negative QRS complexes in leads II, III and aVF during VT, it indicates the site of origin is in:
   a. Apex of left ventricle
   b. Outflow tract VT
   c. Left ventricular free wall VT
   d. Posterior/inferior portion of ventricle

19. In survivor of sudden cardiac death due to hemodynamically compromising ventricular tachycardias with poor LV function, what is the treatment of choice?
   a. Class I antiarrhythmic drug
   b. Amiodarone
   c. Sotalol
   d. ICD

20. In hypertrophic cardiomyopathy, patient with high risk features for sudden cardiac death and with non-sustained VT, the treatment of choice is:
   a. Class I antiarrhythmic drugs
   b. Beta blockers
   c. Amiodarone
   d. ICD

21. An ECG during sinus rhythm exhibiting complete or incomplete RBBB along with presence of Epsilon wave and episode of VT of LBBB contour suggest diagnosis of:
   a. Brugada syndrome
   b. Arrhythmogenic right ventricular cardiomyopathy
   c. Catecholaminergic polymorphic ventricular tachycardia (CPVT)
   d. Brugada syndrome

22. In a patient exercise induced ventricular extrasystoles culminating into monomorphic or bidirectional ventricular tachycardia with a family history of sudden death, the possible diagnosis is:
   a. Hypertrophic cardiomyopathy
   b. Arrhythmogenic right ventricular cardiomyopathy
   c. Brugada syndrome
   d. Catecholaminergic polymorphic ventricular tachycardia (CPVT)

23. What is treatment of choice in a patient with catecholaminergic polymorphic ventricular tachycardia (CPVT):
   a. Class I antiarrhythmic drugs
   b. Class IC antiarrhythmic drugs
   c. Beta blockers and ICD
   d. ICD only

24. Which of the following is the cause of Torsades de pointes (TdP)?
   a. Severe bradycardia
   b. Potassium depletion
   c. Use of QT prolonging medication
   d. All of the above

25. Which of the following is treatment of choice in Torsades de pointes?
a. Class IA antiarrhythmic drugs
b. Class IC antiarrhythmic drugs
c. Class III antiarrhythmic drugs
d. IV magnesium

26. Which of the following should *not* be used in treatment of Torsades de pointes (TdP)?
a. IV magnesium
b. IV isoproterenol
c. Temporary ventricular or atrial pacing
d. IV amiodarone

27. What is the treatment of choice in patient with Torsades de pointes resulting from long QT syndrome?
a. Beta blockers
b. Amiodarone
c. Calcium channel blockers
d. Beta blockades + ICDs

28. What is treatment of choice in patient with long QT syndrome with syncope and aborted sudden death?
a. Beta blockers
b. Permanent pacemaker implantation
c. ICD
d. Beta blocker + ICD

29. Which of the following causes short QT interval?
a. Hyperkalemia
b. Hypercalcemia
c. Hyperthermia
d. All

30. What is treatment of choice in patient with symptomatic short QT syndrome (SQTS)?
a. Flecainide
b. Beta blockers
c. Quinidine
d. Quinidine + ICD

31. "J" wave syndrome includes which of the following?
a. Brugada syndrome
b. Early repolarization syndrome
c. Catecholaminergic polymorphic ventricular tachycardia (CPVT)
d. Both a and b

32. "J" waves or Osborn wave in early repolarization syndrome is seen best in which leads?
a. Lead V_1-V_3
b. Lead II, III, aVF
c. Lead V_4-V_6
d. Lead I, II, III, aVF, aVL and V_4-V_6

33. ST elevation mimicking Brugada type I pattern is seen in:
a. Right bundle branch block
b. Occlusion left anterior descending artery or conus branch
c. ARVC
d. All of the above

34. Which is drug of choice for patient with Brugada syndrome who have frequent or storms of ventricular tachycardia/VF on ICD?
a. Amiodarone
b. Sotalol
c. Beta blockers
d. Quinidine

35. What is treatment of choice for patient with early repolarization syndrome who have recurrent, frequent VT/VF?
a. Quinidine
b. Isoproterenol
c. Phenytoin
d. a or b

36. Which is characteristic electrocardiographic feature of outflow tract ventricular tachycardia?
a. LBBB contour in V_1 and inferior axis in frontal plane
b. LBBB contour in V_1 and superior axis in the frontal plane
c. RBBB contour in V_1 and inferior axis in frontal plane
d. RBBB contour in V_1 and superior axis in frontal plane

37. All the following can terminate outflow tract ventricular tachycardia *except*:
a. Vagal maneuvers
b. Isoproterenol
c. Beta blocker
d. Verapamil

38. Which of the following is a cause of bidirectional ventricular tachycardia?
a. Digitalis intoxication
b. Catecholaminergic polymorphic ventricular tachycardia
c. Both of the above
d. None of the above

39. More than one distinct morphology during the same episode of ventricular tachycardia is labelled as:
a. Monomorphic VT
b. Polymorphic VT
c. VT storm
d. Pleomorphic VT

40. If there is continuously changing morphology of ventricular tachycardia seen from beat to beat, then it is labelled as:
a. Polymorphic VT
b. Pleomorphic VT
c. Repetitive monomorphic VT
d. Sustained VT

41. VT storm is:
a. More than 3 separate episodes of VT in 24 hours requiring intervention to terminate
b. Continuously changing morphology of the VT from beat to beat
c. More than one distinct morphology during the same episode of VT
d. Sustained ventricular tachycardia

42. Which of the following statement is *correct*?
  a. The right ventricular outflow tract is most common site of origin of idiopathic premature ventricular contraction/NSVT
  b. NSVT is seen in 6% of normal population
  c. PVCs occurring in patients with structurally normal heart may not warrant therapy always
  d. All of the above

43. Which of the following statement regarding PVCs and cardiomyopathy is *not* correct?
  a. LV dysfunction can occur when PVCs are present for prolonged time
  b. LV dysfunction occur among patient with high frequency of PVCs
  c. Patient with a PVC induced cardiomyopathy, LVEF does not improve even when PVCs are eliminated
  d. All of the above

44. Which is *not* correct regarding outflow tract VT?
  a. It occurs more commonly in patients without structural heart disease
  b. It is often provoked by exercise and emotional stress
  c. It occurs more frequently during premenstrual, perimenopausal and gestational period
  d. It often leads to sudden cardiac death

45. Which of the following statement is *correct* regarding outflow tract ventricular tachycardia?
  a. It occurs in persons without structural heart disease
  b. It is often provoked by exercise
  c. This arrhythmia can be suppressed by adenosine infusion
  d. All of the above

46. Belhassen (fascicular tachycardia) is characterized by ECG pattern of:
  a. Right bundle branch block pattern with left superior axis
  b. Right bundle branch block pattern with a left inferior axis
  c. Left bundle branch block with left superior axis
  d. Left bundle branch block with left inferior axis

47. Fascicular VT is characterized by all *except*:
  a. It is seen in patient with structural heart disease
  b. The ventricular tachycardia has relatively narrow QRS duration
  c. It is sensitive to verapamil
  d. It can be induced by atrial pacing

48. False tendons in left ventricle are found in most of the patients of which condition?
  a. RVOT tachycardia
  b. Fascicular tachycardia
  c. Noncompaction of left ventricle
  d. Catecholamine sensitive polymorphic ventricular tachycardia (CPVT)

49. All the following are correct regarding ventricular tachycardia in patients with coronary artery disease *except*:
  a. The risk of VT is highest during first year after MI
  b. Risk of sudden cardiac death from ventricular arrhythmia increased with time
  c. The risk of recurrence of VT diminishes when heart failure and coronary ischemia are controlled
  d. All of the above

50. Which is the possible exit site of ventricular tachycardia in ECG pattern of RBBB with dominant R wave in V_1?
  a. Right ventricle
  b. Left ventricle
  c. Apical wall
  d. Basal wall

51. Monomorphic VT in the setting of structural heart disease is suggestive of:
  a. Underlying myocardial fibrosis/scar
  b. Underlying severe LV dysfunction
  c. Electrolyte imbalance
  d. All of the above

52. Accelerated idioventricular rhythm is seen in which of following conditions?
  a. Acute coronary syndrome
  b. Rheumatic heart disease
  c. Acute myocarditis
  d. All of the above

53. Which is *not* correct regarding accelerated idioventricular rhythm?
  a. It is a marker of successful reperfusion after thrombolytic therapy
  b. Incidence of AIVR is affected by the location of MI or infarct size
  c. It's presence after MI is not associated with an increase in the mortality
  d. All of the above

54. The most common clinical diagnosis associated with atrial fibrillation is:
  a. Hyperthyroidism
  b. Obstructive sleep apnea
  c. Obesity
  d. Hypertension

55. Which of the following is most frequent trigger for initiation of atrial fibrillation?
  a. Atrial ectopic
  b. Multifocal atrial ectopics
  c. Rapid spontaneous activity arising in the pulmonary veins
  d. Frequent ventricular ectopics

56. Which of the following forms the base of the triangle of koch?
   a. Septal leaflet of the tricuspid valve
   b. Tendon of Todaro
   c. Coronary sinus ostium
   d. Crista terminalis

57. The blood supply to the left bundle is from:
   a. AV nodal artery
   b. Left anterior descending artery
   c. Posterior descending artery
   d. All of the above

58. Which of the following is *not* a manifestation of sinus node dysfunction (SND)?
   a. Sinus bradycardia of varying severity
   b. Long sinus pauses after electrical cardioversion of AF
   c. Chronic AF with slow ventricular response
   d. All suggests SND

59. Mutations in the cardiac specific sodium channel gene (SCN 5A) is associated with all the following *except*:
   a. Lev or Lenegre's disease
   b. Brugada Syndrome
   c. Long QT syndrome
   d. Short QT syndrome

60. Complete heart block resulting from all the following conditions requires permanent pacemaker *except*:
   a. Endocarditis with ring abscess
   b. Lyme disease
   c. Chagas cardiomyopathy
   d. Lev or Lenegre disease

61. Which of the following is *correct* regarding "laminopathy"?
   a. It is the disorders of mutation in nuclear envelope protein Lamin A and C
   b. It is associated with dilated cardiomyopathy
   c. It is associated with AV conduction defect
   d. All of the above

62. Which is *incorrect* regarding congenital complete AV block?
   a. Often it is not associated with structural heart disease
   b. It is associated with maternal lupus erythematosus
   c. The scape rhythm is a narrow QRS complex
   d. Permanent pacemaker is indicated for all

63. AV dissociation is a manifestation of which of the following conditions?
   a. Sinus bradycardia   b. Complete heart block
   c. Ventricular tachycardia   d. All

64. Tilt table test is contraindicated in all the following *except*:
   a. Known severe cerebrovascular disease
   b. Severe mitral stenosis
   c. LVOT obstruction
   d. Recurrent transient ischemic attacks

65. Tilt table test is indicated in all the following *except*:
   a. Recurrent vertigo
   b. Chronic fatigue syndrome
   c. Recurrent transient ischemic attack
   d. Obstruction to left ventricular outflow

66. Which of the following is an absolute indication for permanent pacemaker implantation?
   a. Asymptomatic sinus bradycardia
   b. Sinus arrhythmia with pauses of 2–3 seconds
   c. Wenckebach 2° AV block, particularly during sleep
   d. Type II 2° AV block with His-Purkinje block even in absence of symptom

67. Which of the following do *not* require permanent pacemaker implantation?
   a. Sinus arrhythmia with pauses of 2–3 seconds
   b. Wenckebach 2° AV block (particularly during sleep).
   c. Wandering atrial pacemaker
   d. All of the above

68. All the following are short 'RP' tachycardia *except*:
   a. AVNRT   b. AVRT
   c. Sinus tachycardia   d. Junctional tachycardia

69. All the following are long RP tachycardia *except*:
   a. Sinus tachycardia   b. Atypical AVNRT
   c. Atrial tachycardia   d. Typical AVNRT

70. During electrophysiological study in patient with reciprocating tachycardia if the ventriculoatrial interval of <70 msec suggests diagnosis of:
   a. AV nodal re-entrant tachycardia
   b. Tachycardia from accessory AV pathway
   c. Atrial tachycardia
   d. Ventricular tachycardia

71. Wide QRS tachycardia in patient with pre-excitation syndrome can be caused by all the following *except*:
   a. Sinus tachycardia with antegrade conduction over accessory pathway
   b. AV nodal re-entry with no antegrade conduction over accessory pathway
   c. Orthodromic tachycardia with preexisting bundle branch block
   d. Antidromic tachycardia over one accessory pathway and retrograde conduction over second pathway

72. Which of the following feature is suggestive of long refractory period in an accessory pathway?
   a. Intermittent pre-excitation
   b. Abrupt loss of conduction over accessory pathway with exercise
   c. Abrupt loss of conduction over accessory pathway after I/V administration of Procainamide
   d. All of the above

73. What is the mechanism of supraventricular tachycardia when the 'P' wave during tachycardia are identical to sinus P wave and along with long RP interval and a short PR interval?
   a. AV nodal re-entrant tachycardia
   b. Atrioventricular re-entrant tachycardia
   c. Ventricular tachycardia
   d. Sinus node re-entry

74. Retrograde (inverted in lead II, III and avF) P wave during episode of supraventricular tachycardia indicates which of the following mechanism?
   a. AV nodal re-entry
   b. Reciprocating tachycardia using a paraseptal accessory pathway
   c. Both of the above
   d. None of the above

75. Depression of ST segment during a narrow complex QRS tachycardia generally signifies:
   a. Sinus node re-entry
   b. Atrioventricular AV nodal re-entry
   c. AV re-entrant tachycardia using an accessory pathway
   d. Ventricular tachycardia

76. Tachycardia without manifest P wave is probably caused by which of the following mechanism?
   a. Sinus node re-entry
   b. AV nodal re-entry
   c. Atrioventricular re-entrant tachycardia by using an accessory pathway
   d. Ventricular tachycardia

77. Supraventricular tachycardia with a RP interval exceeding 90 msec can be caused by:
   a. Sinus node re-entry
   b. AV nodal re-entry
   c. Ectopic atrial tachycardia
   d. Reciprocating tachycardia by accessory pathway

78. AV dissociation or AV block during tachycardia exclude the possibility of:
   a. AV nodal re-entrant tachycardia
   b. Atrioventricular re-entrant tachycardia using accessory pathway
   c. Both of the above
   d. None of the above

79. Which of the following supraventricular tachycardia present with short RP and long PR interval?
   a. Atrial tachycardia
   b. Sinus node re-entry
   c. Atrioventricular re-entrant tachycardia
   d. AV nodal re-entry

80. All the following produces long RP, short PR interval tachycardia *except*:
   a. Atrial tachycardia
   b. Sinus node re-entry
   c. Atypical AV nodal re-entry
   d. AV nodal re-entry

81. Ventricular tachycardia arising from which of the following location can be terminated with vagal maneuver?
   a. Left ventricular outflow tract
   b. Left ventricular apex
   c. Right ventricular outflow tract
   d. Right ventricular apex

82. Probable clinical diagnosis in a young patient with palpitation or near syncope, particularly after squatting or exercise, a jerky pulse and mid systolic ejection murmur is:
   a. Mitral valve prolapse
   b. Valvular aortic stenosis
   c. Hypertrophic cardiomyopathy
   d. Pulmonary stenosis

83. Which of the following arrhythmias are commonly *not* seen in healthy young person?
   a. Sinus arrhythmias with pauses exceeding 3 sec
   b. Type I (Wenckebach) second-degree AV block
   c. Wandering atrial pacemaker
   d. Type II second-degree AV conduction disturbance

84. What frequency of premature ventricular complexes have been shown to produce a cardiomyopathy and heart failure in some people which can be reversed following elimination of PVCs?
   a. 5% of the total
   b. 10% of the total
   c. More than 15% of the total
   d. More than 20% of the total

85. Which of the following statement is *correct*?
   a. Prognosis of even frequent and complex PVCs in asymptomatic healthy patient is good without an increased risk of death.
   b. Frequency and complex PVCs following acute MI are associated with a two to fivefold increased risk of cardiac or sudden death
   c. Treating these PVCs in MI patients improve prognosis
   d. All are correct

86. Which of the following is a measure of intraventricular conduction disturbance during electrophysiological testing?
   a. A-H interval
   b. H-V interval
   c. Sinus node recovery time
   d. Sinoatrial conduction time

87. Which of the following causes of syncope can be evaluated reliably in electrophysiologic laboratory?
   a. Sinus node dysfunction
   b. AV block
   c. Tachyarrhythmia
   d. All of the above

88. Which is *not* correct regarding quinidine?
   a. It shorten QT interval
   b. It is useful for treatment of ventricular arrhythmia in Brugada syndrome
   c. It is useful for treatment of arrhythmias in the fetus
   d. It can cause torsade de pointes

89. Which of the following modality is used for treatment of quinidine induced torsade de pointes?
   a. Intravenous magnesium
   b. Atrial or ventricular pacing
   c. Isoproterenol
   d. All of the above

90. The administration of which of the following drug can results in appearance of Brugada sign in patient with normal resting electrocardiogram?
   a. Quinidine
   b. Procainamide
   c. Flecainide
   d. Ajmaline

91. Which of the following drug infusion can cause sudden loss of pre-excitation in a patient with accessory pathway?
   a. Disopyramide
   b. Quinidine
   c. Sotalol
   d. Procainamide

92. Which is *incorrect* regarding procainamide induced SLE?
   a. Antinuclear antibody develops in majority of patients
   b. Brain and kidneys are extensively involved
   c. Corticosteroid administration may eliminate the symptom
   d. There is no predilection for women

93. Disopyramide is useful in treatment of which of the following conditions?
   a. Ventricular arrhythmias
   b. For prevention of episodes of neurally mediated syncope
   c. In hypertrophic cardiomyopathy
   d. All of the above

94. Which is drug of choice for treatment of digitalis – toxic atrial and ventricular tachyarrhythmias?
   a. Propafenone
   b. Phenytoin
   c. Procainamide
   d. Mexiletine

95. All the following statement are correct regarding flecainide *except*:
   a. Flecainide is useful for treatment of supraventricular arrhythmias only
   b. Flecainide is useful for treatment of fetal arrhythmias and arrhythmias in children
   c. Flecainide administration can produce ST elevation in lead V_1 characteristic of Brugada syndrome
   d. Exercise can precipitate a pro-arrhythmic response in patient receiving flecainide

96. Which of the following is *correct* regarding use of ibutilide in treatment of atrial fibrillation?
   a. Pre-treatment with IV magnesium enhances efficacy of the drug
   b. It should not be used in patient with frequent short paroxysm of AF
   c. The QT prolongation related TdP developed within 4 to 6 hours dosing
   d. Ibutilide cannot be used in patient with AF with accessory pathway

97. Which of the following antiarrhythmic drugs is used for acute conversation of AF to sinus rhythm as well as for chronic suppression of recurrent atrial fibrillation?
   a. Ibutilide
   b. Dofetilide
   c. Calcium channel blocker
   d. Sotalol

98. In addition to its class III effects amiodarone also has:
   a. Class I effect (blocks sodium channel)
   b. Class II effect (antiadrenergic)
   c. Class IV effect (calcium channel blocker)
   d. All of the above

99. Extensive accumulation leading to "blue skin" is an effect seen with which of the following antiarrhythmic drug?
   a. Sotalol
   b. Dronedarone
   c. Amiodarone
   d. Ibutilide

100. All the following drugs are used for acute conversion of atrial fibrillation to sinus rhythm except?
   a. Vernakalant
   b. Ibutilide
   c. Dofetilide
   d. Eleclazine

101. Pulmonary toxicity of amiodarone is uncommon with maintenance dose of:
a. Lower than 100 mg/day
b. Lower than 200 mg/day
c. Lower than 300 mg/day
d. Lower than 400 mg/day

102. Which of the following side effect of amiodarone occurs in almost 100% of patients receiving the drug for longer than 6 months?
a. Pulmonary toxicity
b. Skin discoloration
c. Hypothyroidism
d. Corneal microdeposits

103. Which of the following statement is *not* correct regarding amiodarone pulmonary toxicity?
a. It seen when the doses of 400 mg or more per day is prescribed
b. Exposure to supplemental O2, especially in high concentration alone or combined with mechanical ventilation may potentiate pulmonary toxicity
c. It has predilection for involvement of right lung especially right upper lobe
d. Corticosteroid should be used for 3 to 4 weeks for resolution this toxicity

104. All the following are seen with amiodarone toxicity *except*:
a. Interstitial pneumonitis
b. Hypothyroidism
c. Hepatic dysfunction
d. Renal dysfunction

105. The underlying mechanism of amiodarone induced hypothyroidism is:
a. Coanda effect
b. Wolff–Chaikoff effect
c. Concertina effect
d. Bernheim effect

106. Which of the following statement regarding amiodarone induced thyroid dysfunction is *correct*?
a. Amiodarone induced hypothyroidism is more common in iodine sufficient area
b. Amiodarone induced hyperthyroidism is more common in iodine deficient region
c. The treatment of amiodarone induced hypothyroidism requires higher doses of levothyroxine
d. On cessation of amiodarone hypothyroidism resolves in all patients

107. Which of the following drug is used for treatment of amiodarone induced thyrotoxic crisis?
a. Thionamide
b. Radio iodine
c. Glucocorticoids
d. All

108. Which of the following is the mechanism of amiodarone induced hyperthyroidism?
a. Increased synthesis thyroid hormones
b. Excess release T4 and T3
c. Both of the above
d. None of the above

109. Which of the following statement is *correct* regarding amiodarone induced hyperthyroidism?
a. The clinical manifestation is often masked
b. There is no immediate benefit in stopping amiodarone if hyperthyroidism develops
c. Amiodarone ameliorate hyperthyroidism
d. All of the above

110. Which of the following is a treatment of choice for mixed form of thyrotoxicosis (type 1 or type 2) in amiodarone treated patients?
a. Combination of thionamides and prednisolone
b. Radio iodine and prednisolone
c. Surgery
d. Combination of prednisolone and methimazole

111. Which of the following drug should be used to control digoxin induced atrial tachyarrhythmias?
a. Amiodarone
b. Quinidine
c. Flecainide
d. Phenytoin

112. Which of the following drug should be used for treating digoxin induced infra-nodal tachycardia?
a. Amiodarone
b. Sotalol
c. Lidocaine
d. Flecainide

113. Which of the following statement regarding the use of digoxin is *correct*?
a. It is ineffective in terminating episode of acute or recent onset AF
b. To control ventricular response in patients with permanent AF digoxin should not be used as a single agent to control ventricular rate
c. Electrical DC cardioversion may result in life-threatening VT/VF in digitalis toxic patients
d. All of the above

114. Electrical cardioversion is most effective in terminating:
a. Atrial flutter
b. Parasystole
c. Junctional tachycardia (with or without digitalis toxicity)
d. Accelerated idioventricular rhythm

115. A synchronized shock (DC cardioversion) is used for all cardioversion *except*:
a. AV nodal re-entrant tachycardia
b. Atrioventricular re-entrant tachycardia
c. Atrial flutter
d. Ventricular flutter or VF

116. Most of the supraventricular tachycardias can be terminated with shocks in range of 25–50 joules *except*:
   a. Atrioventricular tachycardia
   b. AV nodal re-entrant tachycardia
   c. Atrial flutter
   d. Atrial fibrillation

117. Which of the following is a favourable candidate for electrical cardioversion of atrial fibrillation?
   a. AF with a large left atrium and long-standing AF
   b. Digitalis toxicity
   c. Antiarrhythmic drug intolerance
   d. Symptomatic AF of <12 months duration

118. Atrial fibrillation is more likely to recur after cardioversion in all the following patients *except*:
   a. Significant COPD
   b. Congestive heart failure
   c. Mitral valve disease
   d. Symptomatic AF of <12 months duration

119. Electrical cardioversion is often the initial treatment of choice for which of the following supraventricular tachyarrhythmias?
   a. Atrial fibrillation
   b. Atrial flutter
   c. AV nodal re-entrant tachycardia
   d. Atrioventricular tachycardia

120. Catheter delivered Cryoablation for treatment of tachyarrhythmias uses which of the following agent?
   a. Hydrogen peroxide   b. Helium
   c. Nitrous oxide   d. Liquid oxygen

121. In which of the following situation, ventricular rate during atrial fibrillation can appear more regular?
   a. When the rate is extremely rapid (>170 beats/min)
   b. Junctional tachycardia
   c. High grade AV block with regular escape rhythm
   d. All of the above

122. Long standing atrial fibrillation refractory to cardioversion is termed as:
   a. Persistent AF
   b. Long standing persistent
   c. Permanent
   d. Any of the above

123. In case of lone atrial fibrillation all are correct *except*:
   a. Occurs in younger people
   b. They do not have any structural heart disease
   c. They are at higher risk of thromboembolic complications
   d. They have familiar or genetic causes

124. Which of the following drug is effective prophylactic for preventing vagotonic paroxysmal atrial fibrillation?
   a. Digoxin
   b. Disopyramide
   c. Beta-blockers
   d. Calcium channel blockers

125. Which of the following is *not* a risk factor for development of atrial fibrillation?
   a. Obesity
   b. Obstructive sleep apnea
   c. Psoriasis
   d. All of the above are risk factors

126. Which is the most common cause of atrial fibrillation?
   a. Hypertension with left ventricular hypertrophy
   b. Ischemic heart disease
   c. Mitral valve disease
   d. Dilated cardiomyopathy

127. Most common correctable cause of atrial fibrillation is:
   a. Hypothyroidism   b. Hyperthyroidism
   c. Pericarditis   d. Pulmonary embolism

128. The strongest predictor of ischemic stroke and systemic thromboembolism in a patient of AF is:
   a. History of stroke
   b. History of transient ischemic episode
   c. Mitral stenosis
   d. All of the above

129. The best-established risk factor for stroke in patients with nonvalvular atrial fibrillation includes all *except*:
   a. Diabetes   b. Hypertension
   c. Age 70 or older   d. All

130. Which of the following is *correct* regarding atrial fibrillation?
   a. The burden of AF is greater in patients with persistent AF than in paroxysmal AF
   b. Risk of stroke is lower in patient with paroxysmal AF than in patient with persistent AF
   c. The recommendation for anticoagulation are the same in patient with paroxysmal or persistent AF
   d. All are correct

131. Subclinical AF is:
   a. Atrial fibrillation which is asymptomatic
   b. Atrial fibrillation which is not associated with failure
   c. AF which is clinically silent but detected by implantable pacemaker and cardioverter defibrillators (ICDs)
   d. Atrial fibrillation which comes in short burst

132. In patients with CHADS2 score greater than 1 who are not able to tolerate anticoagulation with warfarin or NOAC suitable regimen to prevent thromboembolic complication is:
   a. Aspirin alone
   b. Aspirin and platelet inhibitor clopidogrel
   c. Clopidogrel alone
   d. Anyone can be used

133. Which is *not* true regarding NOACs anticoagulant?
   a. There is no need for monitoring of a laboratory test such as INR
   b. The risk of intracranial hemorrhage is 50% lower compared to warfarin
   c. There is no need for bridging therapy with NOACs
   d. NOACs can be used safely in patients with renal disease

134. For initiation of anticoagulation with warfarin in patients with AF, bridging therapy with low molecular weight heparin should be continued until the INR is:
   a. 1.0 or higher
   b. 1.5 or higher
   c. 2.0 or higher
   d. 2.5 or higher

135. For electrical cardioversion of acute atrial fibrillation TEE is must to rule out a left atrial thrombus in which of the following condition?
   a. AF duration longer than 48 hours
   b. If the duration of AF is unclear
   c. Patient not already anticoagulated
   d. All of the above

136. Which is *not* correct regarding pharmacologic cardioversion in atrial fibrillation?
   a. The probability of immediate recurrence of AF is lower with pharmacologic cardioversion
   b. It is not as effective as electrical cardioversion
   c. It is unlikely to be effective if the duration of AF is longer than 48 hours
   d. All are correct

137. All the following drug administered intravenously can be used for cardioversion of AF *except*:
   a. Lidocaine
   b. Ibutilide
   c. Procainamide
   d. Amiodarone

138. The most common oral agent for acute conversion of AF is:
   a. Flecainide
   b. Amiodarone
   c. Procainamide
   d. Ibutilide

139. *Correct* statement regarding electrical cardioversion for AF is:
   a. Biphasic waveform shocks convert AF more effectively than monophasic waveform shocks
   b. Ibutilide administration before cardioversion improves the success rate of cardioversion and prevent immediate recurrence
   c. If there is immediate recurrence of AF within a few second of successful conversion increasing in shocks strength does not help
   d. All are correct

140. Safe cardioversion without anticoagulation can be done for atrial fibrillation of duration:
   a. Less than 24 hours
   b. Less than 48 hours
   c. Less than 3 days
   d. Less than 7 days

141. What is the recommended duration of anticoagulation following cardioversion for atrial fibrillation in a patient with CHA_2DS_2-VASC score '0'?
   a. One week
   b. Two weeks
   c. Three weeks
   d. Four weeks

142. In management of atrial fibrillation, a rate-control strategy comparing to rhythm-control strategy offer benefit in terms of:
   a. Significantly lower rate of hospitalization
   b. Significant reduction of all cause mortality
   c. Significant reduction in stroke
   d. Reduction in worsening heart failure

143. In patient with sinus node dysfunction and atrial fibrillation as a part of Tachy–Brady syndrome, which of the following drug may provide rate control without aggravating sinus bradycardia?
   a. Verapamil
   b. Diltiazem
   c. Metoprolol
   d. Pindolol

144. Which of the following is an appropriate choice for a patient with persistent AF, heart failure and reactive airway disease who has rapid ventricular rate despite treatment with digitalis?
   a. Calcium channel block antagonists
   b. Beta blockers
   c. Flecainide
   d. Amiodarone

145. The risk of torsade de pointes is much lower with which of the following drug?
   a. Sotalol
   b. Dofetilide
   c. Flecainide
   d. Amiodarone

146. Which of the following class of antiarrhythmic drug the ventricular pro-arrhythmia manifest as monomorphic ventricular tachycardia?
   a. Class IA agents
   b. Class IB agents
   c. Class IC agents
   d. Class III drugs

147. In patient with lone atrial fibrillation or minimal heart disease (mild left ventricular hypertrophy) which of the following is first line of drug?
 a. Flecainide
 b. Propafenone
 c. Sotalol
 d. All of the above

148. In patients with substantial left ventricular hypertrophy (left ventricular wall thickness >15 mm), the safest drug to suppress AF is:
 a. Flecainide
 b. Propafenone
 c. Sotalol
 d. Amiodarone/Dronedarone

149. In patients with coronary artery disease with atrial fibrillation which is safest first line option to suppress AF:
 a. Sotalol/Dofetilide
 b. Flecainide
 c. Amiodarone
 d. Quinidine

150. Which of the following drug have neutral effect on survival in patients with heart failure and atrial fibrillation?
 a. Amiodarone
 b. Sotalol
 c. Flecainide
 d. Propafenone

151. Which of the following agents other than antiarrhythmic drugs are known to prevent occurrence of atrial fibrillation?
 a. ACE inhibitors
 b. Angiotensin receptor blockers
 c. Statins
 d. All of the above

152. Which is the most common major complication associated with radiofrequency catheter ablation of AF?
 a. Cardiac tamponade
 b. Pulmonary vein stenosis
 c. Cerebral thromboembolism
 d. All occurs with equal frequency

153. Which is a lethal complication of radiofrequency ablation of atrial fibrillation?
 a. Cardiac tamponade
 b. Pulmonary vein stenosis
 c. Cerebral thromboembolism
 d. Esophageal perforation

154. The most common complication of cryo balloon ablation for AF is:
 a. Esophageal perforation
 b. Cardiac tamponade
 c. Femoral vascular injury
 d. Phrenic nerve injury

155. All the following drugs have been demonstrated to reduce the risk of atrial fibrillation after open heart surgery except:
 a. Colchicine
 b. Atorvastatin
 c. Steroid
 d. Flecainide

156. Which of the following statement regarding postoperative atrial fibrillation is *correct*?
 a. The incidence of AF peaks on second postoperative day
 b. Hypomagnesemia can increase the risk of postoperative AF
 c. Colchicine and steroids reduce the risk of postoperative AF
 d. All of the above

157. All of the following agents are known to decrease the risk of postoperative atrial fibrillation except?
 a. Colchicine
 b. Atorvastatin
 c. Injection of botulinum toxin into the four major epicardial fat pads at operation
 d. Flecainide

158. Which of the following drug has been shown to reduce the risk of atrial fibrillation after major noncardiac surgery?
 a. Sotalol
 b. Amiodarone
 c. Magnesium
 d. Beta blockers

159. Which of the following drug should be used preferably in patient with WPW syndrome who present in AF with a rapid ventricular rate?
 a. Ibutilide
 b. Flecainide
 c. Procainamide
 d. Digitalis

160. Which is *correct* regarding atrial fibrillation in patients with WPW syndrome?
 a. Intravenous procainamide is preferable drug to control atrial fibrillation
 b. Preferred therapy is catheter ablation of accessory pathway
 c. Atrial fibrillation does not recur after successful accessory pathway ablation
 d. All of the above

161. Which of the following is drug of choice for rhythm control in patients with hypertrophic cardiomyopathy and atrial fibrillation?
 a. Sotalol
 b. Beta blockers
 c. Flecainide
 d. Amiodarone

162. The recommended pharmacological agent for rate control AF with pregnancy is:
    a. Intravenous amiodarone
    b. Intravenous magnesium
    c. Intravenous verapamil
    d. Intravenous metoprolol

163. Which of the following drug is safe for conversion to sinus rhythm in pregnant patient with atrial fibrillation?
    a. Amiodarone
    b. Digoxin
    c. Flecainide
    d. Flecainide or sotalol

164. Which of the following is *incorrect* statement?
    a. Transthoracic cardioversion is not safe in the first trimester of pregnancy
    b. Intravenous metoprolol is a drug of choice for acute management of AF and rate control
    c. Flecainide or sotalol can be used safely for conversion to sinus rhythm
    d. In patient with structural heart disease amiodarone is recommended for rhythm control

165. Which of the following drug is most effective to restore sinus rhythm in patient with atrial flutter?
    a. Amiodarone
    b. Sotalol
    c. Procainamide
    d. Ibutilide

166. Which class of drugs slows conduction and prolongs refractoriness in accessory pathway as well as AV node?
    a. Class IA and II
    b. Class II and IV
    c. Digitalis
    d. Class IC and III

167. Which of the following class of drug prolong the refractoriness of accessory pathway and slows the conduction?
    a. Class I a
    b. Class II
    c. Class IV
    d. Adenosine

168. During the episode of tachycardia when the QRS complex is normal and retrograde P wave occurs after completion of QRS complex in ST segment associated with depression of ST segment then which mechanism is possible?
    a. AVNRT
    b. Re-entry over a concealed (retrograde only) accessory pathway
    c. Atrial tachycardia
    d. Atrial flutter

169. Which of the following is *not* a reversible cause of sinus tachycardia?
    a. Hyperthyroidism
    b. Anemia
    c. Hypovolemia
    d. Diabetic neuropathy

170. Bioavailability of which of the following antiarrhythmic drug is three times more after a high fat meal?
    a. Digoxin
    b. Flecainide
    c. Amiodarone
    d. Sotalol

171. Which is mode of pacemaker of choice in patient with normal sinus node function and AV block?
    a. AAI mode
    b. VVI mode
    c. VDD mode
    d. VOO mode

172. In a procedure which requires constant electro-cautery, pacemaker should be programmed to which mode?
    a. AAI mode
    b. VOO mode/AOO mode
    c. VDD mode
    d. DDD mode

173. Which is a pacing mode of choice in patients with sinus node dysfunction and normal AV conduction?
    a. VVI mode
    b. VOO mode
    c. VDD mode
    d. AAI mode

174. Which location of placement of right ventricular lead has been found to be hemodynamically beneficial and prevent left ventricular dysfunction in a dual chamber pacemaker?
    a. RV apex
    b. RVOT
    c. RV septum
    d. High septal pacing near HIS bundle

175. Which is "pacemaker mode" of choice in patients with long standing atrial fibrillation with complete AV block?
    a. DDD
    b. VVI
    c. DDD (R)
    d. VVI (R)

176. A pattern of ST-T segment elevation in right pericardial ECG leads and a high incidence of sudden death in patients with structurally normal heart is named as:
    a. Arrhythmogenic right ventricular dysplasia
    b. Brugada's syndrome
    c. Long QT syndrome
    d. Short QT syndrome

177. The commonest mechanism of paroxysmal supraventricular tachycardia is:
    a. AV nodal re-entrant tachycardia
    b. Atrioventricular re-entrant tachycardia
    c. Atrial tachycardia
    d. All are equally common

178. Epsilon waves are characteristically seen in:
    a. Brugada syndrome
    b. Arrhythmogenic right ventricular dysplasia
    c. Hypothermia
    d. Hypokalemia

179. Ventricular arrhythmias (sustained or non-sustained) of LBBB morphology is characteristics of:
   a. Brugada syndrome
   b. Arrhythmogenic right ventricular dysplasia
   c. Idiopathic ventricular tachycardia
   d. Hypertrophic cardiomyopathy

180. Epsilon waves are best seen in:
   a. Lead II, III, avF
   b. Lead V_4-V_6
   c. Lead avR
   d. Lead V_1-V_3

181. The most serious adverse effect with amiodarone is:
   a. Hypothyroidism
   b. Hyperthyroidism
   c. Interstitial pneumonitis
   d. Peripheral neuropathy

182. Which of the following adverse effect with use of amiodarone is dose related?
   a. Hypothyroidism
   b. Hyperthyroidism
   c. Interstitial pneumonitis
   d. Peripheral neuropathy

183. Torsades de Pointes is rare with:
   a. Sotalol
   b. Ibutilide
   c. Amiodarone
   d. Dofetilide

184. Which of the following drug should be avoided in long QT syndrome?
   a. Ibutilide
   b. Sotalol
   c. Dofetilide
   d. All

185. Atrial fibrillation as proarrhythmic event is seen with injection of which of the following antiarrhythmic drugs?
   a. Digitalis
   b. Adenosine
   c. Amiodarone
   d. Calcium channel blockers

186. The most frequently encountered form of symptomatic sinus node dysfunction is:
   a. Sinus bradycardia
   b. Sino atrial block
   c. Sinus arrest
   d. Tachycardia-bradycardia syndrome

187. Which of the following is *not* a definite manifestation of sinus node dysfunction?
   a. Sinus bradycardia
   b. Sino-atrial block
   c. Sinus arrest
   d. Bradycardia tachycardia syndrome

188. Which of the statements regarding sinus node dysfunction is *correct*?
   a. Syncope is rare in patients with isolated sinus bradycardia
   b. Syncope in patients with isolated sinus bradycardia is usually neurocardiac
   c. Prolonged asystolic period occurring in setting of any form of sinus node dysfunction also implies impaired function of lower (non sinus pacemakers)
   d. All of the above

189. In case with infrequent episode of syncope, which of the following helps in diagnosing sinus node disease accurately:
   a. Random EKG
   b. Prolonged ECG monitoring
   c. Implantable event recorder
   d. All of the above

190. Which of the following drug is known to cause proarrhythmias?
   a. Quinidine
   b. Erythromycin
   c. Astemizole
   d. All

ANSWERS WITH EXPLANATIONS

1. Ans. d. Any of the above

Braunwald 11th Ed; Page 597

Palpitations are the awareness of the heartbeat that may be caused by a rapid heart rate, irregularities in heart rhythm, or an increase in the force of cardiac contraction, as occurs with a post-extrasystolic beat. The onset and offset of palpitations can suggest the etiology of the arrhythmia. A sudden, abrupt, onset, is consistent with a paroxysmal tachycardia such as atrioventricular nodal re-entrant tachycardia, whereas gradual speeding and slowing are more consistent with atrial or sinus tachycardia. Termination by Valsalva maneuver or carotid sinus massage suggests a tachycardia incorporating nodal tissue in the re-entrant pathway, such as sinus node re-entry, atrioventricular re-entrant tachycardia (AVRT), or atrioventricular nodal re-entrant tachycardia.

2. Ans. d. Any of the above

Braunwald 11th Ed; Page 597

Refer to explanation for Q. No 1.

3. Ans. c. Early seizure activity

Braunwald 11th Ed; Page 598

The proper history in case of syncope may help in differentiating syncope of cardiac origin from those of neurological origin. When caused by cardiac arrhythmia the onset of symptoms is rapid and duration is brief, with or without preceding aura, and is not typically followed by a postictal confusional state. It can be associated with bodily injury if the patient falls while unconscious. Palpitations preceding syncope may support an arrhythmic cause of syncope but are often absent if the loss of consciousness is rapid. Seizure activity is uncommon and occurs mostly after prolonged asystole or a rapid ventricular arrhythmia. Therefore, the seizure does not begin with or anticipate the syncope, whereas in epileptic seizures, convulsive movements start within seconds of the onset of syncope. Tongue biting or incontinence is also uncommon in cardiac syncope. Syncope with early seizure activity is frequently caused by epilepsy, whereas later seizure activity is more likely caused by a cardiac arrhythmia with cerebral hypoperfusion.

4. Ans. d. All of the above

Braunwald 11th Ed; Page 598

History taking is very important in arriving at diagnosis of probable cause of sudden cardiac death. History of cardiac disease is important in diagnosis and management as is the family history of sudden cardiac death of significant arrhythmia. The circumstances at the time of sudden cardiac death are often informative. Cardiac symptoms that predate the sudden cardiac death suggest pre-existing structural heart disease. A variety of precipitating factors can provide clues to the etiology of sudden cardiac arrest. Exercise, emotional upset, or stress may precipitate cardiac arrest in the setting of a variety of structural heart diseases, arrhythmogenic cardiomyopathy and primary electrical diseases such as LQTS (types 1 and 2) and CPVT. SCD in LQTS3 or Brugada syndrome is more likely to occur at rest or with sleep. Up to 80% of cases of SCD occurs in some form of structural heart disease, such as CHD, cardiomyopathy or congenital heart diseases. Cardiac causes of SCD, referred to as "autopsy negative" includes primary electrical diseases such as long QT syndrome, Brugada syndrome, catecholaminergic polymorphic ventricular tachycardia (CPVT), idiopathic ventricular fibrillation and sometimes WPW syndrome.

5. Ans. d. Brugada syndrome

Braunwald 11th Ed; Page 598

Refer to explanation for Q. No 4.

6. Ans. c. Both of the above

Braunwald 11th Ed; Page 598

Refer to explanation for Q. No 4.

7. Ans. d. Ventricular tachycardia

Braunwald 11th Ed; Page 599

During the tachycardia obtaining an ECG is a very informative. On physical examination, the presence of regular canon 'a' wave in jugular venous pulse would be consistent with a 1:1 retrograde ventriculo-atrial activation as in tachycardia such as AVRT, AVNRT and some junctional tachycardia and VTs. In contrast, patient may have physical examination feature of AV dissociation, such as intermittent canon 'a' wave, variable intensity of first heart sound, and variable peak systolic blood pressure consistent with arrhythmia including VT and non-paroxysmal AV junctional tachycardia without retrograde capture of atria.

8. Ans. c. Permanent form of AV junctional reciprocating tachycardia

Braunwald 11th Ed; Page 599

Carotid sinus massage (CSM) during the physical examination can be useful to interrupt arrhythmias sensitive to autonomic tone and identify the patient with a hypersensitive carotid sinus reflex. Gentle massage of CSM is usually sufficient to terminate a sensitive tachycardia or produce significant periods of sinus arrest or AV block in susceptible patients. The most definitive responses to CSM are tachycardia termination, as it is observed in AVRT, AVNRT, sinus node re-entry, adenosine-sensitive atrial tachycardia (AT), and idiopathic right ventricular outflow tract tachycardia. Carotid sinus massage can gradually slow a sinus tachycardia without termination and decrease the ventricular response to atrial tachycardia, atrial flutter, and atrial fibrillation without termination. CSM transiently terminates the permanent form of AV junctional reciprocating tachycardia, which then restarts when carotid massage ceases. CSM generally does not affect re-entrant ventricular or junctional tachycardias.

9. Ans. d. Junctional tachycardia

Braunwald 11th Ed; Page 599

Refer to explanation for Q. No 8.

10. Ans. c. Implantable loop recorders

Braunwald 11th Ed; Page 600

Implantable monitors or implantable loop recorders (ILRs) are typically used for the evaluation of suspected serious arrhythmias that occur infrequently and cannot be provoked at diagnostic electrophysiological study. An ILR, a single-lead ECG monitoring device placed subcutaneously, monitors the cardiac rhythm for as long as 24–36 months. These devices have both auto-triggered and patient-activated arrhythmia-recording capabilities.

11. Ans. c. PVCs at rest suppressed by exercise rules out coronary artery disease

Braunwald 11th Ed; Page 601

Cardiac arrhythmias in response to exercise is of helpful in assessing the prognosis. Approximately one-third of individuals without heart disease will have ventricular ectopic associated with exercise. Typically, this manifest as occasional uniform PVCs, more likely to occur at faster heart rate and not reproducible from one stress test to the next. Multiform PVCs, pairs of PVCs, and VT are an infrequent response to exercise in healthy individuals. Ventricular ectopic occurs in about half of patients with CAD and have a higher reproducibility at a lower heart rate (<130 beats/min), than healthy individual. Frequent PVCs (>10/min), polymorphic PVCs and VT are more likely to occur in patients with CAD. PVCs at rest can be suppressed by exercise in patient with CAD, therefore this observation does not necessarily imply a benign prognosis or absence of underlying structural heart disease.

12. Ans. d. All of the above

Braunwald 11th Ed; Page 753

Premature ventricular complex can exhibit fixed or variable coupling interval. Coupling interval is interval between the normal QRS complex and the premature ventricular complex. It can be relatively stable or variable. Fixed coupling can be caused by re-entry, triggered activity or other mechanism. Variable coupling can be caused by parasystole, changing conduction in a re-entrant circuit or changing discharge rates of triggered activity.

13. Ans. d. All of the above

Braunwald 11th Ed; Page 754

Premature ventricular complexes usually have no impact on longevity or limitation of activity. Antiarrhythmic drugs are usually not indicated. If patients are symptomatic, they can be reassured. The predictor of LV dysfunction and future cardiomyopathy are: (a) Frequent PVCs greater than 24% of all beats during 24 hours Holter monitoring; (b) Very wide QRS PVCs; (c) PVCs of epicardial origin. Catheter ablation generally resolves the cardiomyopathy.

14. Ans. d. Septal origin VT

Braunwald 11th Ed; Page 757

The ventricular tachycardia origin or exit site can often be determined on the surface ECG. Ventricular tachycardias from the left ventricular free wall typically exhibit an RBBB contour, whereas those from the right ventricle or septum have an LBBB contour. Septal VTs typically have narrower QRS complexes than free wall VTs. Apical VTs exhibit negative precordial lead concordance, whereas more basal sites typically have positive concordance. Ventricular tachycardias from the posterior (inferior) left or right ventricle often have predominantly negative QRS complexes in leads II, III, and aVF, whereas outflow tract ventricular tachycardias frequently exhibit predominantly positive QRS complexes in these leads.

15. Ans. c. Apical origin VT

Braunwald 11th Ed; Page 757

Refer to explanation for Q. No 14.

16. Ans. c. Basal portion of ventricle

Braunwald 11th Ed; Page 757

Refer to explanation for Q. No 14.

17. Ans. d. Outflow tract ventricular tachycardia

Braunwald 11th Ed; Page 757

Refer to explanation for Q. No 14.

18. Ans. d. Posterior/inferior portion of ventricle

Braunwald 11th Ed; Page 757

Refer to explanation for Q. No 14.

19. Ans. d. ICD

Braunwald 11th Ed; Page 761

For secondary prevention of sustained VT or cardiac arrest in patients with structural heart disease, class I antiarrhythmic drugs produce a worse outcome than do class III antiarrhythmic drugs. An empiric amiodarone results in better survival than EP guided antiarrhythmic drugs, and ICDs provide better survival than amiodarone, particularly in patients with an LVEF <35%.

20. Ans. d. ICD

Braunwald 11th Ed; Page 762

The risk for SCD in patients with hypertrophic cardiomyopathy is increased by the presence of syncope, a family history of SCD in first-degree relatives, septal thickness greater than 3 cm, or the presence of non-sustained VT on 24-hour Holter monitoring. In patients believed to be at high risk for SCD or those with sustained VT or frequent non-sustained VT, an ICD may be indicated.

21. Ans. b. Arrhythmogenic right ventricular cardiomyopathy

Braunwald 11th Ed; Page 762

Arrhythmogenic right ventricular dysplasia is a heterogenous inherited disease that results in fibrofatty infiltration of predominantly the right ventricle. Patients with ARVC have VT that generally has an LBBB contour (because the tachycardia arises in right ventricle).

The ECG during sinus rhythm can exhibit complete or incomplete RBBB and T wave inversions in V_1-V_3. A terminal notch in the QRS, called an epsilon wave, can be present as a result of slowed intraventricular conduction.

22. Ans. d. Catecholaminergic polymorphic ventricular tachycardia (CPVT)

Braunwald 11th Ed; Page 762-763

Catecholaminergic polymorphic VT (CPVT) is an uncommon form of inherited VT that occurs in the absence of overt structural heart disease. Patients typically have syncope or aborted sudden death with highly reproducible, stress-induced VT that is often bidirectional. A family history of sudden death or stress-induced syncope is present in approximately 30% of cases. During exercise, typical responses include initial sinus tachycardia and ventricular extrasystoles, followed by salvoes of monomorphic or bidirectional VT, which eventually lead to polymorphic VT as exercise continues. The treatment of choice is beta blockers and an ICD. Left-sided or bilateral sympathectomy has been reported to be effective in a few cases.

23. Ans. c. Beta blockers and ICD

Braunwald 11th Ed; Page 762-763

Refer to explanation for Q. No. 22.

24. Ans. d. All of the above

Braunwald 11th Ed; Page 763

The most common cause of torsade de pointes are congenital severe bradycardia, potassium depletion and use of QT prolonging medication. The TdP is characterized by QRS complex of changing amplitude that appear to twist around the isoelectric line and occur at rates of 200–250 per minute. Originally described in the setting of bradycardia caused by complete heart block, TdP usually connotes a syndrome, and it can be due to various causes. TdP is common with prolonged repolarization with QT intervals generally exceeding 500 milliseconds. Women, because of long QT intervals are at greater risk than man for TdP.

25. Ans. d. IV magnesium

Braunwald 11th Ed; Page 765

The management of polymorphic ventricular tachycardia as a result of prolonged QT comprises, removal of all offending drugs like Class IA, Class IC, and Class III antiarrhythmic drugs IV Magnesium is the initial treatment of choice for TdP from an acquired cause, followed by temporary ventricular or atrial pacing. Isoproterenol should be given cautiously as it may exacerbate the arrhythmia and can be used to increase the rate until pacing is instituted. Lidocaine, mexiletine, or phenytoin can be tried.

26. Ans. d. IV Amiodarone

Braunwald 11th Ed; Page 765

Refer to explanation for Q. No 25.

27. Ans. d. Beta blockades + ICDs

Braunwald 11th Ed; Page 766

For patients who have long QT syndrome (LQTS) but not syncope, complex ventricular arrhythmias, a family history of SCD, or a QTc interval of 500 milliseconds or more, no therapy or treatment with a beta blocker is generally recommended. In asymptomatic patients with complex ventricular arrhythmias, a family history of early SCD, or a QTc interval of 500 milliseconds or more, beta adrenoceptor blockers such as nadolol at maximally tolerated doses are recommended. Implantation of a permanent pacemaker to prevent the bradycardia or pauses that may predispose to the development of TdP may be indicated. In patients with syncope or aborted sudden death, an ICD is warranted. These patients should also be treated with concomitant beta blockers. Left-sided cervicothoracic sympathetic ganglionectomy that interrupts the stellate ganglion and the first three or four thoracic ganglia, may be helpful.

28. Ans. d. Beta blocker + ICD

Braunwald 11th Ed; Page 766

Refer to explanation for Q. No 27.

29. Ans. d. All

Braunwald 11th Ed; Page 766

Short QT syndrome can be congenital or acquired. Acquired causes are hyperkalemia, hypercalcemia, hyperthermia, acidosis and digitalis.

30. Ans. d. Quinidine + ICD

Braunwald 11th Ed; Page 766

ICD are treatment of choice in symptomatic patient with SQTS to prevent sudden cardiac death. Antiarrhythmic drugs like quinidine which prolongs refractoriness has been found to be effective in some patients.

31. Ans. d. Both a and b

Braunwald 11th Ed; Page 766

The J wave, also referred as the Osborn wave, is the junction of the QRS complex and the ST segment on a surface ECG. The J wave syndromes or a spectrum of pathological early repolarization predisposing to ventricular arrhythmias includes Brugada syndrome and early repolarization syndrome. The main differences between the syndromes lie in the region of the myocardium most affected and thus the ECG leads in which the J wave abnormalities are seen. Brugada syndrome predominantly affects the RV outflow tract and thus ECG leads V_1-V_3. Early repolarization syndrome affects the inferior LV wall and thus ECG leads I, II, III, aVF, aVL, and V_4-V_6.

32. **Ans. d. Lead I, II, III, aVF, aVL and V_4-V_6**

Braunwald 11th Ed; Page 766

Refer to explanation for Q. No 31.

33. **Ans. d. All of the above**

Braunwald 11th Ed; Page 767

Brugada syndrome is characterized by an RBBB and ST-segment elevation in the anterior precordial leads, without evidence of structural heart disease. Findings on ECG are characterized as type 1, type 2, or type 3 patterns. Type 1 changes consist of ST elevation with J wave amplitude >2 mm with negative T wave and ST is elevation. The other causes of ST elevation mimicking Brugada type 1 pattern includes RBBB, pectus excavatum, occlusion of left anterior descending or conus branch and ARVC.

34. **Ans. d. Quinidine**

Braunwald 11th Ed; Page 768

All patients with Brugada syndrome with aborted sudden death or spontaneous VT / VF or history of syncope should receive ICD implantation. Quinidine can normalize the ECG and suppress VT in patients with Brugada by blocking the calcium independent transient outward potassium current or a late sodium current. Quinidine has been effective in patients with frequent or storms of VT/VF on ICD and may also be used for patients who qualify for an ICD but either refuse or are otherwise contraindicated.

35. **Ans. d. a or b**

Braunwald 11th Ed; Page 768

Most patients with early repolarization are not at risk for ventricular arrhythmias. Symptomatic patients with VT/VF, or syncope of presumed arrhythmic origin should undergo ICD implantation. Quinidine and isoproterenol can be used to treat recurrent, frequent VT/VF.

36. **Ans. a. LBBB contour in V_1 and inferior axis in frontal plane**

Braunwald 11th Ed; Page 768

Right ventricular outflow tract VT accounts for about 70% of idiopathic VTs, while 10-15% originate from the LVOT. Outflow tract VTs have a characteristic electrocardiographic appearance of an LBBB contour in V_1 and an inferior axis in the frontal plane.

37. **Ans. b. Isoproterenol**

Braunwald 11th Ed; Page 768

Outflow tract tachycardia can be terminated by vagal maneuvers, including adenosine, whereas exercise, stress, isoproterenol infusion, and rapid or premature stimulation often initiate or perpetuate the tachycardia. Beta blockers and verapamil can suppress this tachycardia.

38. **Ans. c. Both of the above**

Braunwald 11th Ed; Page 769

Bidirectional ventricular tachycardia is an uncommon type of VT characterized by QRS complexes with RBBB pattern, polarity in the frontal plane alternating from −60 to −90 degrees to +120 to +130 degrees, and a regular rhythm. The ventricular rate is between 140 and 200 beats/min. Bidirectional VT is manifestation of digitalis excess, typically seen in older patients and those with severe myocardial disease. Bidirectional VT also seen in context of CPVT.

39. **Ans. d. Pleomorphic VT**

Hurst's 14th Ed; Page 1983

Ventricular tachycardia definitions
- *Sustained VT*: Duration of VT is >30 seconds or <30 seconds associated with hemodynamic collapse
- *Nonsustained VT*: Duration > 3 beats and <30 seconds not associated with hemodynamic collapse
- *Repetitive monomorphic VT*: Episodes of nonsustained VT that continuously repeat
- *VT storm*: More than three separate episode of VT in 24 hours requiring intervention to terminate
- *Monomorphic VT*: All beats have same QRS morphology (some variation may be seen at initiation)
- *Polymorphic VT*: Continuously changing morphology of the VT is seen from beat to beat
- *Pleomorphic VT*: More than one distinct morphology during the same episode of VT

40. **Ans. a. Polymorphic VT**

Hurst's 14th Ed; Page 1983

Refer to explanation for Q. No 39.

41. **Ans. a. More than 3 separate episodes of VT in 24 hours requiring intervention to terminate**

Hurst's 14th Ed; Page 1983

Refer to explanation for Q. No 39.

42. Ans. d. All of the above

Hurst's 14th Ed; Page 1984

The PVCs/NSVT are commonly seen in patient with structurally normal heart. NSVT is also very common occurring in up to 6% of patients in Holter studies. The right ventricular outflow tract is most common site of origin of idiopathic PVCs/NSVT. PVCs/NSVT originating from this region are characterized on 12 lead electrocardiogram by left bundle branch block pattern in V_1 and tall monophasic R wave in inferior leads. In patient without structural heart disease, PVCs are not associated with any excess risk of sudden death. PVCs that occur in patients with a structurally normal heart may not warrant therapy, unless significant symptoms are present or there is concern for PVC-induced cardiomyopathy.

43. Ans. c. Patient with a PVC induced cardiomyopathy, LVEF does not improve even when PVCs are eliminated

Hurst's 14th Ed; Page 1984

There is an association between frequent PVCs and dilated cardiomyopathy. A higher burden of PVCs over a 24-hour period is associated with higher risk, but development of cardiomyopathy associated with a burden as low as 10% has been described. Current studies regarding the role of PVCs in the development of a cardiomyopathy demonstrate: (1) LV dysfunction can occur when PVCs are present for a prolonged period of time; (2) LV dysfunction occurs among patients with a high frequency of PVCs; and (3) among patients with a PVC-induced cardiomyopathy, LVEF improves in the majority of patients when the PVCs can be eliminated with radiofrequency catheter ablation.

44. Ans. d. It often leads to sudden cardiac death

Hurst's 14th Ed; Page 1986

"Outflow tract" VT occurs frequently in young to middle-aged patients without structural heart disease. This arrhythmia is often provoked by exercise and emotional stress. Recurrence may be associated with exercise, stress, or caffeine, and in women, it occurs more frequently during premenstrual, perimenopausal, and gestational periods.

The proposed cellular mechanism of right ventricular outflow tract tachycardia is cyclic adenosine monophosphate (cAMP)–mediated triggered activity from delayed after depolarizations. This mechanism is supported by the sensitivity of the arrhythmia to adenosine infusion, which often terminates the arrhythmia.

45. Ans. d. All of the the above

Hurst's 14th Ed; Page 1986

Refer to explanation for Q. No 44.

46. Ans. a. Right bundle branch block pattern with left superior axis

Hurst's 14th Ed; Page 1987

Fascicular VT is characterized by a right bundle branch block (RBBB) pattern with a left superior axis on a 12-lead ECG. Belhassen described the sensitivity of this tachycardia to verapamil. Patients typically have a structurally normal heart but may present with an incessant VT and a reversible tachycardia mediated cardiomyopathy can develop. The site of origin of the tachycardia is usually in the region of the left posterior fascicle. The ventricular tachycardia has a relatively narrow QRS (<140 milliseconds), a RBBB pattern in V_1, and superior axis. This tachycardia can be induced with atrial pacing and it is sensitivity to verapamil. The arrhythmia usually presents in patients between age group of 15 and 40 years.

47. Ans. a. It is seen in patient with structural heart disease

Hurst's 14th Ed; Page 1987

Refer to explanation for Q. No 46.

48. Ans. a. RVOT tachycardia

Hurst's 14th Ed; Page 1988

False tendons in left ventricle are found in most patients with fascicular VT and their anatomic and functional significant is unknown.

49. Ans. c. The risk of recurrence of VT diminishes when heart failure and coronary ischemia are controlled

Hurst's 14th Ed; Page 1988

Ventricular arrhythmias in patients with coronary disease range from PVCs to NSVT to sustained VT leading to hemodynamic compromise and sudden cardiac death. The anatomic substrate from which ischemic VT originates usually involves a healed scar after an acute MI. A study has demonstrated that risk of VT is highest during first year after acute MI (3–5%), but VT may occur many years later and risk of sudden cardiac death from ventricular arrhythmia may increase with time. Patient with VT have a high risk of recurrence even when heart failure and coronary ischemia are controlled.

50. Ans. b. Left ventricle

Hurst's 14th Ed; Page 1988

ECG features for VT exit site localization
- LBBB pattern in V_1 suggests exit in RV or interventricular septum
- RBBB pattern with dominant R waves in V_1 indicates LV exit
- Superior axis → inferior wall exit
- Inferior axis → anterior wall
- Dominant S waves in V_3, V_4 → apical exit
- Dominant R waves in V_3, V_4 → basal exit

51. Ans. a. Underlying myocardial fibrosis/scar

Hurst's 14th Ed; Page 1988

Ischemia is rarely a cause of monomorphic VT, it often produces polymorphic VT. Monomorphic VT in the setting of structural heart disease suggests underlying myocardial fibrosis or scar.

52. Ans. d. All of the above

Hurst's 14th Ed; Page 1995

Accelerated idioventricular rhythm (AIVR) is an automatic rhythm originating in the ventricle with rates between 40 and 120 bpm. It is often seen gradually accelerating beyond the sinus rate, resulting in isorhythmic atrioventricular dissociation. Fusion beats may be seen at the beginning and end of the arrhythmia. AIVR may be associated with ischemic cardiomyopathy, acute coronary syndromes, rheumatic heart disease, dilated cardiomyopathy, and acute myocarditis. It is even seen in patients with no apparent heart disease. In setting of acute coronary syndromes, AIVR is considered to be a noninvasive but nonspecific marker for successful reperfusion after thrombolytic therapy. The incidence of AIVR is not affected by theocationn of MI or the infarct size. The presence of AIVR after an MI is not associated with an increase in the mortality.

53. Ans. b. Incidence of AIVR is affected by the location of MI or infarct size

Hurst's 14th Ed; Page 1995

Refer to explanation for Q. No 52.

54. Ans. d. Hypertension

Hurst's 14th Ed; Page 1950

In the developed world, the most common clinical diagnosis associated with atrial fibrillation is hypertension. There are risk factors such as obesity and obstructive sleep apnea. Hyperthyroidism is a commonest reversible cause. The presence of heart failure increases the risk of AF. Hypertension, rheumatic valvular heart disease, and congenital heart disease are most commonly related conditions.

55. Ans. c. Rapid spontaneous activity arising in the pulmonary veins

Hurst's 14th Ed; Page 1950

The mechanism of atrial fibrillation is multifactorial including electrophysiologic and structural abnormalities and it is perpetuated by extrinsic factors such as autonomic disturbances. Different mechanisms may initiate (trigger) and maintain atrial fibrillation in an individual. The most frequent triggers are rapid spontaneous activity arising in the pulmonary veins. Pulmonary vein ectopy is often transient, and persistence of AF after this mode of initiation likely depends on atrial substrate factors.

56. Ans. c. Coronary sinus ostium

Hurst's 14th Ed; Page 1876

The AV nodal complex has three related regions: (1) the transitional cell zone, (2) the compact AV node, and (3) the penetrating AV bundle. The transitional zone consists of the main atrial approaches to the compact AV node. The compact AV node is shaped like a half oval and is located beneath the right atrial endocardium at the apex of the triangle of Koch. The triangle of Koch is formed by the base of the septal leaflet of the tricuspid valve and the tendon of Todaro. The coronary sinus ostium is located at the base of this triangle.

57. Ans. d. All of the above

Hurst's 14th Ed; Page 1876

The sinus node receives blood supply from the sinoatrial nodal artery arising from right coronary artery in about 59% of patients, from the left circumflex artery in 38%, and from both arteries with a dual blood supply in 3% patients. The AV node is supplied by the AV nodal artery arising from the right coronary artery in 90% of patients, whereas the left circumflex artery provides it in the remaining 10% of patients. Both the AV nodal artery and branches of the left anterior descending artery supply the bundle of His. The left bundle has a rich blood supply from the AV nodal artery, posterior descending artery, and branches of the left anterior descending artery.

58. Ans. d. All suggests SND

Hurst's 14th Ed; Page 1876

The common manifestation of sinus node dysfunction (SND) is sinus bradycardia interspersed with periods of atrial tachyarrhythmias. The atrial tachyarrhythmias usually range from paroxysmal atrial tachycardia to atrial flutter and atrial fibrillation. Besides sinus bradycardia of varying severity, prolonged sinus arrest and asystole upon termination of the atrial tachyarrhythmias, due to suppression of sinus node and secondary pacemaker is another feature to suggest sinus node dysfunction. Long sinus pauses that occur after electrical cardioversion of atrial fibrillation are another manifestation of sinus node dysfunction. Similarly, chronic atrial fibrillation with a slow ventricular response in the absence of AV nodal-blocking drugs may also be a manifestation of sinus node dysfunction.

59. Ans. d. Short QT syndrome

Hurst's 14th Ed; Page 2016

Mutations in the cardiac specific sodium channel gene (*SCN5A*) have been associated with progressive cardiac conduction system disease referred as Lev or Lenegre disease. It is a common cardiac conduction disorder characterized by age dependent progressive delay in the propagation of cardiac impulse through the His-Purkinje system with right or left bundle branch block, leading to complete AV block. Patients with Lev disease demonstrate fibrosis within the proximal His bundle, whereas those diagnosed with Lenegre disease often demonstrate fibrosis within the more distal bundle branches and Purkinje fibers. SCN5A mutations can produce a variety of other phenotypes, including Brugada syndrome, congenital type 3 long QT syndrome (LQTS), idiopathic ventricular fibrillation, congenital sick sinus syndrome, atrial fibrillation, and dilated cardiomyopathy.

60. Ans. b. Lyme disease

Hurst's 14th Ed; Page 2016

Heart block may result from various conditions. A large variety of infectious diseases may cause Heart block. Heart block associated with endocarditis may be transient or permanent. In patients with endocarditis and ring abscess, the complete AV block may not resolve and pacing may be required. With Lyme disease, cardiac involvement may occur in 8–10% of patients. More than 50% of patients with cardiac involvement may develop advanced heart block requiring temporary pacing. Even complete AV heart block resolves in 1–2 weeks, and permanent pacemaker is rarely needed. Chagas cardiomyopathy may be associated with persistent AV block. Lev or Lenegre disease are progressive cardiac conduction system disorder which requires permanent pacemaker.

61. Ans. d. All of the above

Hurst's 14th Ed; Page 2017

The nuclear envelope proteins Lamin A and C are necessary for structural integrity of the nucleus. In the presence of LMNA mutation, myocardial cells exposed to mechanical stress undergo cell damage. LMNA mutation are associated with dilated cardiomyopathy, with AV conduction defects and is referred to as "laminopathy".

62. Ans. d. Permanent pacemaker is indicated for all

Hurst's 14th Ed; Page 2018

Congenital complete AV block is a rare anomaly that results from abnormal embryonic development of the AV node and is not associated with structural heart disease in 50% of cases. Congenital complete heart block is also associated with maternal lupus erythematosus. Most children with isolated congenital complete AV block have a stable escape rhythm with a narrow QRS complex. Pacing is generally indicated in children with complete heart block if the heart rate in the awake child is <50 bpm or if associated with LV systolic dysfunction or ventricular arrhythmias.

63. Ans. d. All

Hurst's 14th Ed; Page 2023

Atrioventricular dissociation is characterized by atrial and ventricular activity independent of each other. AV dissociation may be secondary to AV block (complete heart block) or physiologic refractoriness. AV dissociation can occur when the sinus rate is slower than the secondary junctional or ventricular pacemaker as in patients with sinus bradycardia, complete heart block and ventricular tachycardia or junctional tachycardia. In patients with complete heart block, the atrial rate is faster than the ventricular rate, whereas in AV dissociation, the ventricular rate is faster than the atrial rate. Although AV dissociation is present in complete heart block, it is not synonymous.

64. Ans. d. Recurrent transient ischemic attacks

Braunwald 11th Ed; Page 602

Tilt table test is used most often in patient with recurrent syncope, although it may be useful in patient with a single syncopal episode with associated injury, particularly in the absence of structural heart disease. In patient with structural heart disease Tilt table test may be indicated in those with syncope in whom other causes of asystole and tachyarrhythmia have been ruled out. Tilt table test is suggested as useful tool in the diagnosis and therapy of recurrent idiopathic vertigo, chronic fatigue syndrome, recurrent transient ischemic attack, and repeated fall of unknown etiology in elderly patients. Tilt table test is relatively contraindicated in the presence of severe CAD with proximal coronary stenosis, known severe cerebrovascular disease, severe mitral stenosis and obstruction to left ventricular outflow tract (aortic stenosis).

65. Ans. d. Obstruction to left ventricular outflow

Braunwald 11th Ed; Page 602

Refer to explanation for Q. No 64.

66. Ans. d. Type II 2° AV block with His-Purkinje block even in absence of symptom

Braunwald 11th Ed; Page 602

Resting and ambulatory ECG is must for diagnosis and management of bradyarrhythmia. Patient presenting with symptomatic bradyarrhythmia may require no further testing. Certain electrocardiographic and electrophysiologic finding may define therapeutic decision in patient without symptoms, e.g., in patients who have type II second-degree AV block the demonstration of His-Purkinje block even in absence of symptom justify implantation of permanent pacemaker, because the risk of progression to complete AV block is high. Asymptomatic sinus bradycardia in patients with heart rate of 35–40 beats/min, sinus arrhythmia with pauses of 2–3 seconds, Wenckebach 2° AV block (particularly during sleep), wandering atrial pacemaker and junctional escape complexes can be completely normal, especially in young people and in well-conditioned athletes.

67. Ans. d. All of the above

Braunwald 11th Ed; Page 602

Refer to explanation for Q. No 66.

68. Ans. c. Sinus tachycardia

Braunwald 11th Ed; Page 603

Supraventricular tachycardias can be classified based on the temporal relationship of the P wave and R wave. When a P wave occurs closer to preceding R wave (i.e., in the first half of the R-R interval), the tachycardia is called a short RP tachycardia, whereas if a P wave occurs in the second half of the RR cycle, the arrhythmia is called a long RP tachycardia. The differential diagnosis of a short RP tachycardia includes typical AVNRT, AVRT, junctional tachycardia, and atrial tachycardia with a markedly prolonged PR interval. Long RP tachycardias include sinus tachycardia, atypical AVNRT, permanent junctional reciprocating tachycardia, and atrial tachycardia.

69. Ans. d. Typical AVNRT

Braunwald 11th Ed; Page 603

Refer to explanation for Q. No 68.

70. Ans. a. AV nodal re-entrant tachycardia

Braunwald 11th Ed; Page 726-727

The method to confirm the participation of accessory pathway in the supraventricular tachycardia is by electrophysiological study. No patient with reciprocating tachycardia from accessory pathway has a VA interval <70 msec—this is measured from onset of ventricular depolarization to the onset earliest atrial activity. In contrast, in most patients with re-entrant AV nodal re-entrant tachycardia interval from onset of ventricular activity to the earliest onset of atrial activity are <70 msec.

71. Ans. b. AV nodal re-entry with no antegrade conduction over accessory pathway

Braunwald 11th Ed; Page 727-728

In patient with pre-excitation syndrome wide QRS tachycardia can be caused by multiple mechanisms: (1) sinus or atrial tachycardia, AV nodal re-entry, an atrial flutter on fibrillation with antegrade conduction over accessory pathway; (2) orthodromic reciprocating tachycardia with functional or preexisting bundle branch block; (3) antidromic reciprocating tachycardia; (4) reciprocating tachycardia with anterograde conduction over one accessory pathway and retrograde conduction over second pathway; (5) tachycardia using nodofascicular or atriofascicular fibre; and (6) ventricular tachycardia.

72. Ans. d. All of the above

Braunwald 11th Ed; Page 728

Accessory pathway can conduct antergradely and retrogradely. Intermittent pre-excitation during sinus rhythm and abrupt loss of conduction over accessory pathway after I/V administration of procainamide and with exercise suggest that refractory period of accessory pathway is long and that the patient is not at risk of rapid ventricular rate during atrial flutter or fibrillation. These are relative specific but not very sensitive approach with a low positive predictive accuracy. Electrophysiological assessment of refractory period of accessory pathway is a more accurate way to assess.

73. Ans. d. Sinus node re-entry

Braunwald 11th Ed; Page 728-729

Relationship between P and QRS can help in differentiating different mechanism of supraventricular tachycardia. P wave during tachycardia that are identical to sinus P wave and that are occur with long RP interval and a short PR interval are most likely caused by sinus node re-entry, sinus tachycardia or an atrial tachycardia arising from right atrium near the sinus node. Retrograde (inverted in Lead II, III, aVF) P wave usually the represent re-entry involving AV junction, either AV nodal re-entry or reciprocating tachycardia using the paraseptal accessory pathway. Depression of ST segment during narrow complex tachycardia generally signifies AV re-entrant tachycardia using an accessory pathway. Tachycardia without manifest P wave is probably caused by AV nodal re-entry (retrograde P wave buried in QRS complex), whereas a tachycardia with RP interval exceeding 90 msec can be caused by accessory pathway. AV dissociation or AV block during tachycardia exclude the participation of AV accessory pathway and makes AV nodal re-entrant tachycardia less likely.

74. Ans. c. Both of the above

Braunwald 11th Ed; Page 728-729

Refer to explanation for Q. No 73.

75. Ans. c. AV re-entrant tachycardia using an accessory pathway

Braunwald 11th Ed; Page 728-729

Refer to explanation for Q. No 73.

76. Ans. b. AV nodal re-entry

Braunwald 11th Ed; Page 728-729

Refer to explanation for Q. No 73.

77. Ans. d. Reciprocating tachycardia by accessory pathway

Braunwald 11th Ed; Page 728-729

Refer to explanation for Q. No 73.

CHAPTER 20 | Cardiac Arrhythmia, Pacing and Electrophysiology

78. Ans. c. Both of the above.

Braunwald 11th Ed; Page 728-729

Refer to explanation for Q. No 73.

79. Ans. d. AV nodal re-entry

Braunwald 11th Ed; Page 728-729

Classification of supraventricular tachycardias based on RP/PR interval

Short RP, long PR interval	Long RP, short PR interval
AV nodal re-entry	Atrial tachycardia
AV re-entry	• Sinus node re-entry • Atypical AV nodal re-entry • AVRT with a slowly conducting accessory pathway (e.g., PJRT)

80. Ans. d. AV nodal re-entry

Braunwald 11th Ed; Page 728-729

Refer to explanation for Q. No 79.

81. Ans. c. Right ventricular outflow tract

Braunwald 11th Ed; Page 602

Significant rhythm disturbances are uncommon in healthy young person. Sinus bradycardia with heart rates of 35-40 beats/min, sinus arrhythmia with pauses exceeding 3 seconds, sinoatrial exit block, type I (Wenckebach) second-degree AV block (often during sleep), wandering atrial pacemaker, junctional escape complexes, and premature atrial complexes and PVCs can be observed and not necessarily abnormal. Frequent and complex atrial and ventricular rhythm disturbances are less frequently observed, however, and type II second-degree AV conduction disturbances are not recorded in normal patients.

82. Ans. c. Hypertrophic cardiomyopathy

Braunwald 11th Ed; Page 602

Refer to explanation for Q. No 81.

83. Ans. d. Type II second-degree AV conduction disturbance

Braunwald 11th Ed; Page 602

Refer to explanation for Q. No 81.

84. Ans. c. More than 15% of the total

Braunwald 11th Ed; Page 652

Long term prognosis of frequent and complex PVCs in asymptomatic healthy patients is very good without an increased risk of death. However, frequent PVCs (>15% of the total) have been shown to produce a cardiomyopathy and heart failure in some people which can be reversed following elimination of PVCs.

85. Ans. c. Treating these PVCs in MI patients improve prognosis

Braunwald 11th Ed; Page 653

The PVCs in asymptomatic healthy patients is very good, without an increased risk of death. Most patients with ischemic heart disease, particularly after MI, exhibit PVCs when they are monitored for 24 hours. The frequency of PVCs progressively increases during the first several weeks and then decreases at about 6 months after myocardial infarction. Frequent and complex PVCs are associated with a two to fivefold increased risk for cardiac or sudden death in patients after MI, but treating these PVCs may not improve the prognosis. The Cardiac Arrhythmia Suppression Trial (CAST) showed that PVCs identified patients at increased risk for sudden death, but that successful suppression of PVCs with flecainide, encainide, or moricizine was associated with increased mortality compared with placebo.

86. Ans. b. H-V interval

Braunwald 11th Ed; Page 656

In patients with AV block, the site of block can be determined from the surface ECG analysis. When the site of block cannot be determined from ECG then invasive EPS is indicated. A-H interval indicates conduction time from sinus node to HIS bundle while the H-V interval provides information about intraventricular conduction disturbance. A prolonged H-V interval (>55 msec) is associated with a greater likelihood for the development of complete AV block. The sinus node recovery time and sinoatrial conduction time gives ideas about sinus node function.

87. Ans. c. Tachyarrhythmia

Braunwald 11th Ed; Page 659

The three common arrhythmic causes of syncope are sinus node dysfunction, AV block and tachyarrhythmias. Of the three, tachyarrhythmia are most reliably evaluated in electrophysiologic laboratory followed by sinus node abnormality and His-Purkinje block.

88. Ans. a. It shorten QT interval

Braunwald 11th Ed; Page 675

Quinidine is a versatile antiarrhythmic drug that was used for treatment of premature supraventricular and ventricular complexes and sustained tachyarrhythmias. Quinidine can slow cardiac conduction manifesting as prolongation QRS duration or sinoatrial or AV nodal conduction disturbance. Quinidine can give rise to syncope in 0.5–2.0% of patients due to self-terminating episode of torsade de pointes. Quinidine prolongs the QT interval in most patients. In recent year there has been renewed interest in the quinidine. It has been found to be useful for treating primary ventricular fibrillation, ventricular arrhythmias in the patients with Brugada syndrome and short QT syndrome. Because it crosses the placenta, quinidine can be used to treat arrhythmias in the fetus.

89. Ans. d. All of the above

Braunwald 11th Ed Page 675

Quinidine prolongs the QT interval leading to syncope due to episodes of torsade de pointes. In patient with quinidine induced syncope significant prolongation (QT interval of 500–600 msec) is often characteristic. Most episodes occur within 2 to 4 days of therapy. Therapy of proarrhythmia requires immediate discontinuation of the drug. Magnesium given intravenously (2 g over 1–2 minutes, followed by an infusion of 3–20 mg/min) is the initial drug of choice. Atrial or ventricular pacing can be used to suppress the ventricular tachyarrhythmia. When pacing is not available, isoproterenol can be given with caution. The arrhythmia gradually dissipates as quinidine is cleared and QT interval returns to baseline.

90. Ans. b. Procainamide

Braunwald 11th Ed; Page 675

Procainamide is used to treat both supraventricular and ventricular tachyarrhythmias. The use of procainamide has diagnostic application when given intravenously (10 mg/kg over 5–10 min). In patients with suspected Brugada syndrome who have a normal resting electrocardiogram (ECG), drug infusion can result in the characteristic "Brugada sign," whereas in patients with WPW syndrome, the drug can cause sudden loss of pre-excitation, a finding indicative of an accessory pathway with a long refractory period and suggesting low risk for a dangerously rapid ventricular rate during atrial fibrillation.

91. Ans. d. Procainamide

Braunwald 11th Ed; Page 675

Refer to explanation for Q. No 90.

92. Ans. c. Corticosteroid administration may eliminate the symptom

Braunwald 11th Ed; Page 677

Patients on procainamide can develop Lupus syndrome characterized by Arthralgia, fever, pleuropericarditis, hepatomegaly, and hemorrhagic pericardial effusion with tamponade. This syndrome occurs more frequently and earlier in patients who are slow acetylators of procainamide and is genetically influenced. Acetylation of procainamide to form NAPA appears to block the SLE-inducing effect. In 60–70% of patients receiving long-term procainamide therapy, ANAs develop, with clinical symptoms occurring in 20–30%, which is reversible when procainamide is stopped. Corticosteroid administration in these patients may eliminate the symptoms. In this syndrome, in contrast to naturally occurring SLE, the brain and kidneys are typically spared, and there is no predilection for women.

93. Ans. d. All of the above

Braunwald 11th Ed; Page 677

Disopyramide has electrophysiologic effects similar to those of quinidine and procainamide. It is used for treatment of ventricular premature complexes and preventing recurrence of VT in selected patients. Disopyramide helps prevent recurrence of atrial fibrillation after successful cardioversion. Because of its vagolytic effects it may be useful in preventing episodes of neurally mediated syncope. It has been used in patients with hypertrophic cardiomyopathy for both AF therapy and its negative inotropic effect.

94. Ans. b. Phenytoin

Braunwald 11th Ed; Page 679

Phenytoin is an antiepileptic drug has antiarrhythmic property of similar to class I-B. Its value as an antiarrhythmic drug is limited to rare cases of digitalis-toxic atrial and ventricular tachyarrhythmias and occasional cases of ventricular arrhythmias when used in combination with other agents.

95. Ans. a. Flecainide is useful for treatment of supraventricular arrhythmias only

Braunwald 11th Ed; Page 679

Flecainide is effective drug in totally suppressing PVCs and short runs of nonsustained VT. Flecainide produces a dose dependent prolongation of VT cycle length which can improve hemodynamic tolerance. Flecainide is also useful in various SVTs, such as atrial tachycardia, atrial flutter, and atrial fibrillation. Flecainide has been used to treat fetal arrhythmias and arrhythmias in children. Flecainide administration can produce ST elevation in lead V_1, characteristic of Brugada syndrome, in susceptible patients and has been used as a diagnostic tool in persons suspected of having Brugada syndrome. Proarrhythmic effects are some of the most important adverse effects of flecainide. Worsening of existing ventricular arrhythmias or the onset of new ventricular arrhythmias can occur in 5–30% of patients, especially in those with preexisting sustained VT, cardiac decompensation, and higher doses of drug. Exercise can amplify the conduction slowing in the ventricle produced by flecainide and in some cases can precipitate a proarrhythmic response. Therefore, exercise testing has been recommended to screen for proarrhythmia before and periodically during treatment.

96. Ans. d. Ibutilide cannot be used in patient with AF with accessory pathway

Braunwald 11th Ed; Page 684

Ibutilide is a class III agents, it prolongs repolarization. Ibutilide is given as an IV IV infusion of 1 mg over 10 minutes. It should not be given in the presence of a QTc interval longer than 440 milliseconds or other drugs that prolong the QT interval or in patients with uncorrected hypokalemia, hypomagnesemia, or bradycardia. Pretreatment with IV magnesium may decrease the risk for ventricular arrhythmias and enhance efficacy in treating some atrial arrhythmias. Ibutilide is indicated for termination of an established episode of atrial flutter or atrial fibrillation. It should not be used in patients with frequent short paroxysms of AF because it merely terminates episodes and is not useful for long-term prevention. Ibutilide prolongs accessory pathway refractoriness and can temporarily slow the ventricular rate during pre-excited atrial fibrillation. The most significant adverse effect of ibutilide is QT prolongation related TdP, which occurs in approximately 2% of patients. This effect develops within the first 4-6 hours of dosing, after which the risk is negligible.

97. Ans. b. Dofetilide

Braunwald 11th Ed; Page 684

Dofetilide is a class III antiarrhythmic drug, which is available only as oral preparation. Dose is from 0.125 to 0.5 mg twice daily and must be initiated in a hospital setting with continuous electrocardiographic monitoring to ensure that inordinate QT prolongation and TDP do not develop. Dofetilide is approved for the acute conversion of AF to sinus rhythm, as well as for chronic suppression of AF.

98. Ans. d. All of the above

Braunwald 11th Ed; Page 681

Amiodarone prolongs the action potential duration and refractoriness of all cardiac fibers without affecting resting membrane potential. Amiodarone noncompetitively antagonizes alpha and beta receptors. Amiodarone also exhibits slow channel blocking effects. The effective refractory period of all cardiac tissues is prolonged. Amiodarone has class I (blocks sodium channel), class II (anti-adrenergic), and class IV (calcium channel blocking effect) in addition to its class III effect.

99. Ans. c. Amiodarone

Braunwald 11th Ed; Page 682

Amiodarone and its active metabolite desethyl amiodarone accumulate extensively in liver, lung, fat "blue skin" and other tissues.

100. Ans. d. Eleclazine

Braunwald 11th Ed; Page 688

Eleclazine hydrochloride is selective blocker of late I_{Na}, which is known to shorten action potential and reduces the dispersion of repolarization. The drug is being developed for use in LQT3 and hypertrophic cardiomyopathy. Vernakalant is a mixed potassium and sodium channel blocker used intravenously for conversion of atrial fibrillation to sinus rhythm. Vernakalant prolongs atrial APD and refractoriness. The safety for IV conversion of AF (initial dose of 3 mg/kg over 10 minutes followed by 2 mg/kg over 15 minutes for persistent arrhythmia) have been demonstrated in the Atrial Arrhythmia Conversion Trials 1 and 3.

101. Ans. c. Lower than 300 mg/day

Braunwald 11th Ed; Page 682

Pulmonary toxicity is the most serious adverse reaction with use of continued therapy with amiodarone on long term at a higher dose. The mechanism is unclear but may involve a hypersensitivity reaction, widespread phospholipidosis, or both. Dyspnea, nonproductive cough, and fever are common symptoms, along with crackles on examination, hypoxia, reduced carbon monoxide diffusion capacity (DLCO), and radiographic evidence of pulmonary infiltrates. Amiodarone must be discontinued and corticosteroids mut be tried. If maintenance dose lower than 300 mg/day is used, pulmonary toxicity is uncommon but can occur.

102. Ans. d. Corneal microdeposits

Braunwald 11th Ed; Page 683

Amiodarone induced pulmonary toxicity is most serious adverse effect of use of amiodarone. The risk of toxicity from this increase with higher plasma concentration. Amiodarone induced pulmonary toxicity correlate better with the cumulative dose rather than with the daily dose or plasma concentration. Although toxicity can occur at any time after treatment is initiated those considered at greatest risks are individual who have received a daily dose of 400 mg or more for >2 months or lower dose commonly 200 mg daily for >2 years. The incidence of amiodarone induced pulmonary toxicity is 5-15% in those who consumes amiodarone 400 mg or more per day. Amiodarone induced pulmonary toxicity is more frequent in men and increases with age. Individual with preexisting lung disease appear to be more susceptible. There is evidence that exposure to supplemental oxygen especially in high concentration alone or when combined with mechanical ventilation may potentiate amiodarone induced pulmonary toxicity. Amiodarone and its metabolite can produce lung damage directly by cytotoxic effect and indirectly by immunological reaction.

Amiodarone induced pulmonary toxicity, the common presentation is that of alveolar or interstitial pneumonitis with subacute onset. Individual usually present with progressive shortness of breath, nonproductive cough, malaise, fever and occasional pleuritic chest pain. The physical examination may be unremarkable in milder cases but in more severely affected individual diffuse rales, hypoxemia and respiratory distress may be noted. The pulmonary function test usually reveals low lung volume and restrictive pattern. A reduced diffusing capacity of lung for carbon monoxide is seen but is nonspecific sign. Variant degree of hypoxemia is seen.

Chest X-ray often reveals patchy or diffuse infiltrates, which are commonly bilateral. Some infiltrates have a ground glass appearance. It has been noted that the right lung especially right upper lobe is more frequently involved than the left lung. Once the diagnosis of amiodarone induced toxicity is considered likely the drug should be discontinued. After stopping amiodarone resolution is likely to be slow and some degree of worsening may occur before improvement is noted. This is due to the long elimination half life of drug and tendency to concentrate in tissue such as lung. Systemic corticosteroids are recommended for treatment of AIPT. Generally, prednisolone is started in dose of 40 mg/day to 60 mg/day orally and tapered slowly. The pharmacodynamic of amiodarone dictate treatment for 4 to 12 months. Cases of relapse on early steroids withdrawal has been reported.

103. Ans. d. Corticosteroid should be used for 3 to 4 weeks for resolution this toxicity

Braunwald 11th Ed; Page 683

Refer to explanation for Q. No 102.

104. Ans. d. Renal dysfunction

Braunwald 11th Ed; Page 682

The three main complication of long-term amiodarone uses are: pulmonary toxicity, thyroid disease and liver toxicity. Pulmonary toxicity progresses slowly in setting of amiodarone used. It can take months to years to develop and occur in about 1-5% of patients taking 200 mg daily and in as many years 15% taking more than 400 mg daily. The pneumonic to remember amiodarone side effect and toxicity are "bitch" *b* for equal to bradycardia/blue man, *i* for interstitial lung disease, *t* for thyroid hypo or hyper; *c* for corneal occlur/cutaneous (skin); *h* for hepatic /hypotension when IV used.

105. Ans. b. Wolff–Chaikoff effect

Ther Adv Endocrinol Metab 2011 Jun 2 (3); 115-126

Wolff-Chaikoff effect is an auto regulatory phenomenon whereby a large amount of ingested iodine acutely inhibits thyroid hormone synthesis within the follicular cell, irrespective of the serum level of thyroid stimulating hormone (TSH). The Wolff-Chaikoff effect is taught to be transient, with the thyroid gland returning to its near normal hormonal synthesis in 26 to 50 hours in normal subjects. It provides temporary protection against thyroid gland synthesizing and excessive quantity of thyroid hormones in states of excess iodine. However, it can also lead to hypothyroidism in susceptible patients with underlying thyroid disease, who can experience a delayed cap from Wolff-Chaikoff effect. The Wolff-Chaikoff effect is an effective means of rejecting a large quantity of imbibed iodide, and therefore, preventing the thyroid from synthesizing large quantities are thyroid hormones.

106. Ans. d. On cessation of amiodarone hypothyroidism resolves in all patients

Ther Adv Endocrinol Metab 2011 Jun 2 (3); 115-126

Amiodarone induced transient changes in thyroid function often occurs in euthyroid individuals. Overt hypothyroidism (TSH >10 mµ/L) develops in 5% of patients and subclinical hypothyroidism (TSH 4.5-10 mµ/L) develops since 25% of patients. Patients with underlying Hashimoto's thyroiditis or positive antithyroid antibodies are more likely to develop persistent hypothyroidism. In iodine sufficient areas, amiodarone induced hypothyroidism is more common than hyperthyroidism and may occur in up to 20% of patients treated with amiodarone. In contrast, amiodarone induced hyperthyroidism is more common than hypothyroidism in iodine deficient reason. Patient should have thyroid function assess several weeks after starting amiodarone and every few months thereafter for development of overt hypothyroidism especially those with evidence of autoimmunity prior to initiating amiodarone. Hypothyroidism should be diagnosed on the basis of screening serum TSH value before the patient has symptom. Small increment in serum TSH (10-20 mµ/L) are seen in euthyroid patients from first 3 to 6 months after amiodarone therapy is initiated. Amiodarone induced hypothyroidism should only be diagnosed when serum T4 concentration are low or mild TSH elevation persist. Thyroid function can be normalized easily by replacement with T4 (levothyroxine) while amiodarone is continued. The goal of therapy is to restore the serum TSH concentration to normal, keeping in mind that a larger than usual dose may be required because of likely effects of amiodarone on intra pituitary T4 metabolism and T3 production and possibility thyroid hormone action. Amiodarone is usually not discontinued unless it fails to control underlying arrhythmia. However, if amiodarone is stopped hypothyroidism in patient with no apparent preexisting thyroid often resolves. In contrast, hypothyroidism may persist after withdrawal of amiodarone in patients who have underlying chronic autoimmune thyroiditis with high titers antithyroid peroxidase (anti TPO) antibodies and goitre and they may require permanent T4 therapy.

107. Ans. d. All

Ther Adv Endocrinol Metab 2011 Jun 2 (3); 115–126

There are two types of amiodarone induced thyrotoxicosis (AIT): In type 1, there is increased synthesis of thyroid hormones, whereby in type 2 there is excess release of T4 and T3 due to a destructive thyroiditis. Type 1 AIT there is hyperthyroidism with increased synthesis of T3 and T4. This type is typically seen in patient with preexisting multinodular goitre or latent grave's disease. The excess iodine from amiodarone provides increase substrate resulting in enhance thyroid production. Type 2 AIT, the hyperthyroidism is a destructive thyroiditis that result in excess release of T4 and T3 without increase hormone synthesis. Atypically occurs in patient without underlying thyroid disease and is caused by a direct toxic effect of amiodarone on thyroid follicular epithelial cells.

108. Ans. c. Both of the above

Ther Adv Endocrinol Metab 2011 Jun 2 (3); 115–126

Refer to explanation for Q. No 107.

109. Ans. d. All of the above

Ther Adv Endocrinol Metab 2011 Jun 2 (3); 115–126

The clinical manifestation of amiodarone hyperthyroidism is often masked because of beta-blocking activity of amiodarone which minimizes many of the adrenergic manifestation of thyroid hormone access and possibly because amiodarone metabolite may block binding of T3 to its nuclear receptor. The amiodarone may be necessary to control a life-threatening arrhythmia and since the half life of elimination from the bodies approximately 100 days, there is no immediate benefit to stopping amiodarone in cases who develop hyperthyroidism. Amiodarone appears to ameliorate hyperthyroidism by blocking T4 to T3 conversion, beta adrenergic receptor and possibly T3 receptor. Stopping amiodarone might actually exacerbate hyperthyroid symptoms and signs. Type 1 AIT is treated with thionamides, radioiodine and surgery while treatment of type 2 AIT requires glucocorticoids or a times surgery for the patients who are refractory to glucocorticoids.

110. Ans. d. Combination of prednisolone and methimazole

Ther Adv Endocrinol Metab 2011 Jun 2 (3); 115–126

Treatment of mechanism unknown patients in amiodarone induced hyperthyroidism where there is a mixed form of thyrotoxicosis is complex. A combination of prednisolone (40 mg/day) and methimazole (40 mg/day) is treatment of choice. A rapid response suggests type 2 hyperthyroidism. The methimazole can then be tapered or stopped and if it indicated iopanoic acid can be added. A poor response suggests type 1 hyperthyroidism. If so steroid can be tapered and depending upon subsequent course, perchlorate, lithium and/or surgery may be necessary.

111. Ans. d. Phenytoin

Braunwald 11th Ed; Page 687

Digoxin related arrhythmia includes bradycardia related to greatly enhance vagal effects (e.g., sinus bradycardia or arrest, AV nodal block) and tachyarrhythmia that may be caused by DAD mediated triggered activity (e.g., atrial, junctional, and fascicular and ventricular tachycardia). The therapy for most bradyarrhythmia consists of withdrawal of digoxin, atropine, or temporary pacing may be needed in symptomatic patients. Phenytoin can be used to control atrial tachyarrhythmias, whereas Lidocaine can be used successfully in treating infra-nodal tachycardia.

112. Ans. c. Lidocaine

Braunwald 11th Ed; Page 687

Refer to explanation for Q. No 111.

113. Ans. d. All of the above

Braunwald 11th Ed; Page 687

Digoxin can be used intravenously to slow the ventricular rate during atrial fibrillation and atrial flutter. Digoxin is not effective in terminating episode of acute or recent onset AF and its conversion to sinus rhythm. The digoxin more often used orally to control ventricular ate in permanent AF. When a patient with atrial fibrillation at rest and vagal tone predominate ventricular rate can be maintained with in 60–100 beats/min in 40–60% cases. However, when patient begin to exercise, decrease in vagal tone and increase in adrenergic tone combined to diminish the beneficial effect of digoxin on AV nodal conduction and therefore, patient can experience a marked increase in ventricular rate even with mild exertion. Digoxin is therefore, rarely use as a single agent to control the ventricular rate in AF. The drug has little ability to prevent episode of paroxysmal AF and to control the ventricular rate during episode and may even provoke episodes in patients with so called vagal AF. The electrical DC cardioversion should be performed only in cases of life-threatening arrhythmia due to digitalis toxicity, only when absolutely necessary because life threatening VT or VF can result and can be difficult to control.

114. Ans. a. Atrial flutter

Braunwald 11th Ed; Page 688

Electrical cardioversion is most effective in terminating tachycardia related to re-entry such as atrial flutter and many cases of atrial fibrillation, AV node re-entry, reciprocating tachycardia associated with WPW syndrome, most form of ventricular tachycardia, ventricular flutter, and ventricular fibrillation. Tachycardias thought to be caused by disorder of impulse formation (automaticity) includes parasystole, some form of tachycardia, junctional tachycardia (with or without digitalis), accelerated idioventricular rhythm and relatively uncommon forms of ventricular tachycardias. Any attempt to cardiovert these tachycardias electrically is not indicated in most cases because they typically recur within second after shock. The mechanism behind this phenomenon is the release of endogenous catecholamine consequent to shock can further exacerbate the arrhythmia. It has not been established whether cardioversion can terminate tachycardia caused by enhance automaticity or triggered activity.

115. Ans. d. Ventricular flutter or VF

Braunwald 11th Ed; Page 688

Synchronized shock is used for all cardioversion except for very rapid ventricular tachyarrhythmias such as ventricular flutter or ventricular fibrillation. For cardioversion of defibrillation energies greater than those for synchronize cardioversion are required, and synchronization is not necessary because there is no vulnerable period of the T wave to avoid.

116. Ans. d. Atrial fibrillation

Braunwald 11th Ed; Page 688

During DC cardioversion the minimum effective electrical shock should be titrated to avoid shock related myocardial damage. Except for atrial fibrillation shock in range of 25-50 joules successfully terminate most of the SVTs. The starting level to terminate atrial fibrillation with monophasic machine should be no <100 joules and with the biphasic system a shock as low as 25 joules may succeed.

117. Ans. d. Symptomatic AF of <12 months duration

Braunwald 11th Ed; Page 689

Favourable candidate for electrical cardioversion of atrial fibrillation includes patients who: (1) have symptomatic AF of <12 months duration; (2) continue to have AF after the precipitating cause has been removed; (3) have a rapid ventricular rate that is difficult to slow and (4) have symptoms of decreased cardiac output (fatigue, light headedness, dyspnea) attributable to lack of atrial contraction contribution to ventricular filling. Unfavourable candidates include patients with: (a) digitalis toxicity; (b) no symptoms and a well-controlled ventricular rate without therapy; (c) sinus node dysfunction, bradycardia, tachycardia syndrome; (d) large left atrium and long standing AF; (e) episodes of AF that revert spontaneously to sinus rhythm; (g) no mechanical atrial systole after the return of electrical atrial systole; (h) AF and complete heart block; (i) antiarrhythmic drug intolerance.

118. Ans. d. Symptomatic AF of <12 months duration

Braunwald 11th Ed; Page 689

AF is more likely to recur after cardioversion in patients who have significant chronic obstructive lung disease, congestive heart failure, mitral valve disease (particularly mitral regurgitation), AF present longer than 1 year and large left atrium (echocardiographic diameter >4.5 cm).

119. Ans. b. Atrial flutter

Braunwald 11th Ed; Page 689

In patients with atrial flutter slowing the ventricular rate by administration of beta or calcium channel blocker or terminating the flutter with antiarrhythmic agent may be difficult and electrical cardioversion is often the treatment of choice. For patients with other types of SVT, electrical cardioversion may be used when: (1) vagal manoeuvre or simple medical management with IV adenosine or verapamil has failed to terminate tachycardia; (2) clinical setting indicate that prompt restoration of sinus rhythm is desirable because of hemodynamic decompensation.

120. Ans. c. Nitrous oxide

Braunwald 11th Ed; Page 691

Catheter deliver cryoablation causes tissue damage by freezing cellular structure. Nitrous oxide is delivered to the tip of catheter where it is allowed to internally boil and cool the tip electrode after which gas is circulated back to the delivery console. Catheter tip temperature can be regulated with cooling as low as (-) 80°. Cooling to 0°C causes reversal loss of function and can be used as a diagnostic test (i.e., termination of a tachycardia when the catheter is in contact with the group of cells critical to its perpetuation, or determining its effect on normal conduction when close to AV node). The catheter tip can then be cooled and mould deeply to produce permanent damage and cure of arrhythmia.

121. Ans. d. All of the above

Braunwald 11th Ed; Page 730

The ventricular rate during untreated atrial fibrillation typically is 100-160 beats/min. Patients with WPW syndrome can experienced ventricular rate during atrial fibrillation exceeding 250 beats/min, because of conduction over the accessory pathway. The ventricular rate during atrial fibrillation can appear more regular when the rate is extremely rapid (>170 beats/min), when a junctional tachycardia independently controls the ventricle, when there is a high degree AV block with a regular escape rhythm or when the QRS complexes are fully paste.

122. Ans. c. Permanent

Braunwald 11th Ed; Page 730

Atrial fibrillation can be classified according to duration. Atrial fibrillation that terminates spontaneously within 7 days is terms "paroxysmal" and atrial fibrillation present continuously for >7 days is called "persistent". Atrial fibrillation that persists for longer than one year is terms "longstanding persistent" whereas longstanding AF refractory to cardioversion is term "permanent".

123. Ans. c. They are at higher risk of thromboembolic complications

Braunwald 11th Ed; Page 730

Lone atrial fibrillation referred to atrial fibrillation that occurs in patients younger than 60 years who do not have hypertension or any evidence of structural heart disease. Patients with lone atrial fibrillation are at lower risk of thromboembolic complication eliminating the necessity for anticoagulation. They also may be more likely to have familiar or genetic causes. In addition, the absence of structural heart disease allows the safe use of rhythm-controlled drug such as flecainide in patients with lone atrial fibrillation.

124. Ans. b. Disopyramide

Braunwald 11th Ed; Page 730

Paroxysmal atrial fibrillation is classified clinically on the basis of autonomic setting in which it most often occurs. In approximately 25% of patients with paroxysmal AF have vagotonic AF during which AF is initiated in the setting of high vagal tone, typically during the relaxing or sleep time. Drug exerting a vagotonic effect (digitalis) can aggravate vagotonic AF and drug with a vagolytic effect (disopyramide) may be particularly appropriate for prophylactic therapy. Adrenergic AF occurs in approximately 10-15% of patients with paroxysmal AF in the setting of high sympathetic tone as during strenuous exertion. In patients with adrenergic atrial fibrillation, beta blocker not only provide rate control but can prevent the onset of AF.

125. Ans. d. All of the above are risk factors

Braunwald 11th Ed; Page 731

The incidence of AF is age and gender related. Congestive heart failure, aortic and mitral valve disease, left atrial enlargement, hypertension and advanced age are independent risk factors for development of atrial fibrillation, as are obesity and obstructive sleep apnea. Another risk factor is psoriasis which when severe triples the risk of AF in patients younger than 50.

126. Ans. a. Hypertension with left ventricular hypertrophy

Braunwald 11th Ed; Page 732

The majority of patients with atrial fibrillation have hypertension (usually with left ventricular hypertrophy) or some other forms of structural heart disease. In addition to hypertensive heart disease, the most common cardiac abnormality associated with atrial fibrillation are ischemic heart disease, mitral valve disease, hypertrophic cardiomyopathy and dilated cardiomyopathy. Less common causes of atrial fibrillation are restrictive cardiomyopathies such as amyloidosis, constrictive pericarditis, cardiac tumor. Severe pulmonary hypertension is often associated with AF.

127. Ans. b. Hyperthyroidism

Braunwald 11th Ed; Page 732

The AF can have causes that are temporary or reversible. The most common temporary causes are excessive alcohol intake (holiday heart), open heart or thoracic surgery, myocardial infarction, pericarditis, myocarditis, and pulmonary embolism. The most common correctable cause is hyperthyroidism.

128. Ans. d. All of the above

Braunwald 11th Ed; Page 733

The strongest predictor of ischemic stroke and systemic thromboembolism in patients with atrial fibrillation are a history of stroke or transient ischemic episode and mitral stenosis. When patients with atrial fibrillation and a prior ischemic stroke are treated with aspirin the risk of another stroke is very high in the range of 10-12% per year. On the other hand, in patients with lone atrial fibrillation, cumulative 15 years of risk of stroke in the range of 1-2%. Besides prior stroke the best-established risk factor for stroke in patient with nonvalvular AF are diabetes, hypertension, heart failure and age 70 or older.

129. Ans. d. All of the above

Braunwald 11th Ed; Page 733

Refer to explanation for Q. No 128.

130. Ans. b. Risk of stroke is lower in patient with paroxysmal AF than in patient with persistent AF

Braunwald 11th Ed; Page 733

By definition the burden of AF is greater in patient with persistent AF than in patient with paroxysmal AF. It may be reasonable to assume that the risk of stroke is lower in patients with occasional episode of self-limited AF than in patients with AF continuously. However, the available data indicate that the risk of thromboembolic complication is the same in patient with paroxysmal and persistent AF. Accordingly, guidelines recommendation for anticoagulation are the same in patient with paroxysmal and persistent AF.

131. Ans. c. AF which is clinically silent but detected by implantable pacemaker and cardioverter defibrillators (ICDs)

Braunwald 11th Ed; Page 734

Current dual chamber pacemaker and implantable cardioverter defibrillator (ICD) are capable of detecting short episodes of asymptomatic AF that otherwise would not have been detected clinically. These subclinical atrial tachyarrhythmias are independently associated with a 2.5 folds increase in the risk of stroke.

132. Ans. b. Aspirin and platelet inhibitor clopidogrel

Braunwald 11th Ed; Page 734

Combination therapy with aspirin and platelet inhibitor clopidogrel is more efficacious than aspirin alone for prevention of thromboembolic complication in patients with CHADS II score >1 and who are not able to tolerate anticoagulation with warfarin or NOAC. The potential benefit of combination therapy with aspirin plus clopidogrel may out way the increased risk of bleeding complication in high-risk patients who are not suitable candidates for warfarin or NOACs.

133. Ans. d. NOACs can be used safely in patients with renal disease

Braunwald 11th Ed; Page 734-735

Direct thrombin inhibitor and factor Xa inhibitors have several advantages over vitamin K antagonist such as warfarin, the most notable being a fixed dose regimen that eliminate the need for monitoring of a laboratory test such as INR. Dabigatran, an oral direct thrombin inhibitor and rivaroxaban and apixaban, factor Xa inhibitors are approved drugs for prevention of stroke/embolism in patients with nonvalvular AF. One of the most serious risks of anticoagulation is intracranial hemorrhage. Recent studies have indicated that the risk of intracranial hemorrhage is about 50% lower with NOACs compared to warfarin. The NOACs in addition to eliminating the need for laboratory monitoring have other advantage over warfarin like fewer drug interaction, no food interaction and rapid onset of action that obviates the need for bridging therapy. However, there are some disadvantages compared to warfarin like higher cost, more gastrointestinal side effects in the case of dabigatran, twice-daily dosing for dabigatran and apixaban, and absence of a readily available laboratory test to verify compliance. Furthermore, these agents cannot be used safely in patients with severe renal disease. Another limitation is that there are no specific reversal agents for all the NOACs.

134. Ans. c. 2.0 or higher

Braunwald 11th Ed; Page 735

Low molecular weight heparin (LMWH) has a longer half life than unfractionated heparin and a predictable antithrombotic effect is attained with a fixed dosage administered subcutaneously twice daily. LMWH is a practical alternative to unfractionated heparin for initiation of anticoagulation with warfarin in patients with AF. Bridging therapy with LMWH be continued until the INR is 2.0 or higher.

135. Ans. d. All of the above

Braunwald 11th Ed; Page 736

The advantages of early cardioversion in case of AF is relief of symptom, avoidance of the need for TEE or therapeutic anticoagulation for 3-4 weeks before cardioversion, if cardioversion is performed within 48 hours of AF onset and possibly a lower risk of early AF recurrence because of less atrial remodeling. A reason to defer cardioversion is the unavailability of TEE and in an unanticoagulated patient with AF of unclear duration or duration >48 hours.

136. Ans. c. It is unlikely to be effective if the duration of AF is longer than 48 hours

Braunwald 11th Ed; Page 736

For management of atrial fibrillation, cardioversion can be performed early in the course of an episode of AF, there is option of either pharmacologic or electrical cardioversion. Pharmacologic cardioversion has advantage of not requiring general anesthesia or deep sedation. Beside this, the probability of an immediate recurrence of AF is lower with pharmacologic cardioversion than with electrical cardioversion. Pharmacological cardioversion is associated with the risk of adverse drug effect and is not as effective as electrical cardioversion. Pharmacologic cardioversion is unlikely to be effective if the duration of AF is longer than 7 days.

137. Ans. a. Lidocaine

Braunwald 11th Ed; Page 736

Drugs that can be administered intravenously for cardioversion of AF consist of ibutilide, procainamide, and amiodarone. For AF episodes >2-3 days in duration, efficacy is approximately 60-70% for ibutilide, 40-50% for amiodarone, and 30-40% for procainamide. Acute pharmacologic cardioversion of AF also can be attempted with oral drugs in patients without structural heart disease. The most common oral agents for acute conversion of AF are propafenone (300-600 mg) and flecainide (100-200 mg).

138. Ans. a. Flecainide

Braunwald 11th Ed; Page 736

Refer to explanation for Q. No 137.

139. Ans. d. All are correct

Braunwald 11th Ed; Page 736

The transthoracic cardioversion is efficacious in 95% of cases of atrial fibrillation. Biphasic waveform shocks convert AF more effectively than monophasic waveform shocks and allow the use of lower energy shocks, resulting in less skin irritation. An appropriate first-shock strength using a biphasic waveform is 150–200 J, followed by higher output shocks if needed. If a 360J biphasic shock is unsuccessful, ibutilide should be infused before another shock is delivered because it lowers the defibrillation energy requirement and improves the success rate of transthoracic cardioversion. Transthoracic cardioversion can fail to restore sinus rhythm. An increase in shock strength or infusion of ibutilide often results in successful repeat cardioversion. Another type of failure is an immediate recurrence of AF within a few seconds of successful conversion to sinus rhythm. This occurs in approximately 25% for episodes <24 hours in duration and 10% for episodes >24 hours in duration. For this type of cardioversion failure, an increase in shock strength is of no value. If the patient has not been receiving an oral rhythm-control agent, infusion of ibutilide may be helpful to prevent an immediate recurrence of AF.

140. Ans. b. Less than 48 hours

Braunwald 11th Ed; Page 736

Therapeutic anticoagulation is necessary for 3 weeks or more before cardioversion to prevent thromboembolic complications if the AF has been ongoing for >48 hours. If the time of onset of AF is unclear, for the sake of safety, AF duration should be assumed to be >48 hours. If the duration of AF is known to be <48 hours, cardioversion can be performed without anticoagulation. To improve the safety margin, it may be appropriate to use a 24-hour cut off for the AF duration that allows safe cardioversion without anticoagulation.

141. Ans. d. Four weeks

Braunwald 11th Ed; Page 736

All the patients who undergo pharmacologic or electrical cardioversion they should be anticoagulated for 4 weeks after successful cardioversion to prevent thromboembolic complications that may occur because of atrial stunning.

142. Ans. a. Significantly lower rate of hospitalization

Braunwald 11th Ed; Page 736

Several randomized studies have compared a rate-control strategy with a rhythm-control strategy in patients with atrial fibrillation. Overall, these studies have demonstrated a significantly lower rate of rehospitalization with a rate-control strategy, but no significant differences in other major outcomes, such as all-cause mortality, strokes, bleeding events, worsening heart failure, or quality of life.

143. Ans. d. Pindolol

Braunwald 11th Ed; Page 737

The oral agents available for long-term heart rate control in patients with AF are digitalis, beta blockers, calcium channel antagonists, and amiodarone. The first-line agents for rate control are beta blockers and the calcium channel blockers verapamil and diltiazem. A combination is often used to improve efficacy and to limit side effects by allowing the use of smaller dosages of the individual drugs. In patients with sinus node dysfunction and tachy-brady syndrome, the use of a beta blocker with intrinsic sympathomimetic activity (pindolol, acebutolol) may provide rate control without aggravating sinus bradycardia.

144. Ans. d. Amiodarone

Braunwald 11th Ed; Page 737

Amiodarone is much less frequently used drug for rate control in patient with atrial fibrillation, because of risk of organ toxicity associated with long-term therapy. Amiodarone can be an appropriate choice for rate control if other agents are not tolerated or are ineffective. Amiodarone is an appropriate choice for a patient with persistent AF, heart failure, and reactive airway disease who cannot tolerate either a calcium channel antagonist or a beta blocker and who has a rapid ventricular rate despite treatment with digitalis.

145. Ans. d. Amiodarone

Braunwald 11th Ed; Page 737

Ventricular proarrhythmia from class 1A agents such as quinidine, procainamide, disopyramide and class III agents like sotalol, dofetilide, dronedarone, amiodarone, manifests as QT prolongation and polymorphic ventricular tachycardia (torsade de pointes). Risk of torsade de pointes appears to be much lower with amiodarone and dronedarone than with other class III drugs.

The ventricular proarrhythmia from class IC agents (flecainide and propafenone) manifests as monomorphic ventricular tachycardia, sometimes associated with widening of the QRS complex during sinus rhythm but not QT prolongation.

146. Ans. d. Class III drugs

Braunwald 11th Ed; Page 737

Refer to explanation for Q. No 145.

147. Ans. d. All of the above

Braunwald 11th Ed; Page 737

The best options for drug therapy to suppress AF depend on the patient's comorbidities. In patients with lone AF or minimal heart disease (e.g., mild left ventricular hypertrophy), flecainide, propafenone, sotalol, and dronedarone are reasonable first-line drugs, and amiodarone and dofetilide can be considered if the first-line agents are ineffective or not tolerated. In patients with substantial left ventricular hypertrophy (left ventricular wall thickness >15 mm), the hypertrophy heightens the risk of ventricular proarrhythmia, and the safest choices for drug therapy are amiodarone and dronedarone. In patients with coronary artery disease, several of the class I agents have been found to increase the risk of death, and the safest first-line options are dofetilide and sotalol, with amiodarone reserved for use as a second-line agent. In patients with heart failure, several antiarrhythmic drugs have been associated with increased mortality, and the only two drugs known to have a neutral effect on survival are amiodarone and dofetilide.

148. Ans. d. Amiodarone/Dronedarone

Braunwald 11th Ed; Page 737

Refer to explanation for Q. No 147.

149. Ans. a. Sotalol/Dofetilide

Braunwald 11th Ed; Page 737

Refer to explanation for Q. No 147.

150. Ans. a. Amiodarone

Braunwald 11th Ed; Page 737

Refer to explanation for Q. No 147.

151. Ans. d. All of the above

Braunwald 11th Ed; Page 738

Experimental studies have indicated that angiotensin-converting enzyme (ACE) inhibitors and angiotensin receptor blockers (ARBs) have favorable effects on electrical and structural remodeling. A meta-analysis demonstrated that the strongest beneficial effects have been observed with ARBs and in patients with heart failure. Some evidence indicates that statins prevent AF, perhaps because of their anti-inflammatory effects. A systematic review of 16 observational studies demonstrated a 12% reduction in the relative risk of new onset AF and a 15% reduction in recurrent AF in patients treated with statins. Similar observation has been there with consumption of omega-3 polyunsaturated fatty acids because of their anti-inflammatory and antioxidant effects and also they are known to have direct ion channel effects.

152. Ans. d. All occurs with equal frequency

Braunwald 11th Ed; Page 739

The risk of major complications from radiofrequency catheter ablation of AF is reported to be 5–6%. The most common major complications are cardiac tamponade, pulmonary vein stenosis and cerebral thromboembolism, each with a prevalence of approximately 1%. The risk of a femoral vascular injury is reported to be 1–2%.

153. Ans. d. Esophageal perforation

Braunwald 11th Ed; Page 739

The risk of esophageal perforation is reported in the range of 0.01–0.02%. This complication is of great concern as it often proves lethal.

154. Ans. d. Phrenic nerve injury

Braunwald 11th Ed; Page 740

The complication associated with cryoablation catheter are cardiac tamponade (~1%), femoral vascular injury (1–2%) and phrenic nerve injury. The incidence of right phrenic nerve injury is approximately 10%, with the injury resolving within 12 months in almost all patients. Injury to the left phrenic nerve is possible but rare.

155. Ans. d. Flecainide

Braunwald 11th Ed; Page 742

Atrial fibrillation is common after open heart surgery and is occurs in 25–40% of patients who undergo coronary artery bypass graft surgery or valve replacement. AF is associated with a twofold increase in the risk of postoperative stroke and is the most common reason for prolonged hospitalization. The incidence of AF peaks on the second postoperative day. The antiarrhythmic drugs that decrease the risk of postoperative AF are amiodarone and sotalol by 50–65%, and beta blockers by approximately 30%. Hypomagnesemia is common after open heart surgery and can increase the risk of AF. Magnesium administration is reported to decreases the risk of postoperative AF by 20–40%. Colchicine, atorvastatin, and steroids also have been demonstrated in randomized studies to reduce the risk of AF after open heart surgery by approximately 35–40%. The main mechanism by which these agents prevent AF probably is an anti-inflammatory effect. A novel approach to the prevention of AF after cardiac surgery is injection of botulinum toxin into the four major epicardial fat pads at operation. This causes temporary autonomic blockade and has been shown to reduce the incidence of AF after CABG to <10%.

156. Ans. d. All of the above

Braunwald 11th Ed; Page 742

Refer to explanation for Q. No 155.

157. Ans. d. Flecainide

Braunwald 11th Ed; Page 742

Refer to explanation for Q. No 155.

158. Ans. d. Beta blockers

Braunwald 11th Ed; Page 743

New-onset AF occurs postoperatively in <5% of patients undergoing major noncardiac surgery. Some of the possible mechanisms are sympathetic activation, electrolyte abnormalities and hypoxia. Beta blockers have been shown to reduce the risk of AF after major noncardiac surgery by approximately 25%.

159. Ans. c. Procainamide

Braunwald 11th Ed; Page 743

Patients with the WPW syndrome and an accessory pathway with a short refractory period can experience a very rapid ventricular rate during atrial fibrillation. Patients with WPW syndrome who present in AF with a rapid ventricular rate should undergo transthoracic cardioversion if there is a hemodynamic instability. If the patient is hemodynamically stable, intravenous procainamide or ibutilide can be used for pharmacologic cardioversion. Procainamide is preferable to ibutilide because it blocks accessory pathway conduction and slows the ventricular rate before AF has converted to sinus rhythm. Digitalis and calcium channel antagonists are contraindicated in patients with WPW syndrome and AF. These agents selectively block conduction in the AV node and can result in acceleration of conduction through the accessory pathway.

160. Ans. d. All of the above

Braunwald 11th Ed; Page 743

The preferred therapy for patients with WPW syndrome and AF with a rapid ventricular rate is catheter ablation of the accessory pathway. The efficacy of catheter ablation is 95% or higher for most types of accessory pathways, and the risk of a major complication is very low. AF typically does not recur after successful accessory pathway ablation, probably because AF in WPW syndrome often is as a result of atrioventricular reciprocating tachycardia (AVRT).

161. Ans. d. Amiodarone

Braunwald 11th Ed; Page 743

Atrial fibrillation occurs in approximately 25% of patients with hypertrophic cardiomyopathy and can cause severe hemodynamic impairment because of an inadequate diastolic filling time and loss of atrioventricular synchrony. Because of a high risk of thromboembolic complications, anticoagulation is indicated in AF patients with HCM, independent of the CHA_2DS_2-VASc score. Severe left ventricular hypertrophy increases the risk of drug-induced torsade de pointes, and the only rhythm-control agents recommended for patients with HCM and a wall thickness >1.5 cm are dronedarone and amiodarone.

162. Ans. d. Intravenous metoprolol

Braunwald 11th Ed; Page 744

Transthoracic cardioversion is considered safe at all stages of pregnancy. The recommended pharmacologic agents for acute management of AF consist of intravenous metoprolol for rate control and flecainide or sotalol for conversion to sinus rhythm. For rate control, digoxin can be used and if it ineffective, a beta blocker can be used, but only after first trimester. If there is no structural heart disease, flecainide and sotalol are recommended for long term rhythm control. In the patient with structural heart disease, amiodarone is recommended for rhythm control.

163. Ans. d. Flecainide or sotalol

Braunwald 11th Ed; Page 744

Refer to explanation for Q. No 162.

164. Ans. a. Transthoracic cardioversion is not safe in the first trimester of pregnancy

Braunwald 11th Ed; Page 744

Refer to explanation for Q. No 162.

165. Ans. d. Ibutilide

Braunwald 11th Ed; Page 744

Short acting drug Ibutilide can be given intravenously to convert atrial flutter. Ibutilide successfully cardiovert approximately 60–90% of episodes of atrial flutter. Other medications, such as procainamide or amiodarone, can be given to convert atrial flutter chemically, but they are generally less effective than ibutilide.

166. Ans. d. Class IC and III.

Braunwald 11th Ed; Page 719

Drugs that slow conduction in and prolong refractoriness of the accessory pathway and atrioventricular node

Affected tissue	Drugs
Accessory pathway	Class IA
AV Node	• Class II • Class IV • Adenosine • Digitalis
Both	• Class IC • Class III (amiodarone)

167. Ans. a. Class I a

Braunwald 11th Ed; Page 719

Refer to explanation for Q. No 166.

168. Ans. b. Re-entry over a concealed (retrograde only) accessory pathway

Braunwald 11th Ed; Page 719

The presence of an accessory pathway that conducts unidirectionally from the ventricle to the atrium but not in the reverse direction is not apparent by analysis of the ECG during sinus rhythm because the ventricle is not pre-excited. Therefore, electrocardiographic manifestations of WPW syndrome are absent, and the accessory pathway is "concealed." During a macroreentrant tachycardia when the anterograde conduction occurs over AV node–His bundle pathway and retrograde conduction over this concealed accessory pathway, it results in AV reciprocating tachycardia. On electrocardiographic examination, a tachycardia resulting from this mechanism can be suspected when the QRS complex is normal and the retrograde P wave occurs after completion of the QRS complex, in the ST segment, or early in the T wave. And sometimes the P wave is not clearly visible and can result in depression of the ST segment. During an episode of reciprocating tachycardia.

169. Ans. d. Diabetic neuropathy

Braunwald 11th Ed; Page 710

Sinus tachycardia is increase in the sinus node discharge, and it is common in infancy and childhood, and it is normal reaction to various physiologic or pathophysiologic stresses such as fever, hypotension, thyrotoxicosis, anemia, anxiety, exertion, hypovolemia, pulmonary emboli, myocardial ischemia, congestive heart failure, and in peripheral neuropathies. The most common reversible cause includes hyperthyroidism, anemia, infection, inflammation and hypovolemia. Diabetic neuropathy is also common but not reversible.

170. Ans. c. Amiodarone

Braunwald 11th Ed; Page 686

The absorption of orally administered drug from the gut lumen to the systemic circulation, and efficiency of this absorption is defined as "bioavailability". Various factors affect the bioavailability of drugs. Many antiarrhythmic drugs have a *food-fast effect*; that is, the bioavailability of a drug may be changed several-fold in presence of food or during fasting. Oral amiodarone is three times more bioavailable after a high-fat meal.

171. Ans. c. VDD mode

Braunwald 11th Ed; Page 784

The basic pacing mode in single chamber is VVI mode. Pacing occurs when the ventricular rate slows below the programmed lower rate limit of pacemaker. There is no atrial sensing, so AV synchrony is not preserved. This mode is indicated in patients with permanent AF and in those in whom AV synchrony is less important than simplicity of the pacing system.

The AAI mode is the corresponding single-chamber atrial pacing mode, it is appropriate for patients with sinus node dysfunction and intact AV conduction. Because it does not provide ventricular pacing, AAI mode should not be used in patients who are at high risk for AV block.

The DDD pacing mode preserves AV synchrony whenever possible. In DDD mode the atrial rate cannot go lower than the programmed lower rate and the AV delay is the maximum permitted time from an atrial event to a ventricular event. If a spontaneous ventricular event does not occur by the time the AV delay elapses, a ventricular paced event occurs. In the setting of AV block, all ventricular events are paced. The special characteristic of the DDD pacing mode is the ability to "track" intrinsic atrial activity so that a ventricular beat follows each P wave in order to maintain AV synchrony. The DDI and VDD pacing modes comprise complementary subsets of DDD functionality. The DDI mode lacks atrial tracking and is suitable for patients with sinus bradycardia, with or without intact AV conduction. Because AV synchrony is lost when the sinus rate exceeds the lower rate limit, the DDI mode is rarely programmed unless atrial sensing problems prevent reliable mode switching in DDD mode. The VDD mode lacks atrial pacing and is suitable for patients with normal sinus node function and AV block. It can be achieved using a single lead with additional atrial sensing electrodes, permitting ventricular tracking of atrial activity to achieve AV synchrony. The VDD mode should not be used in patients with sinus bradycardia, since ventricular pacing without AV synchrony will occur at the lower rate limit, equivalent to the VVI mode.

In DDD mode, there is a provision of automatic mode switch. Automatic mode switching initiates a temporary mode change to a nontracking mode (usually DDI or DDIR) in response to an atrial sensed rate above a specified value. When the atrial rhythm slows sufficiently, the mode switches back to an atrial tracking mode. "Noise" reversion algorithms are intended to prevent pacemaker inhibition during continuous ventricular oversensing, such as that occurring during EMI. They initiate a fixed-rate, asynchronous pacing modes (DOO, VOO) for the duration of oversensing. During procedure which requires constant electrocautery pacemaker should be programmed to be OO or AOO mode.

172. Ans. b. VOO mode/AOO mode

Braunwald 11th Ed; Page 784

Refer to explanation for Q. No 171.

173. Ans. d. AAI mode

Braunwald 11th Ed; Page 784

Refer to explanation for Q. No 171.

174. Ans. d. High septal pacing near HIS bundle

Braunwald 11th Ed; Page 783

Dual chamber pacing in patients with impaired AV conduction ensures that the AV interval is in physiologic range. However, right ventricular apical pacing produces both intraventricular and interventricular dyssynchrony, even if the pacing pulse is synchronized to the atrial impulse. Pacing alternative RV sites such as septum and outflow tract have not reduced dyssynchrony consistently. Pacing-induced dyssynchrony is hemodynamically significant in patients with left ventricular dysfunction, in whom it increases the incidence of heart failure and persistent atrial fibrillation. The alternative approach to achieve maximum hemodynamic effect is to pace HIS bundle using an active fixation RV lead. The paced QRS complex activates the ventricle over the physiologic His-Purkinje system, restoring ventricular electrical synchrony in patients with normal ventricular conduction and in some with bundle branch block. Compared with RV apical pacing, small randomized studies indicate that His bundle pacing improves exercise capacity, ventricular synchrony, and LV ejection fraction. The success rate of HIS bundle pacing is around 80%, and pacing thresholds are more than twice as high as RV thresholds, reducing the generator longevity.

175. Ans. d. VVI (R)

Braunwald 11th Ed; Page 785

In patients with long standing atrial fibrillation with AV block, the pacing mode of choice is VVI (R).

176. Ans. b. Brugada's syndrome

Hurst's 14th Ed; Page 1524 & 1916

Brugada syndrome was introduced as a new clinical entity by Pedro and Josep Brugada in 1992. The syndrome has attracted considerable interest because of its high incidence in many parts of the world and its association with high-risk of sudden death, especially in males as they enter their third and fourth decade of life. Sudden unexplained nocturnal death syndrome (SUNDS), also known as Sudden unexplained death syndrome (SUDS), a disorder most prevalent in south east Asia and Burgada syndrome have recently been shown to be phenotypically, genetically and functionally the same disorder.

177. Ans. a. AV nodal reentrant tachycardia

Hurst's 14th Ed; Page 1967

The term paroxysmal supraventricular tachycardia (PSVT) refers to a clinical syndrome characterized by a rapid, regular tachycardia with abrupt onset and termination. Approximately two-thirds of cases of PSVT result from AV nodal re-entrant tachycardia (AVNRT). Orthodromic AV reciprocating tachycardia (AVRT) which involves an accessory pathway is the second most common cause of PSVT, accounting for approximately one-third of cases. The term Wolff-Parkinson-White syndrome (WPW) designates a condition comprising both pre-excitation and tachyarrhythmias. Atrial tachycardias which arise exclusively from atrial tissue, account for approximately 5% of all cases of PSVT.

178. Ans. b. Arrhythmogenic right ventricular dysplasia

Hurst's 10th Ed; Page 1800

Arrhythmogenic right ventricular dysplasia (ARVD) is characterized by fatty infiltration, fibrosis and thinning of the right ventricle and is associated with ventricular arrhythmias and sudden death. Although most cases appear to be sporadic, approximately 30% of patients have a family history of ARVD. Epsilon waves, or small high frequency deflections found in the terminal portion of the QRS complex in leads V_1-V_3 may be present. The diagnosis of ARVD is challenging in some cases. A task force proposed several criteria for the diagnosis of ARVD. This consensus of experts, several major and minor diagnostic criteria are described. The major criteria include the following:

- Severe dilatation and reduction in RVEF with normal LV function
- Localized RV aneurysms
- Severe segmental dilation of the RV
- Fibrofatty replacement of myocardium on endomyocardial biopsy
- An epsilon wave present on the 12-lead electrocardiogram
- A family history of ARVD confirmed at necropsy or surgery

The minor criteria include the following:
- Mild global RV dilation or EF reduction with normal LV
- Mild segmental dilation of the RV
- Regional RV hypokinesia
- Inverted T waves in the right precordial leads in the absence of a right bundle branch block (RBBB)
- Late potentials on a signal average electrocardiogram
- LBBB morphology ventricular arrhythmias (sustained or nonsustained)
- Frequent ventricular extrasystoles (>1,000/24 h)
- Family history of sudden death at age younger than age 35 years suspected to be caused by RV dysplaia

179. Ans. b. Arrhythmogenic right ventricular dysplasia

Hurst's 10th Ed; Page 1800

Refer to explanation for Q. No 178.

180. Ans. d. Lead V_1 to V_3

Hurst's 10th Ed; Page 1800

Refer to explanation for Q. No 178.

181. Ans. c. Interstitial pneumonitis

IGNOU, MCC 005, Page 44-45

Adverse effects leading to discontinuation of amiodarone occurs in 3-4% of patients. Minor side effects that seldom require drug discontinuation include corneal microdeposits, asymptomatic transient elevation of hepatic enzymes, photosensitivity of the skin, blue-gray skin discoloration, and subjective gastrointestinal side effects. Very few cases of optic neuritis causing blindness have been reported. Amiodarone-induced hypothyroidism occurs in approximately 8% of patients and requires the addition of thyroid replacement. Drug-induced hyperthyroidism (2%) may require discontinuation of therapy. The most serious adverse effect is interstitial pneumonitis or bronchiolitis obliterans. Patients with baseline abnormal chest radiographs or pulmonary function tests have a higher incidence of pulmonary fibrosis. This adverse effect is dose related and occurs rarely if less than 400 mg/day is used. However, acute pneumonitis may occur even after a few weeks of amiodarone therapy. Neurological side effects, including a peripheral neuropathy and myopathy, usually resolve on lowering the dose, but may produce unstable gait in the elderly. Drug-induced bradycardia may require permanent pacing in up to 2% of patients. Torsade de pointes and incessant ventricular tachycardias are rare.

182. Ans. c. Interstitial pneumonitis

IGNOU, MCC 005, Page 44-45

Refer to explanation for Q. No 181.

183. Ans. c. Amiodarone

IGNOU, MCC 005, Page 44-45

Refer to explanation for Q. No 181.

184. Ans. d. All

Hurst's 10th Ed; Page 899-918

All the class III antiarrhythmic drugs (ibutilide, sotalol, amiodarone, dofetilide) prolongs repolarization both in atrial and ventricular myocardium and therefore they prolong QT interval and hence should not be used in long QT syndrome.

185. Ans. b. Adenosine

Braunwald 11th Ed; Page 687

Injection of adenosine may produce serious adverse event like prolonged ventricular asystole, ventricular tachycardia or even ventricular fibrillation. Atrial fibrillation is another proarrhythmic event which may be seen after injection of adenosine.

186. Ans. d. Tachycardia-bradycardia syndrome

Braunwald 11th Ed; Page 615

The various manifestation of sinus node dysfunctions are:
a. sinus bradycardia;
b. sinoatrial block and sinus arrest,
c. bradycardia-tachycardia syndrome.

Bradycardia-tachycardia syndrome is the most frequently encountered form of symptomatic sinus node dysfunction and is associated with the highest incidence of syncope. The syncope is generally associated with the marked pauses following the cessation of paroxysmal supraventricular tachyarrhythmias that occur in the setting of sinus bradycardia (primarily atrial fibrillation), a prolonged asystolic period occurring in the setting of any form of sinus node dysfunction also implies impaired function of lower (nonsinus) pacemakers. The drugs used to prevent atrial fibrillation or control its rare are often responsible for the symptomatic bradycardias following cessation of the arrhythmia and hence, the need for pacemakers. Syncope is much rarer in patients with isolated sinus bradycardia. When these patients are symptomatic, it is usually fatigue or dyspnea on exertion. Syncope in patients with isolated sinus bradycardia is usually neurocardiac. Autonomic reflex abnormalities consistent with neurocardiac syncope are usually present when syncope occurs in patients with isolated sinus bradycardia.

187. Ans. a. Sinus bradycardia

Braunwald 11th Ed; Page 615

Refer to explanation for Q. No 186.

188. Ans. d. All of the above

Braunwald 11th Ed; Page 615

Refer to explanation for Q. No 186.

189. Ans. c. Implantable event recorder

Hurst's 14th Ed; Page 2012

If a random ECG in a patient with episodic symptoms is normal, prolonged (24 h) ECG monitoring is the next step in evaluating sinus node function. Most episodes of syncope or dizziness are paroxysmal and unpredictable, and even 24 hours monitoring may fail to include a symptomatic episode. The use of event recorders has improved ability to correlate symptoms with sinus node dysfunction. In cases with infrequent episodes of syncope, an implantable event recorder is now available.

190. Ans. d. All

Hurst's 14th Ed; Page 2126

The paradox that antiarrhythmic agents can cause arrhythmias has been recognized since quinidine's introduction in 1918. the most common form of proarrhythmia, seen with Vaughan-Williams class I a and class III antiarrhythmics, stems from QT interval prolongation resulting from blockade of repolarizing potassium currents and is accordingly, sometimes referred to as the acquired long QT syndrome. Besides antiarrhythmic drugs, many other commonly used medications with diverse actions have been implicated in ventricular proarrhythmia. Common examples include erythromycin, terfenadine, astemizole, and certain psychotropic drugs, such as tricyclic antidepressants and antipsychotics. A few drugs (cisapride, terfenadine, astemizole) were withdrawn from the US market because of such concerns.

SYNCOPE

1. All the following are correct regarding the syncope *except*:
   a. It is the transient episode of altered consciousness
   b. Noncardiac syncope is the most common
   c. Syncope is more common in women than man
   d. The incidence of syncope increases with age

2. During the head up tilt test the optimal angle should be:
   a. Less than 30°
   b. Less than 45°
   c. Between 60 and 80°
   d. More than 80°

3. Which of the following is *correct* regarding head up tilt test in evaluation of syncope?
   a. Tilt angle <45° sacrifices sensitivity
   b. Angles >80° results in more false positive results
   c. Low dose isoproterenol infusion increases the number of positive response compared to base line
   d. All of the above

4. All the following group of drugs are used in treatment of neurocardiogenic syncope *except*:
   a. Beta adrenoreceptor blockade drugs
   b. Anticholinergic agents
   c. Methylxanthines
   d. Alpha adrenoreceptor blockade drugs

5. The common type of carotid sinus syncope is:
   a. Cardioinhibitory type   b. Vasodepressor type
   c. Mixed form   d. All of equally common

ANSWERS WITH EXPLANATIONS

1. Ans. a. It is the transient episode of altered consciousness

Hurst's 10th Ed; Page 995

Syncope is a sudden loss of consciousness and postural tone caused by transient decreased cerebral blood flow. It is associated with spontaneous recovery. The occurrence of syncope in general population is about 3% in men and 3.5% in women. As a general rule, the incidence of syncope increases with age. The cause of syncope includes cardiovascular disorders, disorder of vascular tone or blood volume and cerebrovascular disorders. The relative incidence of these categories varies with the clinical side from which patients are selected. In hospitalized patients, syncope is most often a result of cardiovascular disorder, whereas in emergency room other causes of syncope predominate. In many cases, the cause of syncope may be multifactorial. In up to 50% of cases, the cause of syncope cannot be determined with certainty even after aggressive evaluation.

2. Ans. c. Between 60 and 80°

Hurst's 10th Ed; Page 997

Head up tilt (HUT) testing has become a useful diagnostic study for the identification of patients with neurocardiogenic syncope. The sensitivity, specificity and reproducibility of HUT testing depends on the patient population studied and HUT protocol employed. HUT at an angle 60–90° for a time period of 20–60 minutes has been found to yield a sensitivity ranging from 20–74%. Longer duration of HUT (45–60 min) leads to improved sensitivity without the significant increase in false positive response. The optimal HUT angle should be between 60–80°. Tilt angle <45° sacrifices sensitivity, whereas angle >80° can result in more false positive result. An average of 63% of patients studied with HUT after a negative electrophysiologic study were found to have a positive HUT response suggesting that significant proportion of patient with unexplained syncope have neurocardiogenic syncope. Isoproterenol infusion during HT testing has been shown to improve sensitivity. Low dose isoproterenol infusion (<2 µg/min) has been shown to nearly double the number of positive response compared with baseline, with an acceptable sensitivity of 93% and reproducibility of 83%. High doses of isoproterenol especially at HUT angle of >80° markedly increase the incidence of false positive response. High dose intravenous isoproterenol, intravenous adenosine and sublingual nitroglycerine during HUT have been shown to increase sensitivity with some reduction in specificity and significant reduction in time required to perform the test.

3. Ans. d. All of the above

Hurst's 10th Ed; Page 997

Refer to explanation for Q. No 2.

4. Ans. d. Alpha adrenoreceptor blockade drugs

Hurst's 10th Ed; Page 997

Therapeutic options for patient with neurocardiogenic syncope include volume expansion, beta adrenergic receptor blockade, anticholinergic agents, serotonin reuptake inhibitors, methylxanthines, alpha agonists and dual chamber cardiac pacing. A stepped approach to pharmacologic therapy is advisable, starting with low initial doses as these patients seem to be more prone to adverse reaction than general population. If one class of drug is ineffective, a combination of drugs each acting on different limbs responsible for neurocardiogenic syncope is beneficial.

5. Ans. a. Cardioinhibitory type

Hurst's 10th Ed; Page 1000-1001

Compression of the carotid sinus in normal person is often associated with transient slowing of the heart rate and mild hypotension. In some patients such stimulation is followed by a profound slowing of heart rate and/or a marked diminution of arterial pressure. This disorder is referred as carotid sinus hypersensitivity. There are three forms of carotid sinus syncope—cardioinhibitory, vasodepressor and mixed type: (1) The cardioinhibitory type of carotid sinus syncope is most common and is associated with slowing of the heart rate secondary to marked sinus bradycardia, sinoatrial block and/or high degree AV block. Syncope in this instance is related to prolonged asystole rather than to a fall in peripheral vascular resistance; (2) Vasodepressor type of carotid sinus syncope is that form of the syndrome in which syncope occur as a result of primary decrease in arterial pressure in the absence of profound bradycardia. Presyncopal signs such as nausea, sweating and pallor are not usually observed and the fall in arterial pressure may be precipitous; (3) Mixed form—in the mixed form of carotid sinus syncope with bradycardia and hypotension, the vasodepressor component may not be evident until after atropine blockade or during cardiac pacing. Under such circumstances carotid sinus massage uncovers the hypotension in absence of bradycardia. Carotid sinus syncope and presyncope are commonly found in elderly patients and is often associated with generalized atherosclerosis.

PACING AND ELECTROPHYSIOLOGY

1. Which of the following is a physiological pacemaker?
   a. Atrial inhibited (AAI)
   b. Ventricular inhibited (VVI)
   c. Ventricular asynchronous pacemaker (VOO)
   d. Ventricular triggered pacemaker (VAT)

2. Which of the following physiological pacemaker is *not* a dual chamber pacemaker?
   a. Atrial synchronous pacer (AAI)
   b. Atrial synchronous, ventricular inhibited type (VDD)
   c. DDD pacemaker
   d. DVI pacemaker

3. Pacemaker syndrome is often seen with which of following pacemakers?
   a. VVI pacemaker   b. VDD pacemaker
   c. DVI pacemaker   d. DDD pacemaker

4. Endless loop tachycardia is a problem often seen with:
   a. VVI pacemaker   b. DDD pacemaker
   c. AAI pacemaker   d. DVI pacemaker

5. Which of the following electromagnetic interference can lead to interference with pacemaker?
   a. Cardioversion and defibrillation
   b. Electrocautery
   c. Magnetic resonance imaging
   d. All of the above

CHAPTER 20 | Cardiac Arrhythmia, Pacing and Electrophysiology

6. Which of the following is a problem peculiar to the dual chamber pacemakers?
   a. Electrical cross talk
   b. Thromboembolism
   c. Atrial fibrillation
   d. None of them

7. Which of the following is a contraindication for implanting a dual chamber pacemakers?
   a. Atrial fibrillation
   b. Presence of AV nodal disease
   c. Retrograde V-A conduction
   d. All of the above

8. Optimal mode of pacemaker for a young active man with chronic atrial fibrillation and complete AV block is:
   a. VVI RR (ventricular inhibited rate responsive)
   b. AAI
   c. DDD pacemaker
   d. VDD (atrial synchronous – ventricular inhibited pacemakers)

9. Optimal mode of pacemaker for a young active man with sinus node disease and normal AV conduction is:
   a. VVI pacemakers
   b. VVIRR pacemakers
   c. DDIRR pacemakers
   d. AAIRR pacemakers

10. Power source in currently used pacemaker pulse generator battery is:
   a. Zinc mercury cell
   b. Nickel cadmium rechargeable battery
   c. Nuclear cells
   d. Lithium iodide cell

11. The appearance of left ventricular stimulation with a right bundle branch block configuration in ECG could be due to?
   a. Right ventricular interventricular septal perforation by a lead
   b. Placement of lead in a left ventricular cardiac venous territory
   c. Epimyocardial left ventricular pacing
   d. All of the above

12. Which of the following indicates pacemaker malfunction?
   a. Fusion beats
   b. Pseudo-fusion beats
   c. Hysteresis
   d. None of the above

13. Which of the following helps in diagnosing acute myocardial infarction in patients with pacemakers?
   a. Intermittent sinus or ectopic rhythm showing changes of myocardial infarction
   b. Inhibition of output of ventricular inhibited pulse generator by chest wall stimulation
   c. ST-qR pattern in ECG
   d. All of the above

ANSWERS WITH EXPLANATIONS

1. Ans. a. Atrial inhibited (AAI)

Braunwald 5th Ed; Page 712

Atrial inhibited pacemaker (AAI) mode is similar to VVI (ventricular demand) mode except that here the pacemaker senses atrial electrical activity and paces the atrium. AAI pacing is use for patient with sick sinus syndrome and intact AV conduction. Because it paces the atria and in presence of intact AV conduction, after a preset interval, there is contraction of ventricle, there is maintenance of atrioventricular synchrony similar to the normal AV sequential contraction. Therefore, this pacemaker is a physiological pacemaker.

2. Ans. a. Atrial synchronous pacer (AAI)

Braunwald 5th Ed; Page 712

Physiological pacemaker is one, which maintains atrioventricular synchrony. All dual chamber pacemakers by design have atrial and ventricular sensing as well as pacing capability and therefore they maintain atrioventricular synchrony and they are called as physiological pacemakers. However, atrial synchronous pacer (AAI) is a single chamber pacemaker where only one lead (atrial lead) is implanted and in presence of intact AV conduction. It maintains atrioventricular synchrony and therefore it is a physiological pacemaker, even though it is a single lead and single chamber pacemaker implantation.

3. Ans. a. VVI pacemaker

Braunwald 5th Ed; Page 722

Pacemaker syndrome is a constellation of clinical sign and symptoms produced by the adverse hemodynamic and electrophysiological response to pacing because of inadequate timing of atrial and ventricular contraction. During VVI (ventricular) single chamber pacing, the pacemaker syndrome is most commonly occurs in patient with normal or near normal LV function and retrograde ventriculoatrial conduction. The prominent symptoms of pacemaker syndrome are due mostly to the reduction in cardiac output, hypotension and higher ventricular filling pressure. Symptom includes orthostatic hypotension, syncope or near syncope, fatigue, exercise intolerance, light headedness, weakness, lethargy, dyspnea, induction of congestive heart failure, cough, patients awareness of beat to beat variation of cardiac response, neck pulsation or pressure sensation and fullness in the chest, neck or head, headache, impaired exercise capacity and disturbed mentation. The mechanism of pacemaker syndrome lies in loss of atrioventricular synchrony. This loss of atrioventricular synchrony decrease the cardiac output by 20–30% at rest. The hemodynamic compromise in the pacemaker syndrome is more complex because retrograde ventriculoatrial conduction causes a negative atrial kick with more profound hemodynamic disadvantage than simple loss of atrioventricular synchrony. Atrial contraction against closed mitral and tricuspid atrioventricular valve causes systemic and pulmonary venous congestion, sometimes leading to the development of congestive heart failure in previously compensated patient. In addition to the marked reduction in cardiac output, retrograde ventriculoatrial conduction leads to atrial distention and activation of stress receptor that produces a reflex vasodepressor effect mediated by autonomic nervous system. Thus, in the face of hypotension due to low cardiac output, compensatory mechanisms that ordinarily increases the peripheral resistance becomes attenuated. The pacemaker syndrome due to single chamber ventricular pacemakers (VVI and VVIR) is an iatrogenic condition and can be eliminated by restoring atrioventricular synchrony either with atrial pacing alone (if AV conduction is normal) or dual chamber pacing with an appropriate atrioventricular delay. Occasionally, restoration of atrioventricular synchrony during ventricular pacing can be achieved by reducing the pacing rate (or using hysteresis) to minimize competition with sinus rhythm. At the time of pacemaker implantation the lack of a drop in blood pressure with VVI pacing testing does not eliminate the potential for pacemaker syndrome.

4. Ans. a. VVI pacemaker

Braunwald 5th Ed; Page 717

Endless loop tachycardia is a well-known complication of dual chamber pacing and it starts with the sensing of a retrograde P wave, usually linked to a ventricular extra systole. Endless loop tachycardia can be sustained or unsustained and often occurs at the programmed upper rate of the pacemaker. Intact retrograde VA conduction occurs in approximately two-thirds or more of patients with sinus node dysfunction and in 15–30% patients with AV block. Thus, 35–50% of all patients receiving dual chamber pacemakers may be susceptible to the endless loop tachycardia. The conversion to asynchronous mode with the magnet over the pacemaker usually terminate the endless loop tachycardia and to prevent the endless loop tachycardia the postventricular atrial refractory period should be programmed to 15 m/sec beyond the duration of retrograde VA conduction time determined non invasively by pacemaker programming.

5. Ans. d. All of the above

Braunwald 5th Ed; Page 728

Cardioversion or defibrillation, electrocautery, radiation therapy and magnetic resonance imaging all can lead to the interference with the function of the pacemaker. These devices or procedures can cause rapid pacing, inhibition, resetting of the pulse generators leading to the transient or permanent malfunction of the pacemaker.

6. Ans. a. Electrical cross talk

Braunwald 5th Ed; Page 715

Electrical crosstalk also known as self-inhibition refers to the inappropriate detection of the atrial stimulus by the ventricular channel and this problem is peculiar to the dual chamber pacemaker. Crosstalk depends on the amplitude of the atrial stimulus and the sensitivity of ventricular channel and is less frequent with bipolar leads. Electrical crosstalk often can be eliminated by reduction of atrial output and/or ventricular sensitivity. The prevention of crosstalk also requires a ventricular blanking (refractory period 10–60 m/sec) that starts coincidently with the atrial stimulus.

7. Ans. a. Atrial fibrillation

Braunwald 5th Ed; Page 725-726

Individual patient considerations: While deciding the type of pacemaker to be used, the physician needs to determine whether the atrium can be paced and/or sensed, whether latent or overt AV block exists and whether atrial chronotropic incompetence is present. The majority of patients with atria that can be paced and/or sensed should be considered for single-chamber atrial or dual chamber pacing (AAI, AAIR, VDD, DDD or DDDR) because VVI or VVIR pacing causes greater morbidity and mortality. Single lead ventricular pacing should be reserved primarily for patients with chronic atrial fibrillation and AV block. A VVI pacemaker programmed to a low rate may be justified in the occasional patient with infrequent episodes of bradycardia. Replacement of a depleted VVI pacemaker with another VVI or VVIR unit is reasonable in many asymptomatic patients. Single lead ventricular pacing is appropriate in patients who are incapacitated and inactive as well as those with a short-life expectancy. VVIR does not improve survival when compared with the VVI mode.

It is important to assess what is best for the patient's level of activity, whether there is underlying coronary artery disease or LV dysfunction, what is affordable, what is the simplest system that will optimize hemodynamics, what is the natural history of the condition for which pacing is being used, and what is the impact of present and future drug therapy? Advanced age is not an indication for a simpler (and cheaper) VVI or VVIR system. Active elderly patients benefit greatly from restoration of AV synchrony because the atrial contribution to cardiac output normally increases with advanced age. Dual-chamber pacemakers in the elderly appear cost-effective on a long-term basis by avoiding or reducing the complications associated with single-lead ventricular pacing.

Patients with angina pectoris generally tolerate DDD, DDDR, or VVIR modes better than the VVI mode, provided the upper rate is not excessively high. The increased MVO2 related to rate increase on exercise is counterbalanced by the increase in MVO2 during fixed-frequency VVI pacing, probably secondary to enhanced contractility (from increased sympathetic activity) and wall tension which increase stroke volume. The DDI or DDD mode with search hysteresis is preferred for carotid sinus hypersensitivity or neutrally mediated syncope. For example, pacing might occur at a relatively fast rate of 100 beats/min when the spontaneous rate drops below a certain value such as 50 beats/min. After a given period of pacing, the pacemaker "searches" for the return of normal rhythm (>50 beats/min) by intermittent prolongation of one or more pacing intervals. Pacing ceases if the spontaneous R-R interval is <1,200 m/sec. This feature avoids continuation of pacing at 100 beats/min until it is inhibited by a spontaneous rhythm >100 beats/min, as with conventional hysteresis function. Patients with paroxysmal supraventricular tachyarrhythmias require a DDD or DDDR system with automatic mode conversion or fall back option to slower paced ventricular rates to avoid tracking of unphysiological atrial rates. A single-lead VDD pacing system may provide a relatively simple and less expensive VDD/VVIR pacemaker for patients with AV block and normal atrial chronotropic function. Cost considerations aside, either a sensor-driven single-chamber or a sensor-driven dual-chamber pacemaker with extensive programability of pacing modes would meet the needs of all patients given the high incidence of atrial chronotropic incompetence in the elderly and its progression or development overtime.

8. Ans. a. VVI RR (ventricular inhibited rate responsive)

Braunwald 5th Ed; Page 725-726

Refer to explanation for Q. No 7.

9. Ans. d. AAIRR pacemakers

Braunwald 5th Ed; Page 725-726

Refer to explanation for Q. No 7.

10. Ans. d. Lithium iodide cell

Braunwald 5th Ed; Page 726

Power source in currently use pacemaker pulse generator battery contains lithium iodide.

11. Ans. d. All of the above

Braunwald 5th Ed; Page 713

The pattern of ventricular activation in cases of right ventricular pacing produces a left bundle branch block pattern of depolarization. During right ventricular pacing, paced beat usually exhibit a typical left bundle branch block pattern in lead I and avL but leads V_5 and V_6 sometime shows deep S wave because of the main electrical forces may be moving away from the horizontal level where V_5 and V_6 are recorded. The mean electrical axis of the paced QRS complex in the frontal plane is oriented superiorly (more often in the left than in the right upper quadrant) because the sequence of activation travels from apex to base away from the inferior leads. As the pacing electrodes moves towards right ventricular outflow tract, activation travels simultaneously to the base superiorly and to the apex inferiorly and the mean axis of the pace QRS complex in the frontal plane may point to the left lower quadrant. Epicardial or endocardial stimulation of the left ventricle produces late activation of right ventricle and therefore a right bundle branch block pattern. Pacing from the distal coronary sinus procedures the same pattern.

12. Ans. d. None of the above

Braunwald 5th Ed; Page 713

Fusion beats or pseudofusion beats are common phenomena during ventricular pacing. Hysteresis is one of the functions found in majority of pacemakers. During ventricular pacing, ventricular fusion beat occur when the ventricles are activated simultaneously by a spontaneous depolarization and a paced impulse. A ventricular fusion beat is often narrower than a pure paced beat and can exhibit various morphologies depending on the relative contribution of the two foci to the ventricular depolarization. Pseudofusion beats consist of the superimposition of an ineffectual pacemaker spike on the spontaneous QRS complex originating from a single focus and represents a normal manifestation of a VVI pacing.

13. Ans. d. All of the above

Braunwald 5th Ed; Page 713

The diagnosis of myocardial infarction in patients with pacemaker is at times difficult. Because the QRS complex during right ventricular pacing resembles that of a spontaneous left bundle branch pattern, the diagnosis of myocardial infarction often can be made during right ventricular pacing by applying the criteria used in complete LBBB. Large unipolar stimuli can mask Q waves. An extensive anteroseptal myocardial infarction can cause a Q wave in lead I, avL, V_5 and V_6 producing a qR pattern following the stimulus. Although the sensitivity of qR change is low, its specificity approaches 100% because it is never seen in lead V_5 and V_6 during uncomplicated pacing. A qR or qR complex in lead II, III and avF is also diagnostic of an inferior wall myocardial infarction. An anterior wall myocardial infarction can be associated with late notching of the ascending limb of the QRS complex in the left precordial leads indicating an extensive infarction. During right ventricular apical pacing the inferior leads and anterior leads (V_1–V_3) often record secondary ST segment elevation. ST segment depression can occur as a normal finding in lead I, avL, V_5, and V_6. Relatively stable ST-T wave changes resembling primary abnormalities occasionally can be seen during uncomplicated right ventricular pacing. Sequential electrocardiograms are often needed to determine the significance of ST-T wave abnormalities. ST-T wave abnormality occur more commonly in acute myocardial infarction than the qR pattern or QRS notching noted as described. Pronounced primary ST segment elevation with convex configuration clinches the diagnosis of myocardial infarction. When less obvious, the diagnosis becomes certain only when the polarity of T wave is opposite to that of ST segment elevation. ST segment depression concordant with QRS complex occasionally can occur in lead V_3–V_6 during uncomplicated RV pacing and rarely in leads V_1 and V_2 and therefore, obvious ST segment depression in lead V_1 and V_2 should be considered abnormal and indicative of anterior or inferior myocardial infarction. Inhibition of pacemaker by chest wall stimulation or by reduction of the rate or output may allow the emergence of the spontaneous rhythm and reveal diagnostic Q wave. Continuous ventricular pacing per second induced striking ST-T abnormality in the underlying spontaneous beats.

CARDIAC ARRHYTHMIA AND PACING

1. **Ventriculophasic sinus arrhythmia is:**
   a. When PP interval cyclically shorten during inspiration
   b. When phasic variation in PP interval is unrelated to the respiratory cycle
   c. When PP interval that contains a QRS complex are shorter than PP cycle without QRS complex
   d. None of the above

2. **During sinus pause, if the PP interval does not equal in multiple of the basic PP interval, then the mechanism is:**
   a. Sinus arrest
   b. Sinoatrial exit block
   c. Wandering pacemaker
   d. Sinus arrhythmia

3. **In electrocardiogram when there is a progressive shortening of PP interval till sinus pause then it is:**
   a. Wenckebach second-degree SA block
   b. Type II SA block
   c. Sinus pause
   d. Sinus arrhythmia

4. **In ECG when the interval without P wave that equals approximately 2, 3, or 4 times than the normal PP cycle then it is called as:**
   a. Type I Wenckebach second-degree SA block
   b. Type II second-degree SA exit block
   c. Sinus pause
   d. Sinus arrest

5. **Which of the following *cannot* be recognized by surface ECG?**
   a. First degree SA exit block
   b. Type I Wenckebach second-degree SA exit block
   c. Type II second-degree SA exit block
   d. Ventriculophasic sinus arrhythmia

6. **During the pacemaker implantation, the minimum current for a pulse of infinite duration that results in depolarization is labelled as:**
   a. Phasing threshold
   b. Rheobase
   c. Chronaxie
   d. None of them

7. **All the following can raise the pacing threshold *except*?**
   a. Hyperkalemia
   b. Hypokalemia
   c. Acidosis
   d. Profound hypothyroidism

8. **Which of the following raises pacing threshold?**
   a. Sodium channel blocking drugs
   b. Hyperkalemia
   c. Alkalosis
   d. All of the above

9. **Subcutaneous ICD performs:**
   a. High voltage cardioversion or defibrillation
   b. ATP
   c. Resynchronization
   d. Long term bradycardia pacing

10. **Which of the following increases the effectiveness of cardiac resynchronization therapy?**
    a. Lower EF
    b. Left bundle branch block morphology
    c. Duration of QRS
    d. All of the above

11. Which of the following modes of resynchronization therapy brings improved left ventricular structure and function with a low and stable pacing threshold?
   a. Biventricular pacing via coronary sinus
   b. HIS bundle pacing
   c. Left bundle branch block pacing
   d. All are equal

12. Leadless pacemakers are implanted in:
   a. Right atrium
   b. Right ventricle
   c. Coronary sinus
   d. Left ventricle

13. Which is the common complication with leadless pacemaker?
   a. Pneumothorax
   b. Hematoma
   c. Pericardial effusion and tamponade
   d. Subcutaneous pocket infection

ANSWERS WITH EXPLANATIONS

1. Ans. c. When PP interval that contains a QRS complex are shorter than PP cycle without QRS complex

Braunwald 11th Ed; Page 772

Sinus arrhythmia: It is a phasic variation in sinus rate due to effect of autonomic system. It is seen in young especially those with slower heart rates or after enhanced vagal tone. It is also seen in athlete and after administration of digitalis. Sinus arrhythmia appears in two forms. In the respiratory form the P-P interval cyclically shortens during inspiration, primarily as a result of reflex inhibition of vagal tone and slows during expiration. Nonrespiratory sinus arrhythmia is characterized by a phasic variation in the P-P interval unrelated to the respiratory cycle and can be the result of digitalis intoxication. Ventriculophasic sinus arrhythmia occurs during complete AV block and a slow ventricular rate, when P-P cycles that contain a QRS complex are shorter than P-P cycles without a QRS complex. This is probably caused by the influence of the autonomic nervous system responding to changes in ventricular stroke volume.

2. Ans. a. Sinus arrest

Braunwald 11th Ed; Page 773

Sinus pause or sinus arrest is recognized by a pause in the sinus rhythm. The P-P interval delimiting the pause does not equal a multiple of the basic P-P interval. Sinus arrest is primarily due to the slowing or cessation of spontaneous sinus node automaticity, and it is a disorder of impulse formation. Contrary to that sinoatrial exit block is an arrhythmia that is recognized electrocardiographically by a pause resulting from absence of the normally expected P wave. The duration of pause is a multiple of the basic P-P interval. Sinoatrial exit block is caused by a conduction disturbance during which an impulse formed within the sinus node fails to depolarize the atria or does so with delay.

3. Ans. a. Wenckebach second-degree SA block

Braunwald 11th Ed; Page 773

Sinoatrial exit block is an arrhythmia that is recognized electrocardiographically by a pause resulting from absence of the normally expected P wave. The duration of the pause is a multiple of the basic P-P interval. SA exit block is caused by a conduction disturbance during which an impulse formed within the sinus node fails to depolarize the atria or does so with delay. An interval without P waves that equals approximately two, three, or four times the normal P-P cycle characterizes type II second-degree SA exit block. During type I (Wenckebach) second-degree SA exit block, the P-P interval progressively shortens before the pause, and duration of the pause is less than two P-P cycles. First-degree SA exit block cannot be recognized on the electrocardiogram because SA nodal discharge is not recorded.

4. Ans. b. Type II second-degree SA exit block

Braunwald 11th Ed; Page 773

Refer to explanation for Q. No 3.

5. Ans. a. First degree SA exit block

Braunwald 11th Ed; Page 773

Refer to explanation for Q. No 3.

6. Ans. b. Rheobase

Braunwald 11th Ed; Page 781

The strength-duration curve plots stimulus strength required for pacing as a function of pulse duration. It is represented by an inverse hyperbolic function. Two parameters, the rheobase and the chronaxie, characterize this curve. The rheobase is the minimum current for a pulse of infinite duration that results in depolarization.

The chronaxie is the pulse duration on the curve that corresponds to twice the rheobase current. The chronaxie is important for design of efficient pacing pulses because a pulse with duration equal to the chronaxie paces with the lowest energy. This is important for generator size and longevity.

7. Ans. b. Hypokalemia

Braunwald 11th Ed; Page 781

The most clinically important metabolic abnormality is hyperkalemia, which raises pacing thresholds and alters sensing by causing conduction delays and local conduction block. Marked acidosis or alkalosis and profound hypothyroidism also raise the pacing threshold.

Pacing threshold is also raised by sodium channel blocking drugs especially class IC drugs like flecainide.

8. Ans. d. All of the above

Braunwald 11th Ed; Page 781

Refer to explanation for Q. No 7.

9. Ans. a. High voltage cardioversion or defibrillation

Braunwald 11th Ed; Page 788

Subcutaneous ICD eliminates many of the drawback associated with transvenous lead insertion, lead-related complications during MRI scans, and hazards of transvenous extraction when lead removal is required. Subcutaneous ICD can deliver high voltage defibrillation stimuli but they cannot perform ATP, resynchronization, or long-term bradycardia pacing.

10. Ans. c. Duration of QRS

JACC EP 2022; May 8(5); Page 662

Based on multiple randomized trial, CRT (with or without defibrillating capabilities) has a class I indication to reduce morbidity and mortality in patients with sinus rhythm, New York Heart Association classification class III or IV, heart failure symptoms, left ventricular ejection fraction (LVEF) <35% and QRS duration of >120 msec. receiving optimal medical therapy. Response to CRT differ widely with approximately 30% of patients having found to be nonresponder. Analysis from major CRT trials has identified subgroups in which CRT is less effective. QRS duration and morphology has been demonstrated to play an important role in response to therapy. CRT is more effective in left bundle branch block compared with non LBBB morphology, and its effectiveness increases with QRS duration.

11. Ans. c. Left bundle branch block pacing

Front. Cardiovasc. Med. 23 Aug 22

Left bundle branch block pacing has been found to be feasible with a high success implantation rate and effective to correct LBBB and improved left ventricular structure and function with a low and stable pacing threshold.

12. Ans. b. Right ventricle

Indian Pacing and Electrophysiology Journal 22 (2022); 87-90

Leadless pacemakers are implanted in the right ventricle and the micra transcatheter pacing system is the only leadless pacemaker currently available in clinical practice. Leadless pacemaker provides benefit over conventional transvenous pacemaker by avoiding a subcutaneous pocket and leads traversing the tricuspid valve.

13. Ans. c. Pericardial effusion and tamponade

Indian Pacing and Electrophysiology Journal 22 (2022); 87-90

With the leadless pacemaker, the implants success rate is around 95–100%. The complication occurs in around 3.1% cases and includes pericardial effusion and cardiac tamponade in 0.96% and 1.47% patients. As the lead is pass through the femoral approach and there is no subcutaneous pocket, so the problem of pocket infection, lead infection and tricuspid regurgitation is not seen with the leadless pacemaker.

Chapter 21: Pulmonary Hypertension

1. What is the mean driving pressure (i.e., the difference between mean blood pressure in pulmonary artery and in the left atrium) between pulmonary circulation and LA:
   a. <5 mm
   b. <10 mm
   c. <20 mm
   d. <40 mm

2. Pulmonary vascular resistance in normal condition is approximately:
   a. Half of the systemic vascular resistance
   b. One-third of systemic vascular resistance
   c. One-fifth of systemic vascular resistance
   d. One-eighth of systemic vascular resistance

3. In normal condition, pulmonary circulation is capable of accommodating how much increase in resting blood flow with no change in pulmonary artery pressure?
   a. Double
   b. Three times
   c. Four-folds
   d. >10 folds

4. What will be the approximate value of pulmonary arterial pressure at an altitude of 50,000 feet?
   a. 20/12 (15)
   b. 25/50 (18)
   c. 30/15 (30)
   d. 38/14 (25)

5. Pulmonary arterial hypertension is rare with which of the following?
   a. Systemic sclerosis
   b. Systemic lupus erythematosus
   c. Mixed connective tissue disorder
   d. Rheumatoid arthritis

6. Which of the following is *not* risk factor for pulmonary arterial hypertension (PAH)?
   a. Fenfluramine
   b. Toxic rapeseed oil
   c. Cocaine
   d. Cigarette smoking

7. The gold standard test for confirmation of suspected pulmonary arterial hypertension is:
   a. Chest radiography
   b. Contrast angiography
   c. Echocardiography and Doppler
   d. Right heart catheterization

8. Which is the commonest segment of pulmonary arterial tree involved in thromboembolic pulmonary hypertension?
   a. Small vessels
   b. Intermediate artery
   c. Large central arteries
   d. All are equally affected

9. Which of the following is of no proven value in treating the pulmonary arterial hypertension associated with interstitial fibrosis?
   a. Oxygen therapy
   b. Inhaled vasodilators such as prostacyclin analogue
   c. Systemically administered vasodilator and glucocorticoids
   d. All of the above

10. The gold standard for diagnosing pulmonary artery hypertension in patients with COPD is?
    a. Echocardiography
    b. Radionuclide study
    c. Right heart catheterization
    d. Electrocardiography

11. The safest and most effective approach to pulmonary vasodilation in obstructive lung disease with arterial hypoxemia is:
    a. Systemic vasodilator
    b. Inhaled prostacyclin analogue
    c. Endothelin antagonist
    d. Supplemental oxygen

12. Which of the following is the cause of alveolar hypoventilation with normal lungs?
    a. Central sleep apnea
    b. Obstructive sleep apnea
    c. Encephalitis
    d. All of the above

13. Which subgroup of pulmonary arterial hypertension have better survival in natural history?
    a. Idiopathic pulmonary arterial hypertension
    b. HIV associated pulmonary arterial hypertension
    c. PAH with coexisting portal hypertension
    d. Eisenmenger syndrome

14. Syncope is exceedingly rare symptoms in which of the following?
   a. Idiopathic PAH
   b. PAH after complete surgical repair of congenital shunt
   c. Eisenmenger syndrome
   d. All of the above

15. Which of the following connective tissue disorder have a highest prevalence of PAH?
   a. Scleroderma
   b. SLE
   c. Mixed connective tissue disease
   d. Rheumatoid arthritis

16. Phlebotomy is recommended for symptoms of hyperviscosity, if the hematocrit is greater than:
   a. 45% b. 55%
   c. 60% d. 65% to 70%

17. The drug Riociguat is a:
   a. PDE-5 inhibitors
   b. Endothelin receptor antagonist
   c. Prostacyclin
   d. Guanylyl cyclase activator

ANSWERS WITH EXPLANATIONS

1. Ans. b. <10 mm

Hurst's 14th Ed; Page 1785

Pulmonary circulation has unique features. Because of its large capacity, great distensibility, its lower resistance to blood flow, and the modest amounts of smooth muscle in the small arteries and arterioles, the pulmonary circulation is not predisposed to become hypertensive usually. In the normal individual lying supine, systolic blood pressure in the pulmonary circuit is approximately 15 to 25 mm Hg; the corresponding diastolic pressure is 5 to 10 mm Hg. The mean driving pressure (i.e., the difference between the mean blood pressure in the pulmonary artery and in the left atrium, the transpulmonary gradient) is usually <10 mm Hg. Because blood flow (cardiac output) is the same in both circulations in the absence of any systemic to pulmonary communications, the pulmonary vascular resistance is approximately one-eighth of systemic vascular resistance. The large cross-sectional surface area of pulmonary circulation, coupled with the distensibility of its thin-walled vessels and the large recruitable vascular reserve, account for these unique characteristics. During exercise, as pulmonary blood flow increases, new regions of the pulmonary vascular bed are open and existing vasculature dilates. Accordingly, the pulmonary circulation is capable of accommodating a fourfold or greater increase in resting blood flow with virtually no change in pulmonary artery pressure, with a concomitant decrease in pulmonary vascular resistance.

2. Ans. d. One-eighth of systemic vascular resistance

Hurst's 14th Ed; Page 1785

Please refer to the answer of Q. No 1.

3. Ans. c. Four-folds

Hurst's 14th Ed; Page 1785

Please refer to the answer of Q. No 1.

4. Ans. d. 38/14 (25)

Hurst's 14th Ed; Page 1786

The pulmonary hemodynamics of adults residing at sea level and above sea level differs. At sea level, a cardiac output of 5 to 6 L/min is associated with a pulmonary arterial pressure of approximately 20/12 mm Hg, with a mean of approximately 15 mm Hg. At an altitude of 15,000 feet, the same level of blood flow is associated with somewhat higher pressures (see the table below). Pulmonary arterial pressures also tend to increase somewhat with age.

	Sea level	Altitude (~15,000 ft)
Pulmonary arterial pressure (PPA), mm Hg	20/12,15	38/14,25
Cardiac output (Q), L/min	6	6
Left atrial pressure (P_{LA}) mm Hg	5	5
Pulmonary vascular resistance (PVR),^{a} (mm Hg/L)/min (R units)	1.7	3.3

5. Ans. d. Rheumatoid arthritis

Hurst's 14th Ed; Page 1788

The prevalence of pulmonary vascular disease is around 2-4% of patients with portal hypertension and an approximately 0.5% of patients with HIV infection. The incidence of PAH in patients with systemic sclerosis ranges from 8 to 12%. PAH has been reported to occur in around 23 to 53% of patients with mixed connective tissue diseases and in 1 to 14% of patients with systemic lupus erythematosus, but it is rare in patients with rheumatoid arthritis, Sjogren syndrome, or dermatomyositis.

6. Ans. d. Cigarette smoking

Hurst's 14th Ed; Page 1788

Risk Factors for Pulmonary Arterial Hypertension (PAH)
- *Definite*:
  - Aminorex
  - Fenfluramine
  - Dexfenfluramine
  - Toxic rapeseed oil
- *Likely*:
  - Amphetamines
  - L-Tryptophan
  - Methamphetamines
- *Possible*:
  - Cocaine
  - Phenylpropanolamine
  - St. John's wort
  - Chemotherapeutic agents
  - Selective serotonin reuptake inhibitors
- *Unlikely*:
  - Oral contraceptives
  - Estrogen
  - Cigarette smoking

7. Ans. d. Right heart catheterization

Hurst's 14th Ed; Page 1789

The gold standard test for confirmation of suspected pulmonary arterial hypertension is right heart catheterization. This helps in the direct determination of right atrial and ventricular pressure, pulmonary arterial pressure, PCWP (as an approximation of pulmonary venous pressure), pulmonary blood flow (cardiac output when there are no systemic to pulmonary shunt) and the response of these parameters to intervention like vasodilator testing, oxygen supplementation and exercise. The echocardiography is a good alternative. However, echocardiography has limitation because it not infrequently overestimates or underestimates RV systolic pressures as a result of poor visualization of tricuspid regurgitant. Contrast angiography has a role in the work up for pulmonary arterial hypertension when chronic thromboembolic disease is suspected.

8. Ans. b. Intermediate artery

Hurst's 14th Ed; Page 1792

It is the occlusion of intermediate pulmonary artery by emboli which is the most commonly seen.

9. Ans. c. Systemically administered vasodilator and glucocorticoids

Hurst's 14th Ed; Page 1794

Oxygen therapy particularly during daily activity or sleep may help in attenuating the hypoxic pulmonary pressor response. Glucocorticoids and other potent immunosuppressive and antifibrotic agents are mainstay of therapy and often effect some symptomatic relief. Systematically administered vasodilators have no proven place in treating the PAH associated with interstitial fibrosis and may worsen intrapulmonary gas exchange. Evidence are in favour of inhaled vasodilators, such as the prostacyclin analogue iloprost. It produces selective pulmonary vasodilation and have antiproliferative effects.

10. Ans. c. Right heart catheterization

Hurst's 14th Ed; Page 1794

The gold standard for diagnosing PH in patients with COPD, as for other forms of PH, is right-heart catheterization. Noninvasive studies, such as echocardiography is useful; however, it frequently overestimates or underestimates the true pulmonary artery systolic pressure. Additionally, RV enlargement the cardinal sign of PH, can be difficult to discern in obstructive airways disease because of hyperinflation and cardiac rotation resulting in poor echo windows.

11. Ans. d. Supplemental oxygen

Hurst's 14th Ed; Page 1794

Vasodilators have been evaluated in PH associated with COPD. However, currently are no data to support treatment of COPD with these therapies. Rather they aggravate arterial hypoxemia by exaggerating ventilation-perfusion abnormalities. The safest and most effective approach to pulmonary vasodilatation in obstructive lung disease with arterial hypoxemia is the use of supplemental oxygen.

12. Ans. d. All of the above

Hurst's 14th Ed; Page 1794

In patients who hypoventilate despite normal lungs, the primary pathogenetic mechanism is alveolar hypoxia potentiated by respiratory acidosis. In individuals with normal lungs, alveolar hypoventilation generally originates from an inadequate ventilatory drive (after encephalitis or in central sleep apnea), covert obstruction of the upper airways (in obstructive sleep apnea), an ineffective chest bellows (after poliomyelitis or polymyositis), lungs entrapped by neoplasm or fibrosis or in morbid obesity.

13. Ans. d. Eisenmenger syndrome

Hurst's 14th Ed; Page 1795

The prognosis in pulmonary arterial hypertension depends on underlying etiology of the disease. The prognosis of patients with associated PAH with connective tissue disease is worse than for idiopathic PAH. Survival in patients with HIV-associated PAH is similar to that of patients with idiopathic PAH. Patient with PAH and coexisting portal hypertension have a worse prognosis as idiopathic PAH. The natural history of Eisenmenger syndrome is relatively better than that of idiopathic PAH, with an overall 75% 5-year survival and a 40% 25-year survival.

14. Ans. c. Eisenmenger syndrome

Hurst's 14th Ed; Page 1797

Dyspnea, is commonest symptom of idiopathic PAH, so is with the Eisenmenger syndrome. Syncope is an exceedingly rare symptom in unoperated patients with the Eisenmenger syndrome, because of the ability to decompress the right heart via an open atrial septal defect, ventricular septal defect, or patent ductus arteriosus. In contrast, patients with idiopathic PAH with an intact atrial septum (without a patent foramen ovale) and patients with elevated PVR after complete surgical repair of congenital shunts may present with syncope.

15. Ans. a. Scleroderma

Hurst's 14th Ed; Page 1800

Screening in patients with connective tissue disorder is important for early identification of pulmonary arterial hypertension in asymptomatic or minimally symptomatic individuals. Patient with scleroderma have high prevalence of PAH as compared with the much lower prevalence in patients with SLE, rheumatoid arthritis and other connective tissue diseases. The general treatment for patients with all form of pulmonary arterial hypertension (PAH) includes avoidance of circumstances or substances that may aggravate the disease state. Exercise should be guided by symptoms, and exposure to high altitude may worsen PAH by producing hypoxia-induced pulmonary vasoconstriction. Pregnancy, oral contraceptives, and appetite suppressants should be avoided. Because anesthesia and surgery of any type pose an increased risk of hemodynamic instability and death, elective procedures should be performed carefully. Phlebotomy with replacement of fluid (e.g., plasma or albumin) is helpful in patients with pulmonary vascular disease and cyanotic congenital heart disease in whom severe hypoxemia has evoked substantial polycythemia. Phlebotomy is recommended for symptoms of hyperviscosity as a result of severe polycythemia, such as headache or blurry vision, or if the hematocrit is greater than 65 to 70%. Caution is required to avoid depletion of iron stores and to avoid reduction in the circulating blood volume. There is a role of nitric oxide and phosphodiesterase inhibitors in management of pulmonary arterial hypertension. Nitric oxide (NO) is synthesized in endothelial cells from one of the guanidine nitrogens of L-arginine by the enzyme NO synthase. It has proved to be the endothelium-derived relaxing factor that contributes to the low initial tone of the pulmonary circulation.

16. Ans. d. 65% to 70%

Hurst's 14th Ed; Page 1800

Refer to the answer of Q. No 15.

17. Ans. d. Guanyly cyclase activator

Hurst's 14th Ed; Page 1803

Riociguat is a guanylyl cyclase activator that is approved for the treatment of PAH and inoperable chronic thromboembolic pulmonary hypertension. Riociguat should not be used in combination with a PDE-5 inhibitor because of the risk of hypotension.

CHAPTER 22: Cardiovascular Changes with Aging

1. Which of the following is more potent predictor of cardiovascular event in middle aged and older adults?
   a. Systolic blood pressure
   b. Diastolic blood pressure
   c. Pulse pressure
   d. Heart rate

2. Which is the commonest valvular lesion seen with aging?
   a. Aortic stenosis
   b. Mitral annular calcification
   c. Mitral regurgitation
   d. Mitral stenosis

ANSWERS WITH EXPLANATIONS

1. Ans. c. Pulse pressure

Braunwald 11th Ed; Page 1735

Due to structural and functional changes in the arterial walls in majority of older adults the systolic blood pressure progresses into the hypertensive range. In contrast, the diastolic blood pressure tends to rise until the sixth decade and declines thereafter because of the reduced elastic recoil from the stiffer large arteries. The pulse pressure, the difference between systolic and diastolic blood pressure also increases, augmenting the pulsatile load on the heart and vasculature. Several studies have suggested that pulse pressure is a potent predictor of cardiovascular events in middle-aged and older adults than either systolic or diastolic blood pressure.

2. Ans. a. Aortic stenosis

Hurst's 14th Ed; Page 1585

The prevalence of symptomatic aortic stenosis increases from 0.2% in patients under age 60 years to nearly 10% in those over 80 years of age. Aortic stenosis is the most common valvular abnormality requiring surgical or percutaneous intervention in elderly age group.

CHAPTER 23

Athlete Heart

1. Which of the following is the most common cause of sudden cardiac death in athletes older than 35 years?
   a. Hypertrophic cardiomyopathy
   b. Arrhythmogenic RV dysplasia
   c. Atherosclerotic coronary artery disease
   d. Congenital coronary artery abnormalities

2. Which of the following is the most common cause of sudden cardiac death in younger athletes?
   a. Hypertrophic cardiomyopathy
   b. Arrhythmogenic right ventricular cardiomyopathy
   c. Congenital coronary abnormalities
   d. Atherosclerotic coronary artery disease

3. Which of the following is *not* a component of athlete's heart?
   a. Chamber enlargement and hypertrophy
   b. Augmented ventricular systolic function
   c. Sinus arrhythmia
   d. Sinus tachycardia

4. The acute cardiovascular response to athletic training includes all the following *except*:
   a. Increase in cardiac output
   b. Increase in stroke volume
   c. Increase in MVO_2
   d. Increase in peripheral vascular resistance

5. Which of the following feature differentiate physiological changes of an athlete heart from hypertrophic cardiomyopathy?
   a. High degree of LV hypertrophy (wall thickness >16 mm)
   b. Asymmetric septal hypertrophy
   c. LV cavity <45 mm
   d. Disappearance of hypertrophy after physical deconditioning

6. The term "Commotio Cordis" is applied to:
   a. Sudden chest pain and breathlessness due to impaction of food particle in esophagus
   b. Sudden palpitation in crowded environments
   c. Blunt nonpenetrating chest blows during athletic or recreational activities causing sudden cardiac death
   d. Breathlessness felt in closed space

7. The mechanism of sudden cardiac death following a blunt nonpenetrating chest blow (Commotio Cordis) is:
   a. Cardiac contusion leading to myocardial ischemia
   b. Cardiac rupture due to nonpenetrating chest blow
   c. Rupture of aorta
   d. Primary electrical event leading to ventricular fibrillation

8. Which of the following sport activity produces a combination of both pressure and volume overload in the heart?
   a. Long distance running   b. Cycling
   c. Weightlifting   d. Basketball

9. Which of the following exercise produces volume overload in the heart and cardiomegaly involving all four chambers?
   a. Long distance running or cycling
   b. Weightlifting
   c. Basketball
   d. All of the above

10. Which of the sport activity produces pressure overload and concentric increase in left ventricular wall thickness?
    a. Long distance running   b. Cycling
    c. Weightlifting   d. Basketball

ANSWERS WITH EXPLANATIONS

1. Ans. c. Atherosclerotic coronary artery disease

Hurst's 14th Ed; Page 1563

Population based data shows that sudden death in young athletes occur with an incidence of 1-2 per 100,000 athletes per year with a frequency eight folds lower in female athletes. In athletes younger than 35 years, inherited diseases such as SCM, arrhythmogenic RV cardiomyopathy and congenital coronary artery abnormalities of wrong sinus origin are the most common cause of sudden death. In athletes older than age 35 years, atherosclerotic coronary artery disease is the most common cause of death. HCM is the single most common cause of cardiac arrest in athletes. HCM accounts for about one-third of sports related sudden fatality.

2. Ans. a. Hypertrophic cardiomyopathy

Hurst's 14th Ed; Page 1563

Refer to explanation for Q. No 1.

3. Ans. d. Sinus tachycardia

Hurst's 14th Ed; Page 1561

The athlete's heart refers to the clinical syndrome of cardiac chamber enlargement, hypertrophy, and normal or augmented ventricular systolic function commonly accompanied by sinus arrhythmia, sinus bradycardia, and a systolic flow murmur. These adaptation to exercise are physiologic and benign. The acute response to training for athletic activities among long-distance runner, swimmer, or bicycling includes substantial increases in maximum oxygen consumption, cardiac output, stroke volume, and systolic blood pressure, associated with decrease in peripheral vascular resistance.

4. Ans. d. Increase in peripheral vascular resistance

Hurst's 14th Ed; Page 1561

Refer to explanation for Q. No 3.

5. Ans. d. Disappearance of hypertrophy after physical deconditioning

Hurst's 14th Ed; Page 1562

The cardiac changes of athletes in response to systemic conditioning are variable, with cardiac remodeling in approximately one-half of trained athletes. The changes include alterations in ventricular chamber dimensions, including increased left and right ventricular and left atrial cavity size and volume, associated with normal systolic and diastolic function. Enlargement of the left ventricular (LV) chamber (> 60 mm) occurs in approximately 15% of highly trained athletes. Occasionally enlargement of the LV is accompanied by a mild increase in absolute LV wall thickness exceeding upper normal limits (range, 13-15 mm). Remodeling of LV mass is dynamic and develops after the initiation of vigorous conditioning. Differentiating the physiological changes resulting from habitual exercise in athletic heart syndrome with hypertrophic cardiomyopathy or dilated cardiomyopathy is challenging situation. Physiologic cardiac adaptation from regular exercise leads to an increase in LV wall thickness. This can be difficult to distinguish from pathologic changes of hypertrophic cardiomyopathy. Criteria favoring hypertrophic cardiomyopathy include a high degree of LV hypertrophy (wall thickness, >16 mm) with an unusual distribution (heterogeneous, asymmetric, or sparing the anterior septum), a small LV cavity (<45 mm), the presence of striking electrocardiographic abnormalities, and the persistence of hypertrophy after physical deconditioning.

6. Ans. c. Blunt nonpenetrating chest blows during athletic or recreational activities causing sudden cardiac death

Hurst's 14th Ed; Page 1564

In the absence of underlying cardiovascular disease blunt nonpenetrating chest blows during athletic or recreational activities that causes sudden cardiac death are known as commotio cordis. It is not uncommon occurrence in the young sports, and it is one of the leading cause of sudden cardiac death in young athletes. The most common sports associated with commotio cordis deaths are those in which projectiles are integral to the game, (e.g., baseball, softball, ice hockey, football).

7. Ans. d. Primary electrical event leading to ventricular fibrillation

Hurst's 14th Ed; Page 1565

The mechanism by which commotio cordis occurs is complex. Sudden impact of the blow delivered directly over the heart and timing within the vulnerable phase of repolarization associated peak LV pressure caused by the blow leads to ventricular fibrillation. Sudden cardiac death is a primary electrical event. The cellular determinants of ventricular fibrillation induced by chest wall blows likely include ion channel activation caused by increased LV pressure.

8. Ans. d. Basketball

Braunwald 11th Ed; Page 1039-1040

Highly trained athletes often exhibit remodeling of the heart. Cardiomegaly is an adaptation to generate the sustained increase in cardiac output required for regular high-intensity exercise. Endurance training such as long-distance running or cycling produces a sustained volume load to the heart, resulting in four chamber enlargement and increased stroke volume at rest and exercise. Strength training such as weightlifting presents a pressure load to the heart that may be accompanied by concentric increase in left ventricular wall thickness. Sports like basketball present a combination of both types of loads.

9. Ans. a. Long distance running or cycling

Braunwald 11th Ed; Page 1039-1040

Refer to explanation for Q. No 8.

10. Ans. c. Weightlifting

Braunwald 11th Ed; Page 1039-1040

Refer to explanation for Q. No 8.

CHAPTER 24

Pericardial Disease

1. Which of the following chemical agent serve as a lubricant to reduce friction between the surfaces of parietal and visceral pericardium?
   a. Prostaglandin
   b. Phospholipids
   c. Nitric oxide
   d. Albumin

2. Which of the following is *true* regarding systolic whoop or pericardial honk?
   a. It is a short musical murmur seen in later part of systole and is often without other evidence of heart disease
   b. It is mostly due to the pathological changes in mitral valve
   c. Cineangiogram demonstrates ballooning of mitral valve into LA during ventricular systole
   d. All are true

3. What is the normal pressure in pericardial cavity?
   a. 0 to +2 cm H_2
   b. −2 to +2 cm H_2
   c. −5 to +5 cm H_2
   d. −5 to +5 mm H_2

4. The ST segment elevation of acute pericarditis can be differentiated from ST segment elevation due to acute myocardial infarction by which of the following criteria?
   a. Absence of ST segment elevation in lead aVR and V_1
   b. The T waves are usually upright in leads with ST segment elevation
   c. The ST segment axis in frontal plane ranges from 30–60°
   d. All of the above

5. Which of the following ECG feature helps in differentiating changes of acute pericarditis from acute myocardial infarction?
   a. T wave inversion associated with loss of R wave voltage
   b. Appearance of Q waves
   c. Depression of PR segment
   d. All of the above

6. Which of the following drug has been shown to be effective in treatment of recurrent pericarditis?
   a. Corticosteroids
   b. Acetylsalicylic acid
   c. Colchicines
   d. Methotrexate

7. A patch of dullness on auscultation beneath the angle of the left scapula (Ewart's sign) suggest diagnosis of:
   a. Aortic aneurysm
   b. Constrictive effusive pericarditis
   c. Pericardial effusion
   d. Pleural effusion

8. All the following are correct regarding echocardiography in pericardial effusion, *except*:
   a. Echocardiography is sufficiently sensitive to detect as little as 20 mL of pericardial fluid
   b. About 8–15% of asymptomatic subjects have small pericardial effusion seen on echocardiography
   c. A substantial number (40% of normal pregnant woman have asymptomatic pericardial effusion)
   d. Echocardiography helps in precise quantification of effusion

9. During pericardiocentesis for cardiac tamponade which hemodynamic changes occurs first:
   a. Disappearance of right atrial collapse
   b. Disappearance of right ventricular collapse
   c. Increase in cardiac output
   d. Decrease in heart rate

10. Pulses paradoxus may be absent in cardiac tamponade in cases with:
    a. Left ventricular hypertrophy
    b. Pulmonary hypertension
    c. Aortic regurgitation
    d. All of the above

11. Which of the following is *not* a component of Beck's Triad used for diagnosis of cardiac tamponade?
    a. A decline in systematic arterial pressure
    b. A rising venous pressure
    c. A small quiet heart
    d. Cardiomegaly as X-ray chest

12. Beck's triad is rarely observed in cardiac tamponade due to:
 a. Idiopathic pericarditis
 b. Penetrating cardiac trauma
 c. Rupture aortic aneurysm
 d. Aortic dissection

13. Which is the most common physical finding in cases with cardiac tamponade?
 a. Jugular venous distention
 b. Pulsus paradoxus
 c. Pericardial friction rub
 d. Diminished heart sounds

14. Pulsus paradoxus is observed in all the following, *except*:
 a. COPD
 b. Massive pulmonary embolism
 c. Hemorrhagic shock and hypovolemia
 d. All of the above

15. Low pressure cardiac tamponade is seen in:
 a. Tuberculosis
 b. Neoplastic pericarditis
 c. Both of the above
 d. None of the above

16. Which of the following drug is used for treatment of recurrent pericardial effusion following cardiac trauma?
 a. Aspirin
 b. Glucocorticosteroids
 c. Nonsteroid anti-inflammatory agents
 d. All of the above

17. Which of the following statement is *correct* regarding right ventricular diastolic collapse in cases of cardiac tamponade?
 a. Right ventricular diastolic collapse is more predictive of cardiac tamponade than pulsus paradoxus
 b. Right ventricular diastolic collapse is absent in presence of right ventricular hypertrophy
 c. Right ventricular diastolic collapse can occur even by presence of large pleural effusion
 d. All of the above

18. Which of the following is the cause of continued elevation of right atrial pressure after successful pericardiocentesis?
 a. Effusive constrictive pericarditis
 b. Cardiac tamponade with left ventricular dysfunction
 c. Tricuspid valve disease
 d. All of the above

19. Cardiac tamponade due to retrograde bleeding is seen with which of the following condition?
 a. Blunt and penetrating trauma
 b. Post MI rupture of LV free wall
 c. Complication of interventional procedure
 d. Aortic dissection

20. Cardiac tamponade can occur without a paradoxic pulse in which of the following condition?
 a. Chronic LV dysfunction
 b. Aortic regurgitation
 c. Dissection of aorta
 d. All of the above

21. Low pressure cardiac tamponade is seen in which of the following condition?
 a. Patients on hemodialysis
 b. Patients with blood loss and volume depletion
 c. Patients with pericardial effusion on diuretics
 d. All of the above

22. X-ray chest in patient with pericardial effusion shows increased cardiothoracic ratio only when quantity of effusion exceeds:
 a. 100 mL   b. 200 mL
 c. 300 mL   d. 500 mL

23. Regional tamponade with left ventricular diastolic collapse is most commonly seen after:
 a. Trauma during cardiac intervention
 b. After cardiac surgery
 c. In case of dissection of aorta
 d. All of the above

24. Triad of hypotension, shock and elevated JVP (jugular venous pressure) is seen in:
 a. Cardiac tamponade
 b. Decompensated heart failure
 c. Pulmonary embolus
 d. All of the above

25. "Oreo Cookie Sign" is characteristic radiological finding in:
 a. Congestive heart failure
 b. Pulmonary embolism
 c. Pulmonary hypertension
 d. Pericardial effusion

26. Closed pericardiocentesis is contraindicated in cardiac tamponade resulting from:
 a. Bacterial pericardial effusion
 b. Uremic effusion
 c. Hemopericardium due to following cardiac intervention
 d. Type A aortic dissection

27. "Gold paint" effusion occurs in:
    a. Tubercular pericarditis
    b. Malignant effusion
    c. Hypothyroidism
    d. Pyogenic bacterial infection

28. Pericardial knock is heard in:
    a. Pericardial effusion
    b. Constrictive pericarditis
    c. Cardiac tamponade
    d. Acute pericarditis

29. Which of the following diagnostic modality is most accurate for measuring pericardial thickness?
    a. Two-dimensional echocardiography
    b. Transesophageal echocardiography
    c. Computed tomography
    d. Magnetic resonance imaging

30. In case of an acute and/or chronic pericarditis with thickened pericardium which of the following diagnostic modality may be useful in identifying patients who are candidates for medical management with anti-inflammatory drugs?
    a. X-ray chest
    b. Two-dimensional echocardiography
    c. Computed tomography
    d. Magnetic resonance imaging

31. Which of the following is drug of choice for rate control in patients with constrictive pericarditis with atrial fibrillation and a rapid ventricular response?
    a. Betablockers
    b. Calcium channel blocker
    c. Amiodarone
    d. Digoxin

32. Which is the most common cause of effusive constrictive pericarditis?
    a. Cancer
    b. Irradiation
    c. Following pericardiectomy
    d. Tuberculosis

33. Which of the following modality is used to prevent constriction in patients with tuberculous pericarditis?
    a. Prompt antitubercular therapy
    b. Intrapericardial urokinase
    c. Adjunctive prednisolone
    d. All of the above

34. All the following are correct regarding tuberculous pericarditis, *except*?
    a. There is a long interval between tuberculous pericarditis and its evolving to constriction
    b. Antitubercular treatment given for 9 months or longer gives no better results
    c. Intrapericardial urokinase and oral prednisolone can prevent evolution to constriction
    d. All of the above

35. Which of the following is *not* correct regarding uremic pericarditis?
    a. Chest pain is infrequent
    b. ECG changes are usually absent
    c. Pericardial effusions are often hemorrhagic
    d. Cardiac tamponade is quite common

36. Trapezius ridge radiation of chest pain points towards diagnosis of:
    a. Acute coronary syndrome
    b. Acute pulmonary embolism
    c. Acute pericarditis
    d. Dissection of aorta

37. The classical finding of "diffuse ST segment elevation" in acute pericarditis is seen in all leads, *except*:
    a. aVR   b. aVL
    c. aVF   d. V_1

38. Which of the following is the earliest ECG changes in acute pericarditis?
    a. PR segment depression
    b. Diffuse ST segment elevation
    c. T inversion
    d. T inversion with ST segment depression

39. What is the recommended duration of therapy with colchicine to improve the response of NSAIDs and reduce the recurrence of pericarditis?
    a. 2 weeks   b. 4 weeks
    c. 8 weeks   d. 12 weeks

40. Which of the following is drug of choice for patients with recurrent pericarditis who are resistant to colchicine and corticosteroids?
    a. Azathioprine
    b. Intravenous immunoglobulin
    c. Anakinra
    d. All of above can be used

41. Which of the following statement regarding recurrent pericarditis is *incorrect*?
    a. Use of high dose of corticosteroid for treating pericarditis is associated with high recurrence
    b. Recurrent pericarditis leads often to constrictive pericarditis
    c. Risk of constriction is associated with etiology, not the number of recurrences
    d. All are incorrect

42. **Knuckle sign (PR elevation in lead aVR) is electrocardiographic features of which of the following condition?**
    a. Dissection of aorta
    b. Acute pulmonary embolism
    c. Acute coronary syndrome
    d. Acute pericarditis

43. **Evolution toward constrictive pericarditis is rare with which of the following etiologies?**
    a. Viral pericarditis
    b. Autoimmune
    c. Neoplastic pericarditis
    d. Tubercular pericarditis

44. **P mitrales (broad, notched P wave in lead II) in the absence of mitral disease has been described as a sign of:**
    a. Acute pulmonary embolism
    b. Acute pericarditis
    c. Constrictive pericarditis
    d. Takotsubo syndrome

ANSWERS WITH EXPLANATIONS

1. Ans. b. Phospholipids

Braunwald 5th Ed; Page 1478

The human pericardium normally contains up to 50 mL of clear fluid. The visceral pericardium is believed to be the source of normal pericardial fluid and excessive fluid in disease states. Normal pericardial fluid appears to be an ultrafiltrate of plasma. Protein concentrations are about 1/3rd those of plasma and albumin is present in higher ratio in pericardial fluid. Pericardial fluid contains phospholipids that serve as a lubricant to reduce friction between the surfaces of parietal pericardium and visceral pericardium.

2. Ans. d. All are true

Hurst's 8th Ed; Page 283

Levine and Harvey described a musical, apical systolic murmur that they called a whoop because it simulated the whoop of whooping cough. These murmurs are loud, high pitched, musical sonorous, and vibratory; are best heard at the apex in late systole and are frequently intermittent. They are often preceded by clicks and originate in the mitral valve. They are associated with ballooning of the mitral valve or MR (or both) and their unusual quality is secondary to the high frequency vibrations of the mitral apparatus. The systolic whoop or honk together with the late systolic murmurs, with or without associated clicks, is part of a continuum representing abnormalities of the mitral valve apparatus of varying etiologies.

3. Ans. c. –5 to +5 cm H_2

Braunwald 5th Ed; Page 1479

The normal pericardium is relatively stiff and the relationship between pressure within the pericardium and total intrapericardial volume which is the sum of the volume of the heart itself and the reserve volume of the surrounding pericardial sac, appears as a steep curve when plotted on a graph. When measured with a fluid filled or micromanometer dipped catheter, pericardial pressure is nearly equal to intrapleural pressure and varies from –5 to +5 cm H_2O during the respiratory cycle.

4. Ans. d. All of the above

Braunwald 5th Ed; Page 1483

Serial electrocardiogram is extremely helpful in confirming the diagnosis of acute pericarditis. Electrocardiographic abnormalities appear in about 90% cases of acute pericarditis. Electrocardiographic changes can occur a few hours or days after the onset of pericardial pain, and the electrocardiographic diagnosis of acute pericarditis is made by detecting the serial appearance of 4 stages of abnormalities of ST segment and T wave. These changes are due to an actual current of injury caused by superficial myocardial inflammation or epicardial injury. There are 4 stages in the evaluation of acute pericarditis. *Stage 1* electrocardiographic changes accompanying the onset of chest pain and is virtually diagnostic of acute pericarditis. These changes comprises ST segment elevation which unlike the pattern of ST segment elevation in acute myocardial infarction is concave upward and usually present in all leads except aVR and V_1. The T waves are usually upright in the leads with ST segment elevation. The ST segment axis in the frontal plane also defers in these two conditions and is ranging from 30–60° in acute pericarditis unlike acute myocardial infarction in which ST segment axis varies from 100 to 120°. *Stage 2* occurs several days later and represents the return of ST segment to baseline accompanied by T wave flattening. These changes in ST segment usually occur prior to the appearance of T wave inversion. In contrast, T wave in acute myocardial infarction often become inverted before the ST segment return to baseline. *Stage 3* is characterized by inversion of T wave so that T wave vector becomes directed opposite to ST segment vector. T wave inversion is generally present in most leads and is not associated with loss of R wave voltage and appearance of Q waves. These feature help to differentiate this stage of nonspecific T wave inversion from changes associated with evolution of transmural or subendocardial myocardial infarction. *Stage 4* represent the reversion of T wave changes to normal, which may occur up to weeks or month later. T wave inversion may occasionally persist indefinitely in patient with chronic pericardial inflammation due to tuberculosis, uremia or neoplastic pericardial disease.

5. Ans. d. All of the above

Braunwald 5th Ed; Page 1483

Refer to explanation for Q. No 4.

6. Ans. c. Colchicines

Braunwald 5th Ed; Page 1485

The most troublesome complication is the development of recurrent episode of pericardial inflammation at interval of weeks or months after the initial episode of pericarditis. It is seen in about 20–28% of patients. The majority of patient can be managed by reinstitution of high dose nonsteroidal anti-inflammatory agents and very gradual tapering over several months to discontinuation or alternate dose therapy. In some patient disabling chest pain associated with fever may recur over a period of years and may require steroid administration. Intravenous methylprednisolone given as pulse therapy may be useful in the management of severe recurrent acute idiopathic pericarditis. Pericardiectomy has been proposed for the relief of refractory relapsing pericarditis but pericardiectomy is not always followed by relief of pain. In new promising approach for the treatment of symptomatic recurrent pericarditis before using corticosteroid is the chronic administration of colchicines. Colchicines therapy at a dose of 1 mg daily is associated with no recurrence in about 75% of patients during the follow-up of 3 years. Pericarditis can also be complicated by development of disabling or life-threatening hemodynamic complication due to cardiac compression. These includes: (1) development of pericardial effusion under pressure resulting in cardiac tamponade; (2) development of fibrosis and/or calcification of pericardium resulting in chronic constrictive physiology; and (3) a combination of both effusive and constrictive pericardial disease.

7. Ans. c. Pericardial effusion

Braunwald 5th Ed; Page 1485

On physical examination, a small pericardial effusion in the absence of an increase in intrapericardial pressure may result in no specific physical finding, whereas a large effusion may produce several characteristic physical finding. The heart sound may be muffled owing to the interposition of fluid between the chest wall and the cardiac chambers. Compression of the base of the left lung by pericardial fluid produces Ewart's sign, i.e., a patch of dullness on auscultation between the angles of left scapula. Rales may be heard over lung field secondary to the compression of left lung parenchyma.

8. Ans. d. Echocardiography helps in precise quantification of effusion

Braunwald 5th Ed; Page 1486

Echocardiogram is the most accurate, rapid and widely used technique for evaluating pericardial effusion, in following the accumulation or resolution of fluid over time, and in assessing the functional status of cardiac valves and myocardium. Accumulation of pericardial fluid results in appearance of an echo free space between the posterior left ventricular wall and posterior parietal pericardium and between the anterior wall of the right ventricle and adjacent echoes of the parietal pericardium and chest wall. Posterior and anterior epicardial fat can simulate this echocardiographic appearance of pericardial effusion. M-mode echocardiography is sufficiently sensitive to detect as little as 20 mL of pericardial fluid. Although the quantification of pericardial effusion by echocardiography is not precise, several guidelines of assessment are helpful. Very small effusion are likely to be image only posteriorly, with separation of the pericardial and epicardial echoes only in systole. A small to moderate size effusion are likely to be imaged only posteriorly with the presence of an echo free space throughout the cardiac cycle. Pericardial effusion of approximately 300 ml can usually be imaged both anteriorly and posteriorly. Moderate to large effusion may be associated with excessive swinging motion of the heart and false positive appearances of mitral valve prolapse and anterior septal motion. Usually, the echo free space represents the pericardial effusion disappears behind the left atrium due to the absence of fluid/pericardial sinus. However, in massive effusion fluid may also collect in the oblique sinus resulting in an echo free spaced behind left atrium as well as the left ventricle.

9. Ans. b. Disappearance of right ventricular collapse

Braunwald 5th Ed; Page 1488

Simultaneous hemodynamic and 2D echocardiographic measurement in patients undergoing pericardiocentesis have shown that the hemodynamic improvement first occurs at the point of disappearance of right ventricular diastolic collapse which is followed by disappearance of right atrium collapse and further improvement in cardiac output and decrease in heart rate during continued pericardiocentesis.

10. Ans. d. All of the above

Braunwald 5th Ed; Page 1488–1489

Mechanism of pulsus paradoxus: Inspiration and the transmission of negative intrathoracic pressure to the pericardial space further alter the dynamics of right and left ventricular filling and are responsible for pulsus paradoxus the inspiratory fall of aortic systolic pressure

>10 mm Hg. The finding of weakening of the arterial pulse during inspiration was described by Kussmaul in 1873 as the apparent paradox of the disappearance of the pulse during inspiration despite persistence of the heart beat. It should be emphasized that pulsus paradoxus is in fact an exaggeration of the normal inspiratory decline of left ventricular stroke volume by about 7% and of systemic arterial pressure by 3%. Inspiration is normally accompanied by an increase in diastolic dimensions of the right ventricle, a small decrease in left ventricular dimension, and increased velocity of flow from the venae cavae into the right atrium. Pulsus paradoxus in cardiac temponade appears to result from an exaggeration of these normal findings.

The nonspecificity of pulsus paradoxus: Pulsus paradoxus has also been observed in severe lung disease and massive pulmonary embolism. Under these circumstances, pulsus paradoxus is probably related to the transmission of excessively negative intrathoracic pressure during inspiration to the aorta, inspiratory pooling of right ventricular stroke volume in the lungs; and exaggerated right heart filling with an associated decrease in left-heart filling during inspiration.

Pulsus paradoxus may be absent in cardiac tamponade when left ventricular hypertrophy or heart failure causes a marked elevation of left ventricular diastolic pressure so that the two ventricles are unequally compressed. This may occur in atrial septal defect when the increase in systemic venous return during inspiration is shared between the two sides of the heart, and in aortic regurgitation when there is a major component of left ventricular filling that is independent of respiratory variation. Pulsus paradoxus may also be absent in the present of pulmonary hypertension and right ventricular hypertrophy that impedes the inspiratory increase in right ventricular filling. In this unusual clinical situation, the depression of left ventricular diastolic filling and cardiac outcome may depend on regional compression of the left ventricle.

11. Ans. d. Cardiomegaly as X-ray chest

Braunwald 5th Ed; Page 1489

The physical finding in cardiac tamponade was described by the thoracic surgeon Claude S Beck in 1935 and it is called as Beck's triad which is used for diagnosis of cardiac tamponade. The triad consists of: (1) decline in systemic arterial pressure; (2) elevation of systemic venous pressure; and (3) a small, quiet heart. These are three components of Beck's triad. These 3 features are typical of cardiac tamponade from sudden intraperitoneal hemorrhage due to penetrating heart wounds from trauma or invasive diagnostic cardiac procedures, aortic dissection and intrapericardial rupture of an aortic or cardiac aneurysm. This syndrome develops when the pericardium is not enlarged or stretched, so that the addition of <200 mL of fluid or blood causes intrapericardial pressure to rise abruptly to above 22–30 mm Hg.

12. Ans. a. Idiopathic pericarditis

Braunwald 5th Ed; Page 1489

Refer to explanation for Q. No 11.

13. Ans. a. Jugular venous distention

Braunwald 5th Ed; Page 1489

The physical examination in patients with cardiac tamponade reveals jugular venous distension which is the most common physical finding. In addition to the absolute elevation of the systemic venous pressure, a characteristic wave form consisting of a prominent systolic X descent and absence of diastolic Y descent can often be appreciated bedside. Other common physical finding includes tachypnea (80%), tachycardia (77%), pulsus paradoxus (77%), pulsus paradoxus with total inspiratory disappearance of brachial pulse and Korotkoff sound (23%), pericardial friction rub (29%), hepatomegaly (55%), and diminished heart sounds (34%). Systolic arterial hypotension consisting of a systolic pressure <100 mm Hg is present in 30–40% of cases. Majority of the patients are alert, with warm extremities and preservation of urine output. Elevated systemic arterial pressure may occur in patient with cardiac tamponade who have pre-existing hypertension. The finding of pulsus paradoxus is crucial in making the diagnosis of cardiac tamponade because most patients with slowly developing cardiac tamponade do not have classical physical findings of a small, quiet heart and severe hypotension. Pulses paradoxus can be detected on physical examination as an inspiratory decrease in the amplitude of the palpated pulse in the femoral or carotid arteries. Total paradox, i.e., complete disappearance of the palpated pulse during inspiration occurs during very severe cardiac tamponade or tamponale combined with hypovolemia. Other disorders with systemic venous distension, pulses paradoxus and clear lung field that can be confused with cardiac tamponade include obstructive pulmonary disease, constrictive pericarditis, restrictive cardiomyopathy and massive pulmonary embolism. Pulsus paradoxus is occasionally noted during severe hypovolemia due to hemorrhagic shock but jugular venous distension is usually absent. Cardiac tamponade may be confused with shock due to right ventricular infarction with jugular venous distension and clear lung fields. The pulsus paradoxus may be absent in cardiac tamponade in cases with left ventricular hypertrophy, chronic renal failure, pulmonary hypertension and aortic regurgitation. These are the whole conditions there is elevated left ventricular end-diastolic pressure which prevents the emergence of pulses paradoxus.

14. Ans. d. All of the above

Braunwald 5th Ed; Page 1488–1489

Refer to explanation for Q. No 10.

15. Ans. c. Both of the above

Braunwald 5th Ed; Page 1490

The low pressure cardiac tamponade occurs in setting of hypovolemia and it represents an early stage in the development of cardiac tamponade in which accumulation of a pericardial effusion causes intrapericardial pressure to rise and equilibrate with low right heart diastolic filling pressure. The clinical finding includes absence of jugular venous distention and the right atrial pressure is low. Pericardiocentesis reduces intrapericardial pressure and causes the separation of right atrial and intrapericardial pressures. Low pressure cardiac tamponade tend to occur in patient with tuberculosis and neoplastic pericarditis complicated by severe dehydration.

16. Ans. d. All of the above

Braunwald 5th Ed; Page 1536

An uncomplicated pericarditis secondary to cardiac trauma usually resolves. Tamponade, however requires emergency operative treatment. Recurrent pericardial effusion is sometime associated with chest pain and fever, i.e., the so called postpericardiotomy syndrome, occurs in small number of patient. Although patient with recurrent effusion usually respond to aspirin or nonsteroidal anti-inflammatory agents occasionally glucocorticosteroids are necessary. Constrictive pericarditis occurs as a rare complication of traumatic pericarditis with or without recurrent effusion.

17. Ans. d. All of the above

Braunwald 5th Ed; Page 1491

Two-dimensional and Doppler echocardiography provides clue about pericardial effusion associated with cardiac tamponade. The presence of pulsus paradoxus is associated with sudden leftward motion of the septum during the inspiration and exaggerated increase in the right ventricular size. This characteristic respiratory variation in ventricular preload can also be detected by Doppler ultrasound findings of exaggerated tricuspid and pulmonary flow velocity and reduction of peak mitral inflow velocity with onset of inspiration and the opposite changes after the onset of expiration. When the inspiratory reduction in the left ventricular filling is extreme, the aortic valve may close prematurely or fail to open and mitral valve opening may be delayed until atrial systole. The presence and magnitude of respiratory variation in mitral flow velocity are usually not predictive of the magnitude of hemodynamic compromise. Cardiac temponade is also associated with "pseudohypertrophy" (an increase in the left ventricular diastolic wall thickness), which correlates inversely with the decrease in the cavity volume, but the independent prognostic value of this sign is not known. Diastolic right atrial and right ventricular compression or collapse can occur early during the development of cardiac tamponade. Left atrial and left ventricular diastolic collapse can occur when regional left heart compression is present. Right ventricular diastolic collapse appears to be more predictive of cardiac tamponade than pulsus paradoxus, particularly during hypovolemia and these echocardiographic signs may be reversed by volume expansion. Right ventricular diastolic collapse may be absent in the presence of right ventricular hypertrophy and can occur when large pleural effusion causes elevation of intrapericardial pressure by external compression. Thus, the echocardiographic finding of pericardial effusion, an inspiratory increase in the right ventricular dimension and right atrial and ventricular diastolic collapse strongly suggests the diagnosis of cardiac tamponade but these changes are not 100% sensitive or specific.

18. Ans. d. All of the above

Braunwald 5th Ed; Page 1493

Aspiration of pericardial fluid in patients with cardiac tamponade results initially in the lowering of the identical intrapericardial, right atrial, right ventricular and left ventricular diastolic pressure, followed by a fall of intrapericardial pressure below right atrial pressure and reappearance of descent in the right atrial wave form. Further aspiration causes intrapericardial pressure to fall to a mean level of zero and fluctuate with changes in intrathoracic pressure. Because the pressure volume curve of the pericardium is steep, the initial aspiration of 50–100 mL of pericardial fluid usually leads to striking reduction in intrapericardial pressure, marked improvement in systemic arterial pressure and cardiac output and abolition of pulsus paradoxus. The reduction of intrapericardial pressure is often followed by diuresis, related both to the augmentation of cardiac output and the release of atrial natriuretic factor. If intrapericardial pressure falls to zero or becomes negative and right atrial pressure remains elevated, effusive—constrictive pericarditis should be strongly considered especially in patients with underlying neoplasm or prior radiation. Other causes of continued elevation of right atrial pressure after successful pericardiocentesis include the coexistence of cardiac tamponade and pre-existing left ventricular dysfunction causing in turn pulmonary hypertension and right atrial hypertension, tricuspid valve disease and restrictive cardiomyopathy. In patients with suspected malignant disease, pulmonary hypertension due to pulmonary microvascular tumor is an important cause of persistent elevation of right atrial pressure and failure to relieve dyspnea after complete drainage of the pericardial space.

19. Ans. d. Aortic dissection

Braunwald 11th Ed; Page 1667

Tamponade can be due to any condition which causes effusion. The tamponade may result from bleeding to pericardial sac after blunt and penetrating trauma, following post MI rupture of LV free wall and as a complication of cardiac interventional procedure. Retrograde bleeding is a major cause leading to death is seen in aortic dissection.

20. Ans. d. All of the above

Braunwald 11th Ed; Page 1668

One of the characteristics finding of cardiac tamponade is pulsus paradoxus. The mechanism of the paradoxic pulse in cardiac tamponade is multifactorial, but respiratory changes in systemic venous return is most important. In cardiac tamponade, the normal inspiratory increase in systemic venous return is present and the normal inspiratory decline in systemic venous pressure is retained (Kussmaul sign is absent). The increase in right heart filling pressure occurs, under conditions where total heart volume is fixed and left heart volume markedly reduced. The interventricular septum shifts to the left in exaggerated fashion on inspiration, encroaching on the left ventricle such that the stroke volume and pressure generation are further reduced. This is called as exaggerated ventricular interaction. Although the inspiratory increase in the right heart volume (preload) increases the right ventricular stroke volume, a few cardiac cycles are required to increase the left ventricular filling and stroke volume and counteract the septal shift. There is also increase afterload caused by transmission of negative intrathoracic pressure to the aorta and traction on the pericardium caused by descent of the diaphragm. Along with these mechanisms, left and right heart pressure and stroke volume variations are exaggerated. When there are preexisting elevations in diastolic pressures and/or volume, tamponade can occur without a paradoxic pulse. This situation is seen in patients with chronic LV dysfunction, aortic regurgitation and atrial septal defect. Similarly in patients with pericardial tamponade due to retrograde bleeding resulting from, tamponade may occur without a paradoxic pulse because of aortic valve disruption and regurgitation.

21. Ans. d. All of the above

Braunwald 11th Ed; Page 1668

The usual mean left, and right sided filling pressure are typically around 20-25 mm Hg in patient with cardiac tamponade. Tamponade can occur at low filling pressure, and it is termed as "low pressure tamponade". Low pressure tamponade occurs when there is a decrease in the blood volume in the setting of pre-existing effusion that would not otherwise cause hemodynamic consequences. A modestly elevated pericardial pressure can then lower that transmural filling pressure to level where the stroke volume is compromised. Because venous pressure is only modestly elevated or even normal, the other diagnosis may be missed. Low pressure tamponade may be observed during hemodialysis, in patients with blood loss, and volume depletion and when diuretics are administered to patients with effusion.

22. Ans. b. 200 mL

Gaillard F, Radiopedia.org 7729

Pericardial effusions occur when excess fluid collects in the pericardial space (a normal pericardial sac contains approximately 30-50 mL of fluid). Small pericardial effusions are often occult on plain X-ray film. Greater than 200 mL of pericardial fluid is usually required to become radiographically visible.

23. Ans. b. After cardiac surgery

Braunwald 11th Ed; Page 1668

Pericardial effusions can be loculated or localized, resulting in regional tamponade, which is most commonly seen after cardiac surgery. Increasing pressure within the compartment of loculated pericardial effusion reaching the limit of pericardial distensibility and consequent transient reversal of transmural left ventricular pressure during diastole are most likely basis for diastolic collapse of the thick wall ventricle in setting of regional cardiac tamponade. Left ventricular diastolic collapse is an infrequent sign of regional cardiac tamponade and is a useful marker of tamponade in postoperative patients.

24. Ans. d. All of the above

Braunwald 11th Ed; Page 1669

The triad of systemic hypotension, shock and elevated JVP can be seen in cardiac tamponade, decompensated heart failure, pulmonary embolism or other causes of pulmonary hypertension and in right ventricular myocardial infarction.

25. Ans. d. Pericardial effusion

Gaillard F, Radiopedia.org 15498

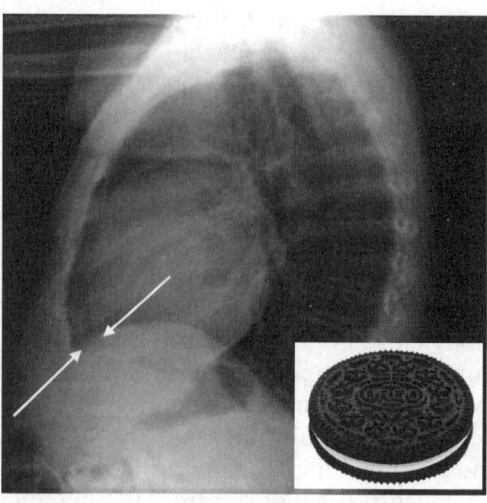

The classical "Oreo cookie sign" is of pericardial effusion seen on lateral chest radiograph. The most anterior radiolucent line is the epicardial fat, the radiopaque line is the pericardial effusion, and the posterior radiolucent line is the pericardial fat.

26. Ans. d. Type A aortic dissection

Braunwald 11th Ed; Page 1671

Closed pericardiocentesis is usually performed in majority of patients with cardiac tamponade who has hemodynamic compromise. The usual danger of closed approach is that lowering intrapericardial pressure will allow more bleeding without affording and opportunity to correct its source and therefore closed pericardiocentesis in patients with hemopericardium due to type A aortic dissection has been considered relatively contraindicated. However, in some patients under strict monitoring of systolic blood pressure, preoperative pericardiocentesis using intermittent cycle of drainage (dictated by systolic blood pressure level) appears to be safe and effective for stabilization in this subset of patients.

27. Ans. c. Hypothyroidism

Braunwald 11th Ed; Page 1672

Normal pericardial fluid has the features of a plasma ultrafiltrate. Lymphocytes are the predominant cell type. Most effusions are exudates, transudate are seen in patients with congestive heart failure and in hypoproteinemia. Sanguineous fluid is nonspecific and does not necessarily indicate active bleeding. Analysis of fluid gives clue about etiology and it is useful in bacterial infection and malignant effusion. Chylous effusions can occur after traumatic or surgical injury to the thoracic duct or obstruction by neoplasms. Cholesterol-rich ("gold paint") effusions occur in hypothyroidism.

28. Ans. b. Constrictive pericarditis

Braunwald 11th Ed; Page 1673

The most notable cardiac physical finding on auscultation in patient with constrictive pericarditis is the presence of pericardial knock. It is an early diastolic sound best heard at the left sternal border and/or the cardiac apex. It occurs slightly earlier and has a higher frequency content than a third heart sound and corresponds to early, abrupt cessation of ventricular filling in patients of constrictive pericarditis.

29. Ans. c. Computed tomography

Braunwald 11th Ed; Page 1674

ECG-synchronized CT and MRI are important diagnostic modality and important adjuncts to the echocardiography-Doppler examinations in evaluating suspected case of constrictive pericarditis. CT is helpful in detecting even minute amounts of pericardial calcification and is the most accurate method for measuring thickness (normal <2 mm). The MRI provides a detailed examination of the pericardium without the need for contrast or ionizing radiation. However, it is less sensitive for detecting calcification than CT and less accurate for measuring thickness.

30. Ans. d. Magnetic resonance imaging

Braunwald 11th Ed; Page 1674

A thickened pericardium indicates acute and/or chronic pericarditis. Late gadolinium enhancement on MRI is more specific for active inflammation and may be useful in identifying patients who are candidates for medical management with anti-inflammatory drugs.

31. Ans. d. Digoxin

Braunwald 11th Ed; Page 1675

In patients with constrictive pericarditis arrhythmias are common. Sinus tachycardia is seen as a compensatory mechanism. β-adrenergic blockers and calcium antagonists that slows the heart rate should be avoided in patients with sinus tachycardia because it is compensatory. In patients with atrial fibrillation and a rapid ventricular response, digoxin is recommended for rate control.

32. Ans. d. Tuberculosis

Braunwald 11th Ed; Page 1676

The common causes of effusive constrictive pericarditis are cancer, irradiation, TB, complication following pericardiectomy and connective tissue diseases. The condition may be idiopathic also. Tuberculosis is leading cause in developing countries.

33. Ans. d. All of the above

Braunwald 11th Ed; Page 1676

Tuberculous pericarditis has a high risk (20–40%) of evolving to constriction often within 6 months. Prompt antibiotic therapy is essential to prevent this. Treatments that may be useful to preventing constriction include intrapericardial urokinase and adjunctive prednisolone for 6 weeks.

34. Ans. a. There is a long interval between tuberculous pericarditis and its evolving to constriction

Braunwald 11th Ed; Page 1676

Tuberculous pericarditis if left untreated carries a high mortality rate (20–40%). Tuberculous pericarditis has a high risk (20–40%) of evolving to constriction, often within 6 months. Prompt antibiotic therapy is essential to prevent this complication. Rifampicin, isoniazid, pyrazinamide, and ethambutol for at least 2 months, followed by isoniazid and rifampicin for a total of 6 months, is recommended therapy. Treatment for 9 months or longer gives no better results. The additional treatment with intrapericardial urokinase and adjunctive oral prednisolone for 6 to 8 weeks may be useful to prevent constriction.

35. Ans. d. Cardiac tamponade is quite common

Braunwald 11th Ed; Page 1677

Pericardial disease in patients with renal failure have three main presentations (1) uremic pericarditis, often with moderate to large effusions, occurring before dialysis or within 8 weeks from its initiation and it is related to retention of toxic metabolites; (2) dialysis pericarditis - occurring 8 weeks or more after initiation of dialysis; and (3) constrictive pericarditis, which is rare. Many of the features of pericardial disease in patients with renal failure are distinctive. Chest pain is relatively infrequent (one third of patients are asymptomatic), ECG changes are usually absent because the myocardium is not involved, and pericardial effusions are often hemorrhagic because of uremic coagulopathy. Tamponade is uncommon because effusions usually develop gradually.

36. Ans. c. Acute pericarditis

Braunwald 11th Ed; Page 1663

The main symptom of acute pericarditis is chest pain, often quite severe. The pain may be retrosternal, it may be localized to anterior chest and radiate to the neck, shoulder and arm. Pericardial pain is pleuritic and worsen by lying down. The trapezius ridge is a classic radiation of pericardial chest pain.

37. Ans. a. aVR

Braunwald 11th Ed; Page 1664

The electrocardiogram in case of acute pericarditis produces "diffuse ST segment elevation". The ST segment vector points left anteriorly and inferiorly, with ST segment elevation in all leads except aVR and often V_1. Usually, the ST segment is coved upwards and resemble the current of injury of transmural ischemia.

38. Ans. a. PR segment depression

Braunwald 11th Ed; Page 1664

The PR segment depression is the earliest ECG sign of acute pericarditis, and it reflects pericardial involvement overlying the atria. PR depression can occur without ST elevation and be the initial or sole ECG manifestation. The typical ECG evolution follows four stages: (1) PR depression and/or diffuse ST-segment elevation, (2) normalization of the ST segment, (3) T-wave inversion with or without ST-segment depression, and (4) normalization.

39. Ans. d. 12 weeks

Braunwald 11th Ed; Page 1666

Colchicine is recommended in treatment of pericarditis for at least 3 months as an adjunct to NSAIDs to improve the response and reduce recurrence. Colchicine exerts an anti-inflammatory effect by blocking microtubule assembly in WBCs. It is recommended in dose of 0.5 to 0.6 mg orally every 12 hours.

40. Ans. d. All of above can be used

Braunwald 11th Ed; Page 1667

For patients with recurrent pericarditis who are resistant to colchicine and corticosteroids additional therapy which are available includes Azathioprine (2 mg/kg/day orally for several months), human intravenous immunoglobulin (400–500 mg/kg/day for 5 days with a repeat course after one month), or Anakinra, an interleukin 1-antagonists (1 to 2 mg/kg/day up to 100 mg daily subcutaneously for several months).

41. Ans. b. Recurrent pericarditis leads often to constrictive pericarditis

Braunwald 11th Ed; Page 1667

Recurrence of pericarditis occurs in 15–30% of patients with idiopathic acute pericarditis. Recurrent pericarditis has never been associated with evolution to constrictive pericarditis. The risk of constriction is associated with etiology, not the number of recurrences. Use of high dose of corticosteroids (prednisolone 1 to 1.5 mg/kg/day) are associated with major side effects and also more recurrences when applied for treatment of initial pericarditis.

42. Ans. d. Acute pericarditis

Hurst's 14th Ed; Page 1598

Electrocardiographic features of acute pericarditis include PR segment depression or diffuse ST elevation except in lead aVR. Another ECG feature of acute pericarditis is PR elevation in lead aVR (Knuckle sign).

43. Ans. a. Viral pericarditis

Hurst's 14th Ed; Page 1601

The most feared complication of pericarditis is the evolution towards constriction. Constrictive pericarditis rarely occurs in idiopathic and viral pericarditis (<1%). It is usually more common for specific etiologies such as autoimmune and neoplastic pericarditis (2 to 5%) and especially tuberculous and purulent pericarditis (20 to 30%).

44. Ans. c. Constrictive pericarditis

Hurst's 14th Ed; Page 1612

The ECG in cases of constrictive pericarditis shows nonspecific ST-T wave abnormalities. Atrial fibrillation occurs commonly in patients with constrictive pericarditis. P mitrales (broad, notched P wave in lead II) in the absence of mitral disease has also been described as a s sign of constrictive pericarditis.

CARDIAC TUMOR

1. Which is the most common primary malignant tumor of the pericardium?
   a. Teratomas
   b. Mesothelioma
   c. Angiosarcoma
   d. Lipomas

2. Which of the following tumor is most likely to spread to pericardium?
   a. Breast cancer
   b. Lung cancer
   c. Haematological malignancy
   d. Melanoma

3. A left ventricular myocardial apical mass that contracts in a manner similar to the surrounding tissue is likely to be a:
   a. LV apical thrombus
   b. Cardiac tumor
   c. Focal hypertrophy
   d. Effusion

4. If a cardiac mass changes in size from one image to next in echocardiography what is the probable pathological lesion?
   a. Cardiac tumor
   b. Left ventricular noncompaction
   c. Focal hypertrophy
   d. LV apical thrombus

5. Which of the following is the most common benign cardiac tumor in children?
   a. Myxoma
   b. Lipoma
   c. Rhabdomyoma
   d. Fibroelastoma

6. Which of the following is *incorrect* regarding carney complex?
   a. It is autosomal recessive condition
   b. Often cardiac myxoma are discovered in atypical location in the heart
   c. Hyperpigmented skin lesions are common
   d. Hyperactivity of adrenal or testicular gland are seen

7. The symptoms of dyspnea that is worse while lying on the left side points toward the possibility of:
   a. Mitral stenosis
   b. Pericardial effusion
   c. Left atrial thrombus
   d. Myxoma

8. Which is the most common auscultatory finding in a patient with left atrial myxoma?
   a. Loud first heart sound
   b. Opening snap
   c. Diastolic murmur
   d. Systolic murmur

9. Which is *not* correct regarding myxoma?
   a. It may be familial
   b. Myxoma cells express a variety of antigens and endothelial markers
   c. Myxoma have fragile extension and tendency to fragment spontaneously
   d. Myxoma do not recur after excision

10. Which of the cardiac tumor may regress with age?
    a. Myxoma
    b. Fibroma
    c. Rhabdomyoma
    d. Lipoma

11. Which of the following tumor arises from valvular structure of the heart?
    a. Rhabdomyoma
    b. Myxoma
    c. Papillary fibroelastoma
    d. Fibroma

12. Which of the following cancer is the most common cause of cardiac metastasis?
    a. Lung cancer
    b. Esophageal cancer
    c. Hematological malignancy
    d. Bone cancer

13. Which is the most common cause of superior vena cava syndrome?
    a. Malignancy
    b. Post pacemaker
    c. Thymoma
    d. Aortic aneurysm

14. Facial edema which is worse in the morning and gets better during the day such as the diagnosis of:
    a. Tricuspid regurgitation
    b. Left atrial myxoma
    c. Superior vena cava syndrome
    d. Aortic aneurysm

ANSWERS WITH EXPLANATIONS

1. Ans. b. Mesothelioma

Hurst's 14th Ed; Page 2321

The most common primary malignant tumor of the pericardium is mesothelioma. It usually presents in middle aged adults and men are more affected than women. Pericardial teratomas or benign tumor are usually occurring in children. Angiosarcomas are the second most common primary pericardial malignancy originating in right atrium or in the pericardium seen in young adults. Pericardial lipomas are usually benign.

2. Ans. d. Melanoma

Hurst's 14th Ed; Page 2322

Metastatic spread of tumor to pericardium is common. Around 10% of all malignancy spread to some portion of heart and 85% eventually involves the pericardium. Lung cancer, breast cancer and hematological malignancy accounts for almost 2/3rd cases of metastatic disease to the pericardium. Melanoma is a tumor most likely to spread to pericardium with 70% of patients with metastatic melanoma having pericardial involvement.

3. Ans. c. Focal hypertrophy

Braunwald 11th Ed; Page 1866

Echocardiography is helpful in assessing the nature of cardiac mass. When one is assessing a cardiac mass to determine the nature of mass, the clinical contact in which images obtained is very important. Cardiac mass can be tumor, thrombi, infection and artifacts. The presence of a severe wall motion abnormality plus mass that appears to be distinct from the myocardial wall, as well as lobulated, strongly suggests that the mass is a thrombus as opposed to a tumor. Motion imaging may be helpful in diagnosing a cardiac tumor. If a tumor is infiltrating the myocardium, it is unlikely to contract in a normal fashion. A left ventricular myocardial apical mass that contracts in a manner similar to the surrounding tissue is likely to be either focal hypertrophy or a left ventricular noncompaction as opposed to a cardiac tumor. Progression of an image over a time may indicate the pathologic process. If a cardiac mass changes in size from one image to the next, suspicion of a cardiac tumor is much higher.

4. Ans. a. Cardiac tumor

Braunwald 11th Ed; Page 1866

Refer to explanation for Q. No 3.

5. Ans. c. Rhabdomyoma

Braunwald 11th Ed; Page 1867

The majority of primary cardiac tumors are benign, and myxoma is by far the most common type seen in adults and only small percentage is seen in children. Rhabdomyoma is the most common benign tumor in children, accounting for 40 to 60% of the cases.

6. Ans. a. It is autosomal recessive condition

Braunwald 11th Ed; Page 1869

Most myxomas are found in left atrium. They are also found in decreasing frequencies in the right atrium, right ventricle, and left ventricle. Most myxomas occur sporadically, but they may be familial. Occasionally myxoma has been described in relation to a particular syndrome called the Carney complex. It is an autosomal dominant condition associated with cardiac myxomas, myxomas in other regions (cutaneous or mammary), hyperpigmented skin lesions, hyperactivity of the adrenal or testicular glands, and pituitary tumors. The Carney complex occurs at a younger age and should be considered when cardiac myxomas are discovered in atypical locations in the heart.

7. Ans. d. Myxoma

Braunwald 11th Ed; Page 1869

Patients with myxomas are usually asymptomatic and the tumor is found on an incidental 2D echocardiography. When symptoms are present, dyspnea, especially dyspnea that is worse while lying on the left side, points towards the possibility of a myxoma. Most of the clinical presentations of myxoma result from mitral valve obstruction (syncope, dyspnea, and pulmonary edema) followed by embolic manifestations. Patients may present with nonspecific symptoms such as fatigue, cough, low-grade fever, arthralgia, myalgia, weight loss, erythematous rash, and laboratory findings of anemia, and raised erythrocyte sedimentation rate (ESR), CRP and gamma globulin. The cardiac auscultation abnormality detected in >60% of patients with myxoma. The most common auscultation findings are systolic murmur (50% of cases) followed by a loud first heart sound (32%), an opening snap (26%), and a diastolic murmur (15%). The underlying reason for the systolic murmur may be damage to the valves, failure of the leaflets to coapt, or narrowing of the outflow tract by the tumor.

8. Ans. d. Systolic murmur

Braunwald 11th Ed; Page 1869

Refer to explanation for Q. No 7.

9. Ans. d. Myxoma do not recur after excision

Braunwald 11th Ed; Page 1869

The most myxoma occurs sporadically but they may be familial. The cardiac myxoma originates from a pluripotential stem cell, and myxoma cells express a variety of antigens and other endothelial markers. Myxomas typically form a pedunculated mass with a short, broad base, but sessile forms can also occur. A villous or papillary form of myxoma has multiple fine or very fine villous, gelatinous, and fragile extensions that have a tendency to fragment spontaneously and are associated with embolic phenomena. The definitive treatment of cardiac myxoma is surgical removal. The lifelong follow up is needed in these patients because myxoma have some tendency to recur, at rates varying from 5 to 14%. The time to recurrence in different series vary from 0.5 to 6.5 years.

10. Ans. c. Rhabdomyoma

Braunwald 11th Ed; Page 1871

Rhabdomyomas are usually found in ventricle and are the most common benign cardiac tumor found in children. The majority of these patients have signs of or a family history of tuberous sclerosis. These tumors may regress with age; they can sometimes grow or appear during puberty only.

11. Ans. c. Papillary fibroelastoma

Braunwald 11th Ed; Page 1871

Valvular structures may have a papillary fibroelastoma, which is often found incidentally. These tumors are small in size, <2 cm, and most commonly occur on the aortic valve, followed by the mitral valve. Rarely they may be found anywhere in the endocardial surface. These fibroelastomas are usually solitary; and they may result in embolic phenomena, and when situated on the aortic valve, can cause coronary ostial occlusion.

12. Ans. a. Lung cancer

Braunwald 11th Ed; Page 1873

A recent review suggests that lung cancer is the most common cause of cardiac metastasis, followed by esophageal cancer and hematological malignancy.

13. Ans. a. Malignancy

Braunwald 11th Ed; Page 1875

The most common cause of superior vena cava syndrome is malignancy of which lung carcinoma is the most common, followed by lymphoma and metastatic cancer. Malignancy accounts for >85% of causes of SVC syndrome. Other causes of SVC syndrome, which are mostly benign, account for 3 to 15% of cases and include thrombosis due to the use of intravascular devices such as catheters or pacemakers, infection, thymoma, substernal thyroid goiter, and aortic aneurysm. The clinical diagnosis is usually made on the basis of a constellation of symptoms and signs. A usual patient present with facial edema, dyspnea, and cough. Facial edema is most frequently seen; it is worse in the morning and gets better during the day as the patient ambulates.

Superior vena cava syndrome results from any inflammatory process in the mediastinum or enlargement of lymph node or ascending aorta, may cause SVC compression resulting in reduce blood flow and eventually complete occlusion. The usual presentation of SVC syndrome involves facial edema, dyspnea and cough. Facial edema is most frequently seen. It is worse in the morning and gets better during the day as the patient ambulates. Other less frequent symptoms include stridor, headache, syncope, dizziness, hoarseness, and confusion. Common findings on examination include facial edema, distended neck and chest veins, arm edema, and facial plethora.

14. Ans. c. Superior vena cava syndrome

Braunwald 11th Ed; Page 1875

Refer to explanation for Q. No 13.

CHAPTER 25

Cardiac Tumor

1. **Constitutional symptoms of left atrial myxoma is attributed to:**
   a. Secretion of prostaglandins
   b. Cell mediated hypersensitivity
   c. Tumor necrosis factor
   d. Interleukin-6

2. **An embolic stroke in a young person without evidence of cerebrovascular disease particularly in presence of sinus rhythm raises the possibility of:**
   a. Intracardiac myxoma
   b. Infective endocarditis
   c. Prolapse of mitral valve
   d. All of the above

3. **Myocardial tumors most commonly results in:**
   a. Myocardial rupture
   b. Congestion heart failure
   c. Disturbance of conduction or rhythm
   d. Systemic embolization

4. **Which statement is *not* correct regarding cardiac tumors?**
   a. Myxoma occurs more commonly in left atrium while sarcoma occurs more commonly in right atrium
   b. Symptoms of left atrial myxoma are often paroxysmal and arise characteristically in a particular body position
   c. The specific signs and symptoms produced by tumors are more closely related to their anatomical location than histological type
   d. All of the above

5. **Left ventricular tumors may clinically stimulates finding of:**
   a. Subaortic stenosis
   b. Hypertrophic cardiomyopathy
   c. Aortic stenosis
   d. All of the above

6. **The most common primary malignant cardiac tumor is:**
   a. Myxoma   b. Sarcoma
   c. Mesothelioma   d. Teratoma

7. **The most common type of primary cardiac tumor is:**
   a. Sarcoma   b. Mesothelioma
   c. Lipoma   d. Myxoma

8. **Which of the following feature characterizes syndrome myxoma or Corney Syndrome?**
   a. Myxoma in other location
   b. Spotty pigmentation like lentigines
   c. Endocrine hyperactivity
   d. All of the above

9. **The most common tumor of cardiac valves are:**
   a. Mesothelioma   b. Papillary fibroelastoma
   c. Myxoma   d. Lambl' excrescence

10. **Which of the following feature helps in differentiating left atrial myxoma from thrombus?**
    a. Mottled appearance
    b. Septal location
    c. Presence of echolucency
    d. All of the above

11. **Which of the following feature differentiates left atrial thrombus from left atrial myxoma?**
    a. Layered appearance   b. Posterior location
    c. Absence of echolucency   d. All

ANSWERS WITH EXPLANATIONS

1. **Ans. d. Interleukin-6**

   Hurst's 8th Ed; Chapter 111; Page 2007–2023

   Cardiac tumors particularly cardiac myxoma can produce a broad range of systemic (i.e., noncardiac) findings include fever, cachexia, malaise, arthralgias, Raynaud's phenomena, rash, clubbing and episodic bizarre behavior as well as systemic and pulmonary emboli. A variety of laboratory findings have been reported including hypergammaglobulinemia, elevated erythrocytes sedimentation rate, thrombocytosis, thrombocytopnea, polycythemia, leukocytosis, anemia. Systemic signs and symptoms are frequently resolved when the tumor is removed. The association of constitutional symptoms with cardiac myxoma is likely to be due to the tumors constitutive synthesis and secretion of interleukin-6 (IL-6). It is an inflammatory cytokine thought to be a major inducer of acute phase response which is associated with fever, leukocytosis and activation of compliment and clotting cascades. High levels of myxoma cell production of IL-6 may be accompanied by elevated serum concentration in patients with cardiac myxoma who have symptoms characteristic of autoimmune diseases.

2. Ans. d. All of the above

Hurst's 8th Ed; Chapter 111; Page 2007-2023

The embolization of tumor fragments are of thrombus from the surface of a myxoma is a frequent and often dramatic clinical occurrence. Although the myxoma are the source of most tumor emboli because of the combination of their friable constituency and intracavitary location other types of cardiac tumor occasionally may embolize. An embolic stroke in a young person without evidence of cerebrovascular disease particularly in the presence of sinus rhythm should raise the possibility of intracardiac myxoma as well as infective endocarditis and prolapse of mitral valve.

3. Ans. c. Disturbance of conduction or rhythm

Hurst's 8th Ed; Chapter 111; Page 2007-2023

Myocardial tumors when clinically apparent most commonly results in disturbance of conduction of rhythm. The precise nature of which is determined by the location of the tumor. Tumors in the area of atrioventricular node typically angiomas and mesotheliomas may produce atrioventricular conduction disturbance including complete heart block and assesesly and can lead to sudden death. A wide variety of arrhythmias may be produced including atrial fibrillation or flutter, paroxysmal atrial tachycardia with or without block nodal rhythm, ventricular premature beats, ventricular tachycardia and ventricular fibrillation. Intramural tumor may also produce symptoms by virtue of their size and location. Impairment of ventricular performance may simulate congestive, restrictive or hypertrophic cardiomyopathy. Tumor infiltration of myocardial wall occasionally causes myocardial rupture.

4. Ans. d. All of the above

Hurst's 8th Ed; Chapter 111; Page 2007-2023

Left atrial tumors are not uncommon. Mobile pedunculated left atrial tumor may prolapse to variable degree into the mitral valve orifice resulting in obstruction to atrioventricular blood flow and frequently mitral regurgitation. The resultant sign and symptoms often mimics those of mitral valve disease especially mitral stenosis and includes dyspnea, orthopnea, paroxysmal nocturnal dyspnea, pulmonary dema, cough, hemoptysis, chest pain, peripheral edema and fatigue. However, weight loss pallor syncope and sudden death manifestation that are common with mitral valve disease also occur. It is not unusual for the symptoms to be sudden in onset, intermittent and related to the patient body position. Although, the majority of symptom produced by left atrial tumor are unspecific. The occurrence of paroxysmal symptom that arise characteristically in a particular body position and are out of proportion to the clinical findings should raise suspicion of a left atrial tumor. The most common primary cardiac tumor presenting in the left atrium is benign myxoma, in which large majority of cases is solitary.

Right atrial tumor frequently produce symptoms of right heart failure including fatigue, peripheral edema, ascites, hepatomegaly and prominence of A wave in jugular venous pressure. The average time interval from the symptomatic presentation to the correct diagnosis of right atrial tumor may be years. The development of right heart failure may be rapidly progressive and often associated with new systolic or diastolic murmur or both.

It is not uncommon to misdiagnosed right atrial tumors as Ebstein anomaly of tricuspid valve, constrictive pericarditis, tricuspid stenosis, carcinoid syndrome, superior vena cava syndrome and cardiomyopathy. Pulmonary embolism and pulmonary hypertension occur and may simulate classical thromboembolic disease. Right atrial hypertension may cause right to left shunt through patent foreman ovale with systemic hypoxia cyanosis clubbing and polycythemia whereas myxoma occurs much more common in the left atrium than in the right atriums are, occurs more commonly in the right atrium. Right ventricular tumors often present with the right heart failure as a result of obstruction to right ventricular filling or outflow tract. Clinical manifestation includes peripheral edema, hepatomegaly, ascites, shortness of breath, syncope and sudden death. The left ventricular tumors are predominately intraluminar location, their often asymptomatic or they may present as conduction disturbance or arrhythmias or them an interfere with ventricular function. However, when the tumor has a significant intracavitary component, there may be obstruction to left ventricular outflow resulting in syncope and finding consistent with left ventricular failure. Atypical chest pain has also been reported and in some cases may reflect obstruction of a coronary artery either directly by a tumor involvement or as a result of tumor embolus to the coronary artery. The types of benign and malignant mesenchymal tumor that may develop in the heart or typical of those occurring in any areas of striated muscle and connective tissue. Although the exit incidence of each specific cardiac tumor type cannot be stated, about 75% of all cardiac tumors are benign histologically and the remainder are malignant. The majority of benign cardiac tumors are myxoma, followed by infrequency by wide range of other tumors. Almost all malignant tumors are sarcoma and of these angiomyosarcoma, and the rhabdomyosarcoma are the most common form.

The specific sign and symptoms produced by cardiac tumors are more closely related to their precise anatomical location than to their histological type.

5. Ans. d. All of the above

Hurst's 8th Ed; Chapter 111; Page 2007-2023

The physical examination in a case with left ventricular tumor reveals a systolic murmur, and both the murmurs and the blood pressure may vary with the position. Left ventricular tumors may simulate the findings of aortic stenosis, subaortic stenosis, hypertrophic cardiomyopathy, endocardial fibroelastosis and coronary artery disease.

6. Ans. b. Sarcoma

Hurst's 8th Ed; Chapter 111; Page 2007-2023

Tumor type	% of group		
	Adults	Children	Infants
Angiosarcoma	33	0	0
Rhabdomyosarcoma	21	33	66
Mesothelioma	16	0	0
Fibrosarcoma	11	11	33
Malignant lymphoma	6	0	0
Extraskeletal osteosarcoma	4	0	0
Thymoma	3	0	0
Neurogenic sarcoma	3	11	0
Leiomyosarcoma	1	0	0
Liposarcoma	1	0	0
Synovial sarcoma	1	0	0
Malignant teratoma	0	44	0

7. Ans. d. Myxoma

Hurst's 8th Ed; Chapter 111; Page 2007-2023

Myxomas are the most common type of primary cardiac tumors comprising 30-50% of the total in most pathological series. Myxomas are common in the age group 3-83 years and not infrequently diagnosed in elderly patients in whom the symptom and sign of cardiac tumor have been attributed to other causes for a substantial time. Approximately 86% of myxoma occur in left atrium and over 90% are solitary. In the left atrium, the usual site of attachment is in the area of fossa ovales. Myxoma also may occur in the right atrium and less often in right or left ventricle. Multiple tumors may occur in the same chamber or in combination of chambers. Although myxomas may occasionally be found on the posterior left atrial wall, tumor presenting in this location should raise suspicion of malignancy. Myxomas of the mitral and tricuspid valves have been reported.

8. Ans. d. All of the above

Hurst's 8th Ed; Chapter 111; Page 2007-2023

Familial cardiac myxomas constitute approximately 10% or less of all myxomas and appears to have an autosomal dominant transmission. Some patients with cardiac myxoma have a syndrome frequently called syndrome myxoma or Carney syndrome that also consist of: (1) myxoma in other location (breast or skin); (2) spotty pigmentation (lentigines, pigmented nevi or both); and (3) endocrine over activity (pituitary adenoma, primary pigmented, nodular adrenocortical disease or testicular tumor involving the endocrine components). Patients with Carney syndrome tends to be younger (mean age 20s) are more likely to have myxoma in location other than the left atrium, sometime have bilateral tumor and are more likely to develop recurrences. Although the etiology of the syndrome myxoma is unknown, it has been proposed to result from a widespread abnormality resulting in excessive proliferation of certain mesenchymal cells.

9. Ans. b. Papillary fibroelastoma

Hurst's 8th Ed; Chapter 111; Page 2007-2023

Papillary fibroelastomas is the most common tumor of the cardiac valve. They are clinically insignificant but they have the potential to embolise to vital structure or cause valvular dysfunction and those on aortic valve can partially obstruct a coronary orifice. These lesions have a characteristic frond like appearance resembling a sea anemone may be single or multiple up to 3 to 4 cm in diameter and may occur on any valve or on papillary muscle, chordae tendineae or endocardium, usually attached by a short pedicle. Most often the ventricular surface of the semilunar valve and the atrial surface of atrioventricular valves are affected. The tricuspid valve is most commonly involved in children and the mitral and aortic valves in adult.

10. Ans. d. All of the above

Hurst's 8th Ed; Chapter 111; Page 2007-2023

2D echocardiography facilitates the differentiation between left atrial thrombus and myxoma. Left atrial thrombus typically produces a layered appearance and is generally situated in the posterior portion of atrium whereas the left atrial myxoma is often mottled in appearance and rarely occurs in the posterior portion of the atrium. In some atrial myxoma, areas of echolucency may be seen within the tumor mass, corresponding to areas of hemorrhage within the tumor. Since these areas of echolucency are not found in thrombotic or infective lesions, this finding may be of value in the differential diagnosis of an intra-atrial mass. Continuous mode Doppler ultrasonography may be useful for evaluating the hemodynamic consequence of valvular obstruction or incompetence caused by cardiac tumor.

11. Ans. d. All

Hurst's 8th Ed; Chapter 111; Page 2007-2023

Refer to explanation for Q. No 10.

NEOPLASTIC HEART DISEASE

1. Which of the following is *not* a feature of Triad characteristics of intracavitary cardiac tumors?
   a. Obstruction
   b. Embolization
   c. Constitutional symptom
   d. New heart murmurs

2. All the following are correct *except*:
   a. More than 75% of cardiac tumors are benign
   b. Myxoma constitutes 50% of all histologically benign tumor of the heart
   c. 75% of the myxoma are located in the left atrium
   d. Right ventricle is the rarest site of myxoma

3. Most of true myxoma arise from:
   a. Cardiac valves
   b. Mural endocardium
   c. Pulmonary vessels
   d. Vena cava

4. Which is *not* a feature with cardiac myxomas?
   a. Familial pattern of tumor development
   b. Recurrence
   c. Multicentric origin
   d. Metastasis

5. All the followings are correct about cardiac myxoma *except*:
   a. Most patients with myxoma are below 30 years of age
   b. Children have a higher incidence of ventricular myxomas than adults
   c. There is higher prevalence of myxoma in females
   d. All are correct

6. Which of the following is *not* a feature of syndrome myxoma or Corney's complex?
   a. Cardiac myxoma
   b. Spotty skin pigmentations
   c. Peripheral and endocranial neoplasm
   d. Occurring in old age

7. Myocardial infarction in myxoma patients with normal coronaries has been ascribed to the secretion by tumor of:
   a. Cytokine
   b. Interleukin-6
   c. Prostaglandins
   d. Immunoglobulin G

8. Which of the following is an unusual feature of cardiac myxoma?
   a. Raynand's phenomenon
   b. Multiple systemic arterial aneurysm
   c. Coronary artery aneurysmal dilatation and myocardial infarction
   d. All of the above

9. Which of the following statement is *correct* regarding cardiac myxomas?
   a. Embolic tumor phenomenon occurs less frequently with RA than LA myxoma
   b. Constitutional symptoms are less frequent with RA myxoma
   c. Calcification is more common in RA myxoma
   d. All are correct

10. Which of the following malignant tumor has tandem metastasis to the heart?
   a. Bronchogenic carcinoma
   b. Leukemia
   c. Malignant melanoma
   d. Breast carcinoma

11. Risk of radiation induced damage to cardiac structure increases if the dose of radiation exceed:
   a. 40 Gy
   b. 75 Gy
   c. 90 Gy
   d. 100 Gy

ANSWERS WITH EXPLANATIONS

1. Ans. d. New heart murmurs

Hurst's 8th Ed; Chapter 111; Page 2007-2023

The heart may be the site of a primary tumor or may be invaded secondarily by malignancies that arise in adjacent or remote organs. Whether the tumors are primary or secondary, neoplastic heart disease can be expressed in only limited ways. In presence of neoplastic disease, pericardial pain, effusion, tamponade, constriction, rapid increase in the heart size, new heart murmur, electrocardiographic changes, atrial or ventricular arrhythmias, atrioventricular block and unexplained heart failure are suggestive of secondary invasion of the heart. The triad of obstruction, embolization and constitutional manifestation characterizes intracavity tumors especially myxoma.

2. Ans. d. Right ventricle is the rarest site of myxoma

Hurst's 8th Ed; Chapter 111; Page 2007-2023

Intracavitary myxoma is the most frequent benign tumor of the heart. Myxomas constitute nearly 50% of all histologically benign tumor of the heart. While most (75%) are located in the left atrium, myxomas are also found in the right atrium (18%), right ventricle (4%) and left ventricle (3%). Cardiac myxoma usually originates from the region of fossa ovalis but may arise from a variety of location within the atria. Approximately 75% occur in left atria. Most true myxomas arise only from mural endocardium despite isolated reports that they arise from the cardiac valves, pulmonary vessels and vena cava.

3. Ans. b. Mural endocardium

Hurst's 8th Ed; Chapter 111; Page 2007-2023

Refer to explanation for Q. No 13.

4. Ans. d. Metastasis

Hurst's 8th Ed; Chapter 111; Page 2007-2023

Most patients with myxomas are 30-60 years of age, although myxoma have been discovered in children, infants and neonates and also in the elderly. Children have a higher incidence of ventricular myxoma than do adults. A high prevalence in females has been found in most of the series. Familial occurrence have been reported more frequently in the males. Tumors are divided equally on both sides of the heart and opposite atria are usually involved in afflicted members. Familial cases are associated with younger age at presentation and a higher recurrence rate. Neoplastic origin of myxoma is supported by the ultrastructural characteristic of the tumor, the result of biochemical analysis, the cultural properties of the tumor cells and DNA analysis of the tumor. Although myxoma can recur because of their incomplete removal and distant growth of embolic myxomatus materials has been observed, the existence of a true malignant cardiac myxoma remains doubtful. The occurrence of multiple tumors within the ventricle, bilaterally in each atrium or simultaneously in atria or ventricle gives the likelihood of a multicentric origin rather than metastasis of the tumor.

5. Ans. a. Most patients with myxoma are below 30 years of age

Hurst's 8th Ed; Chapter 111; Page 2007-2023

Refer to explanation for Q. No 15.

6. Ans. d. Occurring in old age

Hurst's 8th Ed; Chapter 111; Page 2007-2023

Syndrome myxoma or Carney's complex characterizes a subset of patients with cardiac myxoma associated with spotty skin pigmentations and peripheral and endocrinal neoplasm. These patients in contrast to those with sporadic myxoma are usually younger, have a higher frequency of familial myxoma and more frequently have multiple and recurrent tumors.

7. Ans. a. Cytokine

Hurst's 8th Ed; Chapter 111; Page 2007-2023

Coronary artery embolism associated with myxoma has been documented by both angiography in living patients and histology at postmortem studies. Myocardial infarction occasionally is the first manifestation of a myxoma. Coronary angiography may demonstrative vascular flush in the tumor from the branches of both the right and left coronary arteries. Both left and right atrial myxomas and ventricular myxoma have been demonstrated in this manner. Aneurysm and occlusion of the coronary artery caused by tumor emboli have also been demonstrated by coronary angiography.

Myocardial infarction in myxoma patient with normal coronary arteries has been ascribed to cytokine secretion by the tumor.

8. Ans. d. All of the above

Hurst's 8th Ed; Chapter 111; Page 2007-2023

Left atrial myxoma most often present as mitral valvular disease and must be differentiated from it. Characteristically, the clinical course is relatively recent in origin however, it may occasionally span over many years. Fever, constitutional symptoms and embolic phenomena mimic infective endocarditis. On rare occasion, the myxoma itself may be infected. Muscle pain, skin rash and Raynaud's phenomenon may simulate peripheral vasculitis. Multiple systemic arterial aneurysm secondary to myxomatus embolization mimics polyarteritis nodosa. Similarly, coronary artery aneurysmal dilatation and myocardial infarction have been attributed to coronary myxoma embolization.

9. Ans. d. All are correct

Hurst's 8th Ed; Chapter 111; Page 2007-2023

Myxomas in the right atrial cavity constitute about 1/5th of all myxoma and tend to be more solid, have a wider attachment and involve a greater amount of atrial wall or septum than those in left atria. They originate from a variety of location within the right atrium including the inferior margin of foreman ovale, tricuspid valve and posterior wall and characteristically produces tricuspid valve or vena cava obstruction. Clinically, symptoms of low cardiac output and manifestation of systemic venous hypertension are present, with a prominent JVP, hepatomegaly, ascites, edema and cyanosis, which may be episodic and vary with the position of the patient. Persistence of sinus rhythm is common. Intermittent episode of syncope and abrupt onset of dyspnea, features never seen with rheumatic tricuspid stenosis are reported in one-third of these patient. The pendular action of a prolapsing right atrial myxoma (Wrecking ball effect), especially when it is calcified may damage or destroy the tricuspid valve and produce severe tricuspid regurgitation. While embolic tumor phenomena occur less frequently with the right atrial than left atrial myxomas, pulmonary emboli have been reported at times. They may be extensive and produce irreversible pulmonary hypertension. Right atrial myxoma has been incorrectly diagnosed as recurrent pulmonary thromboembolism. Paradoxical embolization may occur if an interatrial communication exist. Constitutional symptoms are less frequent in patient with right atrial myxoma. Anemia, polycythemia and cyanosis have been reported. Polycythemia and cyanosis may be caused by either right to left shunting through a patent foreman ovale or atrial septal defect, low cardiac output and hypoxic stimulation of the bone marrow, intravascular hemoconcentration or erythropoietin production by tumor. Mesenteric vasculitis of a non-embolic, probably autoimmune origin have been reported in patient with right atrial myxoma.

10. Ans. c. Malignant melanoma

Hurst's 8th Ed; Chapter 111; Page 2007-2023

Metastatic tumors involve the heart, the pericardium, or both from a primary origin in some other organ. The heart is a site of metastatic tumor in 5–6% of the cases and heart including the pericardium, is seen in about 13–14% of the cases. In one of the series, cardiac metastasis was reported in patients with malignant tumors in the range as wide as 1.5–21%. The relative infrequency of cardiac metastasis have been attributed to the strong kneading action of the heart, the metabolic peculiarities of the striated muscle, rapid coronary blood flow and lymphatic connection that drain afferently from the heart. Cardiac metastasis occurs with all types of primary tumors. No malignant tumor tends particularly to metastasis to the heart with the possible exception of malignant melanoma which involves the myocardium in more than 50% of cases. Cardiac metastasis are most frequent with bronchogenic carcinoma and carcinoma breast, occurring in one-third of cases. Cardiac infiltration often macroscopic, seen in one half of the cases of leukemia and in one sixth cases of lymphoma.

11. Ans. a. 40 Gy

Hurst's 8th Ed; Chapter 111; Page 2007-2023

The treatment of secondary tumors of the heart involves radiation or chemotherapy. Depending on the cytologic types and radiosensitivity of the tumor, radiation of the cardiac area with or without systemic chemotherapy is the treatment of choice. The heart can tolerate 20–40 Gy, beyond which the risk of radiation induced pericardial, myocardial and valvular damages are increased.

CHAPTER 26

Cardiac Trauma

1. Rupture of which cardiac chamber occurs commonly following cardiac massage:
   a. Right ventricle
   b. Left ventricle
   c. Aorta
   d. Pulmonary artery

2. The cardiac chamber most commonly involved in penetrating cardiac injury is:
   a. Right ventricle
   b. Left ventricle
   c. Left atrium
   d. Right atrium

3. In nonpenetrating chest trauma commonest valve to be involved is:
   a. Mitral valve
   b. Pulmonary valve
   c. Aortic valve
   d. Tricuspid valve

4. The most common cardiovascular traumatic lesion following automobile accident is:
   a. Rupture of aorta
   b. Laceration of right ventricle
   c. Rupture of left ventricle
   d. Rupture of right atrium

5. A diagnostic triad of increased arterial pressure and pulse amplitude in upper limb, decreased arterial pressure and pulse amplitude in lower limb and radiological evidence of widening of superior mediastinum (Symbas Triad) suggests diagnosis of:
   a. Cardiac tamponade
   b. Dissection of aorta
   c. Rupture of aorta
   d. Expanding mediastinal mass

ANSWERS WITH EXPLANATIONS

1. Ans. b. Left ventricle

Hurst's 11th Ed; Page 2225-2229

Closed chest cardiac massage is generally thought to be safe and simple and it is included as a part of cardiopulmonary resuscitation. Rupture of left ventricle is more common complication of cardiac massage than is rupture of right ventricle. However, rupture of either chamber may occur and may be life-threatening if the patient survives the arrhythmia that necessitated massage in the first place. Rupture of right ventricular papillary muscle with acute tricuspid regurgitation has also been reported as a complication of close chest cardiac massage as has rupture of the atria and aorta and dissecting hematoma of a coronary artery. A variety of non-cardiovascular traumatic lesions such as fracture of the sternum, hemothorax, pneumothorax and laceration of abdominal organ may occur.

2. Ans. a. Right ventricle

Hurst's 11th Ed; Page 2225-2229

Penetrating cardiac injuries occurring in civilian life are due to a variety of objects such as bullets, knife, ice picks, etc. Penetrating injuries may also be due to the invert displacement of ribs or sternal fragment accompanying chest injury. The chamber most commonly involved in this type of injury is the right ventricle because of its anterior position followed in descending order of frequency by the left ventricle, the right atrium and the left atrium. Penetrating wounds of pericardium are not only the causes of wound that may result in cardiac injury occasionally wounds of other areas of the chest as well as of the neck and upper abdomen are associated with the penetration of heart. In addition, intravenous or intracardiac catheters may fracture and become impaled within the walls of great vessels or cardiac chamber. Migration of an indwelling venous catheter into pulmonary artery which may ultimately lead to the perforation of the vessel is another complication that has increase in frequency with its wide spirit use in intensive care unit. Perforation of right ventricle with the transvenous pacing electrode is not uncommon but tamponade is rare. During cardiac catheterization perforation of thin wall right atrium or outflow tract of right ventricle has been reported.

3. Ans. c. Aortic valve

Hurst's 11th Ed; Page 2225-2229

Patients with preexisting valvular disease are at higher risk when those with normal valve for developing valvular injury following blunt trauma. In one of the series reported by Parmley, there was a 9% incidence of valvular injury in their report of 540 cases of non-penetrating chest trauma. In most series, damage to the aortic valve is by far the most common of this lesion. Indeed sustained damage of the aortic valve should be suspected in any patient without history of heart disease who has a heart murmur after severe blunt trauma to the chest. Damage to the cardiac valve may also occur as a consequence of penetrating wound of the heart, but in contrast to the damage caused by non-penetrating injury these are rarely solitary lesions. Blunt chest trauma has also been reported to cause bioprosthetic valve dysfunction.

4. Ans. a. Rupture of aorta

Hurst's 11th Ed; Page 2225-2229

Rupture of the aorta is one of the most common traumatic lesions involving the heart or great vessel. It is the most common after automobile accident but can also occur after fall from height, or other type of crashing injury. In automobile accidents, most commonly rupture occurs at the isthmus whether the collagen are head on or broadside.

5. Ans. c. Rupture of aorta

Hurst's 11th Ed; Page 2225-2229

In > 50% of cases of rupture of aorta, the diagnosis is made by a triad reported by Symbas and it consist of: (1) increased arterial pressure and pulse amplitude in the upper extremity; (2) decrease pressure and pulse amplitude in lower extremity; and (3) radiological evidence of widening of superior mediastinum. CT-scanning is not a useful screening procedure but transesophageal echocardiography has become increasingly useful in documenting aortic laceration.

CHAPTER 27

Aortic Disease

1. **Which of the following physical finding is uncommon with proximal aortic dissection?**
   a. Hypertension
   b. Hypotension
   c. Pulse deficits (diminution or absence of pulse)
   d. Aortic regurgitation

2. **A proximal dissection of aorta may involve the ostia of coronary artery and produces EKG feature of acute myocardial infarction commonly of:**
   a. Inferior wall MI
   b. Anterior MI
   c. Inferolateral MI
   d. Anterolateral MI

3. **The calcium sign (separation of the intimal calcification from outer aortic soft tissue border by >1 cm) is suggestive of:**
   a. Dissection of aorta
   b. Coarctation of aorta
   c. Pseudocoarctation of aorta
   d. Severe aortic regurgitation

4. **Which of the following is a disadvantage of using MRI in the diagnosis of aortic dissection?**
   a. It is contraindicated in patients with prosthetic implants
   b. It provides limited images of branch vessels
   c. It does not identify presence of aortic regurgitation
   d. All of the above

5. **Which of the following imaging modality is the gold standard diagnostic for evaluating aortic dissection?**
   a. Aortography
   b. CT imaging
   c. MRI
   d. TEE

6. **Which of the following is *not* correct regarding Takayasu arteritis?**
   a. It often involves aortic arch and its major branches
   b. The lesion of Takayasu arteritis is purely stenotic
   c. The coronary artery is affected in <10% cases
   d. Aortic regurgitation is seen in 25% cases

7. **The rat tall angiographic appearance of thoracic aorta is suggestive of:**
   a. Dissection of aorta
   b. Diffuse atheroma of aorta
   c. Giant cell arteritis
   d. Takayasu's arteritis

8. **Which of the following feature helps in differentiating giant cell arteritis from Takayasu's arteritis?**
   a. Narrowing or occlusion of branch vessel of thoracic aorta
   b. Involvement of aortic valve leading to aortic regurgitation
   c. Presence of aortic dissection
   d. Noninvolvement of renal arteries

9. **Which of the following is included in major criteria for diagnosis of Takayasu's disease?**
   a. Left mid common carotid lesion
   b. Distal brachiocephalic trunk lesion
   c. Right mid subclavian artery lesion
   d. Hypertension

10. **Which of the following is an obligatory criteria for diagnosis of Takayasu's disease?**
    a. High ESR
    b. Hypertension
    c. Left mid subclavian artery lesion
    d. Age below 40 years

11. **What is the pulse wave velocity through the aortic wall?**
    a. 3 m/sec
    b. 2 m/sec
    c. 5 m/sec
    d. 10 m/sec

12. **What is the level of bifurcation of abdominal aorta?**
    a. 12th thoracic vertebrae
    b. 2nd lumbar vertebrae
    c. 3rd lumbar vertebrae
    d. 4th lumbar vertebrae

13. **Which is *not* correct regarding aortic isthmus?**
    a. It is the point where ascending aorta joins the arch of aorta
    b. It is vulnerable point for trauma
    c. It is the point where coarctation of aorta occurs
    d. All are correct

14. Which is the location where aorta can be palpated normally without being enlarged?
   a. 2nd right intercostals space
   b. Suprasternal notch
   c. Abdomen
   d. Interscapular area

15. Which portion of aorta is affected most by atherosclerosis?
   a. Arch of aorta
   b. Thoracic aorta
   c. Suprarenal portion of abdominal aorta
   d. Infrarenal portion of abdominal aorta

16. Which is the most common site of rupture of abdominal aorta?
   a. Left retroperitoneum
   b. Peritoneal cavity
   c. Inferior vena cava
   d. Iliac veins

17. Which is the standard imaging modality to define size and extent of abdominal aortic aneurysm along with status of renal and mesenteric vessels?
   a. CT
   b. Aortography
   c. MRI
   d. Ultrasonography

18. Which portion of thoracic aorta is commonly involved with aneurysm?
   a. Ascending aorta
   b. Isthmus
   c. Arch of aorta
   d. Descending aorta

19. Which is the most common cause of aneurysm of ascending aorta?
   a. Atherosclerosis
   b. Syphilis
   c. Infectious aortitis
   d. Cystic medial degeneration

20. All the following are correct regarding dissection of aorta, *except*:
   a. A dissection presenting <2 weeks is defined as acute
   b. All patients have identifiable intimal tear
   c. Commonest site of intimal tear is ascending aorta
   d. At diagnosis about 2/3 of aortic dissection are acute

21. Which of the following congenital cardiovascular anomaly predisposes to dissection of aorta?
   a. Bicuspid aortic valve
   b. Unicuspid aortic valve
   c. Coarctation of aorta
   d. Turner syndrome

22. Which portion of the aorta is vulnerable to deceleration trauma?
   a. Ascending aorta
   b. Arch of aorta
   c. Aortic isthmus
   d. Descending thoracic aorta

23. Which of the following risk factor is strongly related with the occurrence of abdominal aortic aneurysm?
   a. Hypertension
   b. Hyperlipidaemia
   c. Diabetes
   d. Smoking

24. Abdominal aortic aneurysms are defined by an abdominal aorta dimension of:
   a. >2 cm in diameter
   b. >3 cm in diameter
   c. >4 cm in diameter
   d. >4.5 cm in diameter

25. Elective repair of abdominal aortic aneurysm is recommended in asymptomatic patients with diameter greater than:
   a. 3.0 to 3.5 cm
   b. 4.0 to 4.5 cm
   c. 4.5 to 5.0 cm
   d. 5.0 to 5.5 cm

26. "Tree bark" or Wrinkled appearance of aortic intima is characteristics of:
   a. Marfan's syndrome
   b. Ehler–Danlos syndrome
   c. Syphilitic aortitis
   d. Takayasu syndrome

27. Which of the following is a drug of choice for blood pressure reduction in patient with dissection of aorta?
   a. IV beta blocker
   b. IV sodium nitroprusside
   c. IV nitroglycerine
   d. IV ACE inhibitor

ANSWERS WITH EXPLANATIONS

1. Ans. a. Hypertension

Braunwald 6th Ed; Page 1434

The finding on physical examination generally reflect the location of aortic dissection and extent of associated cardiovascular involvement. Hypertension is seen in >80-90% of patients with distal aortic dissection but is less common in proximal dissection. Hypotension on the other hand occur more commonly among those with proximal than distal aortic dissection. True hypotension usually is the result of cardiac tamponade, intrapleural rupture or intraperitoneal rupture. Dissection involving the brachiocephalic vessel may result in pseudohypertension, an inaccurate measurement of blood pressure due to compromise or occlusion of the brachial arteries. The physical finding most typically associated with aortic dissection, i.e., pulse deficit, the murmur of aortic regurgitation and neurological manifestation are more characteristic of proximal than of distal dissection. The presence of pulse deficit (diminution or absence) in patients with acute chest pain strongly suggests presence of aortic dissection. Pulse deficit are present in about 50% of proximal aortic dissection and occurs throughout the arterial tree but are seen in only 15% of distal dissection, where they usually involve the femoral or left subclavian arteries. Such pulse deficit result from extension of dissection flap into an artery with compression of the true lumen by false channel or from proximal obstruction of flow due to a mobile portion of intimal flap overlying the vessel orifice. Aortic regurgitation is an important feature of proximal aortic dissection with the murmur of aortic regurgitation detected in 16-67% of cases. When aortic regurgitation is present in patients with distal dissection, it generally antedates the dissection and may be the result of the pre-existing dilatation of the aortic root due to the underlying aortic pathology such as cystic medial degeneration. Neurological manifestation occurs in as many as 6-19% of all aortic dissection but are more common with proximal dissection. Cerebrovascular accident may occur in 3-6% when there is a direct involvement of innominate or left common carotid arteries, less frequently patient may present with altered consciousness or even coma. In a small minority about 1-2 % of cases, a proximal dissection flap may involve the ostium of coronary artery and cause acute myocardial infarction. The dissection more often affects the right coronary artery than the left explaining why this myocardial infarction tends to be inferior in location.

2. Ans. a. Inferior wall MI

Braunwald 6th Ed; Page 1434

In a small minority of cases of dissection, about 1-2% of cases, a proximal dissection flap may involve the ostium of a coronary artery and cause acute myocardial infarction. The dissection more often affects the right coronary artery than the left, explaining why these myocardial infarctions tend to be inferior in location. Unfortunately, when secondary myocardial infarction does occur, its symptoms may complicate the clinical picture by obscuring the symptoms of the primary aortic dissection. Most worrisome is the possibility that in the setting of electrocardiographic evidence of myocardial infarction, the underlying aortic dissection may go unrecognized. Moreover, the consequences of such a misdiagnosis in the era of thrombolytic therapy can be catastrophic.

3. Ans. a. Dissection of aorta

Braunwald 6th Ed; Page 1435

The most common abnormality seen on chest X-ray in aortic dissection is a widening of aortic silhouette, apparent in 80-90% of cases and sometime with a localized bulge overlying the site of origin. Less often, nonspecific widening of superior mediastinum is seen. If the calcification of aortic knob is present, separation of intimal calcification from outer soft issue border by >1 cm, i.e., the calcium sign is suggestive although not diagnostic of aortic dissection.

4. Ans. d. All of the above

Braunwald 6th Ed; Page 1438

The use of MRI has particular appeal for diagnosing aortic dissection in that it is entirely noninvasive and does not require the use of intravenous contrast material or ionizing radiation. MRI produces high quality images in the transverse, sagittal and coronal planes as well as in left anterior oblique view that displace the entire thoracic aorta in one plane. The availability of multiple views facilitates the diagnosis of aortic dissection and the determination of its extent and also reveals the presence of branch vessel involvement. MRI is ideal for evaluation of patient with pre-existing aortic disease such as those with thoracic aortic aneurysm or prior aortic graft repair because it provides sufficient anatomical detail to distinguish aortic dissection from other aortic pathology. MRI has sensitivity and specificity of 98% and it has a sensitivity of 88% for identifying the site of intimal tear, 98% for the presence of thrombus and 100% for the presence of pericardial effusion. The use of the cine MRI technique in a subset of patient has shown 88% sensitivity for detecting aortic regurgitation. The remarkably high accuracy of MRI has made it the current gold standard for diagnosing the presence or absence of aortic dissection. However, MRI have a number of disadvantages: (a) it is contraindicated in patients with pacemaker; (b) certain type of vascular clips; and (c) certain older type of metallic prosthetic heart valve.

MRI provides early limited images of the branch vessel and does not consistently identify the presence of aortic regurgitation.

5. Ans. c. MRI

Braunwald 6th Ed; Page 1438

Contrast enhance CT scanning is helpful in diagnosing aortic dissection. Aortic dissection is diagnosed by the presence of two distinct aortic lumens, either visibly separated by an intimal flap or distinguished by a differential rate of contrast opacification. Indirect sign of aortic dissection may also be evident. In two large prospective series of patients with suspected aortic dissection, contrast enhanced CT scanning have been found to have a sensitivity of 83% with specificity of 100%. Newer techniques such as ultrafast CT scanning with electron beam which provides superior image resolution and helical CT scanning which permits a three-dimensional display of the aorta and its branches has improved the accuracy of CT in diagnosing aortic dissection as well as better defining anatomical features. CT scanning has the advantage that unlike aortography it is noninvasive, however, it does require the use of an intravenous contrast agents. Most hospitals are equipped with readily accessible CT scanner, available on emergency basis. CT is also helpful in identifying the presence of thrombus in the false lumen and detecting the presence of a pericardial effusion. A disadvantage of CT scanning is that its sensitivity for aortic dissection lower than that for other available modalities. Moreover, an intimal flap is identified in only 2/3rd of cases and site of intimal tear is really identified. CT scanning also cannot reliably detect the presence of aortic regurgitation or involvement of the branch vessel.

6. Ans. b. The lesion of Takayasu arteritis is purely stenotic

Braunwald 8th Ed; Page 152-1574

Takayasu's arteritis is a chronic inflammatory disease of unknown etiology involving the aorta and its major branches which was first noted in 1908 by the Japanese Ophthalmologist Takayasu. Takayasu arteritis occurs worldwide, although the large majority of cases are seen in Asia and Africa. A specific cause has not been found, although the bulk of evidence favors an autoimmune etiology. It has been linked to rheumatic fever, streptococcal infection, rheumatoid arthritis and other collagen vascular diseases. An association between the disease and certain HLA subtypes have been reported. In the early stage of disease, there is active inflammation involving granulomatous arteritis of the aorta and its branches, with secondary alteration in the media and adventitia. The disease progresses at a variable rate to a later sclerotic stage in which there is intimal hyperplasia, medial degeneration and adventitial fibrosis. The proliferative process leads to obliterative luminal changes in the aorta and other involved arteries.

Takayasu's arteritis most often involves the aortic arch and its branches, with changes that are usually most marked at branch points in the aorta. It may present as multisegmental aortic disease with areas of normal wall between the affected sites, as diffuse involvement of the aorta, or as disease of individual arteries arising from the aorta. The pulmonary artery may also be involved. The lesions are purely stenotic in 85% of patients, purely dilatative into 2% and mixed in 13%. The coronary arteries are affected in <10% of patients. Aortic regurgitation as a consequence of disease of the proximal ascending aorta is seen in about one quarter of cases. Ueno, et al have subdivided the disease into three types depending upon the predominant site of involvement. Type 1 involves primarily the aortic arch and its branches Type 2 spares the aortic arch involving the thoracoabdominal and its branches, Type 3 combine the features of both. Lupi-Herrera et al. have suggested a fourth category Type 4 in which there is a pulmonary arterial involvement.

7. Ans. d. Takayasu's arteritis

Braunwald 8th Ed; Page 152-1574

The laboratory diagnosis of aortoarteritis during the acute phase includes an elevated sedimentation rate, a low grade leukocytosis and mild anemia of chronic disease. These returns towards normal when the systemic phase is resolved. IgG and IgM levels are elevated in >1/2 of the patients. Chest X-rays are usually unrevealing, although rim of calcification is sometime visible in the wall of involved arteries. Arteriography typically reveals finding of an irregular intimal surface in which stenosis of aorta or its branch vessel, post stenotic dilatation, aortic or arterial aneurysm and even complete occlusion of the vessel. The affected thoracic aorta has been described as having a narrowed, rat-tail angiographic appearance.

8. Ans. d. Noninvolvement of renal arteries

Braunwald 8th Ed; Page 152-1574

Giant cell arteritis is one of the most common forms of vasculitis occurring predominately among older people and characteristically involving medium size arteries. The aorta and its branches are affected in about 15% of the cases. The disease is also referred as granulomatous arteritis, temporal arteritis and cranial arteritis. The disease has a special predilection for the branches of the proximal aorta, especially those supplying the head and neck, extracranial structures and upper extremity. End-arteritis is not an important feature but the mural involvement can lead to obstruction of involved arteries. Involvement of the aorta and its major branches usually coexist with the more classic and prevalent syndrome of temporal arteritis and polymyalgia rheumatica, although the aorta may rarely serve as primary target of the disease. Infrequently, the inflammatory process may weaken the aortic valve leading to the localized aneurysm formation, aortic annular dilatation and aortic regurgitation. Narrowing or occlusion of the branch vessel of the thoracic aorta often referred to as aortic arch syndrome may be found in 9-14% of cases, producing symptoms similar to those of Takayasu's arteritis such as decreased upper extremity pulses and blood pressure, or leg claudication, Raynaud's phenomena, transient ischemic attacks, coronary ischemia and abdominal angina. Interestingly in contrast with Takayasu's arteritis, renal artery involvement is almost never seen. Aortic aneurysm, aortic regurgitation and aortic dissection occur less commonly.

9. Ans. c. Right mid subclavian artery lesion

Braunwald 8th Ed; Page 1575

Proposed criteria for the clinical diagnosis of takayasu's disease

Criterion	Definition
Obligatory criterion Age ≤ 40 years	Age ≤ 40 years at diagnosis or at onset of characteristic signs and symptoms of 1 month duration in patient history
Two major criteria	
Left mid subclavian artery lesion	The most severe stenosis or occlusion present in the mid portion from the point 1 cm proximal to the left vertebral artery orifice to that 3 cm distal to the orifice determined by angiography
Right mid subclavian artery lesion	The most severe stenosis or occlusion present in the mid portion from the right vertebral artery orifice to the point 3 cm distal to the orifice determined by angiography
Nine minor criteria	
High ESR	Unexplained persistent high ESR > 20 mm/h (Westergren) at diagnosis or presence of the evidence in patient history
Carotid artery tenderness	Unilateral or bilateral tenderness of common carotid arteries by physician palpation: Neck muscle tenderness is unacceptable
Hypertension	Persistent blood pressure > 140/90 mm Hg brachial or > 160/90 mm Hg popliteal at age < 40 years or presence of the history at age < 40 years
Aortic regurgitation	By auscultation or Doppler echocardiography or angiography
or Annuloaortic ectasia	By angiography or two-dimensional echocardiography
Pulmonary artery lesion	Lobar or segmental arterial occlusion or equivalent determined by angiography or perfusion scintigraphy; or presence of stenosis, aneurysm, luminal irregularity of any combination in pulmonary trunk or in unilateral or bilateral pulmonary arteries determined by angiography

Continued

Continued

Criterion	Definition
Left mid common carotid lesion	Presence of the most severe stenosis or occlusion in the mid portion of 5 cm in length from the point 2 cm distal to its orifice determined by angiography
Distal brachiocephalic trunk lesion	Presence of the most severe stenosis or occlusion in the distal third determined by angiography
Descending thoracic aorta lesion	Narrowing dilation or aneurysm, luminal irregularity, or any combination determined by angiography: Tortuosity alone is unacceptable
Abdominal aorta lesion	Narrowing dilation or aneurysm, luminal irregularity, or any combination and absence of lesion in aortoiliac region consisting of 2 cm of terminal aorta and bilateral common iliac arteries determined by angiography: Tortuosity alone is unacceptable

10. Ans. d. Age below 40 years

Braunwald 8th Ed; Page 1575

Refer to explanation for Q. No 9.

11. Ans. c. 5 m/sec

Braunwald 8th Ed; Page 1546

Abdominal aorta is also called the greatest artery by the ancient. The aorta is a conductance vessel and is composed of three layers—the thin inner layer or intima, a thick middle layer or media and a rather thin outer layer or adventitia. The strength of the aorta lies in the media which is composed of laminated but intertwining sheets of elastic tissue arranged in a spiral manner that offers maximum tensile strength. During ventricular systole, the aorta is distended by the force of the blood ejected into it by the left ventricle and in this manner part of the kinetic energy generated by the contracting left ventricle is converted into potential energy stored in the aortic valve. Then during diastole, the potential energy is transformed back into kinetic energy as the aortic walls recoil, propelling the blood into the aortic lumen distally into the arterial bed. Thus, the aorta plays an essential role in maintaining forwards circulation of the blood in diastole after it is delivered into aorta by the left ventricle during systole. The pulse wave itself with its milking effect is transmitted along the aorta to the periphery at a speed of about 5 m/sec. This is much faster than the velocity of intraluminal blood itself, which travels at only 40-50 cm per second. The aorta is divided anatomically into thoracic and abdominal component. The thoracic aorta is further divided into ascending, arch and descending segments while the abdominal aorta consist of suprarenal and infrarenal segment. The ascending aorta is 5 cm long and has two distinct segments. The lower segment is aortic root beginning at the level of aortic valve and extending to the sinotubular junction. This is a wider portion of ascending aorta, measuring about 3.3 cm in the width. The bases of the aortic leaflets are supported by aortic root from which the three sinuses of Valsalva bulge outwards to allow for the full excursion of aortic valve leaflet during systole. In addition, the two coronary arteries arise from these sinuses of Valsalva. The upper tubular segment of ascending aorta rises to join the aortic arch. Normally, the ascending aorta sits just to the right of the midline with its proximal portion lying within the pericardial cavity. The arch of aorta give rise to all the brachiocephalic arteries. From the ascending aorta, it courses slightly leftward in front of trachea and then proceed posteriorly to the left of the trachea and esophagus. The pulmonary artery bifurcation and right pulmonary artery lie inferior to arch, as thus the left lung. The descending thoracic aorta begins in the posterior mediastinum to the left of vertebral column and gradually courses in front of vertebral column as it descends occupying a position immediately behind the esophagus. Distally, it passes through diaphragm usually at level of the 12th thoracic vertebra. The point at which the aortic arch joins the descending aorta is the aortic isthmus. The aorta is especially vulnerable to trauma at this site because it is here that relatively mobile portion of the aorta, i.e., the ascending aorta and arch becomes relatively fixed to the thoracic cage by the pleural reflection, the paired intercostal arteries and left subclavian arteries. This is also where coarctation of the aorta are located. The abdominal aorta continues from thoracic aorta giving off the important splanchnic arteries and ending at its bifurcation at the level of 4th lumbar vertebra. Unless the aorta is abnormally enlarged, the only location in which it can be palpated is the abdomen. The ease with which it can be felt depends largely on the body habitus and pulse pressure. It is readily felt in thin individual. It may be quite sensitive to palpation.

12. Ans. d. 4th lumbar vertebrae

Braunwald 8th Ed; Page 1546

Refer to explanation for Q. No 11.

13. Ans. a. It is the point where ascending aorta joins the arch of aorta

Braunwald 8th Ed; Page 1546

Refer to explanation for Q. No 11.

14. Ans. c. Abdomen

Braunwald 8th Ed; Page 1546

Refer to explanation for Q. No 11.

15. Ans. d. Infrarenal portion of abdominal aorta

Braunwald 6th Ed; Page 1423

Abdominal aortic aneurysms are much more common than the thoracic aortic aneurysm. Age is an important risk factor, as the incidence rises rapidly after 55 years of age in men and 70 years of age in women and abdominal aortic aneurysm occur 4 to 5 times more frequently in men than in women. Abdominal aortic aneurysm arises as a consequence of multiple interacting factors. Classically atherosclerosis has been considered the common underlying etiology. The infrarenal abdominal aorta is most affected by the atherosclerotic process and is similarly most common site of abdominal aneurysm formation. Only a fraction of abdominal aortic aneurysm are suprarenal with these tending to arise only as an extension of thoracic aneurysm (thoracoabdominal). The atherosclerotic process less often involve the descending thoracic aorta and involvement of ascending aorta is distinctly uncommon. Although the mechanism by which atherosclerosis result in aortic aneurysm is obscured, a recent hypothesis account for the disease predilection for the infrarenal abdominal aorta over the other segment. The media of the infrarenal aorta in human has no vasa vasorum and as a consequence at least the inner media must receive the oxygen and nutrients by diffusion from the aortic lumen. Atherosclerotic disease cause thickening of the intima and may thereby compromise the diffusion of such oxygen and nutrients to the medial layer. Exacerbated by increased in aortic wall stress from hypertension, this hypoxemia may lead to ischemic injury of the media, thus initiating a process of degeneration of the media and its elastic elements. The damage produces a weakening of the aortic wall which over a time allows the formation of fusiform or less commonly secular dilatation of aorta.

16. Ans. a. Left retroperitoneum

Braunwald 6th Ed; Page 1423

The abdominal aortic aneurysm are often complicated by intraluminal thrombus formation or rupture. As a result of flow turbulence through the aneurysmal aortic segment, blood may stagnate along the walls and thus allow the formation of mural thrombus. Such thrombus as well as atherosclerotic debris may embolize distally and compromise the circulation of tributaries of arteries. However, the major risk posed by the abdominal aortic aneurysm is that of aneurysm rupture. When rupture occurs 80% of rupture into the left retroperitoneum, which may contain the rupture whereas most of the remainder rupture into the peritoneal cavity causing uncontrolled hemorrhage and rapid circulatory collapse. Rarely an aneurysm may rupture into the inferior vena cava, iliac vein or renal vein.

17. Ans. b. Aortography

Braunwald 6th Ed; Page 1424

Several diagnostic imaging modalities are currently used for detecting, sizing and serially following abdominal aortic aneurysm, as well as for precisely defining the aortic anatomy preoperatively. Abdominal ultrasonography is the most practical way to screen for abdominal aortic aneurysm. It can visualize an aneurysm in the transverse and longitudinal planes, has a sensitivity of nearly 100% and can accurately define aneurysm size within ± 0.3 cm. Its major advantages are that it is inexpensive and noninvasive and does not require the use of a contrast agent. However, ultrasonography is limited by its inability to visualize the cephalad or pelvic extent of the disease or to define the associated mesenteric and renal arterial anatomy. Therefore, it is insufficient for planning operative repair. Computed tomography (CT) is an extremely accurate method for both diagnosing aortic aneurysm and sizing them to within ± 0.2 cm. CT has the advantage over ultrasonography that it can better define the shape and extent of the aneurysm as well as the local anatomical relationship of the visceral and renal vessel. Disadvantages are that the procedure is more expensive and less widely available than ultrasonography and it also requires the use of ionizing radiation and intravenous contrast. Although CT may therefore be less practical than ultrasonography as a screening tool, its high accuracy in sizing aneurysm makes it an excellent modality for serially following changes in aneurysm size. It is important to note that CT measurement of aneurysm size tend to be larger than ultrasound measurement by an average of 0.27 cm. Aortography has long been the standard imaging modality for the preoperative definition of abdominal aortic aneurysm anatomy. Aortography may underestimate aneurysm size in the presence of nonopacified mural-thrombus lining the aneurysm wall. However, it remains an excellent technique for defining the suprarenal extent of aneurysm and any associated iliofemoral disease. It is also excellent for defining renal and mesenteric arterial anatomy. Magnetic resonance imaging (MRI) angiography is an alternative to aortography for preoperative evaluation of aortic aneurysm.

18. Ans. d. Descending aorta

Braunwald 6th Ed; Page 1427

Thoracic aortic aneurysm are much less common than the aneurysm of the abdominal aorta and their incidence has remains static over period of time that saw a marked increase in the incidence of abdominal aortic aneurysm. Thoracic aneurysms are classified by the portion of aorta involved, i.e., ascending, arch or descending thoracic aorta. This anatomical distinction is important because the etiology, natural history and therapy of the thoracic aneurysm differ for each of this segment. Aneurysm of the descending aorta occurs most commonly, followed by aneurysm of the ascending aorta, whereas arch aneurysm occurs much less often. In addition, descending thoracic aneurysm may extent distally to involve abdominal aorta creating what is known as thoracoabdominal aortic aneurysm. Sometimes, the entire aorta may be ectatic with localized aneurysm seen at sites in both the thoracic and abdominal aorta. Aneurysm of the ascending thoracic aorta most often results from the process of cystic medial degeneration (or cystic medial necrosis). Cystic medial degeneration is found in virtually all cases of the Marfan's syndrome and may be associated with other connective tissue disorder as well such as Ehlers–Danlos syndrome. Atherosclerotic aneurysm infrequently occurs in the ascending aorta and tends to be associated with diffuse aortic atherosclerosis. Aneurysm in the aortic arch are often contiguous with aneurysm of ascending or descending aorta. They may be due to atherosclerotic disease, cystic medial degeneration, syphilis or other infections. The predominate cause of aneurysm of the descending thoracic aorta is atherosclerosis. These aneurysm tend to originate just distal to the origin of left subclavian artery and may be either fusiform or saccular. Syphilis was once a common cause of ascending thoracic aortic aneurysm but today it has become a rarity as a result of aggressive antibiotic treatment of the disease in its early stages. Infectious aortitis is a rare cause of aortic aneurysm and may result from a primary infection of aortic wall causing aortic dilatation with formation of fusiform or saccular aneurysm. More commonly, infected or mycotic aneurysm may arise secondarily from an infection occurring in a pre-existing aneurysm of another etiology. When an infected aneurysm involves the ascending aorta it is often the consequence of direct spread from aortic bacterial endocarditis.

19. Ans. d. Cystic medial degeneration

Braunwald 6th Ed; Page 1427

Refer to explanation for Q. No 18.

20. Ans. b. All patients have identifiable intimal tear

Braunwald 6th Ed; Page 1431

Acute aortic dissection is an uncommon but potentially catastrophic illness that occurs with an incidence of at least 2000 cases per year in the United States. Early mortality is as high as 1% per hour if untreated, but survival may be significantly improved by the timely institution of appropriate medical and/or surgical therapy. Prompt clinical recognition and definitive diagnostic testing are therefore essential in the management of patients with aortic dissection.

Aortic dissection is believed to begin with the formation of a tear in the aortic intima that directly exposes an underlying diseased medial layer to the driving force (or pulse pressure) of the intraluminal blood. This blood penetrates the diseased medial layer and cleaves the laminar plane of the media in row, thus dissecting the aortic wall. Driven by persistent intraluminal pressure, the dissection process extends a variable length along the aortic wall, typically antegrade (driven by the forward force of aortic blood flow) but sometimes retrograde from the site of intimal tear. The blood filled space between the dissected layers of the aortic wall becomes the false lumen. Shear forces may lead to further tears in the intimal flap (the inner portion of the dissected aortic wall), producing exit sites or additional entry sites for blood flow in the false lumen. The false lumen may become distended with blood, causing the intimal flap to bow into the true lumen, thereby narrowing its caliber and distorting its shape.

It has also been suggested that aortic dissection may begin instead with the rupture of the vasa vasorum within the aortic media, i.e., with the development of an intraluminal hematoma. Local hemorrhage then secondarily ruptures through the intimal layer, creating the intimal tear and aortic dissection. The fact that in autopsy series as many as 13% of aortic dissections do not have an identifiable intimal tear argues that at least in this minority of cases, independent medial hemorrhage is the primary cause of dissection. On the other hand, one might argue that the lack of an intimal tear in these patients indicates that they do not, in fact, have classic aortic dissection, but rather suffer intramural hematoma of the aorta, a closely related condition.

Most classification schemes for aortic dissection are based on the fact that the vast majority of aortic dissections originate in one of two locations: (1) the ascending aorta, within several centimeters of the aortic valve; and (2) the descending aorta, just distal to the origin of the left subclavian artery at the site of the ligamentum arteriosum. 65% of intimal tears occur in the ascending aorta, 20% in the descending aorta, 10% in the aortic arch, and 5% in the abdominal aorta.

There are 3 major classification systems to define the location and extent of aortic involvement, as defined in table below and depicted as: (1) DeBakey types I, II, and III; (2) Stanford types A and B; and (3) anatomical categories 'proximal' and 'distal'. All three schemes share the same basic principle of distinguishing these aortic dissections with or without ascending aortic involvement for prognostic and therapeutic reasons. In general, surgery is indicated for dissections involving the ascending aorta, whereas medical management is reserved for those dissections without ascending aortic involvement. Accordingly, because both DeBakey types I and II involve the ascending aorta, they are grouped together for simplicity in the Stanford (type A) and anatomical (proximal) classification systems. Aortic dissections confined to the abdominal aorta, although quite uncommon, are best categorized as type B or distal dissections. Proximal or type A dissections occur in about two-thirds of cases, with distal dissections composing the remaining one-third.

Type	Site of origin and extent of aortic involvement
DeBakey	
Type I	Originates in the ascending aorta, propagates at least to the aortic arch and often beyond it distally
Type II	Originates in and is confined to the ascending aorta
Type III	Originates in the descending aorta and extends distally down the aorta or rarely, retrograde into the aortic arch and ascending aorta
Stanford	
Type A	All dissections involving the ascending aorta, regardless of the site of origin
Type B	All dissections not involving the ascending aorta
Descriptive	
Proximal	Includes DeBakey types I and II or Stanford type A
Distal	Includes DeBakey type III or Stanford type B

In addition to its location, aortic dissection is also classified according to its duration, defined as the length of time from symptom onset to medical evaluation. The mortality from dissection and its risk of progression decreases progressively overtime, making therapeutic strategies for long standing aortic dissections quite different from those for dissections presently acutely. A dissection present <2 weeks is defined as 'acute', whereas those present 2 weeks or more are defined as 'chronic' because the mortality curve for untreated aortic dissections begins to level off at 75–80% at this time. At diagnosis, about two-thirds of aortic dissections are acute and the remaining third are chronic.

21. Ans. a. Bicuspid aortic valve

Braunwald 6th Ed; Page 1433

The peak incidence of aortic dissection is in the 6th and 7th decade of the life, with man affected twice as often as women. A coexisting history of hypertension is found in almost 80% of cases in a recent series. Bicuspid aortic valve is a well-established risk factor for proximal aortic dissection and histologically has been found in 17–14% of all aortic dissection. Interestingly, the risk of aortic dissection appears to be independent of severity of bicuspid valve stenosis. Certain other congenital cardiovascular abnormalities predispose the aorta to dissection, including the unicuspid aortic valve and possibly coarctation of the aorta. Aortic dissection has also been reported to occur in association with Noonan syndrome and Turner's syndrome. Rarely aortic dissection complicates arteritis involving the aorta particularly giant cell arteritis. A number of reports describe aortic dissection in association with cocaine abuse among younger man but no direct causal relationship has yet been established.

22. Ans. c. Aortic isthmus

Braunwald 11th Ed; Page 1295

The ascending aorta joins arch of aorta and then arch of aorta joins the descending aorta at a point which is marked by presence of ligamentum arteriosum. This is called as aortic isthmus. The aortic isthmus is vulnerable to deceleration trauma because this site marks the transition between the mobile ascending aorta and arch and the descending aorta, which is relatively fixed to the thoracic cage.

23. Ans. d. Smoking

Braunwald 11th Ed; Page 1296

Abdominal aortic aneurysms (AAAs) are approximately 5 times more prevalence in men than women and are strongly associated with age and most occurring in above the age of 60 years. AAAs are strongly associated with cigarette smoking. Current and former smokers have a five-fold increased risk compared to nonsmokers. Other risk factors include emphysema, hypertension, and hyperlipidaemia. Up to 20% of patients with AAAs describe a family history of AAA, indicating a heritable component.

24. Ans. b. 3 cm in diameter

Braunwald 11th Ed; Page 1296

AAAs are defined by an abdominal aorta >3 cm in diameter. Most AAAs arise in the infrarenal aorta, but up to 10% may involve the pararenal or visceral aorta and may extend into the thoracoabdominal segment.

25. Ans. d. 5.0 to 5.5 cm

Braunwald 11th Ed; Page 1298

Patients with small AAAs can be observed safely with imaging surveillance. In general, repair should be considered for asymptomatic aneurysms >5.0 to 5.5 cm in diameter. Symptomatic aneurysms and those with rapid growth (>1 cm/yr) require more urgent consideration.

26. Ans. c. Syphilitic aortitis

Braunwald 11th Ed; Page 1302

Cardiovascular syphilis occurs in the tertiary stage and typically involves the ascending aorta and arch. Pathologic features include lymphocytic and plasma cell inflammation in the adventitia, with the classical appearance of a "tree bark" or wrinkled appearance of the aortic intima. Ascending aortic aneurysm formation occurs in 40% of cases. Tertiary syphilis may cause aortic valvulitis, aortic regurgitation, and coronary ostial stenosis.

27. Ans. a. IV beta blocker

Braunwald 11th Ed; Page 1314

Reduction of systolic BP to levels of approximately 100 to 120 mm Hg or the lowest level necessary for adequate perfusion and a heart rate of 60 to 80 beats/min is recommended. Beta blockers should be administered even if the patient does not have hypertension. For rapid administration of agents to reduce the rate of rise in ventricular force (dP/dt) and stress on the aorta, IV beta blockers should be given. Esmolol or Labetalol is a drug of choice. Sodium nitroprusside also leads to rapid reduction in BP but may result in an increase in dP/dt. Thus, it must be used together with a beta blocker in the setting of acute aortic dissection. IV ACE inhibitors and IV nitroglycerine may be a time useful.

CHAPTER 28

Collagen Diseases and Heart

1. Which of the following statement is *incorrect* regarding Marfan's syndrome?
   a. The most common cardiovascular features are MVP and dilatation of sinus of Valsalva
   b. Children tend to be more severity affected by mitral valve disease, while aortic problems are more likely in adolescence and beyond
   c. Majority of aortic dissection begins just above coronary ostia (Type A)
   d. Repair of mitral valve is often unsuccessful in Marfan's with severe MR

2. In cases of Marfan's syndrome with pregnancy:
   a. There is 50% risk of child inheriting the condition
   b. There is high incidence of dissection
   c. Beta-blockers which are shown to reduce the rate of aortic dilatation and risk of complication in Marfan's syndrome, should be administered
   d. In women with aortic dilatation, abdominal delivery by cesarean section should be preferred mode of delivery

3. Spontaneous rupture of large and medium caliber vessel is seen in:
   a. Pseudoxanthoma elasticum
   b. Ehlers–Danlos syndrome
   c. Aminoacidopathies
   d. Sphingolipidosis

4. Endocardial fibroelastosis without a restrictive cardiomyopathy is found often with:
   a. Pseudoxanthoma elasticum
   b. Sphingolipidoses
   c. Aminoacidopathies
   d. SLE

5. CAD with myocardial ischemia and infarction is a major problem with which of the following collagen disease:
   a. Ehlers–Danlos syndrome
   b. Pseudoxanthoma elasticum
   c. Rheumatoid arthritis
   d. SLE

6. All the following are correct regarding pseudoxanthoma elasticum *except*:
   a. Radial and ulnar artery involvement is seen initially
   b. Bypassing the arterial stenosis is difficult
   c. The basic defect involves the gene for elastin
   d. There is positive association with dietary calcium intake

7. Myocardial infarction is a common manifestation with:
   a. Pseudoxanthoma elasticum
   b. Homocystinuria
   c. Mucopolysaccharidoses
   d. All of the above

8. Which is *incorrect* regarding acute MI in women?
   a. Women are more likely to have history of hypertension, diabetes mellitus and unstable angina
   b. Have higher incidence of transmural MI
   c. There is higher prevalence of tachycardia, rales and heart block on initial presentation
   d. Usually have less benefit when treated with ACE inhibitor post infarction

ANSWERS WITH EXPLANATIONS

1. Ans. d. Repair of mitral valve is often unsuccessful in Marfan's with severe MR

Braunwald 5th Ed; page 1670–1671

Marfan's syndrome is an autosomal dominant disorder and affects skeleton system, eye, cardiovascular system, skin and central nervous system. The most common cardiovascular features of Marfan's syndrome are mitral valve prolapse and dilatation of the sinus of Valsalva. Associated clinical problem of mitral regurgitation, aortic regurgitation and aortic dissection is responsible for most of the early mortality that results in an average age of death in the fourth and fifth decades. Children tend to be more severely affected by mitral valve disease, whereas aortic problems are progressive and more likely in adolescence and beyond. Mitral valve prolapse is a age dependent and more common in women with Marfan's syndrome. The incidence reaches 60–80% when patients are studied by 2D echocardiography. The mitral valve leaflets are elongated and redundant. Progression of severity as judged by appearance or worsening of mitral regurgitation by clinical and echocardiographic criteria occurs in at least one quarter of patients, a much higher rate than in mitral valve prolapse found in the general population. While treating patients with mitral valve prolapse for chronic mitral regurgitation, the coexistent aortic root dilatation may require treatment. Repair of the mitral valve is often successful and durable in patients with Marfan's syndrome. Repair is less easily accomplished when cusps are extremely redundant, there is a marked chordal damage or annulus is heavily calcified. Aorta may be enlarged enough to permit concomitant replacement. The aortic dissection is common in patients with Marfan's syndrome. This complication usually begins just above the coronary ostia (Type A in Stanford scheme) and extends the entire length of aorta (Type 1 in the DeBakey scheme). About 10% of dissection begins distal to the left subclavian (Type B or III). But rarely is dissection limited to the abdominal aorta. Angiography, magnetic resonance imaging and transesophageal echocardiography have a prominent role in the diagnosis of aortic dissection in the patients with Marfan's syndrome.

2. Ans. c. Beta-blockers which are shown to reduce the rate of aortic dilatation and risk of complication in Marfan's syndrome, should be administered

Braunwald 5th Ed; Page 1850–1851

Pregnancy in women with Marfan's syndrome poses a two fold problems: (a) a potential catastrophic and often lethal acute aortic dissection; and (b) a risk of having a child who will inherit the condition. The majority of patients develop complication in form of aortic regurgitation and heart failure and proximal and distal aortic dissection in the later phase of pregnancy. Aortic dissection results in maternal death and in some cases live babies are delivered before successful surgery. The management of pregnancy in women with Marfan's syndrome should include preconception counseling to discuss potential maternal and fetal risk. Women with significant cardiac involvement—in particular, dilatation of aorta are at high-risk for complication during gestation and should be advised against conception or if they are already pregnant, to have an early abortion. In contrast, the risk is significantly lower in patients without cardiac complications and a normal aortic diameter. Preconceptual echocardiographic assessment of aorta and periodic follow-up during pregnancy are highly recommended. Since aneurysm and dissection of aorta can occasionally involved descending aorta, the use of transesophageal seems preferable to transthoracic echocardiography. During pregnancy, physical activity should be limited. Beta-blockers which have been shown to reduce the rate of aortic dissection and risk of complication in patient with Marfan's syndrome should be administered. In case of substantial dilatation of aorta during pregnancy, therapeutic abortion or surgical intervention should be considered. In women with aortic dilatation, aortic dissection or other cardiac complications, abdominal delivery by cesarean section should be preferred mode of delivery to minimize hemodynamic changes associated with vaginal delivery.

3. Ans. b. Ehlers–Danlos syndrome

Braunwald 5th Ed; Page 1672–1673

Ehlers–Danlos syndrome is a group of heterogeneous condition linked by variable involvement of the knee and other joints with hyperelasticity and fragility of the skin occurring with hyper mobility of the joints. Mitral valve prolapse is increased in frequency in majority of the clinical types but aortic root dilatation is an uncommon finding. The most serious cardiovascular problems occurs in the severe form of Ehlers–Danlos syndrome (Type IV) in the form of spontaneous rupture of large and medium caliber arteries. Various defects of type III collagen are the cause of phenotype in virtually all patients so far studied. In the classical syndrome, true aneurysm rarely formed rather a rupture without dissection usually occurs as a catastrophic event. Most prone for spontaneous rupture are the abdominal aorta and its branches, the great vessel of aortic arch and the large arteries of the limbs. False aneurysm and fistula may results in some of the patients.

4. Ans. a. Pseudoxanthoma elasticum

Braunwald 5th Ed; Page 1673

Pseudoxanthoma elasticum is a clinically variable and genetically heterogeneous disorder of unknown cause. Histopathological examination of affected tissue shows fragmentation and calcification of elastic fiber. The skin, eye, the gastrointestinal system and cardiovascular system are the organs most severely affected. The skin shows highly characteristic raised yellow papules (pseudoxanthoma) overlying areas of flexural stress such as neck, cubital and popliteal fossae and groin. Breaks in the elastic laminae produces fundoscopy finding of angioid stricks. Gastrointestinal hemorrhage is common and potential fatal. Mucosal arterioles bleed and because the calcified elastic fiber prevent effective vessel retraction, hemostasis is difficult. The heart is affected in number of ways. Endocardial fibroelastosis is common but because primarily the atria are involved, a restrictive cardiomyopathy is uncommon. Mitral valve prolapse may be increased in frequency but is rarely a clinical problem. Coronary artery disease with myocardial ischemia and infarction is the major problem and common cause of early death.

5. Ans. b. Pseudoxanthoma elasticum

Braunwald 5th Ed; Page 1673

Please refer to the answer of Q. No 4.

6. Ans. c. The basic defect involves the gene for elastin

Braunwald 5th Ed; Page 1673

Elastic and muscular arteries including the coronaries develop a type of arteriosclerosis similar to Monckeberg's sclerosis. Progressive, luminal narrowing occurs and can produce complete occlusion. Initially, this is the most evident at the radial and ulnar arteries where absence of pulse and positive Allen's tests are noted early in the course. Because narrowing progresses slowly collaterals forms and peripheral ischemia is a late complication. Because the arterial stenosis tends to be diffused, bypassing them often involves extensive surgery. Because the basic defect is unknown (but does not involve the gene for elastin) no specific treatment is available. Because of a positive association between phenotypic severity and dietary calcium intake, patient can be advised to restrict consumption dairy products and to avoid calcium supplements. Hypertension and all risk factor for arteriosclerosis should be aggressively controlled.

7. Ans. d. All of the above

Braunwald 5th Ed; Page 1668–1669

Mendelian errors of metabolism with manifestations in the CV system

Disorder	Eponym or common name	MIM no.	Pathogenesis	Cardiovascular involvement	Biochemical defect	Gene lucus	Animal model
• Aminoacido-pathies • Alkaptonuria	Ochronosis	203500	Deposition of homogentisic acid in connective tissue	AS: Atherosclerosis			
Cystinosis, nephropathic type		219800	Lysosomal storage	Hypertension from renal failure, vascular wall thickening	?	?	
Homocystinuria		236200	Unknown	Early CAD: Venous thrombosis: Pulmonary embolism	Cystathionine β-synthase	CBS: 21q21-q22.1	
Oxalosis I	Hyperoxaluria	259900	Vascular and tissue accumulation of oxalate	Conduction defect: Vascular occlusions: Raynaud phenomenon	Peroxisomal alanine: Glyoxylate aminotransferase	AGT	
Details in fatty acid metabolism							
Carnitine transport defect	Primary carnitine deficiency	212140	Lipid myopathy: Defective energy generation	DCM:ECF	?	?	Syrian hamster
MCAD deficiency		201450	Lipid myopathy: Defective energy generation	DCM	Medium-chain acyl-CoA dehydrogenase	ACADM, 1p	
LCAD deficiency		201460	Lipid myopathy: Defective energy generation	DCM	Long-chain acyl-CoA dehydrogenase	ACADL.7	
Glycogen storage disorders							
GSD I	Pompe's	252300	Lysosomal storage	Pseudohyp-ertrophic CM: Short P-R interval, ECF	α-1,4-glucosidase	GAA:17q 21-q25	Canine and bovine

Continued

Continued

Disorder	Eponym or common name	MIM no.	Pathogenesis	Cardiovascular involvement	Biochemical defect	Gene lucus	Animal model
GSD II	Adult acid maltase deficiency	232300	Lysosomal storage	Primary skeletal muscle, respiratory insufficiency: Cor pulmonale	α-1,4-glucosidase		
GSD III	Forbes; debrancher deficiency	232400	Intracellular glycogen accumulation fibrosis	Pseudohypertrophic CM	Amylo 1,6-glucosidase		
Phosphorylase kinase deficiency	GSD of the heart			DCM	Phosphorylase kinase		
Glycoproteinoses							
Fucosidosis, severe		230000	Lysosomal storage	Myocardial thickening	α-fucosidase	FUCA1; 1p34	
Fucosidosis, mild		230000	Lysosmal storage	Angiokeratoma	α-fucosidase	FUCA1; 1p34	
Mannosidosis		248500	Lysosomal storage	Myocardial thickening: Valvular thickening; conduction disturbance	α-mannosidase	MANB, 19p13.2-12	
Aspartylglucosaminuria		208400	Lysosomal storage	Valvular thickening	Aspartylglycosylamine amino hydrolase	AGA, 4q21-qter	
Mucolipidoses ML II	I-cell	252500	Lysosomal storage	Same as MPS IH	Acetylglucosamine-1-phosphotransferase	GNPTA; 4q21-q23	
ML III	Pseudo-Hurler Poliodystrophy	252500	Lysosomal storage	Valvular thickening and dysfunction, especially AS, AR	Acetylglucosamine-1-phosphotransferase	GNPTA; 4q21-q23	
Mucopolysaccharidoses							
MPS IH	Hurler	252800	Lysosomal storage	Early CAD; PH and OAD →CP; valvular dysfunction, especially MR, AR: pseudohypertrophic CM	α-L-iduronidase	IDUA, 22q11-pter	Canine and feline
MPS IS	Scheie	252800	Lysosomal storage	Valvular dysfunction, especially AS	α-L-iduronidase	IDUA, 22q11-pter	
MPS IH/S	Hurler–Scheie	252800	Lysosomal storage	Same as MPS IH	α-L-Iduronidase	IDUA, 22q11-pter	
MPS II	Hunter	209900	Lysosomal storage	Same as MPS IH; less severe in mild MPS II variant	Sulfoiduronate sulfatase	IDS, Xq28	
MPS IIIA	Sanfilippo A	252900	Lysosomal storage	Valvular thickening and occasional dysfunction	Heparin sulfate sulfatase	?	

Continued

Continued

Disorder	Eponym or common name	MIM no.	Pathogenesis	Cardiovascular involvement	Biochemical defect	Gene locus	Animal model
MPS III B	Sanfilippo B	252920	Lysosomal storage	Valvular thickening and occasional dysfunction	N-acetyl-α-D-glucosaminide	?	
MPS III C	Sanfilippo C	252930	Lysosomal storage	Valvular thickening and occasional dysfunction	Acetyl-CoA: alpha-glucosaminide N-acetyltransferase	?	
MPS III D	Sanfilippo D		Lysosomal storage	Valvular thickening and occasional dysfunction	N-acetylglucosamine-6-sulfatase	G6S, 12q14	
MPS IV A	Morquio A	253000	Lysosomal storage	Valvular dysfunction, especially AR	Galactosamine-6-sulfatase		
MPS IV B	Morquio B	253010	Lysosomal storage	Milder than MPS IV A	β-Galactosidase		
MPS VI	Maroteaux–Lamy	253200	Lysosomal storage	Same as MPS IH	Arylsulfatase B	5p11-qter	Feline
MPS VII	Sly	253220	Lysosomal storage	Valvular thickening	β-glucuronidase	GUSB; 7q	Mouse and canine
Sphingolipidoses							
α-galactosidase A deficiency	Fabry	301500	Cellular accumulation of trihexyl ceramide, especially endothelium	Early CAD, valvular thickening and dysfunction; pseudohypertrophic CM; short P-R interval; arteriolar occlusion; angiokeratoma	α-galactosidase A	GLA; Xq22	
Ceramidase deficiency	Farber	228000	Histiocytic infiltration	Nodular thickening of valves	Ceramidase	?	
Glucocerebrosidase deficiency	Gaucher, adult form	230800	Cellular accumulation of glucocerebroside	PH→CP; interstitial infiltration of myocytes by Gaucher cells; constrictive pericarditis	β-glucocereb-roside	GBA; 1q21	
Miscellaneous disorders							
Acidlipase deficiency	Wolman	278000	↑Cholesterol; foam cell infiltration	Atherosclerosis	Lysosomal acid lipase	LIPA, 10q	
Acid lipase deficiency	Cholesteryl ester storage disease	278000	↑Cholesterol, foam cell infiltration	Atherosclerosis, PH	Lysosomal acid lipase	LIPA, 10q	
Geleophysic dysplasia		231050	Lysosomal storage	Valvular dysfunction	?		

8. Ans. b. Have higher incidence of transmural MI

Braunwald 5th Ed; Page 1710

Acute myocardial infarction in women: Although little is known of pathophysiology underlying gender differences in acute MI, it is clear that women have a different clinical presentation and respond differently to both medical and procedural therapies. Women suffering from acute MI are likely to be older and more likely to have a history of hypertension, diabetes, unstable angina, hyperlipidemia and congestive heart failure and are less likely to be smoker than their male counterparts. Women are also more likely to experience neck and shoulder pain, abdominal pain, nausea, vomiting, fatigue and dyspnea in addition to chest pain and or more likely to have silent infarction. Perhaps due in part to these more atypical symptoms women seek medical attention more slowly and even after hospital arrival may experience greater delay in receiving care. Women are more likely to suffer nontransmural infarction. Women with infarction have more serious presentation with greater prevalence of tachycardia, rales, heart block and higher Killip class on initial presentation. Women are less likely to receive thrombolysis and receive it later than do man. Most but not all women with acute infarction are less likely to undergo diagnostic catheterization during their hospital stay. Women have higher rate of in-hospital complication from infarction including bleeding, stroke, shock, myocardial rupture and recurrent chest pain than do men. Although early or in hospital mortality in women appears to be greater than in men, most studies have shown that adjustment for age and clinical characteristics serve to reduce these differences but not to eliminated fully. Mortality 1-3 years after hospital discharge is similar in men and women and when adjustment are made for age and other baseline characteristics women may actually do better. Comparison of benefit from thrombolysis in men and women with acute MI are difficult but it appears that reductions in mortality are similar. The efficacy of thrombolysis are also similar in men and women with similar rate of infarct related artery patency and left ventricular function. However, complication rate particularly hemorrhagic stroke and recurrent myocardial infarction appears to be higher in women. Medical treatment after hospital discharge appears to carry out somewhere different benefit for men and women. Aspirin has not yet proved to prevent reinfarction in women and calcium channel blockers have not been evaluated. Two studies have suggested that men may experience more benefit than women when treated with angiotensin converting enzyme inhibitors postinfarction. In contrast, beta blockers clearly provide a substantial improvement in postinfarction survival in women, i.e., equal to if not greater than that's seen in men.

Chapter 29: Cardiovascular Related Disorders

1. All the following increases during normal pregnancy *except*:
   a. Blood volume
   b. Heart rate
   c. Cardiac output and stroke volume
   d. Systemic vascular resistance

2. The increase in the blood volume during pregnancy is attributed to:
   a. Stimulation of renin–aldosterone system
   b. Excess of prolactin
   c. Deoxycorticosterone and growth hormone
   d. All of the above

3. Which is *incorrect* about hemodynamic changes during postpartum phase in a pregnant woman?
   a. Increase in venous return and increase in the cardiac output
   b. The heart rate and cardiac output return to prelabor values within 24 hours after delivery
   c. Blood pressure and stroke volume takes 24 hours to return to pre labor values
   d. All are correct

4. The hyperkinetic circulation of pregnancy leads to which of the following auscultatory finding?
   a. Cervical venous hum
   b. Mammary souffle
   c. Innocent systolic murmur
   d. Short diastolic murmur

5. Exposure embryo to radiation do *not* cause any adverse effect, if exposure is:
   a. During first 10 days after conception
   b. During first 20 days after conception
   c. During first month after conception
   d. During first 3 months after conception

6. Mother who expose to the radiation on third month of pregnancy may lead to:
   a. Intrauterine growth retardation
   b. Increased incidence of childhood cancer
   c. Teratogenic effect
   d. Both a and b

7. Teratogenic effect in fetus is seen if mother is exposed to radiation during:
   a. One week after conception
   b. 10–50 days after conception
   c. 3 months after conception
   d. During the mid trimester

8. Which of the following limit of radiation exposure does not lead to any risk or is associated with low risk during pregnancy?
   a. Less than 5 rads
   b. 5–10 rads
   c. 10–15 rads
   d. More than 20 rads

9. Termination of pregnancy is advised if mother is expose to the radiation in the range which of the following?
   a. 5 rads
   b. 5–10 rads
   c. 10–15 rads
   d. More than 20 rads

10. Mother needing balloon mitral valvuloplasty for rheumatic mitral stenosis during pregnancy can be managed by which of the following method to avoid radiation exposure?
    a. The abdomen is shielded by protective lead material during the procedure
    b. Procedure can be done under Echocardiographic guidance
    c. Resort to closed mitral valvotomy
    d. Both a and b

11. Which of the following ECG changes are *not* seen in a pregnant woman?
    a. QRS axis shift to left
    b. Small Q wave and inverted P wave in lead 3 that may vary with respiration
    c. Decrease R wave amplitude in right precordial lead
    d. ST segment depression may making myocardial ischema

12. Which is the most common arrhythmia seen during pregnancy?
    a. Sinus tachycardia
    b. Atrial and ventricular premature beats
    c. Paroxysmal supraventricular tachycardia
    d. Ventricular tachycardia

13. Which of the following is *not* an uncommon echocardiographic finding during normal pregnancy?
    a. Progressive increase in all cardiac chamber dimensions
    b. Early and progressive dilatation of mitral, tricuspid and pulmonary annulus
    c. Mild valvular regurgitation (functional)
    d. Small pericardial effusion

14. Which of the following is noted pharmacotherapeutic effect during normal pregnancy?
    a. Increase absorption of the drug administered
    b. Altered volume of distribution of some drugs leading to the higher loading dose
    c. Decrease protein binding of some drugs
    d. All of the above

15. Congenital malformation generally caused by drug toxicity during:
    a. First trimester
    b. Second trimester
    c. Third trimester
    d. Risk is uniform throughout pregnancy

16. Which is *correct* regarding use of beta-blocker during pregnancy?
    a. Avoid initiating beta-blocker during first trimester
    b. Lower doses need to be used
    c. Neonates born to mothers receiving betablockers need to monitored for 72–96 hours
    d. All of the above

17. Which is *not* correct regarding Digitalis preparation?
    a. Do cross the placenta
    b. Teratogenic effects has not been reported
    c. Digitalis preparation are drug of choice for treating fetal arrhythmias
    d. It is drug of choice for treating arrhythmias due to WPW syndrome during pregnancy

18. Which of the following drug block potassium channels?
    a. Metoprolol   b. Atenolol
    c. Timolol   d. Sotalol

19. All the following anti-arrhythmic drugs prolonged action potential duration *except*:
    a. Quinidine   b. Phenytoin
    c. Procainamide   d. Disopyramide

20. Long-term therapy with which of the following drug during pregnancy may cause lupus like syndrome?
    a. Quinidine   b. Procainamide
    c. Disopyramide   d. Mexeletine

21. Respiratory tract anomaly and hernias in the newborn have been reported with use of which of the following drug during pregnancy?
    a. Lidocaine   b. Mexeletine
    c. Flecanide   d. Propafenone

22. The drug of choice for treating fetal supraventricular tachycardia refractory to digitalis is:
    a. Quinidine   b. Flecanide
    c. Propafenone   d. Sotalol

23. The recommendation regarding use of aspirin to prevent pre-eclampsia during pregnancy is:
    a. Low dose aspirin 60–80 mg/day after 12th week of gestation
    b. Low dose aspirin 60–80 mg/day after 20th week of gestation
    c. High dose aspirin 160–325 mg/day after 20th week of gestation
    d. None of the above

24. Which is *not* correct regarding use of Warfarin during pregnancy?
    a. Warfarin embryopathy occurs with first trimester exposure
    b. Central nervous system abnormalities and fetal bleeding with exposure after first trimester
    c. No incidence of embryopathy have been reported by some inpatient taking oral anticoagulation in the first trimester or throughout pregnancy
    d. All are correct

25. Which of the following is safe option of anticoagulation in pregnant woman with prosthetic valve?
    a. Heparin or low molecular weight heparin throughout pregnancy
    b. Warfarin throughout pregnancy
    c. Warfarin throughout pregnancy changing to Heparin or low molecular weight heparin at 38 weeks gestation with planned labor induction at approximately 40 weeks
    d. Heparin or low molecular weight heparin in the first trimester of pregnancy, switching over to warfarin in the second trimester, continuing until approximately. 38 weeks then switch over to heparin or LMWH with planned labor induction at 40 weeks

26. The most common medical complication of pregnancy is:
    a. Hypertension
    b. Cardiac failure
    c. Cardiac arrhythmia
    d. Venous thromboembolism

27. Hypertension with proteinuria 20 weeks after gestation is a:
a. Chronic hypertension
b. Pre-eclampsia
c. Chronic hypertension with super impose pre-eclampsia
d. Gestational hypertension

28. Which of the following *not* a regular component of HELLP syndrome?
a. Hemolysis
b. Hypertension
c. Elevated liver enzymes
d. Low platelet count

29. Which of the following antihypertensive drug is contraindicated during pregnancy?
a. Labetolol
b. Clonidine
c. Hydralazine
d. Angiotensin II receptor blocker

30. Which of the following condition is a contraindication for pregnancy?
a. Primary pulmonary hypertension
b. Eisenmenger's syndrome
c. Marfan's syndrome with dilatation of ascending aorta
d. All of the above

31. Which of the following is a contraindication for pregnancy?
a. Coarctation of the aorta
b. Hypertrophic cardiomyopathy
c. Woman with prosthetic valve
d. Cardiac failure

32. Which is *incorrect* about peripartum cardiomyopathy?
a. It is a restrictive form cardiomyopathy
b. Cardiac failure develops usually in the last month of pregnancy or within 5 months after delivery
c. There is absence of demonstrable heart disease before pregnancy
d. There is documented systolic dysfunction

33. Peripartum cardiomyopathy is uncommon in:
a. Multiparous women
b. Twin pregnancy
c. With pre-eclampsia
d. Women younger than 30 years of age

34. Which is *not* correct regarding peripartum cardiomyopathy?
a. About 50–60% of patients shows complete or near complete recovery within first 6 months postpartum
b. Women with peripartum cardiomyopathy often develop relapse with subsequent pregnancy
c. Relapse is more common with persistent abnormal cardiac function
d. Relapse is not seen in women in whom left ventricular function is restored after the first episode

35. The dominant cause of systolic heart failure during pregnancy is:
a. Myocarditis
b. Peripartum cardiomyopathy
c. Idiopathic dilated cardiomyopathy
d. Valvular heart disease

36. Dominant cause of diastolic heart failure during pregnancy is:
a. Hypertension
b. Aortic stenosis
c. Hypertrophic cardiomyopathy
d. Restrictive cardiomyopathy

37. The most frequently encountered physical finding in patients with pulmonary embolism is:
a. Tachypnea
b. Sinus tachycardia
c. Unexplained pallor
d. Fatigue

38. The most sensitive diagnostic modality for suspected acute pulmonary embolism is:
a. D-dimer assay
b. Magnetic resonance pulmonary angiography
c. Computed tomogrpahic pulmonary angiography
d. Ventilation perfusion scan

39. What is the usual arterial blood gas (ABG) finding in patients with acute pulmonary embolism?
a. Low PO_2, Low CO_2 and respiratory acidosis
b. Low PO_2, Low CO_2 and respiratory alkalosis
c. Low PO_2, High CO_2 and respiratory acidosis
d. Low PO_2, High CO_2 and respiratory alkalosis

40. Which of the following is an indication for thrombolysis in patient with pulmonary embolism
a. Patient with massive pulmonary embolism presenting as a life-threatening emergency
b. Patients with sub massive pulmonary embolism and demonstration of right ventricular dysfunction on Echocardiography
c. Patient who develop recurrent pulmonary embolism despite treatment with heparin
d. All of the above

41. Catheter based intervention is indicated for treatment of pulmonary embolism in which of the following condition?
a. Persistent arterial hypotension (systolic pressure < 90 mm Hg)
b. Systemic hypoperfusion and hypoxemia
c. Severe right ventricular dysfunction
d. All of the above

42. What is the recommended dose of rtPA for treatment of pulmonary embolism?
   a. 40 mg over ½ hour
   b. 50 mg over 1 hour
   c. 100 mg over ½ hour
   d. 100 mg over 2 hours

43. Which of the following electrocardiographic finding is indicative of significant right ventricular dysfunction in patients with acute pulmonary embolism?
   a. S1S2S3
   b. S1Q3T3
   c. Right bundle branch block with right axis deviation
   d. All of the above

44. Most sensitive auscultatory sign for PAH is:
   a. Accentuated pulmonary component of S2
   b. Presence of S4
   c. Systolic murmur at left sternal edge
   d. Presence of pulmonary diastolic murmur

45. The commonly screening test for venous thromboembolism is:
   a. D-dimer assay
   b. Troponin assay
   c. Myoglobin assay
   d. APTT

46. Elevated D-dimer level is finding:
   a. DVT
   b. Pulmonary infection
   c. Malignancy
   d. All of the above

PREGNANCY AND HEART DISEASE

47. All of the following cardiovascular condition calls for avoidance or interruption of pregnancy *except*:
   a. Prosthetic valve
   b. Pulmonary hypertension
   c. Marfan's syndrome with dilated root
   d. Dilated cardiomyopathy with congestive heart failure

48. In all of the following conditions pregnancy can be continued with counseling and close clinical follow-up *except*:
   a. Prosthetic valve
   b. Obstructive lesions
   c. Marfan's syndrome
   d. Dilated CMP with CHF

49. Which of the following is *correct* regarding exercise and pregnancy?
   a. Maximal exercise by swimming causes less fetal bradycardia than same level of cycling
   b. Regular aerobic endurance exercise during pregnancy is associated with reduction in birth weight
   c. Infants born to mothers who work in standing position may be small at birth
   d. All are correct

50. Which of the following parameter does *not* change during pregnancy?
   a. Total body water
   b. Sodium content
   c. Ejection fraction
   d. Stroke volume

ANSWERS WITH EXPLANATIONS

1. Ans. d. Systemic vascular resistance

IGNOU, MCC 007, Page 47

Pregnancy is a physiological condition, but presence of heart disease is an important cause of maternal morbidity and mortality and also influences the outcome of the fetus. Significant cardiocirculatory changes occur during pregnancy and peripartum period which can lead to deterioration in patients with heart disease.

During normal pregnancy there are changes in various cardiocirculatory system and hemodynamics theory as follows:

1. **Blood volume:** The blood volume increases substantially starting at sixth week of pregnancy which rapidly rises till mid pregnancy and continues to rise slowly later. The increase in blood volume varies from 20 to 100% with an average of 50%. Higher increases occur in multigravidas and in multiple pregnancies. The increase in blood volume has some correlation with fetal weight, placental mass and weight of products of conception. The changes in blood volume has been attributed to estrogen medicated stimulation of the rennin–aldosterone system resulting in sodium and water retention. Other hormones like deoxycorticosterone, prolactin, growth hormone may also be involved in water retention during pregnancy.

2. **Heart rate, cardiac output, stroke volume:** Heart rate increases during pregnancy and peaks during third trimester with an average increase of 10–20 beats/min. In come, it may increase still higher particularly in pregnancy with multiple fetuses. The cardiac output increases by 50%, starts to rise from 50th week, reaches plateau at 24th week and may rise slightly thereafter. In the third trimester, the cardiac output is more in lateral position than in supine position, owing to vena cava compression by gravid uterus in supine position. The increase in cardiac output is due to increase in stroke volume in the early pregnancy while in the third trimester; it is due to increase in heart rate.

3. **Blood pressure:** The systemic arterial pressure starts to fall during first trimester maximum fall in mid pregnancy and returns to pregestational levels before term. The pulse pressure widens because of greater fall in diastolic pressure. Reduction in systemic vascular

resistance due to reduce vascular tone is responsible for fall in blood pressure.

2. Ans. d. All of the above

IGNOU, MCC 007, Page 47

Refer to explanation for Q. No 1.

3. Ans. b. The heart rate and cardiac output return to prelabor values within 24 hours after delivery

IGNOU; MCC 007; Page 48

Hemodynamic changes: During labor and delivery changes in hemodynamics occur due to anxiety, pain and uterine contractions. Oxygen consumption is increased by three times, cardiac output increases, blood pressure increases markedly during uterine contractions particularly in second stage of labor. Cesarean section is frequently recommended for pregnant women with heart disease to avoid hemodynamic changes due to pain and anxiety. But significant hemodynamic changes can occur during intubation and by drugs used for anesthesia and analgesia, blood loss, relief of caval compression, extubation and postoperative awakening. Hemodynamic changes also occur during postpartum. Increase in venous return from relief of caval compression, shift of blood from contracting uterus to systemic circulation. This occurs in spite of blood loss during delivery, leading to clinical deterioration in a cardiac patient from increase in cardiac output, ventricular filling pressure and heart rate. The heart rate and cardiac output, ventricular return to prelabor values by one hour after delivery, but blood pressure and stroke volume takes 24 hours to return to prelabor values. It usually takes 12–24 weeks after delivery to return to prepregnancy levels.

4. Ans. c. Innocent systolic murmur

IGNOU; MCC 007, Page 48

Murmurs in Pregnancy

A. Innocent systolic murmur is heard in post pregnant women as a result of hyperkinetic circulation of pregnancy. It is usually mid systolic, soft heard at the lower left sternal edge and pulmonary area radiating to suprasternal region and to left side of neck.
B. Cervical venous hum heard over right supra clavicular fossa.
C. Mammary soufflé systolic or continuous heard over the breast, late in gestation or in lactating period caused by increased flow in mammary arteries, may decrease or vanish when pressure is applied by the stethoscope or when patient moves to erect position.
D. Short diastolic murmur may be heard because of increased flow across with ventricular valves.

5. Ans. a. During first 10 days after conception

IGNOU; MCC 007, Page 49

Chest X-ray during pregnancy: With the advent of echocardiography, most of the cardiovascular lesions can be assessed and hence the need for chest X-ray during pregnancy for cardiac evaluation is practically not needed. The radiation dose associated with routine chest X-ray is minimal, but the potential for adverse biological effects from any amount of exposure to radiation during pregnancy need to be avoided. However, if chest X-ray is a must, the abdomen and pelvic area need to be covered with lead material. The findings in the chest X-ray during normal pregnancy may simulate cardiac diseases and should be interpreted with caution. Strengthening of the left upper cardiac border, horizontal position of the heart secondary to elevated diaphragm, increased lung markings may be seen. Small pleural effusions may be found postpartum, which may reabsorb within 1–2 weeks after delivery. Exposure of the embryo to radiation during first 10 days after conception would most likely cause no effect or leads to resorption. Exposure from 10 to 50 days radiation may have teratogenic effect. Later, time of exposure may cause intrauterine growth retardation, central nervous system abnormalities and increased incidence of childhood cancer. Direct radiation to fetus needs to be avoided. Current recommendations are < 5 rads exposure—no risk or low-risk, 5–10 rads counsel regarding risk, 10–15 rads and beyond, termination of pregnancy is advised.

Radiation exposure can also occur during balloon mitral valvuloplasty for rheumatic mitral stenosis during pregnancy. The abdomen is shielded by protective lead material during the procedure. Alternatively, the procedures can be done under Echo guidance which will avoid radiation exposure.

6. Ans. d. Both a and b

IGNOU; MCC 007, Page 49

Refer to explanation for Q. No 5.

7. Ans. b. 10–50 days after conception

IGNOU; MCC 007, Page 49

Refer to explanation for Q. No 5.

8. Ans. a. Less than 5 rads

IGNOU; MCC 007, Page 49

Refer to explanation for Q. No 5.

9. Ans. c. 10–15 rads

IGNOU; MCC 007, Page 49

Refer to explanation for Q. No 5.

10. Ans. d. Both a and b

IGNOU; MCC 007, Page 49

Refer to explanation for Q. No 5.

11. Ans. c. Decrease R wave amplitude in right precordial lead

IGNOU; MCC 007; Page 49

Electrocardiogram (ECG): The electrocardiography is simple non-invasive patient friendly, reproducible technique that has stood the test of time for more than hundred years. It is most useful:
1. In the diagnosis and prognosis of acute coronary syndromes;
2. In the diagnosis of arrhythmias;
3. In heart failure in assessing QRS width and resynchronization therapy; and
4. Genetic arrhythmology, e.g., long AT syndrome. ECG is safe and inexpensive investigation. There are some changes in the ECG that can occur in normal pregnancy. These are:
   i. QRS axis may shift to the left or right but usually is within normal limits;
   ii. A small Q wave and an inverted P wave in Lead III that may vary with respiration;
   iii. A greater R wave amplitude in Lead V2;
   iv. ST segment depression mimicking myocardial ischemia but not associated with all motion abnormalities by echo, at the end of pregnancy in patients undergoing cesarean section; and
   v. Increased susceptibility to arrhythmias during pregnancy as manifested by sinus tachycardia and atrial or ventricular premature beats. Paroxysmal supraventricular tachycardia has been reported during normal pregnancy and also ventricular in otherwise healthy women.

12. Ans. a. Sinus tachycardia

IGNOU; MCC 007; Page 49

Refer to explanation for Q. No 11.

13. Ans. d. Small pericardial effusion

IGNOU, MCC 007; Page 49-50

Use of echocardiography during pregnancy both for mother and for fetus is considered safe. Transesophageal echocardiography has been increasingly used in pregnancy and appears to be well tolerated by both mother and the fetus. Certain changes that occur during normal pregnancy have been reported. These echocardiographic changes are:
1. Progressive increase in all cardiac chamber dimensions with about 20% increase in the size of right atrium and right ventricle, 12% in left atrial size and 6% in left ventricular size. These changes return to normal after delivery, but may persist for several months;
2. Early and progressive dilation of mitral, tricuspid and pulmonary annuli which may be associated with valvular regurgitation (functional);
3. Small pericardial effusion.

Use of echocardiography is safe for fetus and used to diagnose congenital heart disease during intrauterine life. Many abnormalities can be detected in first and second trimester of pregnancy.

14. Ans. d. All of the above

IGNOU; MCC 007; Page 50-51

Factors Affecting Pharmacotherapy During Pregnancy

Maternal Factors

Absorption
The intestinal motility is reduced due to increased plasma progesterone level resulting in about 30-50% decrease in gastric and intestinal emptying and hence increases absorption of the drug administered. The gastric pH is also increased.

Distribution
During pregnancy the increase in plasma volume expansion can result in altered volume of distribution of some drugs. Hence higher loading doses may be needed to produce expected serum concentration.

Protein binding
Dilutional hypoalbuminemia occurs during pregnancy resulting in decreased protein binding of some drugs. This will affect the estimation of serum concentration of total drug in pregnant women, which may lead to unnecessary increase in drug dosage. Greater fluctuation in the unbound concentration within a dosing interval can produce toxic effects at the beginning of a dosing interval and hence frequent dosing without change in daily dosage may required.

Elimination
Progesterone and other endogenous substances can increase or decrease in hepatic metabolism of certain drugs, e.g., phenytoin metabolism is increased while theophylline metabolism is decreased. Similarly crease in renal plasma flow and glomerular filtration rate can increase renal metabolism of drugs.

Placental fetal unit

Absorption: Unbound free drug only can cross the placental barrier. Non-ionized lipid soluble molecules can cross placenta than less lipid soluble ionized molecules. Maternal and fetal pH influences the crossing of placenta.

Distribution: Nearly 50% of fetal circulation directly reaches the heart and brain by passing the liver. The affinity of drug to bind to fetal plasma proteins may be different from that of maternal protein and hence can influence the concentration of free drug.

Elimination: Most of drugs are primarily eliminated by diffusion of the drug back to the maternal compartment, although there is evidence of metabolism in placenta and fetus to some extent.

15. Ans. a. First trimester

IGNOU; MCC 007; Page 51

Congenital malformations are generally caused by drug toxicity during the first trimester and depend on the nature of drug, duration of fetal exposure and the genetic susceptibility of the fetus. Hence, drug administration in the first trimester should be avoided as much as possible. In the second and third trimesters, interference with fetal growth and development is the major potential hazard of drug exposure.

16. Ans. d. All of the above

IGNOU; MCC 007; Page 53

In general, beta-blockers are relatively safe to be used in pregnancy. However, the following factors need to be considered:

A. Try to avoid initiating beta-blockers if possible, during first trimester.
B. Lower doses need to be used.
C. It is preferable to discontinue beta-blockers 2–3 days before delivery to limit drugs effect on uterine contraction.
D. Neonates born to mothers receiving beta-blockers need to be monitored for 72–96 hours.
E. Beta-blockers with intrinsic sympathomimetic activity or with alpha-blocking properties may be preferred. Better to avoid blocking of two mediated uterine relaxation and peripheral vasodilation.
F. Avoid breastfeeding 3–4 hours after the dose of beta-blockers at the time of expected peak concentration of the drug.

17. Ans. d. It is drug of choice for treating arrhythmias due to WPW syndrome during pregnancy

IGNOU; MCC 007; Page 53

Digitalis: Digitalis preparations cross the placenta but no teratogenic effects are reported. However, adverse effects on the fetus have been reported in the fetus of the mothers who developed digitalis toxicity. Electrocardiographic changes and subsequent death of infants has been reported with maternal digitalis intoxication, miscarriage and low birth weight of newborn have also been reported. Digitalis preparations are the mainstay in the treatment of fetal arrhythmias providing nearly 80% of success rates in supraventricular tachycardias and considered by some as the routine drug of choice in treating fetal arrhythmias. In pregnancy with fetal hydrops higher doses of digitalis is needed because of reduced transplacental passage of digitalis but needs close monitoring of maternal toxicity. The efficacy of digitalis in atrial flutter diminishes and Wolf–Parkinson–White syndrome could worsen with digitalis. Digitalis is indicated in congestive cardiac failure particularly associated with atrial fibrillation. Digitalis preparations are excreted in breast milk in similar concentrations as that found in maternal serum. However, the total amount of daily maternal excretion is minute and do not cause significant effect on the breast fed infant. Hence, digitalis is considered safe in lactating mothers.

18. Ans. d. Sotalol

IGNOU; MCC 007; Page 53–54

Antiarrhythmic Drugs

According to Vaughan–Williams, antiarrhythmic drugs are classified as follows:

- *Class IA:* Drugs that reduce the rate of rise of action potential upstroke and prolong action potential duration, e.g., quinidine, procainamide, disopyramide.
- *Class IB:* Drugs that shorten action potential duration do not reduce rate of rise of action potential, e.g., mexiletine, phenytoin and lidocaine.
- *Class IC:* Drugs that reduce the rate of rise of action potential, primarily slow conduction and can prolong refractoriness minimally, e.g., flecanide, propafenone, and moricizine.
- *Class II*: Drugs that block beta-adrenergic receptors, e.g., propranolol, timolol, metoprolol, atenolol.
- *Class III*: Drugs that block potassium channels, e.g., sotalol, amiodarone, bretylium.
- *Class IV:* Drugs that block slow calcium channels, e.g., verapamil, diltiazem. The use of some of the commonly prescribed drugs during pregnancy is discussed.

19. Ans. b. Phenytoin

IGNOU; MCC 007; Page 53–54

Refer to explanation for Q. No 18.

20. Ans. b. Procainamide

IGNOU; MCC 007; Page 54

Procainamide: Its action is similar to that of quinidine, used to prevent or terminate supraventricular and ventricular arrhythmias and to maintain sinus rhythm after cardioversion of atrial fibrillation. Both procainamide and its metabolic N-acetylprocainamide (NAPA) are excreted in milk but the amount ingest by infant is low and hence safe. It does not cause any teratogenic effect. However, long-term therapy may cause lupus like syndrome.

CHAPTER 29 | Cardiovascular Related Disorders

21. Ans. a. Lidocaine

IGNOU; MCC 007; Page 54

Lidocaine: Lidocaine has been used primarily for epidural or local anesthesia during pregnancy and data of its use as antiarrhythmic agent in pregnancy is scanty. No teratogenic effect reported. It is excreted in milk but the amount reaching the infant is low and safe. Respiratory tract anomalies, hernias in the newborn have been reported. Cautious use with hepatic dysfunction is advocated as it is metabolized in the liver.

22. Ans. b. Flecanide

IGNOU; MCC 007; Page 54-55

Flecanide: It has been used with clinical effectiveness to treat maternal tachyarrhythmias. It readily crosses placenta and has been used to treat fetal tachycardias. It has been found that the fetus can metabolize the drug to avoid accumulation to produce toxicity. Flecanide has been considered by some as treatment of choice in fetal supraventricular tachycardia, particularly refractory to digitalis. Use of flecanide is compatible with breastfeeding. It is proarrhythmic drug in that it may aggravate existing arrhythmia and may cause new ventricular arrhythmias.

23. Ans. a. Low dose aspirin 60-80 mg/day after 12th week of gestation

IGNOU; MCC 007; Page 58

During pregnancy, low dose aspirin 60-80 mg/day after 12th week of gestation, has been suggested to prevent pre-eclampsia. The collaborative low dose aspirin study in pregnancy (CLASP) compared 60 mg aspirin per day with placebo for prevention and early treatment of pre-eclampsia. This involved 9,364 women taking aspirin from 12-13th week of pregnancy. Aspirin reduced the odds of occurrence of pre-eclampsia, reduced fetal growth retardation and there was 12% reduction in premature delivery. The high-risk women benefited more and there were no significant side effects.

24. Ans. d. All are correct

IGNOU; MCC 007; Page 58-59

Anticoagulation during pregnancy (for prosthetic valves): Warfarin crosses the placenta and can produce characteristic embryopathy with first trimester exposure and less commonly central nervous system abnormalities and fetal bleeding with exposure after first trimester. Warfarin can cause spontaneous abortion, prematurity or still birth due to hemorrhage in the placenta or in the fetus. If continued throughout the pregnancy, spontaneous abortion occurs in about 4.2-18%. The incidence of warfarin embryopathy (fetal abnormalities) varies from 5-67% but an estimate of 4-10% appears reasonable based on recent reports. However, no incidence of embryopathy has been reported by some in patients taking oral anticoagulation in the first trimester or throughout pregnancy. The manifestations of embryopathy are telecanthus, hypoplasia of the nose, small nasal bones, depressed nasal bridge, hypoplastic alae nasi, choanal stenosis with upper airway obstruction and punctate dysplasia of epiphysis of long bones as well as the cervical and lumbar vertebral end plates. Also there is high-risk of cerebral hemorrhage in the newborn.

25. Ans. d. Heparin or low molecular weight heparin in the first trimester of pregnancy, switching over to warfarin in the second trimester, continuing until approximately 38 weeks then switch over to heparin or LMWH with planned labor induction at 40 weeks

IGNOU; MCC 007; Page 59

In pregnancy with prosthetic valve, three options of anticoagulation are available:
1. Heparin or low molecular weight heparin (LMWH) throughout pregnancy.
2. Warfarin throughout pregnancy changing to heparin or LMWH at 38 weeks gestation with planned labor induction at approximately 40 weeks.
3. Heparin or LMWH in the first trimester of pregnancy, switching over to warfarin in the second trimester, continuing until approximately 38 weeks then switch over to heparin or LMWH with planned labor induction at approtimately 40 weeks.

26. Ans. a. Hypertension

IGNOU; MCC 007; Page 61-62

Hypertension is seen in about 10% of all pregnancies. It is the most common medical complication of pregnancy and a major cause of both fetal and maternal mortality, the most serious problems being associated with pre-eclampsia and eclampsia. In general, hypertension in pregnancy is defined as blood pressure greater than 140 mm Hg systolic and 90 mm Hg diastolic in at least two occasions six hours apart.

Classification: (Joint national committee—7th report)

Chronic hypertension	BP 140 mm Hg systolic and 90 mm Hg diastolic prior to pregnancy or before 20 weeks of gestation. Persists > 12 weeks postpartum.
Pre-eclampsia	BP 140 mm Hg systolic and 90 mm Hg diastolic with proteinuria > 100 mg/24 h, after 20 weeks of gestation, can progress to eclampsia (seizures). More common in nulliparous women multiple gestations, common with hypertension 4 years, family history of pre-eclampsia, hypertension in previous pregnancy and renal disease
Chronic hypertension with superimposed pre-eclampsia	New onset of proteinuria after 20 weeks in a women with hypertension, sudden 2- to 3-fold increase in proteinuria, sudden increase in BP, thrombocytopenia, elevated alanine aminotransferase or aspartate aminotransferase

Continued

Continued	
Gestational hypertension	Hypertension without proteinuria 20 weeks after gestation. Temporary diagnosis: It may be proteinuric phase of preeclampsia or recurrence of chronic hypertension abated in mid pregnancy, may evolve to pre-eclampsia. If severe may result in higher rates of premature delivery and growth retardation than mild pre-eclampsia
Transient hypertension retrospective diagnosis	Blood pressure normalizes by 12 weeks postpartum, may recur in subsequent pregnancies, predictive of future primary hypertension

27. Ans. d. Gestational hypertension

IGNOU; MCC 007; Page 61-62

28. Ans. b. Hypertension

IGNOU; MCC 007; Page 62

HELLP syndrome: It is a variant of pre-eclampsia, can occur as deceptively benign with minimal or no rise of blood pressure, decreased platelets count, elevation in liver enzymes. This form may progress rapidly to life-threatening symptoms, characterized by hemolysis, marked abnormality of liver function and coagulation. This is termed HELLP (hemolysis, elevated liver enzymes, and low platelet count) syndrome is an emergency and requires prompt termination of pregnancy.

29. Ans. d. Angiotensin II receptor blocker

IGNOU; MCC 007; Page 65

Angiotensin-converting enzyme inhibitors (ACEI) and angiotensin II receptor blockers (ARB) are contraindicated in pregnancy as they can cause fetal toxicity and death.

Antihypertensive drugs in pregnancy

Drugs	Dosage
Methyl dopa	250 mg orally thrice a day
Clonidine	0.1–0.3 mg twice a day
Nifedipine	10 mg 6th or 8th hourly
Atenolol	50–100 mg once a day
Labetolol	50–100 mg two to three times a day
Hydrochlorothiazide	25 mg once a day

30. Ans. d. All of the above

IGNOU; MCC 007; Page 86-87

Apart from social and psychological reasons, pregnancy need to be avoided in certain cardiac diseases, mainly based on maternal conditions. The absolute indications for avoidance of conception are:
1. Primary pulmonary hypertension (PPH), where the reported maternal mortality is around 50–60%. It is also important to realize that even though preconceptional symptoms are mild, progression is rapid during pregnancy. High incidence of prematurity of fetus, fetal growth retardation and fetal loss are associated with PPH.
2. Eisenmenger's syndrome, which is due to development of pulmonary hypertension in patients with pre-existing left to right shunt, which becomes either bidirectional or right to left shunt. The maternal mortality, in this situation is around 40%. It is associated with poor fetal outcomes with fetal loss, prematurity, fetal growth retardation and premature death.
3. Complex congenital heart disease. Although there are recent reports of successful management of pregnancies with repaired or unrepaired complex congenital heart diseases, there is increased risk to the mother as well as to the fetus. Individual patients need to be evaluated and proper advise given.
4. Diseases like Marfan's syndrome particularly when there is significant dilatation of aortic root, pre-conceptional counseling is required and risk to mother and fetus assessed and advised.
5. Other situations including advanced valvular heart diseases, advanced heart failure and previous history of peripartum cardiomyopathy. Proper preconceptional counseling is needed and advised against pregnancy.

31. Ans. d. Cardiac failure

IGNOU; MCC 007; Page 86-87

Refer to explanation for Q. No 30.

32. Ans. a. It is a restrictive form cardiomyopathy

IGNOU; MCC 007; Page 88

Peripartum cardiomyopathy is a form of dilated cardiomyopathy of uncertain etiology with:
1. Development of cardiac failure in the last month of pregnancy or within 5 months after delivery;
2. Absence of demonstrate cause for cardiac failure;
3. Absence of demonstrate heart disease before pregnancy; and
4. Documented systolic dysfunction. The symptoms appear during last month of pregnancy but usually the diagnosis is made in the early peripartum period.

33. Ans. d. Women younger than 30 years of age

IGNOU; MCC 007; Page 88

Peripartum cardiomyopathy is more common in multiparous women, twin pregnancies, in those with pre-eclampsia and in women older than 30 years. The exact etiology is unknown though myocarditis as a cause has been suggested by some investigators documented by myocardial biopsy, but other investigators did not find this association. Low selenium levels and autoantibodies have also been implicated in the pathogenesis of peripartum cardiomyopathy.

34. Ans. d. Relapse is not seen in women in whom left ventricular function is restored after the first episode

IGNOU; MCC 007; Page 88-89

The clinical course of peripartum cardiomyopathy is variable with 50-60% of patients showing complete or near complete recovery, usually within first 6 months postpartum. Mortality varies from 7-50% from small series. The usual causes are progressive heart failure, arrhythmia and thromboembolism. Acute maternal hypoxia can cause fetal distress. Women with peripartum cardiomyopathy often develop relapse with subsequent pregnancies, leading to left ventricular dysfunction, symptomatic deterioration and even to death. Relapse is more common in patients with persistent abnormal cardiac function, but can occur in women in whom, left ventricular function is restored after the first episode. The reported mortality is 0-2% in patients with normal left ventricular ejection fraction before the subsequent pregnancy and 8-17% in patients with depressed ventricular ejection fraction. Hence subsequent pregnancies should be discouraged in patients with peripartum cardiomyopathy with persistent cardiac dysfunction. However, women with recovered cardiac function also can get relapse but the risk of mortality appears to be less and hence in them also subsequent pregnancies are to be discouraged.

35. Ans. b. Peripartum cardiomyopathy

IGNOU; MCC 007; Page 94-95

Dominant systolic heart failure:
1. Peripartum cardiomyopathy
2. Other forms of cardiomyopathy—diabetic, idiopathic, alcoholic
3. Myocarditis
4. Valvular heart disease—especially rheumatic mitral, aortic, tricuspid valve diseases
5. Congenital heart disease with severe pulmonary hypertension
6. Ischemic myocardial disease, coronary artery disease.

Dominant diastolic heart failure:
1. Hypertension
2. Severe aortic stenosis
3. Hypertrophic cardiomyopathy
4. Restrictive cardiomyopathy.

Acute heart failure:
1. Acute mitral or aortic regurgitation
2. Rupture of valve leaflets or supporting structures
3. Infective endocarditis with acute valve incompetence
4. Myocardial infarction.

High output failure:
1. Anemia
2. Hyperthyroidism
3. Systemic arteriovenous fistula
4. Pregnancy
5. Glomerulonephritis
6. Cor pulmonale
7. Polycythemia vera
8. Carcinoid syndrome.

36. Ans. a. Hypertension

IGNOU; MCC 007; Page 94-95

Refer to explanation for Q. No 35.

37. Ans. a. Tachypnea

IGNOU; MCC 007; Page 100-101

Pulmonary embolism depends on its severity. The following clinical presentations are common and include:
1. Acute unexplained dyspnea
2. Pulmonary infarction or hemorrhage
3. Acute right ventricular failure
4. Chronic pulmonary arterial hypertension.

Acute unexplained dyspnea is often the presenting symptom of pulmonary embolism. The most frequency encountered physical finding is tachypnea, with a respiratory rate at rest greater than 16/min. Sinus tachycardia often accompanies dyspnea and can be a clue to the diagnosis of PE. Unexplained pallor, fatigue, apprehension can be other associated symptoms. The diagnosis of PE in this group of patients is many times missed and requires a high index of suspicion in potential clinical situation.

38. Ans. c. Computed tomogrpahic pulmonary angiography

IGNOU; MCC 007; Page 104-105

Computed tomographic (CT) pulmonary angiography (PA): CTPA has gained acceptance as a first-line imaging study in cases of suspected acute PE, replacing traditional V/Q scintigraphy at many institutions. CTPA has also reduced the need for invasive pulmonary angiography.

CTPA provides visualization of the pulmonary arterial system in the axial plane, and multiplanar and three dimensional reconstruction can be generated from raw data to enhance diagnostic accuracy. The cardinal sign of acute PE on CTPA is an intravascular filling defect in a pulmonary artery that partially or completely occludes the vessel and is often associated with increased diameter of the affected vessel. The most specific sign of acute PE is a filling defect that forms acute angles with the vessel wall.

39. Ans. b. Low PO_2, Low CO_2 and respiratory alkalosis

IGNOU; MCC 007; Page 103

Arterial blood gases (ABG): Analysis of ABG is helpful in supporting the diagnosis of PE. Finding of low PO_2, low CO_2 and respiratory alkalosis area pointers to the diagnosis of PE in a patient with risk factors for its development. It should be remembered that conditions which mimic PE like pneumonia, severe chest infections or chronic obstructive lung disease (COPD) can also cause low PO_2.

40. Ans. d. All of the above

IGNOU; MCC 007; Page 107–108

Systemic IV infusion of thrombolytic agents have been proven superior to anticoagulation for treatment of PE. Compared with heparin in hemodynamically stable patients with large PE, systemic thrombolytic therapy reduced mortality (11% vs. 4.7%) and recurrent PE (18.7% vs 7.7%, $p = 0.016$) but was associated with higher rates of bleeding complications. In view of the higher incidence of bleeding thrombolysis is not indicated in all patients with large PE.

The use of thrombolysis should be reserved for following category of patients: (a) Patients with massive PE presenting as a life-threatening emergency; (b) Patients with submassive PE and demonstration of right ventricular dysfunction on echocardiography; (c) Patients who develop recurrent PE despite treatment with heparin. The thrombolytic agents and their dosage schedule are shown in Table. In some centers thrombolytic agents are directly injected into pulmonary arteries (catheter-directed thrombolysis) to facilitate clot lysis.

Thrombolytic protocols for treatment of PE

Drug Name	Protocol
Streptokinase	250,000 U over 30 minutes followed by 100,000 U/h 000 for 24 hours
Urokinase	4,400 U/Kg over 10 minutes followed by 4,400 U/h for 12 hours
rtPA	100 mg over 2 hours

Newer Interventional and Surgical Treatment

There are patients who fail to improve despite all available treatment. For these patients interventional (catheter-directed thrombolysis, clot fragmentation or thrombus aspiration) techniques used in catheterization laboratories or surgical techniques such as embolectomy are indicated. These techniques are available in some advanced tertiary care hospitals.

The indications for use of these interventions are:
1. Persistent arterial hypotension (systolic blood pressure <90 mm Hg or a rapid decrease of >40 mm Hg);
2. Systemic hypoperfusion and hypoxemia;
3. Need for cardiopulmonary resuscitation;
4. Severe right ventricular failure; and
5. Contraindication to anticoagulation or thrombolysis.

41. Ans. d. All of the above

IGNOU; MCC 007; Page 107–108

Refer to explanation for Q. No 40.

42. Ans. d. 100 mg over 2 hours

IGNOU; MCC 007; Page 107–108

Refer to explanation for Q. No 40.

43. Ans. d. All of the above

IGNOU; MCC 007; Page 102

The presence of right ventricular abnormality, as demonstrated by S1Q3T3, right bundle branch block, right axis deviation, or atrial abnormality, are seen in only 26% of patients with PE. Atrial fibrillation, supraventricular arrhythmias and ST-T changes in anterior and inferior leads are also seen.

44. Ans. a. Accentuated pulmonary component of S2

IGNOU; MCC 007; Page 110–111

The physical findings in secondary PAH are usually mixed and reflect the findings of primary cause and of PAH. The most sensitive sign for PAH is an accentuated pulmonary component of S2, which also may be palpable in the pulmonic area, and right ventricular lift of the sternum may be seen. With very high PAP, characteristic diastolic and systolic murmurs of pulmonary valvular and tricuspid valvular regurgitation may be heard together with a systolic ejection sound and right ventricular S3. Elevation of jugular venous pressure, hepatomegaly and peripheral edema are seen when congestive cardiac failure supervenes.

45. Ans. a. D-dimer assay

IGNOU; MCC 007; Page 104

D-dimer assay: D-dimer is a blood test which can be rapidly performed and is utilized these days as a screening test for venous thromboembolism (deep venous thrombosis, or PE). D-dimer is a fibrin specific degradation produce that detects cross-linked fibrin resulting from endogenous fibrinolysis. In the presence of an acute thromboembolic event (like DVT or PE) the simultaneous activation of coagulation factors and fibrinolytic enzymes leads to increased concentration of D-dimer.

Normal values of this protein have high negative predictive value, that is a patient whose D-dimer is < 500 µg is unlikely to have PE. On the other hand, elevated D-dimer levels do not necessarily indicate PE and can be elevated in DVT, infections, inflammation, necrosis, trauma and cancer, etc.

46. Ans. d. All of the above

IGNOU; MCC 007; Page 104

47. Ans. a. Prosthetic valve

Hurst's 11th Ed; Chapter 92; Page 2212–2213

Cardiovascular abnormalities placing a mother and infants at high-risk Advice avoidance or interruption of pregnancy
1. Pulmonary hypertension
2. Dilated cardiomyopathy with congestive failure

3. Marfan's syndrome with dilated aortic root
4. Cyanotic congenital heart disease.

Pregnancy counseling and close clinical follow-up required
1. Prosthetic valve
2. Coarctation of the aorta
3. Marfan's syndrome
4. Dilated cardiomyopathy in asymptomatic women
5. Obstructive lesions.

48. Ans. d. Dilated CMP with CHF

Hurst's 11th Ed; Chapter 92; Page 2212-2213

Refer to explanation for Q. No 47.

49. Ans. d. All are correct

Hurst's 11th Ed; Chapter 92; Page 2212-2213

Exercise during pregnancy is not clearly any more dangerous or beneficial to the mother with heart disease than when she is not pregnant. It does affect the fetus. In animal models, maternal exercise has been associated with a falling uterine blood flow. In humans, it is known that the type of exercise affects maternal hemodynamics and uterine perfusion. Maximal exercise by swimming causes less fetal bradycardia (a marker of uterine blood flow) than the same level of cycling. Regular aerobic endurance exercise during pregnancy has been associated with a reduction in birth weight. Since most of the reduction is due to a decrease in neonatal fat mass, it is not clear if this is detrimental. Infants born to the mother who work in standing position may be abnormally small at birth. Although the long-term effect of these are not clear the implication and relation to exercise and work in the upright position are likely greater for women with heart disease.

50. Ans. c. Ejection fraction

Hurst's 11th Ed; Chapter 92; Page 2212-2213

The mechanism evoking the hemodynamic adaptation to pregnancy are not fully understood. They may in part be due to volume changes. Total body water increases steadily throughout the pregnancy by 6-8 L. Sodium retention results in excessive accumulation of 500-900 mEq by the time of delivery. As early as 6 weeks after conception, plasma volume increases approaching its maximum of 1½ to 2 times normal by the second trimester where it stays throughout the pregnancy. The red blood cell mass also increases but not to the same degree as the increase in plasma volume and as a result the hematocrit falls though rarely to < 30%. Vascular alteration also contributes to the hemodynamic changes of pregnancy. Arterial compliance is increased. Venous capacitance increases as well. Although, there is an increase in venous vascular tone. Intrinsic cardiac changes can also explain some of the hemodynamic changes. The stroke volume increases by approximately 25%. The ejection fraction does not change thus the heart has to enlarge (since the ejection fraction is the stroke volume divided by end diastolic volume). Since the increase in the left ventricular end diastolic and systolic volumes are small and not adequate to explain the constant ejection fraction. Heart must become reconfigured as well. The ultimate cause of these changes is uncertain. Complex interaction of the renin-angiotensin-aldosterone system, the reproductive hormones, prostaglandin, nitric oxide and atrial natriuretic factor contribute to the fluid and sodium changes.

CHAPTER 30: Preventive Cardiology

1. What is the probability of developing recurrent fatal or nonfatal MI in a patient with a prior history of MI?
   a. 5–10%
   b. 15%
   c. 15–20%
   d. About 26%

2. What is the probability of 10 years risk for acute MI in a patient with stable angina?
   a. 5–10%
   b. 15%
   c. 20%
   d. > 25%

3. What is the absolute risk of MI in a patient with noncoronary atherosclerosis viz. carotid or peripheral vascular disease?
   a. 5–10%
   b. 15%
   c. 20–25%
   d. > 30%

4. A CHD risk equivalent is defined when the absolute 10 years risk for hard CHD events (nonfatal and fatal MI) exceeds:
   a. 5%
   b. 10%
   c. 15%
   d. 20%

5. In Framingham point score for estimation of 10 years risk for CAD in men, all the following factors are included, *except*:
   a. Age
   b. Total cholesterol
   c. LDL-C
   d. HDL-C

6. In Framingham point score for estimation of 10 years risk for CAD in women, all the following factors are included, *except*:
   a. Age
   b. Total cholesterol
   c. Systolic BP
   d. Diabetes mellitus

7. Interventions have been proved to lower the risk of CHD for all the following risk factors, *except*:
   a. LDL
   b. Cigarette smoking
   c. Hypertension
   d. Lipoprotein (a)

8. Interventions have been proved to lower the risk of CHD for which of the following risk factors:
   a. Lipoprotein (a)
   b. Hyperhomocysteinemia
   c. Smoking
   d. The metabolic syndrome

9. Which of the following statement is *not* correct regarding CAD and statins?
   a. LDL reduction by statins stabilizes coronary lesion by causing substantial enlargement of coronary lumen
   b. For the lesion causing < 50% stenosis, progression of atherosclerosis can be associated with a paradoxical increase in the lumen cross-sectional area (positive remodeling)
   c. The greatest regression of atherosclerosis among statin treated patient is seen when there is reduction of LDL-C and CRP both
   d. When patient treated with a statin develops CHD, the initial presentation is more likely to be stable angina and less likely to be an acute MI

10. What is the average duration of statin therapy, prior to the development of symptoms in case of statin induced myopathy?
   a. 1 month
   b. 2 months
   c. 6 months
   d. 12 months

11. The incidence of rhabdomyolysis is highest for monotherapy with which of the following statins?
   a. Pravastatin
   b. Atorvastatin
   c. Cerivastatin
   d. Simvastatin

12. All of the following are a risk factor for severe myopathy from statin therapy, *except*?
    a. Use of large quantities of grapefruit juice
    b. Use of alcohol
    c. Use of plant sterols
    d. Verapamil

13. Which of the following statement is *correct*?
    a. The magnitude of benefit attributable to statin therapy is greater among those with elevated CRP levels
    b. For every doubling of dose of statin, LDL-C falls only approximately 6%
    c. The addition of ezetimibe to statin therapy will result in an approximately 25% additional LDL-C lowering
    d. All are correct

14. Which of the following statement is *not* correct?
    a. Immediate release niacin is better tolerated than extended release or slow release niacin
    b. Statin-niacin combination has low risk of severe myopathy
    c. Statin-niacin therapy produces marked clinical and angiographic benefits in patients with low HDL-C and CHD
    d. Niacin in long-term use cause rise of blood glucose

15. Which of the following is *not* a component of atherogenic dyslipidemia?
    a. Elevated TG
    b. Elevated LDL-C
    c. Elevated small, dense LDL-C
    d. Low levels of HDL-C

16. Which of the following is the important mechanism by which high density lipoprotein (HDL) is thought to play a protective roles against atherosclerosis?
    a. Reverse cholesterol transport
    b. Initiation of LDL-oxidation
    c. Both of the above
    d. None of the above

17. Which of the following class of drugs are known to effectively modify atherogenic dyslipidemia?
    a. Statins
    b. Statins and ezetimibe
    c. Fibrates
    d. Fibrates and niacin

18. *True* statement regarding fibrates are?
    a. The risk of severe myopathy is increased in patients treated with statins and fibrates
    b. Fenofibrates and bezafibrates are less likely to cause myopathy when used in combination with statins than is gemfibrozil
    c. Fenofibrate can be safely combined with ezetimibe in patients with atherogenic dyslipidemia
    d. All are correct

19. Which class of the antihypertensive drugs is known to offer maximal reduction in LV mass?
    a. ACE inhibitors
    b. Calcium channel blockers
    c. Beta-blockers
    d. Diuretics

ANSWERS WITH EXPLANATIONS

1. **Ans. d. About 26%**

   Hurst's 8th Ed; Page 1205–1206

   Primary prevention refers to strategies to prevent clinical manifestation of disease in asymptomatic individuals. Secondary preventions refer to the efforts to prevent recurrent clinical events in patients with established disease. Prevention of coronary artery disease require identification and treatment of risk factor and the judicious use of medication that have demonstrated efficacy in clinical trials. Risk factor management prevents and treats coronary atherosclerosis and should be included as an integral part of any management plan for the many acute and chronic manifestation of this disease. The intensity of preventive intervention should correspond to the patient level of absolute risk. The approach to risk assessment and management is based on the American Heart Association guidelines for primary prevention, American Heart Association/American College of Cardiology guidelines for secondary prevention and recommendation of the National Cholesterol Education program (NCEP), adult treatment panel III (ATP III) and the American Diabetic Association. In most current risk algorithms absolute risk is divided into three categories, i.e., high, intermediate and low. Patient at high-risk deserve intensive risk reduction therapy. Those an intermediate risk are also candidate for clinical intervention to the extent that therapy is effective, safe and cost effective. Finally, most lower-risk persons should be encouraged by their physician to follow public health recommendation for primary prevention of coronary artery disease, but some may benefit from risk reducing drug therapy. Each category of absolute risk can be expressed in quantitative term such that those with less than a 10% 10-year risk are considered low-risk, those with a 10–20% 10-year risk are considered intermediate-risk and those with greater than 20% 10-year risk are considered high-risk.

Risk categories

Risk category	10-year absolute risk for myocardial infarction (nonfatal + fatal)
High	>20%
Intermediate	10–20%
Low	<10%

Patients without coronary artery disease whose absolute 10-year risk for CHD equals that of patients who already manifest clinical coronary artery disease are said to have coronary artery disease risk equivalent.

Identification of high-risk patients:

a. **Clinical coronary artery disease:** In this category included are patients with history of acute coronary syndrome, stable angina and coronary revascularization procedure. Evidence from clinical trials of cholesterol lowering therapy indicates that patients with a prior history of myocardial infarction have a 10-year risk for recurrent nonfatal or fatal MI of about 26%. Patients with stable angina pectoris have a 10-years risk of acute MI of approximately 20%.

b. **Noncoronary atherosclerosis:** Patient in this group include those with peripheral artery disease, abdominal aortic aneurysm and symptomatic carotid artery disease or asymptomatic disease with greater than 50% stenosis. The absolute risk for MI in patients with noncoronary atherosclerosis equals that for recurrent MI in patients with established coronary artery disease.

c. **Diabetes mellitus:** Patient with diabetes particularly middle age and older patients with type 2 diabetes mellitus (T2DM) who do not manifest coronary artery disease commonly carry a risk for major coronary event equivalent to that of nondiabetic patients with established coronary artery disease. Moreover, many patients with T2DM have a silent MI and many others have silent ischemia. Thus, most patients with diabetes are a high-risk and ATP III has designated diabetes as a CAD equivalent.

d. **Multiple risk factors without clinical coronary artery disease:** Persons without known atherosclerosis who have multiple risk factors (other than diabetes) often have risk that is equivalent to CAD. The absolute risk for development of CAD over the next decade can be estimated by Framingham risk tables.

Estimate of 10-year risk for men (framingham point scores)

Age	Points
20–34	–9
35–39	–4
40–44	0
45–49	3
50–54	6
55–59	8
60–64	10
65–69	11
70–74	12
75–79	13

Total cholesterol	Points at ages 20–39	Points at ages 40–49	Points at ages 50–59	Points at ages 60–69	Points at ages 70–79
<160	0	0	0	0	0
160–199	4	3	2	1	0
200–239	7	5	3	1	0
240–279	9	6	4	2	1
≥ 280	11	8	5	3	1
Nonsmoker	0	0	0	0	0
Smoker	8	5	3	1	1

HDL	Points
≥ 60	–1
50–59	0
40–49	1
>40	2

Systolic blood pressure	If untreated	If treated
<120	0	0
120–129	0	1
130–139	1	2
140–159	1	2
≥ 160	2	3

Point total	10-year risk	Point total	10-year risk
<0	<1%	9	5%
0	1%	10	6%
1	1%	11	8%
2	1%	12	10%
3	1%	13	12%
4	1%	14	16%
5	2%	15	20%
6	2%	16	25%
7	3%	≥ 17	≥ 30%
8	4%		

10-Year risk estimates for women (framingham point scores)

Age	Points
20–34	–7
35–39	–3
40–44	0
45–49	3
50–54	6
55–59	8
60–64	10
65–69	12
70–74	14
75–79	16

Total cholesterol	Points at ages 20–39	Points at ages 40–49	Points at ages 50–59	Points at ages 60–69	Points at ages 70–79
<160	0	0	0	0	0
160–199	4	3	2	1	1
200–239	8	6	4	2	1
240–279	11	8	5	3	2
≥ 280	13	10	7	4	2
Nonsmoker	0	0	0	0	0
Smoker	9	7	4	2	1

HDL	Points
≥ 60	–1
50–59	0
40–49	1
<40	2

Systolic blood pressure	If untreated	If treated
<120	0	0
120–129	1	3
130–139	2	4
140–159	3	5
≥ 160	4	6

Point total	10-year risk	point total	10-year risk
<9	<1%	17	5%
9	1%	18	6%
10	1%	19	8%
11	1%	20	11%
12	1%	21	14%
13	2%	22	17%
14	2%	23	22%
15	3%	24	27%
16	4%	≥ 25	≥ 30%

These tables show absolute risk for hard CAD (nonfatal and fatal MI) and exclude soft CAD (stable and unstable angina). A CAD risk equivalent is defined when the absolute 10-year risk for hard CAD event exceeds 20%.

2. Ans. c. 20%

Hurst's 8th Ed; Page 1205–1206

Refer to explanation for Q. No 1.

3. Ans. c. 20–25%

Hurst's 8th Ed; Page 1205–1206

Refer to explanation for Q. No 1.

4. Ans. d. 20%

Hurst's 8th Ed; Page 1205–1206

Refer to explanation for Q. No 1.

5. Ans. c. LDL-C

Hurst's 8th Ed; Page 1205–1206

Refer to explanation for Q. No 1.

6. Ans. d. Diabetes mellitus

Hurst's 8th Ed; Page 1205–1206

Refer to explanation for Q. No 1.

7. Ans. d. Lipoprotein (a)

Hurst's 8th Ed; Page 1210–1215

Risk factors for which intervention has proven to lower risk of coronary artery disease:
- Lipid disorder
- Atherogenic diet
- Cigarette smoking
- Hypertension

Risk factors for which interventions are likely to lower risk of coronary artery disease:
- Left ventricular hypertrophy
- Metabolic syndrome
- Diabetes mellitus
- Physical inactivity
- Obesity

Risk factors for which interventions have not been shown to lower risk of coronary artery disease:
- Lipoprotein (a)
- Hyperhomocysteinemia
- Oxidative stress
- Alcohol intake

8. Ans. c. Smoking

Hurst's 8th Ed; Page 1210–1215

Refer to explanation for Q. No 7.

9. Ans. a. LDL reduction by statins stabilizes coronary lesion by causing substantial enlargement of coronary lumen

Hurst's 8th Ed; Page 1208

Lipid disorder, statin therapy and coronary artery disease: LDL-cholesterol is a major cause of coronary artery disease and controlled clinical trials show that lowering LDL-cholesterol reduces risk of coronary artery disease. Accordingly, the NCEP has identified LDL-cholesterol as the primary target of lipid lowering therapy. Numerous cholesterol lowering trials have used dietary and drug intervention. Primary and secondary prevention trials with older cholesterol lowering drugs demonstrated reduced risk of CAD but fail to reduce total mortality. The introduction of statins, i.e., a more powerful LDL lowering drug, made possible a more effective test of cholesterol hypothesis. Since 1993, several large primary and secondary prevention trials with statins using clinical endpoint have been completed and as a whole these trials documents convincingly that cholesterol lowering therapy with statins is both safe and effective for reducing CAD risk. The mechanism by which LDL-cholesterol lowering reduces clinical endpoint is suggested by angiographic studies and more recently, by study using intravascular ultrasound. Most statins trials with immediate endpoint demonstrated that marked reduction of LDL-cholesterol slows progression, and in some cases induced regression of coronary lesions. Although measurable changes in lesion size is small in angiographic studies the incidence of major coronary events was reduced strikingly. This observation enlarged the concept that LDL reduction stabilizes coronary lesion by changing their composition rather than causing them to substantially enlarge the coronary lumen. Intravascular ultrasound studies have demonstrated that for lesion causing less than 50% stenosis, progression of coronary atherosclerosis can be associated with a paradoxical increase in the luminal cross-sectional area (so called positive remodelling), whereas regression is not associated with any change in the lumen area. The greatest regression in atherosclerosis among statin treated patients appears to be among those who not only reduce LDL-cholesterol but who also reduce CRP levels. When a patient treated with statins develop coronary artery disease, the initial presentation is more likely to be stable angina and less likely to be an acute myocardial infarction.

10. Ans. c. 6 months

Hurst's 8th Ed; Page 1214–1215

Statin safety: No increase in noncardiovascular mortality has been observed in subjects randomized to active treatment in any of the large statin trials. Furthermore, none of these trials suggest a lower boundary below which LDL-cholesterol lowering is ineffective or dangerous. Most patients tolerate statins with few side effects. Occasionally, patients will have a mild rise in liver transaminases, but these changes are not believed to be an indication of hepatotoxicity. Statin induced myopathy defined as a serum creatinine kinase level of more than 10 times of the upper limit of normal has been observed in 0.1–0.5% of patients treated with statin during randomized controlled trials. In one of the studies, it was found that in case of statin induced myopathy, the average duration of statin therapy prior to symptom onset was 6 months and muscle pain resolved after an average of 2 months of stopping statins. Some patients receiving statin develops muscle symptom but have normal creatinine kinase levels. Biopsy confirmed myopathy has been documented in such patients. Consequently, normal creatinine kinase levels do not rule out statin induced myopathy in patients with muscle symptoms. However, the frequency of this condition is unknown. Rhabdomyolysis characterized by muscle weakness, myoglobinuria and renal failure is a rare complication of statin therapy. In a series of patient with statin associated myopathy, 13% develop rhabdomyolysis requiring hospitalization. Analysis of 2,50,000 patients database found the average incidence of rhabdomyolysis for monotherapy with atorvastatin, pravastatin or simvastatin was 0.44/10000 person—years. The average incidence rose to nearly 6/10000 person—years when these statins were combined with a fibrate. The rate for monotherapy with cerivastatin which has been withdrawn from the market was greater than 5/10000 person years and risk rose to approximately 1 in every 10 patients per year who were treated with cerivastatin plus a fibrate.

Risk factors for severe myopathy from statin therapy:
- Age > 80 years
- Small body frame and frailty
- Multisystem disease (e.g., chronic renal insufficiency, especially as a result of diabetes)
- Multiple medications
- Specific concomitant medications or consumptions (with various statins, check package insert for warnings):
  – Fibrates (especially gemfibrozil, but other fibrates too)
  – Nicotinic acid (rarely)
  – Cyclosporine
  – Azole antifungals
  – Itraconazole and ketoconazole
  – Macrolide antibiotics
  – Erythromycin and clarithromycin
  – HIV protease inhibitors
  – Nefazodone (antidepressant)
  – Verapamil
  – Large quantities of grapefruit juice (>1 quart per day)
  – Alcohol abuse (independently predisposes to myopathy)
- Perioperative periods
- Acute illnesses.

11. Ans. c. Cerivastatin

Hurst's 8th Ed; Page 1214–1215

Refer to explanation for Q. No 10.

12. Ans. c. Use of plant sterols

Hurst's 8th Ed; Page 1214–1215

Refer to explanation for Q. No 10.

13. Ans. d. All are correct

Hurst's 8th Ed; Page 1215

Statin may confer benefits that go beyond LDL cholesterol lowering. These potential benefit known as pleiotropic effects include anti-inflammatory, vascular and immune altering properties. Of these proposed pleiotropic effects, data are stronger for anti-inflammatory effects and all statins lower C-reactive protein in a manner only partially related to LDL cholesterol reduction. In all clinical trials, both primary and secondary prevention, the magnitude of benefit attributable to statin therapy is greater among those with elevated CRP levels. For every doubling of dose of statin, LDL cholesterol will fall by only approximately 6%. Another strategy to achieve LDL cholesterol goal is to add another agents to a statin, namely ezetimibe, niacin or a bile acid sequestrants. Another rationale for combining other lipid medications with statins, is that statin monotherapy reduces the relative risk of coronary event by approximately 30%. Improving other elements of disordered lipid metabolism beyond LDL cholesterol such as remnant lipoproteins or low HDL cholesterol may improve clinical outcomes and this hypothesis has already been tested in large clinical study. Ezetimibe is primarily effective in lowering LDL cholesterol. It is well tolerated and has an excellent safety profile when combined with statins. When patients are already taking a statin, the addition of ezetimibe will result in an approximately 25% additional LDL cholesterol lowering. The addition of ezetimibe to statin therapy also leads to a further reduction in CRP even though ezetimibe on its own has no effect on this inflammatory biomarker.

14. Ans. a. Immediate release niacin is better tolerated than extended release or slow release niacin

Hurst's 8th Ed; Page 1216

Niacin is a potent drug used in treatment of hyperlipidemia. Niacin should be considered in combination with a statin when triglycerides are elevated and/or HDL-C is reduced in combination with high LDL cholesterol. Only about 3/4th of patients can remain on niacin in the long-term because of flushing, itching, skin rash, rise in plasma glucose, uric acid and liver transaminases and rarely, frank hepatotoxicity. Extended release and slow release niacin is better tolerated than immediate release niacin but the dose should not exceeds 2,000 mgm/day. In the long-term follow up of coronary drug project, niacin reduced total mortality. Niacin is attractive for combined drug therapy with statins because the combination has a very low-risk of severe myopathy and statin niacin therapy produces marked clinical and angiographic benefits in patients with low HDL cholesterol and coronary artery disease.

15. Ans. b. Elevated LDL-C

Hurst's 8th Ed; Page 1216

Although high low density lipoprotein (LDL) is the primary lipid risk factor, other lipid parameters also increases the risk of CAD in person with or without an elevated LDL cholesterol. Specifically, the combination of elevated concentration of triglyceride, small, dense LDL-C and low level of HDL-C is referred as atherogenic dyslipidemia. This is a complex dyslipidemia that usually results from a generalized metabolic disorder related to insulin resistance. Patient with insulin resistance often have the metabolic syndrome. Although, an elevated LDL cholesterol deserves primary emphasis for management, atherogenic dyslipidemia is assuming increasing importance as a contributor to CAD because of growing prevalence of obesity, diabetes and metabolic syndrome. Patient with atherogenic dyslipidemia often have concomitant abnormalities of inflammation (elevated CRP) and hypofibrinolysis [elevated plasminogen activator inhibitor I (PAI – I)].

16. Ans. c. Both of the above

Hurst's 8th Ed; Page 1216

Two important mechanism by which high density lipoprotein (HDL) is thought to play protective role against atherosclerosis are reverse cholesterol transport and inhibition of LDL oxidation.

17. Ans. d. Fibrates and niacin

Hurst's 8th Ed; Page 1216–1217

The drug that most effectively modify atherogenic dyslipidemia are fibrates and niacin. Several trials with fibrates have shown a significant reduction of major coronary events. The role of fibrates as add on therapy to statin is also evaluated in ongoing trials. The risk for severe myopathy is increased in patient treated with statins and fibrates. Fenofibrates and bezafibrates are less likely to cause myopathy when used in combination with statins than is gemfibrozil. The use of statins and fibrates combination should be reserved for high-risk patients. Fenofibrates can be combined safely with ezetimibe in patient with atherogenic dyslipidemia. Niacin lowers triglycerides, lowers the concentration of small, dense LDL particles and raises HDL concentration. Niacin has more side effect than fibrates.

18. Ans. d. All are correct

Hurst's 8th Ed; Page 1216–1217

Refer to explanation for Q. No 17.

19. Ans. a. ACE inhibitors

Hurst's 8th Ed; Page 1217–1218

Left ventricular hypertrophy (LVH), defined either by electrocardiography or echocardiography is a potent independent risk factor for CAD, roughly doubling the risk of cardiovascular death in both men and women. Most antihypertensive drugs can reduce left ventricular hypertrophy. Although, not all drugs are equally effective in this regard despite their equipotent blood pressure lowering capability. An analysis of double blind randomized, controlled studies with parallel group design indicates that ACE inhibitors reduce left ventricular mass by 12%, calcium channel blockers by 11%, beta-blockers by 5% and diuretics by 8%.

Index

A

A wave, abnormalities of 27
Abdomen 371
Abdominal aorta 127, 140
  aneurysm of 242
  bifurcation of 366
  dimension 367
  infrarenal portion of 371
  rupture of 367
Abdominal aortic aneurysm 367
  elective repair of 367
Abdominal jugular reflux 106
Abscess
  formation, perivalvular 282
  periannular 283
Absorption 386
Accelerated idioventricular rhythm 297
Acetazolamide 124
Acid
  lipase deficiency 379
  maltase deficiency 378
Acoustic neuroma 107
Actin 16
Acute coronary syndrome 82, 257
  diagnosis of 132
Acute heart failure 82, 101, 390
  development of 101
Acute pulmonary embolism 288, 292, 383, 384
  feature of 42
Adenoma, adrenal 251
Adenosine 328
Adrenergic nervous system, activation of 108
Adrenogenital syndrome 251
Adult respiratory distress syndrome 275
AIDS 262
Airways, obstructive disease of 278
Akinesis 41
Alagille 212
Alcohol 262
  consumption 256
  septal ablation, complication of 258
Aldosteronism
  primary 88, 251
  secondary 78
Alirocumab 92
Alkaptonuria 377

Allen test 68
Allergic reaction 169
Alpha-adrenoceptor blockers 231
Alpha-agonists 85
Alpha-galactosidase A deficiency 379
Alport syndrome 251
Altered mental status 292
Ambulatory blood pressure monitoring 67, 86
Aminoacidopathies 377
Aminorex fumarate 278
Amiodarone 230, 266, 269, 300, 301, 306, 309, 317, 323-326, 328
  hypothyroidism 318
  pulmonary toxicity of 301
  side effect of 301
  toxicity 301
Amlodipine 89
Amniotic fluid 278
Amoxicillin 216, 264
Ampicillin 173
Amyl nitrite inhalation 23, 24, 29, 227
Amyloidosis 48, 118
  cardiac 46, 104, 115, 118
Anaphylactoid purpura 251
Anemia 162, 181
  treatment of 104
Aneurysm, rupture of 202
Angina
  early recurrence of 145
  nocturnal 179
  pectoris 177
Angiodysplasia 175
Angiography 68
  coronary 68
Angiokeratoma corporis diffusum 251
Angiolipomas 251
Angiotensin 109
  converting enzyme inhibitor 87, 88, 112, 193, 399
  receptor blockers 88, 193, 389
Ankle edema 81
Ankylosing spondylitis 27, 182
Anomalous pulmonary venous drainage, high incidence of 208
Anrep effect 10, 13, 19, 60
Anthracycline 271
  cardiomyopathy 252, 259
  trastuzumab 105

Antiarrhythmic drugs 34, 253, 300, 303-306, 382, 387
  suppress symptomatic arrhythmia 264
Anticoagulation 119, 186, 388
Antidigoxin immunotherapy 107
Antihypertensive drugs 79, 81, 82, 89, 383, 389
Anti-inflammatory drugs 347
Antimicrobial therapy 160
Antiplatelet drug 293
Aorta 372
  ascending 367
  coarctation of 7, 24, 30, 199, 202, 205, 209, 210, 239, 251
  dissection of 367, 368
  proximal dissection of 366
  rupture of 365
Aortic allograft 154
Aortic aneurysm 30
Aortic arch 70, 203, 206, 230
  complete interruption of 228
  interruption 200, 202, 236
  variety of 205
Aortic atresia 8, 238
Aortic dilatation 184, 376
Aortic disease 366
Aortic dissection 83, 351, 353, 366
  diagnosis of 366
Aortic ejection click 176
Aortic impedance 10
Aortic incompetence 183
Aortic intima, wrinkled appearance of 367
Aortic isthmus 200, 366, 374
Aortic pressure 12, 13, 52, 272
  waveforms 59
Aortic regurgitation 27, 28, 60, 170, 175-177, 205, 220, 234, 252
  causes of 206
  severity of 177
  water-hammer pulse of 23
Aortic sinus, congenital aneurysm of 235
Aortic stenosis 60, 176, 177, 187, 188, 190, 341
  isolated 184
  low gradient 187
  murmur of 187
Aortic stiffness 80
Aortic systolic murmur, presence of 181

Index

Aortic valve 48, 171-174, 285, 364
  closure of 12
  disease 187
    staging of 192
  infective endocarditis 42
  replacement 188
  thickening of 236
Aortic valvular disease 192
Aorticopulmonary septal defect 199, 205
Aortography 372
Apert syndrome 214
Apixaban 293
Apnea
  central 279
  hypopnea index 121
  mixed 279
  obstructive 279
Arginine vasopressin 109
Arrhythmia 145, 253, 254, 299, 381
  cardiac 294, 334
  supraventricular 316
Arrhythmogenic cardiomyopathy 41, 255, 266
  diagnosis of 255, 266
Arrhythmogenic right ventricular dysplasia 39, 211, 246, 253, 254, 263, 327, 328
  diagnosis of 255
Arterial blood
  gas 198, 218, 383, 390
  pressure 13
Arterial wall, primary diseases of 278
Arteriovenous fistula
  congenital pulmonary 239
  pulmonary arterial 206, 238, 239
Arteriovenous pressure 71
Arteritis, gestational 278
Artery 132
  disease 138
    atherosclerotic coronary 343
    intermediate 339
    posterior descending 1
    pulmonary 143, 147, 336
Arthritis 162
Aschoff bodies 187
Aschoff nodule 159
Ashman phenomenon 25, 31
Ask-Upmark syndrome 251
Aspartylglucosaminuria 378
Aspergillus 285
Aspirin 129, 138, 277, 322
  low dose 388
Atherogenicity 142
Atherosclerosis 92, 97, 125, 125, 132, 135, 257, 367
  accelerated 196
  advance lesion of 134
  lesion of 135
  noncoronary 393, 395
Athlete's heart 342
Atresia 69, 74
  pulmonary 8

Atrial fibrillation 59, 105, 126, 153, 186, 269, 297, 302-306, 320, 332
  acute conversion of 300
  causes of 302
  development of 302
  electrical cardioversion of 302, 303
  management of 303
  nonvalvular 302
  postoperative 304
  prevalence of 186
  recurrent 300
  treatment of 258, 300
Atrial flutter 133, 305, 319, 320, 331
Atrial septal defect 42, 146, 229
  common variety of 208
  types of 208
Atrial septum, atrioventricular portion of 1
Atrial switch operation 146, 158
Atrial tachyarrhythmias, digoxin induced 301
Atrial thrombus 358
Atrioventricular asynchrony 57
Atrioventricular node 325
Atrioventricular septal defect 214
Atrioventricular valve regurgitation 225
Augment murmur 31
Autoimmune disease, treatment of 257
Azilsartan 89

B

Bacteremia 281
  high grade 281, 283
Bainbridge reflex 14
Ball and cage valve 194
Balloon
  angioplasty 73, 222
  atrial septostomy 22
  mitral valvuloplasty 381
  pulmonary valvotomy 156
Baseline long QT syndrome 266
Bazett formula 34
Beck's triad 345, 346
Bempedoic acid 95
Benzathine penicillin G 164
Beriberi, infantile 250
Bernheim effect 10, 52
Beta-adrenergic agonist 141, 275
Beta-blockers 81, 88, 120, 123, 130, 137, 259, 265, 309, 325, 374, 376, 382
Bezold–Jarisch reflex 14, 131
Bicuspid aortic valve 4, 9, 30, 170, 188, 228, 286, 373
Bicuspid valve, congenital 5
Bicycle ergometer 37
Bidirectional ventricular tachycardia 295, 296
Bifid pulmonary artery waveform 52
Bile-acid binding resins 95
Bileaflet valve 194
Biochemical defect 377

Biological valve 145, 154
Bioprosthetic valves 155
Bisferiens pulse 23
Blalock–Taussig shunt 147
  modified 143
Blood
  gas 218
  pressure 22, 67, 78, 336, 384
    control 80
    diastolic 79, 84, 85
    high 112
    systolic 85, 292, 395, 396
  pump 147
  salvage 149
  urea nitrogen 112
  volume 384
    sensor 12
Bloodless open heart surgery 149
Borrelia burgdorferi 264
Bounding arterial pulse 201, 225
Bovine pericardium 195
Bowditch effect 13, 60
Bowditch phenomenon 12, 60
Brain abscess 204, 232
Broadbent's sign 30
Brockenbrough phenomenon 258
Bronchial circulation 70
Bronchitis, chronic 278
Bronze skin 254
Brugada sign 300
Brugada syndrome 255, 296, 307, 327
Bubble oxygenators 148
Burns 251

C

Cachexia, cardiac 99, 106
Calcification 155, 260
Calcium channel
  antagonist 132
  blockers 81, 88, 89, 258, 259
Cancer 355
  colonic 168
  therapy 105
Canon A wave 51
Carcinoid
  crisis, acute 268
  syndrome 255
Cardiac
  allograft rejection, monitoring of 262
  anatomy 1, 5
  catheterization 68, 216, 261
  decompensation, causes of 197, 203
  defect, congenital 208, 210
  failure 389
  magnetic resonance 254, 287
  resynchronization therapy 334
  silhouette 208, 260
  tamponade 59, 60, 345, 346, 354
    diagnosis of 345
  teratogen 203

transplantation 71
troponin 133
tumor, primary 358
valve 177
 tumor of 358
Cardiologic systole 18
Cardiomyopathy 105, 252, 253, 257, 270, 295, 297, 299, 389
 alcoholic 253, 257
 dilated 41, 252-254, 263
 diphtheritic 249
 functional classification of 261
 hypertrophic 3, 212, 252, 253, 256, 260, 295, 304, 315, 342, 343
  obstructive 26, 59, 60, 257, 272
 iatrogenic 257
 idiopathic dilated 253
 ischemic 117, 252, 262
 mitochondrial 264
 nonischemic dilated 253
 peripartum 120, 383, 390
 restrictive 252, 253, 261, 262, 375
 tachycardia induced 255
 valvular 252
Cardioplegia 144
 solutions 2
Cardiovascular anomaly, congenital 367
Cardiovascular defects 244
Cardiovascular disease 121
 atherosclerotic 93, 98
Cardiovascular disorders 381
Cardiovascular surgery 143
Cardiovascular traumatic lesion 364
Cardioversion 301
 transthoracic 325
Cardioverter defibrillators 322
Carditis 161, 165, 167
Carey Coombs murmur 164
Carney complex 355
Carnitine
 deficiency, primary 377
 parenteral 249
 transport defect 377
Carotid pulse 179
Carotid sinus
 massage 294, 298, 307
 syncope 329
Carpentier classification 189
Carpentier dysfunction 186
Carpentier-Edwards valve 154
Carvedilol 262
Catecholaminergic polymorphic ventricular tachycardia 295, 309
 diagnosis of 255
Caudal angulation 72
Ceftriaxone 173
 high dose 173
Central aortic pressure 80
Central nervous system disorder 99
Central sleep apnea 104, 121-123
Central venous pressure 111

Centrifugal pump 148
Ceramidase deficiency 379
Cerebral artery, middle 285
Cerebral edema 251
Cerebral thrombosis 231
Cerebrovascular disease 358
Cerivastatin 398
Chest
 lateral film projections of 75
 pain 127, 132
  acute 50
  elements of 132
  syndrome 129
 radiogram 252
 roentgenogram 99, 261
 systolic retraction of 24
 trauma, nonpenetrating 364
 wall 278
 X-ray of 99, 346, 350, 385
Chlamydia 137
Cholesterol 251, 395, 396
 absorption inhibitor 92
 biosynthesis pathway 92
Chorea 162, 165, 167
Chromosome 245
Chronic obstructive pulmonary diseases 278
Chylomicrons 96, 143
Circulatory assist device 144
Circumflex coronary artery, occlusion of 128
Cirrhosis, classical triad of 254
Clinical coronary artery disease 395
Clonidine 79
Clopidogrel 130
Closed heart surgery 147, 156
Cocaine abuse 256
Cohen system 69
Colchicines 349
Collagen diseases 375
Colon, malignancy of 286
Commotio Cordis 342
Complete heart block 240, 249, 273, 298
Computed tomographic pulmonary angiography 390
Conduction
 abnormality 264
 defect 377
Congenital anomaly 7, 74, 196, 206, 220
Congenital coronary
 anomaly 69, 74
 stenosis 69, 74
Congenital heart disease 2, 7, 170, 197, 203, 204, 209
 types of 210
Congestion, pulmonary 186
Congestive heart failure 99, 102, 204, 207
 history of 205
 treatment of 232
Connective tissue 377
 disorders 159, 212, 274, 338

Conotruncal malformation 210, 211
Constrictive pericarditis 30, 40, 246, 265, 347, 348, 353, 354
 pericardiectomy for 145
Continuous positive air pressure ventilation 119
Coombs-positive hemolytic anemia 78
Cor pulmonale 274, 275, 278
Cor triatriatum 236
Corkscrew tortuosity 24
Corneal microdeposits 317
Corney's complex 358, 361
Coronary arteriovenous fistula 221
Coronary artery 2, 69, 132
 aneurysm 126, 250
 bypass surgery 69, 133, 144
  indications for 152
 congenital anomaly of 7, 74
 disease 68, 125, 127, 130, 297, 304, 308, 395, 397
  high risk 54
 fistula 69
Coronary atherosclerosis 105
 extent of 50
Coronary blood flow 10
 measurement of 52
Coronary collaterals 69, 135
 circulation 74
Coronary fistula
 drainage of 69
 origin of 69
Coronary revascularization, indications for 130
Coronary sinus 4, 6, 49, 150
 ostium of 2, 312
 type 241
Corrigan's sign 30
Corticosteroid 318, 347
 administration 316
 therapy 163
Cough, nonproductive 11
Coxiella burnetii 170
Coxsackie
 A 248
 B 248
Crista
 supraventricularis 5
 terminalis 3, 5
Cushing's syndrome 251
Cutis laxa 212
Cyanosis 70, 197, 204, 218
 cardiac cause of 204
 respiratory cause of 204
Cystic fibrosis 212, 278
Cytokines 287, 362

D

Dabigatran 120
Dacron 152
Dash diet pattern 88

D-dimer
    assay 391
    level 288
Deafness 254
    familial 212
Debrancher deficiency 378
Deep hypothermia 144
Deep vein thrombosis 289
Degeneration 155
Diabetes mellitus 95, 132, 251, 395, 397
Diabetic neuropathy 326
Diastolic dysfunction 260, 263
Diastolic pressure gradient 183
Diastolic ventricular interaction 14, 61
Dietary potassium intake 85
DiGeorge syndrome 202, 206, 235
Digitalis 275, 382, 387
    toxicity, management of 100
Digitoxin toxicity 99
Digoxin 115, 117, 198, 273, 353
    therapeutic level of 198, 204
Dihydropyridines 89
Dilantin 214
Diltiazem 89, 139
Direct thrombin inhibitor 105
Disopyramide 300, 321
Disseminated lupus erythematosus 251
Distal right coronary artery 3
Diuretics 90, 124
Dobutamine 128, 292
    stress echocardiography 41, 187
Dofetilide 317, 324
Doppler
    echocardiography 40, 62
    velocity probes 60
Double vessel disease 153
Down syndrome 210, 213
Doxorubicin 54
    therapy 50
Doxycycline 264
Dronedarone 324
Drug abuse, intravenous 278
Dual chamber pacemakers 330, 331
Ductal artery 2
Ductus arteriosus 2, 7, 197, 203
    functional closure of 200, 203
    patency of 199
Ductus dependent lesion 203
Duke criteria 171
    modified 168, 172
Duroziez's murmur 183
Dynamic auscultation 29, 227, 257
Dysautonomia, familial 251
Dysbetalipoproteinemia 93
Dyslipidemia, atherogenic 394
Dysplasia
    arteriohepatic 212
    triangle of 254
Dyspnea 15, 178, 183, 260
    causes of 104
    mechanism of 15
    symptoms of 355

E

Early repolarization syndrome 296
Ebstein's anomaly 59, 206, 208, 237, 240
    clinical diagnosis of 207
    diagnosis of 238
Ebstein's malformation 233
Echocardiogram 145, 180, 261
Echocardiography 40, 41, 45, 62, 281, 345, 349, 355
    transthoracic 44
Ectopic fat deposition 93
Edema
    acute pulmonary 99
    interstitial 15
    neurogenic pulmonary 107
    peripheral 112
Effusive constrictive pericarditis, causes of 347
Ehlers–Danlos syndrome 226, 251, 376
Eisenmenger syndrome 339, 340
Either 98
Ejection fraction 43, 392
EKG 32
Eleclazine 317
Electrical cardioversion 301-303
Electrocardiogram 261, 300, 334, 386
Embolic disorders 278
Embryology 1, 7
Endocardial cushion defect 245
Endocarditis 169, 280-282
    feature of 42, 281
    nonbacterial thrombotic 282
    noninfective 42
    nosocomial infective 281
    staphylococcal 171
    treatment of 48
Endomyocardial biopsy 253
    clinical indications for 262
Endomyocardial fibrosis 46, 254
Endothelin 1 antagonist ambrisentan 124
Endothelium, arterial 141
Enzyme neprilysin 11
Ephedrine 251
Epicardial fat pad sign 70
Epinephrine 251
Eponym Steidele's complex 202
Epsilon waves 305, 306
Ergonovine 60
Erythema
    marginatum 165
    migrans 254
Erythromycin 164
Esophageal perforation 324
Ethanol 244, 245
Evolocumab 92
Ewart's sign 345
Exercise
    capacity 38
    pressor reflex 36
    stress test 266
Extracardiac anomaly 199, 229

Eyeballs, pulsation of 22
Ezetimibe 95

F

Fabry's disease 251
Facial edema 355
Fallot's tetralogy 23, 25, 28, 206, 221
Fascicular tachycardia 297
Fatty acid metabolism 377
Femoral artery 23, 170
Ferric carboxymaltose, intravenous 119
Fetal
    alcohol syndrome 196, 210, 245
    cardiac output 203, 215
    circulation 196
        intrinsic component of 200
    ductal artery 4
    echocardiography 224, 233
    heart in utero 198, 204
    movements 215
    rubella
        effect 211, 246
        infections 229
Fever 168, 282
Fibrates 399
Fibrillation following cardiac surgery 133
Fibrinogen labeled iodine scanning 277
Fibroelastoma, papillary 357, 360
Fibroelastosis, endocardial 208, 375
Fibromuscular disease 80
Fibrosis, interstitial 337
Fibrotic scar, formation of 100
Flecainide 300, 316, 323-325
Fluvastatin 97
Fondaparinux 127
Fossa ovalis 241
Framingham point scores 393, 395, 396
Frank–Starling effects 14
    component of 12
Fredrickson classification 142, 143
Friedreich's ataxia 212
Fucosidosis
    mild 378
    severe 378
Fungal infection 47
Furosemide 120

G

Gallop rhythm 231
Gastroepiploic artery graft 144
Gastrointestinal bleeding 175
Gastrointestinal procedure 281
    regimens for 217
Geleophysic dysplasia 379
Geneva score, revised 291
Genitourinary procedure 197
    regimens for 217
Giant cell arteritis 366
Gingival hyperplasia 81
Glucocerebrosidase deficiency 379

Glucocorticoids 339
Glutaraldehyde fixation 194
Glycogen storage
 disease 247
 disorders 377
Glycoproteinoses 378
Goiter, retrosternal 251
Gonadal dysgenesis 251
Goose neck deformity 198
Graham Steel murmur 187
Granuloma
 eosinophilic 278
 noncaseating 255
Granulomatous diseases 278
Great artery
 corrected transposition of 201
 disease 196
 transposition of 49, 158, 201, 233
Guanyly cyclase activator 340
Guillain-Barré syndrome 251

H

Haemophilus influenzae 288
Head up tilt test 329
Healthy mature infants ductus
 arteriosus 197
Heart 61, 375
 artificial 150
 block, congenital complete 201
 boot-shaped 198
 conduction system of 265
 congenital anomaly of 200
 disease 100, 163, 311, 384
  atherosclerotic coronary 138
  carcinoid 256
  congenital 2, 7, 170, 197, 203, 204, 209
  coronary 88
  cyanotic congenital 22, 204
  dynamic congenital 200
  hypertensive 80, 252
  ischemic 126, 190
  minimal 304
  neoplastic 361
  rheumatic 159, 186, 187, 190
  stable ischemic 126
  valvular 175, 186, 187
 failure 11, 40, 99-106, 115, 119, 121, 122,
  125, 169, 174, 197, 254, 281, 285, 288,
  299, 303, 304, 311
  acute 82, 101, 123, 390
  assessment of 100
  chronic 104
  congestive 99, 102, 204, 207
  diastolic 99, 383
  exacerbation 11
  fetal 197
  high risk of 105
  management of 104
  manifestation of 197
  severe symptoms of 116
  symptomatic severity of 121
  systolic 99, 383
  treatment of 103
 lung machine 143
 murmurs 361
 neonatal 197, 198, 204
 rate 10, 32, 34, 255, 384, 385
 sound 12
 transplantation 143
  heterotropic 39
 valvular structure of 355
 venting of 149
Heartbeat, awareness of 294
Heat exchangers 148
HELLP syndrome 383, 389
Hemochromatosis 264
Hemodialysis catheter 286
Hemofiltration 149
Hemolytic uremic syndrome 251
Hemopericardium 46
Hemorrhage, intracranial 243
Henle loop 102
Heparin 388
 therapy 292
 unfractionated 293
Hepatic failure 116
Hepatojugular reflux 23, 99
High altitude pulmonary edema 99, 107
Highly active antiretroviral therapy 270
His-Purkinje block 313
Histiocytic infiltration 379
Holiday heart syndrome 253
Holt-Oram syndrome 246
Homocystinuria 213, 377
Homogentisic acid, deposition of 377
Homograft 154
Hourglass appearance 70
Human atherosclerotic lesion 133
Human embryo 203
Hyaline degeneration 161
Hydantoin 244
Hydralazine 120
Hydrochlorothiazide 86
Hydronephrosis 251
 unilateral 251
Hypercalcemia 251
Hypercapnia 232
Hypercholesterolemia 25, 96, 175
 management of 92
Hypercyanotic spells 231
Hyperglycemia, treatment of 105
Hyperinsulinemia 84
Hyperkalemia 103
Hyperlipidemia 92, 142
 Fredrickson classification of 142, 143
Hyperlipoproteinemia 22, 26
Hypernatremia 251
Hyperoxaluria 377
Hyperparathyroidism, primary 251
Hyperplasia 251
Hypertension 78-80, 85, 110, 188, 228, 251,
 312, 321, 368, 377, 383, 388-390
 acute pulmonary arterial 274
 causes of 80
 diagnosis of 79
 diuretics therapy for 80
 essential 251
 gestational 78, 389
 hyperkinetic pulmonary 30
 isolated systolic 79
 management of 81
 paradoxical 222
 primary pulmonary 274, 278
 pulmonary 122, 180, 220, 274, 337
  arterial 337, 339
 renovascular 80, 83, 88
 severe 78
 systemic 248
 thromboembolic pulmonary 337
 treatment of 81
Hypertensive emergencies 78, 85
Hypertensive heart disease 80, 252
 classification of 87
Hyperthyroidism 251, 321
 amiodarone induced 301
Hypertriglyceridemia 92, 95, 96
Hypertrophic cardiomyopathy 3, 212, 252,
 253, 256, 260, 295, 304, 315, 342, 343
 treatment of 258
Hypertrophic obstructive cardiomyopathy
 26, 59, 60, 257, 272
 maneuver amplifies murmur of 24
 murmur of 29
Hypertrophy
 disappearance of 343
 focal 356
Hyperventilation 37
Hyperviscosity 338
Hypokalemia 34, 336
 excessive 80
Hypokinesis 41
Hyponatremia 100
Hypoplastic left heart syndrome 211
Hypotension
 postprandial 82
 triad of 346
Hypothermia 149, 206
Hypothyroidism 353
 amiodarone induced 301
Hypoventilation
 alveolar 274, 337
 idiopathic 278
Hypovolemia 59
Hypovolumia 136
Hypoxemia, arterial 337
Hypoxic spells, treatment of 197, 204

I

Ibutilide 300, 317, 325
Implantable pacemaker 322

Infection, fetal 246
Infective endocarditis 7, 42, 159, 168-171, 188, 280-283
   community acquired 168
   complex 170
   complication of 281
   diagnosis of 168, 171, 172
   fungal 174
   location of 202
   positive blood culture for 171
Inferior myocardial wall infarction 125
Infiltration, malignant 278
Inflammation 290
Infra-nodal tachycardia, digoxin induced 301
Infundibular septum 220
Injury, cardiac 364
Inlet septal defects 219
Intact ventricular septum 8
Intra-aortic balloon pump 150
Intracavitary cardiac tumors 361
Intracellular glycogen accumulation fibrosis 378
Intracoronary thrombolytic therapy 250
Intramyocardial sinusoids 7
Intrathoracic pressure 123
Intravenous gamma globulin, high dose 249
Ischemia, myocardial 69, 74, 375
Isoproterenol 251, 310
Isovolumic contraction 18, 19

J

J curve
   hypothesis 78
   phenomenon 79
J wave syndrome 63, 296
Janeway lesion 168171
Jones criteria 164
Jugular venous
   distention 350
   pressure 22, 24, 99, 111

K

Kartagener's syndrome 210
Kawasaki disease 247, 248, 250, 251
Kerley B lines 186
Kidney
   abnormal 251
   disease, chronic 91
   injury, acute 80, 87
Klinefelter syndrome 244
Knuckle sign 348
Koch triangle 3, 298
Kussmaul's sign 23, 27, 52, 99, 125
Kyphoscoliosis 278
Kyrgyzstan 166

L

Labetalol 91
Laminopathy 298
Lao view 72, 73
Laplace law 10, 12
Left anterior descending artery 73, 152
Left bundle branch block 34
   pacing 336
   pattern 238
Left circumflex artery 54, 68, 72
   origin of 74
   proximal segment of 68
Left coronary artery, anomalous origin of 221
Left internal
   jugular vein 22
   mammary artery 136
Left subclavian artery 243
Left ventricular
   diastolic dysfunction 40
   end diastolic pressure 52
   hypertrophy 321
      maximum regression of 81
   right atrial shunt 214
   systolic function, recovery of 102
   tumors 358
   wall thickness 304
Licorice 251
Lidocaine 319, 322, 388
Ligamentum arteriosum 2
Lipid
   disorder 397
   myopathy 377
Lipid research clinics coronary primary prevention trial 143
Lipoprotein 92, 93, 397
   atherogenic 93
   fractions 139
   high density 95, 394
   low density 95
   very low density 95
Lithium 244
   carbonate 207
   iodide cell 333
Little syndrome 251
Liver disease, chronic 278
Low cardiac output syndrome 133
Low molecular weight heparin 388
Lower limb pain, unilateral 291
Lumbar vertebrae 371
Lung
   cancer 357
   disease, interstitial 122
Lupus erythematosus, maternal 200
Lyme disease 254, 264, 313
Lysosomal storage 377, 378, 379

M

Magnesium 309
Magnetic resonance imaging 279, 353, 369
Malformation, congenital 209, 382
Malignancy 286, 357
Mammary soufflé 200
Mannosidosis 378
Marfan's syndrome 210, 375, 376
McConnell sign 42, 291
Mean arterial pressure 32
Mechanical prosthetic valves 56, 145, 155
Medtronic-Hancock valve 154
Melanoma 356
   malignant 363
Membrane oxygenator 148, 150
Mesothelioma 356
Metastasis 362
   cardiac 355
Methimazole 319
Methyldopa 79, 83, 91
Metoprolol 90
   intravenous 325
Microalbuminuria 87
Mitochondria 214
Mitral annulus 186
Mitral chordae 174
Mitral disease, absence of 348
Mitral E point-septal separation 62
Mitral E wave velocities 47
Mitral prostheses 44
Mitral regurgitation 186, 202, 257
   acute 31
   chronic 31
   severity of 62
Mitral stenosis 31, 166, 186, 187, 214
   congenital 240
   isolated 187
   juvenile 186
   M mode echocardiographic hallmark of 62
   moderate 155
   severe 186
Mitral valve 41, 44, 145, 173, 186
   abnormality 204
   anterior leaflet of 179
   feature of 177
   involvement 174
   position 170
   premature closure of 62, 184
   prolapse 226, 287
      degenerative 170
      murmur of 29
   regurgitation, pathophysiologic triad of 189
   repair of 375
   replacement 155
   surgery 186
Mixed connective tissue disease 278
M-mode echocardiography 40
Monotherapy 79
Monounsaturated fatty acids 96
Mucocutaneous lymph node syndrome 250
Mucopolysaccharidoses 213, 214, 378
Mulibrey nanism, syndrome of 211
Muller's maneuver 24
Multiple septic emboli 281

Mural endocardium 362
Murmur
    duration of 182, 183
    intensity of 191
    systolic 257, 357
Muscle
    cardiac 11
    papillary 5, 207
Muscular dystrophy 212
Mycotic aneurysm 281
Myocardial abscess 284
Myocardial fibrosis 312
Myocardial infarction 34, 79, 134, 361, 375
    acute 34, 127, 134, 257, 331, 345, 366, 380
    perioperative 145, 153
Myocardial oxygen consumption 135
Myocardial stretch, degree of 12
Myocarditis 247
    active 247
    chronic 247
    diphtheric 247
    infective 247
Myocardium 14, 53, 255
    direct invasion of 249
    myocyte component of 100
Myopathy, severe 394, 398
Myosin 16
Myxoma 355-357, 360-362
    cardiac 361

N

Native valve endocarditis 146, 156
Natriuretic peptide 100, 101, 109
    degradation of 109
Nausea, occurrence of 126
Nebivolol 113
Neck pain, bilateral 177
Necrosis 110
Negative predictive value 126
Nephritis 251
    familial 251
Nephropathy, hyperuricemic 251
Nephrotic syndrome 93
Neprilysin inhibition 100
Neuroblastoma 251
Neurofibromatosis 251
Neuromuscular apparatus, diseases of 278
Niacin 399
Nicoladoni-Branham sign 99
Nitrate 120, 131
Nitric oxide 276
Nitroprusside 91
Nitrous oxide 320
Nocturia 86
Nonsteroidal anti-inflammatory drugs 80, 89, 116
    therapy 81
Noonan syndrome 209
Norepinephrine 292
Normal apnea-hypopnea index 121
Nuclei 214

O

Obesity 140
Oblique sinus 1, 2
Obstruction, severity of 75
Obstructive sleep apnea 78, 85
Ochronosis 377
Open heart surgery 148, 304
Oral anticoagulant 130
Oreo cookie sign 346
Orthopnea 11, 15, 185
Osteogenesis imperfect 213
Ostium secundum 158, 241, 237
Outflow tract
    obstruction, site of 206
    ventricular tachycardia 296, 297, 308
Oxalate, tissue accumulation of 377
Oxygen
    hemoglobin for 131
    supplemental 339
    therapy 280
Oxygenators 147, 148
    types of 148

P

Pacemaker
    malfunction 331
    syndrome 330
Palpitation 294
Pancreatitis, acute 93, 345, 347, 354
Pansystolic murmur 205
Parachute mitral valve 239
Paradoxic pulse 346
Paradoxical embolism 158
Parasitic diseases 278
Paroxysmal nocturnal dyspnea 11, 15
Patent ductus arteriosus 215, 229, 231, 235
Patent foramen ovale 242
PCSK9 inhibitor 95, 192
Pectus excavatum 23
Penicillin 160, 169, 283
Percutaneous balloon coronary
    angioplasty 70
Percutaneous transluminal angioplasty,
    technique of 70
Periannular complication 168
Pericardial calcification 25
Pericardial disease 345
Pericardial effusion 41, 52, 76, 215, 336,
    345, 346, 349, 352
    recurrent 346
Pericardiocentesis 345, 346
Pericarditis 34, 132, 347
    acute 345
    chronic 347
        constrictive 26
    idiopathic 350
    recurrent 345, 347, 354
    tuberculous 347, 353
    viral 354
Pericardium 70, 347, 355

Perimount valve 154
Permanent pacemaker 298, 313
    implantation 298
Pharyngitis, streptococcal 159, 160
Phenoxybenzamine 90
Phenylalanine 244
Phenylephrine 268
Phenytoin 316, 319, 387
Pheochromocytoma 81, 251
Phlebotomy 338
Phospholipids 348
Phosphorylase kinase deficiency 378
Phrenic nerve injury 324
Pindolol 323
Pistol shot sound 23, 30
Plant sterols, use of 398
Platelet
    count 284
    derived growth factor 127, 135
    inhibitor clopidogrel 322
Pleural fibrosis 278
Pneumoconiosis 278
Pneumoniae 137
Pneumonitis, interstitial 328
Poliomyelitis 251
Polycystic kidney disease 251
Polymyositis 278
Polyps 286
Polysomnography 279
Pompe's disease 213, 249, 250
Porphyria 251
Positive predictive value 126
Positron emission tomography 10, 268
Postmyocardial infarction 146
Post-streptococcal reactive arthritis 165
Potassium sparing diuretic 115
Pravastatin 136
Predicted cardiac index 52
Prednisolone 319
Pre-excitation syndrome 298
Pregnancy 381, 384
    counseling 392
    interruption of 384
    medical complication of 382
    murmurs in 385
    termination of 381
Premature ventricular
    complex 295
    contraction 257
Primitive cardiac tube 203
Proarrhythmias 306
Procainamide 316, 325, 387
Propranolol 39
Prostaglandin, blocking synthesis of 87
Prosthetic valve 145, 154, 155, 173, 175,
    194, 382, 388, 391
    endocarditis 146, 169, 281, 282
    hemodynamics 155
Protamine sulfate 144
Protein binding 386
Proteinuria 84, 383

Pseudoaneurysm 40, 134
Pseudocoarctation 202, 244
Pseudoxanthoma elasticum 214, 251, 253, 375-377
Pulmonary artery 143, 147, 336
  absence of 236
  banding 146, 158
  hypertension 337
  obstruction 288
  pressure 70, 280, 337
    waveforms 58
  stenosis 242, 251
Pulmonary capillary wedge pressure 51, 52, 186, 276
  waveforms 58
Pulmonary embolism 274, 275, 288, 289, 291, 377, 383, 384
  diagnosis of 47
  echocardiographic hallmark of 41
  severity index 289, 292
  treatment of 289
Pulmonary hypertension 122, 180, 220, 274, 337
  diagnosis of 274
  toxin-induced 278
Pulmonary outflow tract 198, 204
Pulmonary stenosis
  causes of 145
  quantification of 156
Pulmonary valve 145, 196
  arterial aspect of 42
  disease 155
  leaflets 264
Pulmonary vascular obstructive disease, appearance of 220
Pulmonary veins 2, 3
  confluence of 2
Pulmonic stenosis 64, 202, 242
  occurrence of 208
Pulsatile exophthalmos 22
Pulse
  pressure 341
  tonometry 86
  wave velocity 366
Pulsus
  alternans 22, 99
  bisferien's 52, 175
  paradoxus 22, 52, 346
    mechanism of 349
      nonspecificity of 350
  parvus et tardus 52
Pumps, types of 148
Pure mitral stenosis 258
Purple toes syndrome 289
Pyelonephritis
  chronic 251
  unilateral 251

Q

Quinidine 300, 309, 310

R

Radial artery 151, 152
Radiation 278
  nephritis 251
Radiology, cardiac 50
Radionuclide studies 261
Raynaud phenomenon 377
Regional myocardial perfusion, absolute measurement of 50
Regurgitation
  moderate-to-severe 56
  pulmonary 176
  severe aortic 41, 64, 187
Renal arteritis 251
Renal artery 141
  aneurysm 251
  fibromuscular dysplasia of 251
  noninvolvement of 369
  stenosis 251
    bilateral 87
Renal cortical necrosis 251
Renal cyst, solitary 251
Renal disease 322
Renal dysfunction 318
  acute 70
Renal failure 377
  acute 78
  chronic 292
Renal fistula 251
Renal transplantation 80
Renal trauma 251
Renal tuberculosis 251
Renal tumors 251
Renal vein thrombosis 251
Renin-angiotensin-aldosterone system 88, 110, 111
Renovascular hypertension 80, 83, 88
  causes of 78
Repetitive ventricular premature, prevalence of 32
Respiratory rate 292, 382
Retinal artery, beading of 22
Retinoic acid 244
  embryopathy 246
Retinoids, use of 93
Retrosternal notching 202
Rhabdomyolysis
  incidence of 393
  statin induced 92
Rhabdomyoma 356, 357
Rheobase 335
Rheumatic arthritis 159
Rheumatic carditis 159, 160
  pathognomonic of 161
Rheumatic disease 187
Rheumatic fever 159, 160, 164, 166, 177, 182
  acute 159, 160, 164, 165, 167
  recurrent 165
  secondary prevention of 160, 164

Rheumatic mitral
  stenosis 381
  valvular disease 178
Rheumatoid arthritis 176, 278, 338
Rib
  lower 202, 209
  notching 228
    unilateral 209
Rickettsial organism 170
Right atrial pressure waveforms 57
Right bundle branch block 137, 140, 240, 311
Right coronary artery 4, 6, 73, 221
  catheterization of 69
  proximal occlusion of 128
  reperfusion of 129
Right heart catheterization 276, 339
Right internal jugular vein 22
Right mid subclavian artery lesion 370
Right subclavian artery, anomalous origin of 243
Right upper quadrant abdominal pain 177
Right ventricle 6, 7, 31, 74, 336, 361, 364
Right ventricular
  collapse, disappearance of 349
  dilatation 47
  failure 123
  hypertrophy 221, 275
  outflow tract 315
Riley-Day syndrome 251
Rivaroxaban 293
Roller pump 148
Ross procedure 154
Rubella 244
  infection 208
    maternal 203
  syndrome 251
  virus 248

S

Salicylates 162, 163
Saline 75
Salmonella 285
Saphenous vein 151
Sarcoid
  cardiomyopathy 265
  granulomas 254
Sarcoidosis 46, 156, 278
  cardiac 265
Sarcoma 360
Sarcomere 17
Schistosomiasis 278
Scimitar syndrome 208
Scleroderma 278, 340
Secundum atrial septal defect 25, 245
Segmental renal artery dysplasia 251
Seizures 232
Selective coronary angiography 70, 143
Senning and Mustard operation 146, 158
Sepsis 251

Septal aneurysm, formation of 234
Septal rupture 156
Serpentine pulsations 24
Serum cholesterol 139, 248
Serum insulin 131
Shock, vardiogenic 56
Shone's complex 239
　component of 207
Short QT syndrome 312
Shunt nephritis 251
Sickle cell
　anemia 212
　diseases 278
Simplified pulmonary embolism severity index 289, 292
Sinoatrial node artery 69
Sinus
　arrest 335
　arrhythmia, ventriculophasic 334
　bradycardia 303, 328
　node
　　artery 5
　　disease 306
　　dysfunction 298, 303, 305, 306
　　re-entry 314
　rhythm 186, 300, 305, 358
　tachycardia 136, 305, 314, 343, 386
　venosus 234, 241
Skeletal muscle injury 134
Skin infection, streptococcal 166
Sleep apnea
　diagnosis of 275
　syndromes 275, 278
Sleep disorder breathing 121, 122
Sodium
　consumption, low 88
　cromoglycate 244
　nitroprusside 84
Somatostatin analogue 268
Sotalol 324, 325, 387
Sperm hypermotility 245
Sphericity index 46
Sphingolipidoses 379
Spironolactone 81, 115, 116
Sporadic disorders 213
Square root sign 253
Stable angina 126, 393
Staphylococcus
　aureus 170, 172, 280, 282, 284, 286-288
　epidermidis 157, 284, 286
Starr–Edwards valve 155
Statin therapy 393, 394, 397
Stenosis 64, 71, 187
　congenital pulmonary 145
　moderate pulmonary 156
　peripheral pulmonic 196, 278
　subaortic 206, 214, 236
　subpulmonic 239
Stentless devices 154
Steroids, adrenal 251

Stevens-Johnson syndrome 251
Still's murmur 200
Straight back syndrome 30
Streptococcal infection 160
Streptococcus
　bovis endocarditis 280, 282
　gallolyticus 170
　pneumoniae 280
　viridans 172, 185
Stress
　echocardiography 40
　　specificity of 41
　myocardial perfusion imaging 126
　test 32, 33, 126
Stroke 79, 84
　embolic 358
　hemorrhagic 82
　ischemic 302
　risk of 321
　volume 36, 224, 384
Subacute infective endocarditis 164
Subclavian artery 143, 147
Subclavian flap aortoplasty 222
Subclavian steal syndrome 22
Sudden cardiac death 252, 256, 294, 295, 311, 342, 343
　mechanism of 342
　survivor of 295
Sulfonamides 164
Superior vena cava 42
　obstruction 23
　syndrome 357
　causes of 355
Supravalvular aortic stenosis 203, 245
Supraventricular tachycardia 299, 302
　classification of 315
Surgery
　cardiac 133, 352
　indications for 156
Symbas triad 364
Sympathetic nervous system 110, 111
Sympathomimetics 251
Symptomatic short QT syndrome 296
Symptomatic sinus node dysfunction 306
Syncope 290, 296, 329, 338
　causes of 300
　evaluation of 329
　infrequent episode of 306
　mechanism of 257
　neurocardiogenic 329
Syphilis 176
Syphilitic aortitis 374
Systemic arterial pressure 274
Systemic arteriovenous fistula 107
Systemic lupus erythematosus 47, 224, 276, 278
Systemic vascular resistance 215, 384
Systolic mammary soufflé 223
Systolic pulmonary artery pressure 187

T

Tachyarrhythmia 315
　supraventricular 302
　treatment of 302
　ventricular 300
Tachy-Brady syndrome 303
Tachycardia 266, 298, 299, 305
　bradycardia syndrome 328
　episode of 294
　junctional 26, 307
　monomorphic ventricular 303
　paroxysmal supraventricular 305
　supraventricular 299, 302
　transient termination of 298
Tachypnea 390
Tafamidis 102
Takayasu's arteritis 366, 369
　lesion of 369
Takayasu's disease, diagnosis of 366, 370
Takotsubo cardiomyopathy 254
Telangiectasia 207
　mucocutaneous 207
Tension 15
Teratogenic disorders 214, 230
Thallium imaging 53
Thebesian valve 3-5
Thebesian vein drain 7
Theophylline, cardiovascular effects of 275
Thiazide 115
Thoracic aorta 367
　rat tall angiographic appearance of 366
Thoracoplasty 278
Thoracotomy 143
Thrombocytopenia 172
　heparin induced 289
Thromboembolism 278
　systemic 302
Thrombolysis, use of 138
Thrombolytic therapy 50
Thrombosis 135
Thrombotic disorders 278
Thymic aplasia 202
Thyroid dysfunction 301
Thyrotoxic crisis, amiodarone induced 301
Thyrotoxicosis 180
Tilt table test 298
Torsades de Pointes 265, 296, 306
　causes of 295
　quinidine induced 300
　treatment of 296
Tortuous internal mammary artery 228
Toxemia, incidence of 228
Transaortic ventricular septal myectomy 269
Transcatheter aortic valve implantation 194
Transesophageal echocardiography 40, 42, 172
Transthyretin amyloidosis 104
Trauma, cardiac 346, 364

Treadmill stress test 32
Trepopnea 11, 15
Treppe effect 13, 60
Tricuspid annular plane systolic
 excursion 40
Tricuspid atresia 208, 232, 242
 variety of 209
Tricuspid disease, primary 186
Tricuspid endocarditis 178
Tricuspid insufficiency 178
 pressure gradient 288
Tricuspid regurgitation 23, 59, 105, 175, 176
 severe 25, 59, 175, 185
Tricuspid stenosis 23, 178, 186, 190
 organic 175
Tricuspid valve 5, 42, 180, 185, 284, 287
 disease 185
 septal leaflet of 174
Triglycerides 248, 251
Trihexyl ceramide, cellular accumulation
 of 379
Trimethadione 244
Triple vessel coronary artery disease 46
Triptans 270
Trisomy 213
Troponin 139
Truncus arteriosus 201, 225, 226, 239
 persistence 239
 repair of 199
 variety of 201
Trypanosoma cruzi 249
Tuberculosis 353
Tuberoeruptive xanthoma 22
Tuberous sclerosis 212, 251
Tumor
 carcinoid 48
 cardiac 355, 356, 358
 embolism 278
 malignant 361
 myocardial 358
 necrosis factor 106
Turner syndrome 196, 210, 251

U

Ultrasonography 54
Upper airways obstruction 278
Upper respiratory tract
 infection, streptococcal 160
 procedures 216
Uremic pericarditis 347
Ureteral occlusion, unilateral 251

V

V wave, abnormalities of 28
Vaginal bleeding 103
Vagotonic paroxysmal atrial fibrillation 302
Valproic acid 244
Valsalva maneuver 30, 294
Valsalva sinus 2, 7, 205
Valsartan 89
Valve
 closure, absence of 64
 replacement 256
 tissue 191
 types of 154
Valvular aortic stenosis 175, 176, 179, 181
Valvular lesion 341
Valvulitis 162
Vancomycin 169, 173
Vasa vasorum 132
Vascular cells adhesions molecule 135
Vascular disease, peripheral 393
Vascular wall thickening 377
Vasoconstriction 135
Vasodilation, pulmonary 337
Vein grafts 152
Vena cava 2
 filters 289
 inferior 40, 44
 superior 42, 76
Venography 277
Venous thromboembolism 289, 384
 management of 289
 treatment of 289
Ventricle, basal portion of 308
Ventricular aneurysm 145
Ventricular arrhythmia 32, 306
 suppression of 36
Ventricular assist devices 150
Ventricular fibrillation 343
Ventricular muscle contraction 20
Ventricular pressure waveforms 58
Ventricular septal
 defect 1, 146, 170, 211, 214, 215, 219, 220, 234, 242
 musculature 7
Ventricular septum 198
Ventricular tachyarrhythmia, recurrent 253
Ventricular tachycardia 254, 295-297, 299, 307, 310
 feature of 295
Ventricular wall thickness 263
Verapamil 89, 269, 273
Viral myocarditis, acute 247
Virchow triad 288
Viremia, maternal 229
Visceral pericardium 345
Vitamin
 D 244
 K antagonists 289, 293
Vomiting, occurrence of 126
von Recklinghausen's disease 251

W

Wall motion score index 40
Warfarin 244
 teratogenicity of 194
Waterston shunt 147
Well's score 291
White coat hypertension 67, 79, 86
Williams syndrome 210, 229, 245
 component of 210
Willis circle 221, 235
Wolff-Chaikoff effect 318
Wolf-Parkinson-White syndrome 207, 240

X

X wave, abnormalities of 28
Xanthoma
 eruptive 22
 striatum palmare 22
 tendinosum 25